VOLUME ONE

NEUROLOGICAL SURGERY

*a comprehensive reference guide to the
diagnosis and management
of neurosurgical problems*

EDITED BY

JULIAN R. YOUMANS, M.D., Ph.D.

Professor and Chairman, Department of Neurological Surgery,
School of Medicine, University of California,
Davis, California

1973

W. B. Saunders Company · Philadelphia · London · Toronto

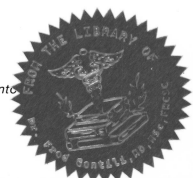

W. B. Saunders Company: West Washington Square
Philadelphia, Pa.   19105

12 Dyott Street
London, WC1A   1DB

833 Oxford Street
Toronto 18, Ontario

Neurological Surgery — Volume One   ISBN 0-7216-9655-4

Print Number: 9   8   7   6   5   4   3   2   1

The Editor dedicates this book
to his parents and to

Nancy Alice
Reed Nesbit
John Edward
Julian Milton

CONTRIBUTORS

OTMAR W. ALBRAND, M.D., Assistant Professor of Neurological Surgery, School of Medicine, University of California at Davis, Davis, California. Associate Neurological Surgeon, Sacramento Medical Center, Sacramento, California.

MARSHALL B. ALLEN, Jr., M.D., F.A.C.S., Professor of Neurological Surgery, Chief of the Section of Neurological Surgery, School of Medicine, Medical College of Georgia. Chief of Neurological Surgery, Eugene Talmadge Memorial Hospital; Consultant in Neurological Surgery, University Hospital, Veterans Administration Hospital and United States Army Specialized Treatment Center at Fort Gordon Army Hospital, Augusta, Georgia. Consultant in Neurological Surgery, Central State Hospital, Milledgeville, Georgia.

H. THOMAS BALLANTINE, Jr., M.D., F.A.C.S., Associate Clinical Professor of Neurological Surgery, School of Medicine, Harvard University. Neurological Surgeon to the Massachusetts General Hospital, Boston, Massachusetts.

H. J. M. BARNETT, M.D., F.R.C.P.(C.), Professor of Neurology, Chairman of Division of Neurology, School of Medicine, University of Western Ontario. Chief of Neurology, University Hospital, London, Ontario.

FRANK BATLEY, M.B., Ch.B., F.R.C.P.(C.), Professor of Radiology, College of Medicine, Ohio State University. Director of Radiation Therapy, Ohio State University Hospitals, Columbus, Ohio.

JOHN R. BENTSON, M.D., Assistant Professor of Radiology, School of Medicine, University of California at Los Angeles. Radiologist, University of California at Los Angeles Center for the Health Sciences; Consultant in Radiology, Wadsworth Veterans Administration Hospital, Los Angeles, California.

ROGER BOLES, M.D., F.A.C.S., Associate Professor of Otorhinolaryngology, School of Medicine, University of Michigan. Attending Otorhinolaryngologist, University Hospital; Consultant, Otorhinolaryngology, Veterans Administration Hospital; Active Medical Staff, St. Joseph Mercy Hospital, Ann Arbor, Michigan. Consultant in Otorhinolaryngology, Wayne County General Hospital, Eloise, Michigan.

CHARLES E. BRACKETT, M.D., F.A.C.S., Professor of Surgery (Neurosurgery), Chairman of Section of Neurological Surgery, School of Medicine, University of Kansas. Neurological Surgeon–in–Chief, University of Kansas Medical Center, Kansas City, Kansas. Consultant in Neurological Surgery, Veterans Administration Hospital, Kansas City, Missouri.

CHARLES LEON BRANCH, M.D., F.A.C.S., Clinical Associate Professor of Neurological Surgery, School of Medicine, University of Texas at San Antonio. Attending Neurological Surgeon, Southwest Texas Methodist Hospital, Baptist Memorial Hospital, Santa Rosa Medical Center, and Nix Memorial Hospital, San Antonio, Texas.

VERNE L. BRECHNER, M.D., F.A.C.A., Professor of Anesthesiology, Vice Chairman of Department of Anesthesiology, School of Medicine, University of California at Los Angeles. Anesthesiologist, University of California at Los Angeles Center for the Health Sciences, Los Angeles, California.

ROBERT W. BRENNAN, M.D., Associate Professor of Medicine, Chief of Division of Neurology, College of Medicine, Pennsylvania State University. Chief of Neurology Service, The Milton S. Hershey Medical Center, Hershey, Pennsylvania.

ALBERT B. BUTLER, M.D., Assistant Professor of Neurological Surgery, School of Medicine, University of Virginia. Attending Neurological Surgeon, University of Virginia Hospital, Charlottesville, Virginia.

FERNANDO CABIESES, M.D., Ph.D., F.A.C.S., Professor of Neurological Surgery (Ret.), School of Medicine, Universidad de San Marcos. Chief, Neurological Surgery Unit, Peruvian Armed Forces, Anglo-American Hospital, and Hospital 2 de Mayo, Lima, Peru.

ROBERT L. CAMPBELL, M.D., F.A.C.S., Professor of Neurological Surgery, Chairman of Department of Neurological Surgery, School of Medicine, University of Indiana. Neurological Surgeon–in–Chief, Indiana Medical Center, Indianapolis, Indiana.

SHELLEY N. CHOU, M.D., Ph.D., F.A.C.S., Professor of Neurological Surgery, School of Medicine, University of Minnesota. Attending Neurological Surgeon, University of Minnesota Hospitals; Consultant, Neurological Surgery Service, Veterans Administration Hospital, Minneapolis, Minnesota.

WILLIAM KEMP CLARK, M.D., F.A.C.S., Professor of Neurological Surgery, Chairman of Division of Neurological Surgery, Southwestern Medical School, University of Texas at Dallas. Director of Neurological Surgery Service, Parkland Memorial Hospital, Presbyterian Hospital, Children's Medical Center, and Veterans Administration Hospital; Consultant in Neurological Surgery, St. Paul's Hospital, Texas Scottish Rite Hospital for Crippled Children, and Baylor University Medical Center, Dallas, Texas.

WILLIAM F. COLLINS, M.D., F.A.C.S., Harvey and Kate Cushing Professor of Surgery, Chairman of Section of Neurological Surgery, School of Medicine, Yale University. Neurological Surgeon–in–Chief, Yale–New Haven Medical Center, New Haven, Connecticut; Consultant in Neurological Surgery, Veterans Administration Hospital, West Haven, Connecticut.

WILLIAM SAUNDERS COXE, M.D., F.A.C.S., Professor of Neurological Surgery, School of Medicine, Washington University. Assistant Neurological Surgeon, Barnes Hospital and St. Louis Children's Hospital; Consultant, Neurological Surgery, Veterans Administration Hospital; Attending Neurological Surgeon, St. Louis City Hospital, St. Louis, Missouri.

THOMAS K. CRAIGMILE, M.D., F.A.C.S., Associate Clinical Professor of Neurological Surgery, School of Medicine, University of Colorado. Attending Neurological Surgeon, Colorado General Hospital, Veterans Administration Hospital, and St. Joseph's Hospital, Denver, Colorado.

COURTLAND HARWELL DAVIS, Jr., M.D., F.A.C.S., Professor of Neurological Surgery, Bowman Gray School of Medicine, Wake Forest University. Attending

Neurological Surgeon, North Carolina Baptist Hospital, Winston-Salem, North Carolina.

IRA C. DENTON, Jr., M.D., Assistant Professor of Neurological Surgery, School of Medicine, West Virginia University. Attending Neurological Surgeon, West Virginia University Medical Center Hospital, Morgantown, West Virginia.

ALBERT D'ERRICO, M.D., F.A.C.S., Clinical Professor of Neurological Surgery, Southwestern Medical School, University of Texas at Dallas. Attending Neurological Surgeon, Baylor University Medical Center, Presbyterian Hospital, Children's Medical Center, and Parkland Memorial Hospital, Dallas, Texas.

ROBERT D. DICKINS, Jr., M.D., F.A.C.S., Teaching Staff in Neurological Surgery, School of Medicine, University of Arkansas. Attending Neurological Surgeon, Baptist Medical Center, St. Vincent's Infirmary, Little Rock, Arkansas.

REED O. DINGMAN, M.D., D.D.S., F.A.C.S., Professor of Surgery, Head of Section of Plastic Surgery, School of Medicine, University of Michigan. Chief of Plastic Surgery, University of Michigan Medical Center and St. Joseph Mercy Hospital; Consultant in Surgery, Veterans Administration Hospital, Ann Arbor, Michigan; Consultant in Plastic Surgery, Sinai Hospital, Detroit, Michigan.

DONALD D. DIRKS, Ph.D., Associate Professor of Head and Neck Surgery (Audiology), School of Medicine, University of California at Los Angeles, Los Angeles, California.

DONALD F. DOHN, M.D., F.A.C.S., Head of Department of Neurological Surgery, Cleveland Clinic. Head of Neurological Surgery Service, Cleveland Clinic Hospital, Cleveland, Ohio.

CHARLES G. DRAKE, M.D., F.R.C.S.(C.), F.A.C.S., Professor of Neurological Surgery, Head of Department of Clinical Neurological Sciences, School of Medicine, University of Western Ontario. Chief of Neurological Surgery Service, University Hospital, London, Ontario.

PETER DYCK, M.D., F.A.C.S., Assistant Clinical Professor of Neurological Surgery, School of Medicine, University of Southern California. Attending Neurological Surgeon, Hospital of the Good Samaritan, St. Vincent's Hospital, Queen of Angels Hospital, Orthopedic Hospital, and Los Angeles County General Hospital, Los Angeles, California.

ROBERT G. FISHER, M.D., Ph.D., F.A.C.S., Professor of Neurological Surgery, Chairman of Department of Neurological Surgery, School of Medicine, University of Oklahoma. Chief of Neurological Surgery, University of Oklahoma Medical Center, Oklahoma City, Oklahoma.

ELDON L. FOLTZ, M.D., F.A.C.S., Professor of Neurological Surgery, Chairman of Division of Neurological Surgery, School of Medicine, University of California at Irvine, Irvine, California. Chief of Neurological Surgery, Orange County Medical Center, Orange, California; Consultant, Veterans Administration Hospital, Long Beach, California.

LYLE A. FRENCH, M.D., Ph.D., F.A.C.S., Professor of Neurological Surgery, Head of Department of Neurological Surgery, School of Medicine; Vice President for Health Sciences, University of Minnesota. Chief of Neurological Surgery, University Hospital and Veterans Administration Hospital, Minneapolis, Minnesota.

JAMES GARBER GALBRAITH, M.D., F.A.C.S., Professor of Neurological Surgery, Director of Division of Neurological Surgery, School of Medicine, University of Alabama. Chief of Neurological Surgery Service, University of Alabama Hospitals and Clinics, Birmingham, Alabama.

W. JAMES GARDNER, M.D., F.A.C.S., Formerly Head of Department of Neurological Surgery, Cleveland Clinic Foundation and Hospital. Neurological Surgeon to Fairview General Hospital, Huron Road Hospital, and St. Alexis Hospital, Cleveland, Ohio.

CORNELIUS P. GOETZINGER, Ph.D., Professor of Audiology, School of Medicine, University of Kansas. Chief of Audiology, University of Kansas Medical Center, Kansas City, Kansas. Consultant in Audiology, General Hospital and Veterans Administration Hospital, Kansas City, Missouri.

FRANK P. GOLDSTEIN, M.D., F.A.C.S., Assistant Professor of Neurological Surgery, School of Medicine, Medical College of Wisconsin. Attending Neurological Surgeon, Milwaukee County General Hospital, Milwaukee, Wisconsin; Attending Neurological Surgeon, Veterans Administration Hospital, Wood, Wisconsin.

ALBERT LOUIS GOODGOLD, M.D., Associate Professor of Clinical Neurology, School of Medicine, New York University. Associate Attending Neurologist, University Hospital and Bellevue Hospital Center; Attending Neurologist, Veterans Administration Hospital, New York, New York.

JACK K. GOODRICH, M.D., F.A.C.R., Professor of Radiology, School of Medicine, Duke University. Director, Division of Nuclear Medicine, Duke University Medical Center and Veterans Administration Hospital, Durham, North Carolina.

JAMES GREENWOOD, Jr., M.D., F.A.C.S., Clinical Professor of Neurological Surgery, College of Medicine, Baylor University. Chief of Neurological Surgery, Methodist Hospital, Houston, Texas.

GERALD A. GRONERT, M.D., Assistant Professor of Anesthesiology, Mayo Graduate School of Medicine, University of Minnesota. Consultant, Department of Anesthesiology, Mayo Clinic, Rochester, Minnesota.

E. STEPHEN GURDJIAN, M.D., Ph.D., F.A.C.S., Emeritus Professor of Neurological Surgery, School of Medicine, Wayne State University. Consulting Neurological Surgeon, Grace Hospital, Detroit, Michigan.

VOIGT R. HODGSON, Ph.D., Associate Professor of Biomechanics, Department of Neurological Surgery, School of Medicine, Wayne State University, Detroit, Michigan.

EDGAR M. HOUSEPIAN, M.D., F.A.C.S., Associate Professor of Clinical Neurological Surgery, College of Physicians and Surgeons, Columbia University. Associate Attending Neurological Surgeon, New York Neurological Institute and Columbia–Presbyterian Medical Center, New York, New York.

WILLIAM E. HUNT, M.D., F.A.C.S., Professor of Neurological Surgery, Director of Division of Neurological Surgery, College of Medicine, Ohio State University. Chief of Neurological Surgery, Ohio State University Hospitals; Consultant in Neurological Surgery, Children's Hospital, Columbus, Ohio.

EDGAR A. KAHN, M.D., F.A.C.S., Emeritus Professor of Neurological Surgery, Emeritus Chairman of Section of Neurological Surgery, School of Medicine, University of Michigan. Attending Neurological Surgeon, University of Michigan Medical Center and St. Joseph Mercy Hospital, Ann Arbor, Michigan.

STEPHEN A. KIEFFER, M.D., Professor of Radiology, School of Medicine, University of Minnesota. Neuroradiologist, University of Minnesota Hospitals. Chief of Diagnostic Radiology Service, Veterans Administration Hospital, Minneapolis, Minnesota.

E. LEON KIER, M.D., Associate Professor of Radiology, Chief of Section of Neuro-radiology, School of Medicine, Yale University. Chief of Neuroradiology, Yale–New Haven Medical Center, New Haven, Connecticut.

GLENN W. KINDT, M.D., F.A.C.S., Associate Professor of Neurological Surgery, School of Medicine, University of Michigan. Attending Neurological Surgeon, University Medical Center and Veterans Administration Hospital, Ann Arbor, Michigan; Attending Neurological Surgeon, Wayne County General Hospital, Wayne, Michigan.

ROBERT B. KING, M.D., F.A.C.S., Professor of Neurological Surgery, Chairman of Department of Neurological Surgery, School of Medicine, State University of New York, Upstate Medical Center. Chief of Neurological Surgery, State University Hospital of the Upstate Medical Center; Attending Neurological Surgeon, Crouse-Irving Memorial Hospital; Consultant, Neurological Surgery, Veterans Administration Hospital, Syracuse, New York.

DAVID G. KLINE, M.D., F.A.C.S., Associate Professor of Neurological Surgery, Chairman of Division of Neurological Surgery, School of Medicine, Louisiana State University. Chairman of Louisiana State University Neurological Surgery Service, Charity Hospital; Visiting Neurological Surgeon, Southern Baptist Hospital, Touro Infirmary, and Hotel Dieu; Academic Staff in Neurological Surgery, Ochsner Foundation Hospital; Consultant in Neurological Surgery, United States Public Health Service Hospital, New Orleans, Louisiana. Visiting Investigator, Delta Regional Primate Center, Covington, Louisiana. Consultant in Neurological Surgery, Keesler Air Force Base Hospital, Biloxi, Mississippi.

THEODORE KURZE, M.D., F.A.C.S., Professor of Neurological Surgery, Chairman of Department of Neurological Surgery, School of Medicine, University of Southern California. Chief of Neurological Surgery, Los Angeles County Medical Center; Attending Neurological Surgeon, Hospital of the Good Samaritan, White Memorial Hospital, and Children's Hospital, Los Angeles, California.

EDWARD H. LAMBERT, M.D., Ph.D., Professor of Physiology, Mayo Graduate School of Medicine, University of Minnesota, Head of Section of Clinical Electromyography, Mayo Clinic, Rochester, Minnesota.

THOMAS WILLIAM LANGFITT, M.D., F.A.C.S., Charles Frazier Professor of Neurological Surgery, Chairman of Division of Neurological Surgery, School of Medicine, University of Pennsylvania. Chief of Neurological Surgery, Philadelphia General Hospital; Consultant Neurological Surgeon, Children's Hospital and Veterans Administration Hospital, Philadelphia, Pennsylvania.

KENNETH E. LIVINGSTON, M.D., F.A.C.S., Associate Professor of Neurological Surgery and Assistant Professor (Research) of Pharmacology, Faculty of Medicine, University of Toronto. Chief of Division of Neurological Surgery, The Wellesley Hospital, Toronto, Ontario.

DON M. LONG, M.D., Ph.D., F.A.C.S., Associate Professor of Neurological Surgery, School of Medicine, University of Minnesota. Associate Neurological Surgeon, University of Minnesota Hospitals; Consultant, Neurological Surgery Service, Veterans Administration Hospital, Minneapolis, Minnesota.

WILLIAM McMURRAY LOUGHEED, M.D., F.R.C.S.(C.), Associate Professor of Neurological Surgery, Faculty of Medicine, University of Toronto. Associate Neurological Surgeon, Toronto General Hospital; Chairman, Division of Neurosciences, Sunnybrook Hospital; Consultant in Neurological Surgery, Toronto East General Hospital and Scarborough General Hospital, Toronto, Ontario.

J. A. McCRARY III, M.D., Associate Professor of Ophthalmology, Assistant Professor, Neurological Surgery and Neurology, School of Medicine, University of Texas at Galveston. Attending Ophthalmologist, University of Texas Medical Branch Hospitals, Galveston, Texas.

ROBERT L. McLAURIN, M.D., F.A.C.S., Professor of Surgery (Neurosurgery), Chairman of Division of Neurological Surgery, College of Medicine, University of Cincinnati. Chief of Neurological Surgery, Cincinnati General Hospital, Children's Hospital, and Holmes Hospital; Consultant in Neurological Surgery, Veterans Administration Hospital, Cincinnati, Ohio.

VERNON H. MARK, M.D., F.A.C.S., Associate Professor of Neurological Surgery, School of Medicine, Harvard University. Director of Neurological Surgery Service, Boston City Hospitals, Boston, Massachusetts.

BRIAN McQ. MARSHALL, M.D., F.R.C.P.(C.), Assistant Professor of Anesthesiology, Faculty of Medicine, University of Toronto. Senior Anesthesiologist, Toronto General Hospital, Toronto, Ontario.

FRANK H. MAYFIELD, M.D., F.A.C.S., Clinical Professor of Neurological Surgery, College of Medicine, University of Cincinnati. Director of Neurological Surgery, The Christ Hospital and Good Samaritan Hospital, Cincinnati, Ohio.

WILLIAM F. MEACHAM, M.D., F.A.C.S., Clinical Professor of Neurological Surgery, Chairman of Department of Neurological Surgery, School of Medicine, Vanderbilt University, and Clinical Professor of Neurological Surgery, School of Medicine, Meharry Medical College. Chief of Neurological Surgery, Vanderbilt University Hospital; Attending Neurological Surgeon, Nashville General Hospital, St. Thomas Hospital, and Baptist Hospital, Nashville, Tennessee.

JOHN D. MICHENFELDER, M.D., Associate Professor of Anesthesiology, Mayo Graduate School of Medicine, University of Minnesota. Consulting Anesthesiologist, Department of Anesthesiology, Mayo Clinic, Rochester, Minnesota.

WILLIAM H. MORETZ, M.D., F.A.C.S., Professor of Surgery, Chairman of Department of Surgery, School of Medicine, Medical College of Georgia. Chief of Surgery, Talmadge Memorial Hospital; Consultant in Surgery, Veterans Administration Hospital and Fort Gordon Army Hospital, Augusta, Georgia.

DONALD E. MORGAN, Ph.D., Assistant Professor of Head and Neck Surgery (Audiology), School of Medicine, University of California at Los Angeles. Director of Audiology Clinic, University of California at Los Angeles Center for the Health Sciences, Los Angeles, California.

T. P. MORLEY, M.D., F.R.C.S.(C.), F.R.C.S. (ENG.), Associate Professor of Neurological Surgery, Chairman of Division of Neurological Surgery, Faculty of Medicine, University of Toronto. Head of Division of Neurological Surgery, Toronto General Hospital, Toronto, Ontario.

SEAN F. MULLAN, M.D., F.A.C.S., Professor of Neurological Surgery, Director of Division of Neurological Surgery, School of Medicine, University of Chicago. Chief of Neurological Surgery, University of Chicago Hospitals and Clinics; Consulting Neurological Surgeon, Illinois Central Hospital, Chicago, Illinois, Consulting Neurological Surgeon, Great Lakes Naval Station, Great Lakes, Illinois.

JOHN J. MURPHY, M.D., F.A.C.S., Professor of Urology, Chief of Division of Urology, School of Medicine, University of Pennsylvania. Chief of Urology, Hospital of the University of Pennsylvania, Philadelphia, Pennsylvania.

MARTIN G. NETSKY, M.D., Professor of Neuropathology, School of Medicine, University of Virginia. Chief of Neuropathology, University of Virginia Hospital, Charlottesville, Virginia.

HORACE A. NORRELL, Jr., M.D., F.A.C.S., Professor of Neurological Surgery, Chairman of Department of Neurological Surgery, School of Medicine, University of Kentucky. Chief of Neurological Surgery, University Hospital and Veterans Administration Hospital; Consultant in Neurological Surgery, The United States Public Health Service Clinical Research Center, Lexington, Kentucky. Consultant in Neurological Surgery, Veterans Administration Hospital, Huntington, West Virginia.

FRANK E. NULSEN, M.D., F.A.C.S., Harvey Huntington Brown, Jr. Professor of Neurological Surgery, Chairman of Division of Neurological Surgery, School of Medicine, Western Reserve University. Chief of Neurological Surgery Service, University Hospital; Consulting Neurological Surgeon, Veterans Administration Hospital; Senior Consultant in Neurological Surgery, Cleveland Metropolitan Hospital, Cleveland, Ohio.

SIXTO OBRADOR, M.D., Professor of Neurological Surgery, Chairman of Department of Neurological Surgery, Faculty of Medicine, Madrid Autonomous University. Chief of Neurological Surgery Services of the Spanish Social Security (Residencia La Paz) and Jimenez Diaz Foundation, Madrid, Spain.

GUY L. ODOM, M.D., F.A.C.S., Professor of Neurological Surgery, Chairman of Division of Neurological Surgery, School of Medicine, Duke University. Chief of Neurological Surgery, Duke University Hospital, Durham, North Carolina.

GEORGE A. OJEMANN, M.D., Associate Professor of Neurological Surgery, School of Medicine, University of Washington. Attending Neurological Surgeon, University Hospital and Harborview Medical Center; Consultant in Neurological Surgery, Veterans Administration Hospital, Seattle, Washington.

ROBERT G. OJEMANN, M.D., F.A.C.S., Associate Clinical Professor of Neurological Surgery, School of Medicine, Harvard University. Associate Visiting Neurosurgeon, Massachusetts General Hospital, Boston, Massachusetts.

AYUB KHAN OMMAYA, M.D., F.R.C.S. (ENG.), F.A.C.S., Associate Clinical Professor of Neurological Surgery, School of Medicine, Georgetown University, Washington, D.C. Associate Neurological Surgeon, Branch of Surgical Neurology, National Institute of Neurological Disease and Blindness, National Institutes of Health; Consulting Neurological Surgeon, The Clinical Center, Bethesda, Maryland.

FRED PLUM, M.D., Anne Parrish Titzell Professor of Neurology, Chairman of Department of Neurology, College of Medicine, Cornell University. Neurologist-in-Chief, The New York Hospital, New York, New York.

G. O'NEIL PROUD, M.D., Professor of Otorhinolaryngology, School of Medicine, University of Kansas. Chief of Otorhinolaryngology, University of Kansas Medical Center, Kansas City, Kansas.

ANTHONY J. RAIMONDI, M.D., F.A.C.S., Professor of Neurological Surgery, Chairman of Division of Neurological Surgery, School of Medicine, Northwestern University. Chairman of Division of Neurological Surgery, Children's Memorial Hospital, Chicago, Illinois.

ROBERT W. RAND, M.D., Ph.D., F.A.C.S., Professor of Neurological Surgery, School of Medicine, University of California at Los Angeles. Attending Neurological Surgeon, University of California Center for the Health Sciences; Consultant in Neurological Surgery. St. John's Hospital and Veterans Administration Hospital, Los Angeles, California.

JOSEPH RANSOHOFF, M.D., F.A.C.S., Professor of Neurological Surgery and Chairman of Department of Neurological Surgery, School of Medicine, New York University. Director of Neurological Surgery, Bellevue Hospital Center, University Hospital, and Veterans Administration Hospital, New York, New York.

ROBERT A. RATCHESON, M.D., Instructor in Neurological Surgery, School of Medicine, Washington University. Assistant Neurological Surgeon, Barnes Hospital, St. Louis, Missouri.

BRONSON S. RAY, M.D., F.A.C.S., Emeritus Clinical Professor of Neurological Surgery, Emeritus Chairman of Department of Neurological Surgery, College of Medicine, Cornell University. Attending Neurological Surgeon, New York Hospital–Cornell Medical Center, New York, New York.

KAI REHDER, M.D., Assistant Professor of Anesthesiology, Mayo Graduate School of Medicine, University of Minnesota. Anesthesiologist, Department of Anesthesiology, Mayo Clinic, Rochester, Minnesota.

RALPH M. REITAN, Ph.D., Professor of Neurological Surgery, School of Medicine, Professor of Psychology, School of Arts and Science, University of Washington. Consulting Psychologist, University Hospital, Seattle, Washington.

ALAN E. RICHARDSON, M.B., B.S., F.R.C.S. (ENG.), F.R.C.S.(E.), Teacher in Neurological Surgery, School of Medicine, London University. Attending Neurological Surgeon, St. George's Hospital and Atkinson Morley's Hospital; Director, Wolfson Medical Rehabilitation Centre, London, England.

JAMES T. ROBERTSON, M.D., F.A.C.S., Associate Professor of Neurological Surgery, Acting Chairman of Department of Neurological Surgery, College of Medicine, University of Tennessee. Attending Neurological Surgeon, City of Memphis Hospitals, Baptist Memorial Hospital, Memphis, Tennessee.

DAVID A. ROTH, M.D., F.A.C.S., Assistant Clinical Professor of Neurological Surgery, School of Medicine, Harvard University. Associate Director of Neurological Surgery Service, Boston City Hospital, Boston, Massachusetts.

SÜLEYMAN SAGLAM, M.D., Assistant Professor of Neurological Surgery, School of Medicine, Hacettepe University. Attending Neurological Surgeon, Hacettepe University Medical Center, Ankara, Turkey.

MARTIN PETER SAYERS, M.D., F.A.C.S., Associate Professor of Neurological Surgery, College of Medicine, Ohio State University. Chief of Division of Neurological Surgery, Columbus Children's Hospital; Attending Neurological Surgeon, University Hospitals and Riverside Methodist Hospital, Columbus, Ohio.

MANNIE M. SCHECHTER, M.D., Professor of Radiology, Albert Einstein College of Medicine, Yeshiva University. Director of Neuroradiology, Hospital of the Albert Einstein College of Medicine and Bronx Municipal Hospital Center, New York, New York.

ROBERT S. SCHWAB, M.D., Late Emeritus Associate Clinical Professor of Neurology, School of Medicine, Harvard University. Late Neurologist and Director Emeritus, Brain Wave Laboratory, Massachusetts General Hospital, Boston, Massachusetts.

EDWARD L. SELJESKOG, M.D., Ph.D., Associate Professor of Neurological Surgery, School of Medicine, University of Minnesota. Attending Neurological Surgeon, University of Minnesota Hospitals and Hennepin County General Hospital, Minneapolis, Minnesota.

JOHN SHILLITO, Jr., M.D., F.A.C.S., Associate Professor of Neurological Surgery, School of Medicine, Harvard University. Senior Associate in Neurological Surgery, Children's Hospital Medical Center, Peter Bent Brigham Hospital, Boston, Massachusetts.

J. LAWTON SMITH, M.D., Professor of Ophthalmology and Neurological Surgery, School of Medicine, University of Miami. Attending Ophthalmologist, Jackson

Memorial Hospital; Consulting Ophthalmologist, Veterans Administration Hospital, Miami, Florida.

W. EUGENE STERN, M.D., F.A.C.S., Professor of Surgery (Neurosurgery), Chairman of Division of Neurosurgery, School of Medicine, University of California at Los Angeles. Chief of Neurosurgery Service, University of California at Los Angeles Center for the Health Sciences, Los Angeles, California.

O. RHETT TALBERT, M.D., F.A.C.P., Professor of Neurology, Chairman of Department of Neurology, School of Medicine, Medical University of South Carolina. Chief of Neurology, Medical University Hospital, Charleston, South Carolina.

ARTHUR TAUB, M.D., Ph.D., Associate Professor of Neurophysiology in Neurological Surgery and Associate Professor of Neurology, School of Medicine, Yale University. Associate Neurologist, Yale–New Haven Medical Center, New Haven, Connecticut.

L. M. THOMAS, M.D., F.A.C.S., Professor of Neurological Surgery, Chairman of Department of Neurological Surgery, Associate Dean for Hospital Affairs, School of Medicine, Wayne State University. Senior Attending Neurological Surgeon, Detroit General Hospital; Attending Neurological Surgeon, Grace Hospital; Consulting Neurological Surgeon, Harper Hospital, Children's Hospital of Michigan, and Veterans Administration Hospital, Detroit, Michigan.

ROBERT L. TIMMONS, M.D., F.A.C.S., Formerly, Associate Professor of Neurological Surgery, School of Medicine, University of North Carolina; Attending Neurological Surgeon, North Carolina Memorial Hospital, Chapel Hill, North Carolina. Presently, Clinical Professor of Surgery (Neurosurgery), School of Medicine, East Carolina University. Attending Neurological Surgeon, Pitt Memorial Hospital, Greenville, North Carolina.

GEORGE T. TINDALL, M.D., F.A.C.S., Professor of Neurological Surgery, Chairman of Division of Neurological Surgery, School of Medicine, The University of Texas at Galveston. Chief Neurological Surgeon, University of Texas Medical Branch Hospitals, Galveston, Texas.

JAMES TITCHENER, M.D., Professor of Psychiatry, College of Medicine, University of Cincinnati. Attending Psychiatrist, Cincinnati General Hospital, Cincinnati, Ohio.

STEPHEN L. TROKEL, M.D., F.A.C.S., Instructor in Ophthalmology, College of Physicians and Surgeons, Columbia University. Assistant Ophthalmologist, Institute of Ophthalmology and Columbia–Presbyterian Medical Center, New York, New York.

CHARLES W. TRUE, M.D., Associate Pathologist, Good Samaritan Hospital, Cincinnati, Ohio.

JOHN S. TYTUS, M.D., F.A.C.S., Clinical Associate Professor of Neurological Surgery, School of Medicine, University of Washington. Chief of Section of Neurological Surgery, The Mason Clinic and Virginia Mason Hospital; Attending Neurological Surgeon, Harborview Medical Center and Children's Orthopedic Hospital, Seattle, Washington.

JOHN M. VAN BUREN, M.D., Ph.D., Clinical Professor of Surgical Neurology, School of Medicine, George Washington University, Washington, D.C. Chief of Branch of Surgical Neurology and Clinical Director, National Institute of Neurological Diseases and Stroke, National Institutes of Health, Bethesda, Maryland.

A. EARL WALKER, M.D., F.A.C.S., Professor Emeritus of Neurological Surgery, School of Medicine, Johns Hopkins University, Baltimore, Maryland. Visiting Professor of Neurological Surgery, School of Medicine, The University of New Mexico, Albuquerque, New Mexico.

JAMES ALLAN WALTERS, M.D., D.P.M., F.R.C.P.(C.), F.A.C.P., Associate Professor of Psychiatry and Medicine, Faculty of Medicine, University of Toronto. Psychiatrist and Physician, The Wellesley Hospital; Consulting Psychiatrist, Toronto General Hospital, Toronto, Ontario.

ARTHUR A. WARD, Jr., M.D., F.A.C.S., Professor of Neurological Surgery, Chairman of Department of Neurological Surgery, School of Medicine, University of Washington. Chief of Neurological Surgery, University Hospital and Harborview Medical Center; Consulting Neurological Surgeon, Veterans Administration Hospital, Seattle, Washington.

CLARK C. WATTS, M.D., Assistant Clinical Professor of Neurological Surgery, Southwestern Medical School, University of Texas at Dallas. Attending Neurological Surgeon, Parkland Memorial Hospital, St. Paul's Hospital, and Children's Medical Center; Consultant in Neurological Surgery, Veterans Administration Hospital, Dallas, Texas.

ALAN J. WEIN, M.D., Instructor in Urology, School of Medicine, University of Pennsylvania. Fellow, Harrison Department of Surgical Research, Philadelphia, Pennsylvania.

KEASLEY WELCH, M.D., F.A.C.S., Franc D. Ingraham Professor of Neurological Surgery, School of Medicine, Harvard University. Neurological Surgeon–in–Chief, Children's Hospital Medical Center; Attending Neurological Surgeon, Peter Bent Brigham Hospital, Boston, Massachusetts.

JAMES C. WHITE, M.D., F.A.C.S., Professor of Surgery, Emeritus, School of Medicine, Harvard University. Senior Consulting Staff in Neurological Surgery, Massachusetts General Hospital, Boston, Massachusetts.

LOWELL ELMOND WHITE, Jr., M.D., Professor of Neuroscience (Neurological Surgery), Chairman of Division of Neuroscience, College of Medicine, University of South Alabama. Attending Neurological Surgeon, Mobile General Hospital, Mobile, Alabama.

ROBERT JOSEPH WHITE, M.D., Ph.D., F.A.C.S., Professor of Neurological Surgery, School of Medicine, Case Western Reserve University. Director of Neurological Surgery and Brain Research Laboratories, Cleveland Metropolitan Hospital; Attending Neurological Surgeon, University Hospitals; Senior Consulting Neurological Surgeon, Veterans Administration Hospital; Neurological Surgery Staff, Lakeside Hospital and Fairview Park General Hospital, Cleveland, Ohio.

ROBERT H. WILKINS, M.D., F.A.C.S., Formerly, Assistant Professor of Neurological Surgery, Duke University. Chief of Neurological Surgery, Veterans Administration Hospital, Durham, North Carolina. Presently, Chairman of Department of Neurological Surgery, Scott and White Clinic, Temple, Texas.

ROBERT H. WILKINSON, Jr., M.D., Associate Professor of Radiology, School of Medicine, Duke University. Staff Radiologist, Duke University Medical Center and Veterans Administration Hospital, Durham, North Carolina.

CHARLES B. WILSON, M.D., F.A.C.S., Professor of Neurological Surgery, Chairman of Department of Neurological Surgery, School of Medicine, University of California at San Francisco. Chief of Neurological Surgery Service, Moffitt Hospital; Attending Neurological Surgeon, San Francisco General Hospital; Consulting Neurological Surgeon, Public Health Service Hospital and Veterans Administration Hospital, San Francisco, California.

EARL F. WOLFMAN, Jr., M.D., F.A.C.S., Professor of Surgery, Chairman of Division of Surgical Sciences, Chairman of Department of Surgery, Associate Dean for Clinical Affairs, University of California at Davis, Davis, California. Chief of Surgical Services, Sacramento Medical Center, Sacramento, California; Consultant in Surgery, United States Air Force Medical Center, Travis Air Force Base, California, and United States Public Health Service Hospital, San Francisco, California.

R. LEWIS WRIGHT, M.D., F.A.C.S., Assistant Clinical Professor of Neurological Surgery, School of Medicine, Medical College of Virginia. Attending Neurological Surgeon, St. Mary's Hospital and Richmond Memorial Hospital; Consulting Neurological Surgeon, Veterans Administration Hospital, Retreat Hospital, and Stuart Circle Hospital, Richmond, Virginia.

DAVID YASHON, M.D., F.A.C.S., Associate Professor of Neurological Surgery, College of Medicine, Ohio State University. Attending Neurological Surgeon, The University Hospitals and Children's Hospital, Columbus, Ohio.

JULIAN R. YOUMANS, M.D., Ph.D., F.A.C.S., Professor of Neurological Surgery, Chairman of Department of Neurological Surgery, University of California School of Medicine at Davis, Davis, California. Chief of Neurological Surgery, Sacramento Medical Center, Sacramento, California; Consultant in Neurological Surgery, United States Air Force Medical Center, Travis Air Force Base, California.

GILBERT F. YOUNG, M.D., Professor of Neurology and Pediatrics, School of Medicine, Medical University of South Carolina. Attending Neurologist and Pediatrician, Medical University Hospital, Charleston, South Carolina.

ROBERT R. YOUNG, M.D., Associate Professor of Neurology, School of Medicine, Harvard University. Associate Neurologist and Director of the Clinical Neurophysiology Laboratories, Massachusetts General Hospital, Boston, Massachusetts.

LAWRENCE H. ZINGESSER, M.D., Associate Professor of Radiology, Albert Einstein College of Medicine, Yeshiva University. Radiologist, Hospital of the Albert Einstein College of Medicine and Bronx Municipal Hospital Center, New York, New York.

PREFACE

Like other medical sciences, neurological surgery has undergone rapid changes in recent years. New techniques and entire areas of new knowledge have been developed. The knowledge that a competent neurosurgeon must master has increased vastly. As a result, no individual or small group can be expert in all areas. The only means of making a book authoritative in every area, and especially in the paraneurosurgical areas in which a neurosurgeon must be knowledgeable, is to use multiple authors from all over the world. The concept of *Neurological Surgery* came with the recognition of this problem and the need for a comprehensive reference volume that would include the more usual areas of concern to a neurosurgeon and also the allied areas in which he must be informed if he is going to give his patients the best care that is possible.

Neurological Surgery is intended for use by the surgeon in practice, the trainee who is beginning to assume responsibility for patient care, and the allied specialist who works with neurosurgical patients. Emphasis is placed on fundamental knowledge concerning etiology, pathogenesis, diagnosis, treatment, and prognosis for each disease entity of concern to the neurosurgeon. Essentials of operative technique are discussed and special techniques are evaluated and put into perspective with the more usual ones. Where appropriate, special sections or chapters are devoted to the basic aspects of neurobiology.

In addition to attempting to fill the need for a comprehensive reference source, *Neurological Surgery* has been set up so as to recognize ongoing problems and divergent views within our specialty. Wherever there are major differences in the points of view concerning methods of diagnosis or treatment, each viewpoint is presented by a recognized proponent. This approach avoids the inevitable dilution that occurs when a conflicting view is evaluated and summarized by an individual, regardless of his fairness and integrity, who does not believe in the merits of the opposing view. A perusal of the chapter titles will show numerous examples of this approach.

Many chapters are included that usually have not been present in previous texts of neurological surgery. Examples are chapters that discuss the psychological evaluation of the neurosurgical patient, neuro-otology, mechanisms of coma, hyperextension-flexion injuries of the neck, the post-traumatic syndrome, cerebral blood flow in clinical problems, the biology of brain tumors, affective disorders, the physiological and the psychiatric aspects of pain, and the principles of stereotaxic surgery. Special emphasis is given to preoperative evaluation and prevention and treatment of complications.

Like the shakedown cruise of a ship, the first edition of a text such as *Neurological Surgery* will have omissions and errors that will be revealed as the book is put to the scrutiny of those interested in our queen specialty. Mr. John Dusseau and his staff at the W. B. Saunders Company have been dedicated to producing a publication of quality, and the editor wishes to give his wholehearted expression of appreciation to them. In particular, Mr. Raymond Kersey has given care and attention to reproducing the illustrations with accuracy and clarity, and Miss Ruth Barker has worked with enthusiasm and dedication throughout the years from inception to the publication. To her, I owe especial thanks for her patient help in the editing and indexing and otherwise shepherding of this book to publication.

A book such as *Neurological Surgery* can be produced only with capable secretarial help. Miss Georgene Pucci has been invaluable to me in handling the thousands of pages of manuscripts, galley proofs, page proofs, and correspondence. Only with assistance of the type given by Miss Barker in Philadelphia and Miss Pucci in Davis could *Neurological Surgery* have become a reality. Finally, I would like to thank the contributors to *Neurological Surgery* for their cooperation and help in achieving for our joint effort the degree of success that it may enjoy.

JULIAN R. YOUMANS

CONTENTS

VOLUME I

III.   SPECIAL TESTS AND EVALUATION

IV. PHYSIOLOGY AND HOMEOSTASIS

V. ANESTHESIA AND OPERATIVE TECHNIQUE

VI. DEVELOPMENTAL AND ACQUIRED ANOMALIES

VOLUME II _____

VII.   VASCULAR DISEASE

VIII. TRAUMA

IX.   BENIGN EXTRADURAL SPINE LESIONS

VOLUME III

X. TUMORS

XI. INFECTIONS

XIII.   ABLATIVE AND NEUROPHYSIOLOGICAL PROCEDURES

XIV. GENERAL CARE AND REHABILITATION

I

History and Examination

GENERAL METHODS OF CLINICAL EXAMINATION

With the continuing development of more precise technical diagnostic procedures and instrumentation, the trend over the years has been to displace the conventional methods of the history and physical examination in diagnosis and management of the sick. This trend has been especially prevalent, and perhaps more justified, in the neurological fields. The past two decades have seen phenomenal progress in the application of modern physical science and engineering to new procedures and the refinement of old ones for probing previously denied reaches of the nervous system. Certainly the caricature of the traditional neurologist with his armamentarium of forbidding tools putting the patient through bizarre gyrations and absurd postures is as anachronistic as the old country doctor. Nevertheless, he did have among his odd manipulations some procedures for eliciting useful information that retain their value in modern diagnosis and treatment. In fact, even today the neurological history and examination remain the diagnostic procedures of primary importance. No single technical procedure matches the neurological history in permitting the clinician to focus on the correct area of etiology; none, for the time and effort invested, matches the neurological examination in giving an overview of the functioning of the nervous system at the moment and its dysfunctions salient to the clinical problem at hand.

The properly conducted and evaluated history and examination permit the most productive choice of technical diagnostic procedures at the least expense, discomfort,

and hazard to the patient. Recognition of the proper relationship of the history and examination to these procedures is the mark of the mature clinician. The planning of technical procedures prior to availing oneself of the information from the history and examination is rarely justified. The distinction between the technician and the physician is fundamentally determined by the rapport each establishes between himself and the patient. No better opportunity exists for the development of that rapport, that is so essential to superlative care of the sick, than the required hour that the physician spends listening to his patient's problem and systematically exploring its physical manifestations. In the age of technology and superspecialization, we must constantly and consciously avoid the tendency to impersonalization inherent in the system of patient care that has evolved.

In arriving at a clinical diagnosis, four essential steps are involved, in the order enumerated:

1. *Eliciting the clinical information* by conducting the history and physical examination. This is the keystone of consistently accurate diagnosis.

2. *Localizing the lesion or disease process* (i.e., establishing the anatomical diagnosis), accomplished in the first instance, and often without the necessity of additional procedures, by correlating the findings on the physical examination with one's knowledge of the anatomy and physiology of the nervous system.

3. *Arriving at an etiological diagnosis or differential diagnosis,* accomplished by correlating one's knowledge of the whereabouts of the lesion with the information elicited in the history as to the onset and subse-

O. R. TALBERT

quent course of the patient's present complaints and previous health data.

4. Utilizing additional diagnostic technical and laboratory procedures necessary to refine anatomical localization and etiological diagnosis and to plan management of the patient's ailment.

CONDUCTING THE HISTORY AND EXAMINATION

For an outline of the procedure for neurological history and examination, one may consult any of a number of textbooks on basic neurology. The emphasis here is to be on more general aims: the approach to the patient and the significance of individual findings.

In diagnosing the immediate neurological ailment presented by the patient, information as to his general state of health, pertinent previous illnesses, and the condition of the other organ systems is essential. The clinical data pertaining to the nervous system must be evaluated in the light of such general information about the patient. The method of obtaining it will vary with the circumstances in which the neurosurgeon practices, but it is his responsibility as a competent clinician to obtain the information in one way or another and to apply it in his undertaking of the neurosurgical diagnosis.

While the conventional separation of the history and physical examination into two distinctive exercises has value in teaching physical diagnosis to students, the mature clinician may find it expedient to modify so pedantic an approach to his patient. The history and examination is best considered a single exercise, which Adams has cogently designated *elicitation of the clinical data*.[1]

The technique of the clinical examination will necessarily vary with the patient's general condition. The following is a suggested approach in examining the ambulatory, cooperative, and fully conscious patient.

The neurological examination virtually begins when the examiner first greets the patient; it is then that he begins making observations of the patient's speech, movements, and mannerisms that often give clues leading to the correct localization and cause of the patient's disorder. Even when the patient is incapable of providing a reliable history, it is informative to give him the opportunity and to observe his deficiencies.

At the termination of the history it is convenient to continue with questions aimed at evaluating the patient's mental function. This requires tact and a demeanor of objectivity. It is usually advisable to begin with a frank inquiry such as: "Do you feel that you have difficulty remembering things or keeping track of events?" This can be elucidated by phrasing questions that require informative answers as to the date, recent news events, and the like, which test orientation, memory, general fund of knowledge, and ability to calculate and think abstractly. This line of questioning usually will not be resented by the patient. If it is, reassurance that this is your attempt to give him a thorough examination should suffice. Resentment, of itself, may betray a lack of insight or abnormal irritability that is of diagnostic significance, and the matter should be explored further with the patient's relatives. After sufficient questioning to elicit the information sought, proceed directly with tests of language function by presenting the patient with pencil and paper and a passage to read.

For the remainder of the examination, the patient should be moved to the examining table or asked to sit on the side of the bed. He should be clad only in shorts and, in the case of a woman, a loosely fitting garment covering the bust and leaving the shoulder girdle and upper limbs bare. No elaborate collection of gadgets is necessary in the examiner's armamentarium; however, there are a few simple aids that are necessary for the neurological examination:

An aromatic agent for testing sense of smell (tobacco, oil of peppermint, cloves)

A sharp pin with round white head 3 to 5 mm in diameter

Ophthalmoscope—otoscope

Visual testing card with graduated print size

Tuning fork, C–256

Tongue blade

Cotton wisp or cotton tip applicator

Reflex hammer

Two stoppered test tubes

The patient should be seated comfortably on the table or bed, legs dangling freely. The first step in the examination proper is to direct attention to the body part to which the patient has referred complaints. This is reassuring and logical to the patient, and frequently will uncover diagnostic information from the start.

One should then return to an orderly procedure of examination, beginning with the eyes. Holding the index finger approximately 18 inches in front of his eyes, have him follow the moving finger to either side, upward and downward. Observe the pupils, lid and brow movements, and the details of ocular movements, which are elaborated upon in Chapter 14. Terminate by having the patient converge vision on the finger as it is moved in toward the nose, observing the pupillary constriction of convergence-accommodation.

Next, perform ophthalmoscopic examination of the fundus, paying particular attention to the optic discs and maculae. With the otoscope light, test the pupillary light reflex in each eye separately. While this light is handy, examine the oropharynx, using a tongue blade to elicit the gag reflex on each side and observing for abnormality of pharynx and palate movements. Have the patient protrude the tongue for inspection. Finally, attach the ear speculum and inspect the auditory canals before dispensing with this instrument.

Returning to the eyes, test visual acuity of each eye separately with the reading card. If the patient uses corrective glasses he should wear them for this test. Using the white pinhead, test the visual fields quadrant by quadrant in each eye by the confrontation method (see Chapter 14). While the pin is handy, test pain sensation over both sides of the face.

Have the patient close the eyes and test smell sensation, each nostril separately, by passing the test object (peppermint, cloves, or tobacco) under the nose and asking for perception of the odor.

Have the patient whistle to observe function of the orbicularis oris muscle. This often provokes a spontaneous smile, offering the opportunity to observe emotional facial movements. Palpate the masseter and temporalis muscles bilaterally while the patient repetitively clenches his teeth. Test

hearing by rubbing the thumb against the fingers near each of the patient's ears. The tuning fork may be used if further testing of auditory function is indicated. Palpate the sternocleidomastoid muscle on either side with the patient's head turned to the opposite side, then inspect the upper borders of the trapezius muscles and test them for strength by having the patient shrug his shoulders.

Examine the neck by having the patient extend his head, then flex it, touching the chin on the chest. Look for limitation of neck motion or pain on motion.

Now, have the patient sit erect, close his eyes, and extend his arms straight forward, palms downward and fingers spread apart. While this posture is maintained for 90 seconds, a number of valuable observations can be made. Tremors and other abnormal involuntary movements are readily evident during maintenance of this posture. It also affords an excellent opportunity to inspect the musculature of trunk and upper limbs for evidence of atrophy. Inspect the shoulder girdle front and rear. Look for abnormal curvature of the spine and other trunk deformities. Keep an eye on the arms to see if one or the other sags to betray a motor weakness or wavers about to betray a deficit in coordination or position sense. Proprioceptive sensation and cerebellar function can be tested further by having the patient touch the tip of his index finger to his nose while the eyes remain closed, then with the eyes open.

Next, have the patient rest his arms in his lap. Move each arm passively, feeling for alteration of muscle tone. With his arms symmetrically relaxed in his lap and his legs dangling freely, test the tendon reflexes in all four limbs, comparing the two sides.

Now, have the patient lie supine on the examining table. Test the plantar, cremasteric, and cutaneous abdominal reflexes. Test sensory function beginning with position sensibility, light touch, and the discriminatory (cortical) sensibilities. Testing for light touch with the cotton wisp should include the extremities and trunk, the corneal reflexes, and the face. Pinprick, being the most unpleasant, is usually best reserved until last. The detail to which sensory testing is carried will vary depending on the nature of the individual problem.

However, minimum testing should include proprioceptive (vibratory and position), cutaneous (light touch and pain) and discriminatory — or "cortical" — modalities. Suspicion of a cerebral lesion will require detailed testing of the discriminatory modalities, whereas information regarding the proprioceptive and cutaneous modalities will be more helpful when disease at lower levels is suspected.

The patient is queried regarding disturbance of sphincter function. Rectal examination for sphincter tone should be done if there is a history of incontinence or if one suspects spinal cord disease.

Finally, the examination should always be terminated by having the patient stand and walk. Observation of gait, posture, swinging of the arms while walking, heel-to-toe (tandem) walking, change of direction in walking, and ability to stand on a narrow base provides evaluation of motor and cerebellar functions that cannot be obtained as readily or reliably by any other technique. Having the patient sit in a low chair and rise, squat and rise, and flex the trunk from the erect posture are easy methods of evaluating strength and function of pelvic girdle and lower limb musculature and motility of the lower spine.

This technique of examination, while lengthy in description, can be carried out within a period of 15 to 20 minutes after brief experience. More prolonged examination at the initial exercise is not likely to be profitable because of fatigue on the part of both patient and examiner. When a particular system or function requires more meticulous evaluation than is afforded by the procedure described, it is best carried out in subsequent examinations.

LOCALIZING THE LESION (ANATOMICAL DIAGNOSIS)

From the body of clinical information obtained from the history and examination, one should next attempt to define the location of the lesion or disease process affecting the nervous system. Rarely can this be done on the basis of one individual finding. Accurate anatomical localization nearly always requires consideration of the *totality of physical findings* rather than any single

one. Multiple findings sometimes constitute a syndrome that signifies impairment of a specific function mediated by a structurally distinct and functionally related system of neurons. In other instances, the combination of findings indicates a lesion confined to a restricted region or level of the nervous system, perhaps involving multiple structures. In still other instances, the findings indicate diffuse disease. It is a helpful step in diagnosis to consider whether the aggregate of findings constitutes a pattern signifying one of these three categories of localization.

Syndromes of Specific Functions

Upper Motor Neuron Paralysis

The "upper motor neuron" system is more a physiological than an anatomical entity. Originally, it was defined anatomically as identical with the pyramidal (corticospinal) tract, which was thought to arise from the Betz cells in the precentral gyrus of each frontal lobe and to form the pyramids on the ventral surface of the medulla oblongata. The signs ascribed to injury to this tract were, therefore, called pyramidal signs. Subsequent investigations have led to the recognition that this concept of the pyramidal tract was inadequate, and some observers have maintained that individual components of this syndrome are due to injury to the extrapyramidal neuronal system rather than the pyramidal. Much of the controversy that has ensued is of little consequence in clinical diagnosis, but one area of disagreement seems to involve different usage of terms that denote the clinical state of muscle tone. The terms "spasticity" and "rigidity" have quite separate and distinct meanings to most clinicians, whereas they seem to be used interchangeably by some writers. Clinically it is useful and conventional to regard spasticity as synonymous with the "clasp knife" phenomenon (lengthening reaction). It is a state of altered tone of skeletal muscle that is elicited most readily when the involved limb is passively moved suddenly. At the beginning and through the initial phase of the movement there is palpable resistance of the muscle being lengthened, then toward the end of the movement there is an abrupt disappearance of the muscle resistance and the limb gives readily to the movement. Its resemblance to the "catch" and "give" of a spring-loaded knife blade being closed is the source of the term "clasp knife reaction." This disorder of muscle tone is to be distinguished from *rigidity*, which is described later.

While the older concept of the pyramidal tract is no longer adequate, a system of which the corticospinal-corticobulbar pathway is the predominant anatomical component consists of neurons arising largely in the cortex of each cerebral hemisphere and transmitting impulses more or less directly—i.e., without synaptic interruption—to its target cells in the contralateral anterior gray column of the spinal cord. A convenient, if not anatomically precise, term by which this system can be designated is "upper motor neuron." The term "pyramidal tract" is so entrenched in clinical parlance, however, that its use is likely to continue. When this system is damaged anywhere along its course, from cerebral cortex through the internal capsule and brain stem to the termination of its axons along the lateral white columns of the spinal cord, there results a syndrome of altered motor function consisting of the following elements:

1. Motor paralysis affecting functionally related groups of muscles rather than individual muscles is usually only partial (paresis) and largely transient and affects mostly the discrete movements of the distal limb segments.

2. Clasp knife phenomenon (spasticity, in the clinical sense) occurs in the involved limb or limbs, but in acute lesions there may be a transient phase of flaccidity or hypotonia ("neuronal shock") lasting a few days or weeks.

3. Hyperactive tendon reflexes are present in the involved limb or limbs, but there may be transient areflexia for the duration of neuronal shock in acute lesions.

4. The cutaneous abdominal and cremasteric reflexes are lost on the paretic side.

5. Babinski's toe sign (extensor plantar response) is present on the paretic side.

6. There is lack of atrophy of the involved muscles, except late from disuse. No muscle fasciculations occur.

In its early stages or milder degrees the only sign of the syndrome may be a Babinski sign or a slight increase in tendon reflexes as compared to the opposite (normal) side. When the lesion is a progressive one, the other signs gradually appear. Lesions that affect both this system and the extrapyramidal system at cerebral hemisphere, brain stem, or spinal cord levels will produce rigidity accompanying, and perhaps overshadowing, the clasp knife reaction in the involved parts.

Lower Motor Neuron Paralysis

The concept of the "lower motor neuron" is likewise a physiological one; however, its anatomy is more precise. The term refers to the aggregate of the neurons of the motor nuclei of the cranial nerves and the anterior gray horn (column) of the spinal cord, each of which, along with the group of somatic muscle fibers innervated by it, constitutes a motor unit. Each neuron of the system is the final common pathway whereby all the multiple influences of the nervous system on motor function are integrated and transmitted to the effector muscle. At the spinal level the aggregate of lower motor neurons at a given spinal cord segment constitutes the efferent limb of the spinal reflex arc. A lesion affecting this system, anywhere from the parent neurons of the anterior horn (column) along their axons coursing through anterior spinal roots, spinal nerves, plexus, peripheral nerves or their synaptic junction with the muscle (motor end-plate) produces a motor syndrome consisting of the following:

1. Motor paralysis of the individual muscle or groups of muscles innervated by them is of variable distribution. The degree of paralysis varies also, depending on the proportion of total motor supply impaired.

2. Loss of muscle tone (flaccidity or hypotonia) is persistent.

3. Tendon reflexes are diminished or absent in the involved limb or limbs; cutaneous reflexes are preserved except where their effector muscles are totally paralyzed.

4. Muscle atrophy begins early, is marked, and increases for the duration of the lesion.

5. There is no Babinski sign or other pathological reflex.

6. Muscle fasciculations occur in some cases.

Since it is the final pathway, the manifestations of lower motor neuron involvement will predominate when the lesion involves it along with other pathways that influence it. Thus when both upper and lower motor neuron supplies to a limb are completely interrupted, the findings will be those of lower motor neuron paralysis; however, when the involvement of the lower motor neuron is only partial, one may find manifestations of both in the same limb. An important point in determining the level of the lesion of lower motor neuron is whether its motor manifestations are accompanied by sensory deficit in the same part. If so, the lesion must be in a mixed nerve bundle in which motor and sensory axons coexist (both anterior and posterior roots, spinal nerve, plexus, or proximal part of peripheral nerve); if not, the lesion must be in anterior gray horn of spinal cord, or anterior root or roots, or distal enough in peripheral nerve to involve only a motor branch.

The cranial nerves present a unique situation with regard to differentiation of upper and lower motor neuron involvement and presence or absence of accompanying sensory deficits. Those which receive supranuclear (corticobulbar) influence from both sides (upper half of the face, pharynx, larynx, tongue, and some of the respiratory muscles) will show little or no paralysis from a unilateral upper motor neuron lesion, except transiently following an acute lesion. Since the only other manifestation of upper neuron paralysis testable in the cranial nerves is the jaw jerk, this can be an important reflex to test in determining the level in the neuraxis of an upper neuron lesion. In some of the cranial nerves (e.g., the fifth and seventh) the arrangement and type of sensory nerve fibers related to the motor fibers is peculiar to the individual nerve. One may consult a textbook of neuroanatomy for the anatomical details.

The Extrapyramidal Syndrome

The older anatomical concept of the extrapyramidal system has, like that of the pyramidal system, undergone modification in recent years; however, as a physiological or functional entity — or more exactly, a system the dysfunction of which is manifested by a consistent set of clinical findings — it has retained its identity over the years. The basal ganglia are still accepted as the anatomical "core" of this system.

These have extensive connections with the cerebral cortex, primarily the premotor area of the frontal lobe. They are also interconnected with one another and with parts of the thalamus and hypothalamus, olivary nuclei, and brain stem reticular formation. Unlike the direct corticospinal-corticobulbar system, the extrapyramidal system is a multisynaptic system of neurons with short-chain axons and feedbacks that indirectly project to the lower motor neuron system by several scattered pathways descending the brain stem and the spinal cord; these, for the most part, cross to the side opposite from their origin at multiple levels. Their clinical manifestations are, therefore, like the corticospinal-corticobulbar system, mainly contralateral.

The cardinal clinical findings indicating involvement of the extrapyramidal system are:

1. Rigidity, a type of increased tone of skeletal musculature in which resistance to passive movement of the limb remains constant throughout the range of the movement and is present regardless of the speed at which the limb is moved. It may be of either the plastic (lead-pipe) or the cogwheel variety.

2. Hyperkinesias (dyskinesias), which are abnormal involuntary movements of several varieties including tremor at rest (or rather partial rest, since it tends to subside not only during the use of the trembling part for volitional movements but also when the part is completely relaxed as during sleep), chorea ("St. Vitus dance"), athetosis, and ballismus (usually occurring unilaterally as hemiballismus).

3. Bradykinesia (hypokinesia) consisting of both a paucity of spontaneous movements and slowness (inhibition) of volitional movements. Spontaneous movements that become impaired include: "automatic movements," which are carried out as accompaniments of volitional movements (e.g., swinging of arms while walking, or expressional facial movements during conversation); and the several components of a complexity of simultaneously performed movements (e.g., walking, talking, and gesticulating simultaneously).

4. Dystonia, an alteration of posture of the body or its parts due to imbalance of tone in antagonist muscle groups that ordinarily maintain the trunk and appendages in their normal posture. Such abnormal

postures are mobile, develop during volitional motor activity, and tend to melt away with cessation of activity. Later, especially those that are maintained for long periods at a time, such as flexion of the trunk in parkinsonism, tend to become fixed.

5. Tendon reflexes that are normal or slightly hyperactive; no Babinski sign or other pathological reflexes present.

The extrapyramidal syndrome is most frequently encountered with nonsurgical diseases, parkinsonism being the most common. However, it sometimes occurs in pure form with focal lesions situated deep in the cerebral hemisphere; and extrapyramidal manifestations are frequently seen in conjunction with upper motor neuron ones when lesions in the central nervous system involve both systems. An important fact in neurosurgical diagnosis is that *unilateral extrapyramidal signs do not necessarily signify a focal operative lesion.* More often than not, the progressive diseases of this system such as parkinsonism begin unilaterally.

Rarely does one encounter all the extrapyramidal manifestations in the same patient. The hyperkinesias, other than tremor, and the bradykinesias especially are unlikely to occur together. In fact, there is some clinical and biochemical evidence that the two are inversely related. Although rigidity is characteristic of the syndrome, chorea may actually be accompanied by hypotonia and laxity of the limbs instead.

Ataxia

The syndromes of the cerebellum are described later in this chapter. Ataxia (incoordination) is a cardinal manifestation of involvement of the cerebellum or its connecting pathways in the brain stem; however, ataxia is not necessarily of cerebellar origin. It may occur as a major manifestation in any of the following four situations:

1. Cerebellar ataxia (discussed later) including the flocculonodular (midline) syndrome and the lateral (cerebellar hemisphere) syndrome.

2. Frontal lobe ataxia (also discussed later).

3. Proprioceptive sensory ataxia in which there is loss of sense of position

in one or more extremities from a lesion involving the posterior white columns of spinal cord or the proprioceptive fibers in the peripheral nervous system. In impairment of proprioceptive sensation, the defect is compensated for by substituting visual and tactile information. Ataxia characteristically develops in the part deprived of sense of position when the eyes are closed and tactile clues to the body are removed. The entire syndrome thus consists of: positive Romberg sign, loss of proprioceptive (position and vibratory) sensation and ataxia.

4. Vestibular (labyrinthine) ataxia in which a lesion involves the labyrinth in the inner ear, the vestibular component of the eighth cranial nerve peripherally, or the vestibular nuclei and pathways within the brain stem. The syndrome consists of the combination of vertigo, nausea and vomiting, horizontal or rotary nystagmus, and a reeling type of ataxia. It is sometimes also referred to as "vertiginous ataxia" because of the prominence of vertigo. In view of the interconnections between the vestibular nuclei in the brain stem and the midline cerebellar structures, this form of ataxia may be difficult to distinguish from the midline cerebellar syndrome; indeed, the two may coexist by simultaneous involvement of both structures by a properly situated lesion in the posterior cranial fossa.

The finding and differentiation of these disorders of specific functions of the nervous system usually permits only an approximate anatomical diagnosis. Most of the syndromes just described could indicate a lesion at any of several levels. The location of a lesion can be determined more precisely by attempting to define the level or *region* to which the combination of abnormal findings points. This approach is discussed next.

Localization of Lesions by Regions

There is a priority of specificity for regional localization among individual clinical findings and syndromes. Some findings (e.g., aphasia) are highly specific indicators of the region involved, whereas others, as just discussed, are specific for particular neuronal systems or pathways traversing more than one region (e.g., upper motor neuron paralysis). By combining these two types of findings it is possible to arrive at an accurate anatomical localization and often simultaneously to determine etiology. The five major regional levels into which most syndromes of focal neurological deficit may be localized readily are the *supratentorial intracranial, the infratentorial intracranial (posterior cranial fossa), the spinal canal, the peripheral nervous system, and the skeletal musculature.* These are discussed in order.

Manifestations of Supratentorial Intracranial Lesions

Lesions localized to the anterior or middle cranial fossa are manifest neurologically by signs of cerebral, visual, olfactory, or endocrine dysfunction depending on the precise location and nature of the lesion. Cerebral manifestations include motor, sensory, or certain mental disturbances, which may present as isolated findings but more often as symptom-complexes (syndromes), each of which has its value in anatomical diagnosis. Either irritative or destructive (deficit-producing) cerebral manifestations or both may constitute such a syndrome. The most useful of these syndromes will be considered individually.

Epileptic Seizures

Epileptic attacks physiologically are irritative phenomena in which abnormal synchronous activation of aggregates of cerebral neurons occurs, usually originating in a restricted area of brain. They manifest themselves in various patterns of clinical change in the victim depending primarily upon the function normally subserved by the originally activated cellular aggregate, its anatomical relation to other functional areas of the nervous system, and the facility and speed with which the discharge is propagated within the nervous system. Epilepsy may be divided into two categories clinically: *generalized* or diffuse seizures and *focal* seizures. The first category includes "grand mal" and "petit mal" seizures believed to arise from deep within the central brain — Penfield's centrencephalic system — and propagated rapidly to activate cerebral neurons generally. These types, beginning in childhood or adolescence, recurring over a period of

months or years, and constituting the patient's only neurological abnormality ("idiopathic epilepsy") seldom are a problem for the neurosurgeon. However, two precautions need to be taken into account here. In the first place, seizures that at first blush may seem to be of grand mal type may be revealed on further information to have additional features clearly signifying that they, in fact, have a focal onset followed by rapid spread to generalized activation. This is especially true of those attacks the very onset of which is missed by the witness-historian, those occurring during sleep, and those in which amnesia for the onset prohibits the patient's recalling the initial focal phenomena. Secondly, not all brief attacks or those in which loss of consciousness is dubious constitute petit mal epilepsy.

Focal epilepsy is the category of seizures of major importance in neurosurgical diagnosis. Seizures of this category may be regarded as invariably arising in a focus of cerebral cortex and therefore always indicating that their causative lesion is within the cranial cavity above the tentorium. They may occur alone or in company with other neurological signs that serve to further localize the lesion. An individual focal seizure may remain focal in its clinical manifestations throughout the duration of the attack (even for long spans of time in occasional cases, i.e., epilepsia partialis continua), or it may spread with varying rapidity and over varying extent of the brain with attendant progressing somatic manifestations (jacksonian march), or it may abruptly proceed from its focal manifestations to a generalized convulsion closely simulating grand mal epilepsy.

The specific patterns of clinical events signifying focal seizures are of almost infinite diversity.[10] *Any paroxysmal experience that can be ascribed, on either experimental or clinical grounds, to synchronous activation of neurons in any focal area of brain should be regarded as potentially signifying a focal seizure.* The potential is enhanced if the experience recurs wholly or in part as a stereotyped pattern and if it is brief in duration. While the two generally recognized characteristics of epilepsy are abnormal or inappropriate motor activity and impairment of consciousness, neither of these is indispensable to the diagnosis of focal epilepsy. Depending on the nature of brain function to which the activated neuronal focus contributes, the clinical manifestations of a focal seizure may be motor, sensory, or mental.[10, 14] In the history, one must inquire as to subjective experiences and, *specifically, whether emotional or sensory experiences occur in association with attacks.* Not only is the patient unlikely to realize that such experiences constitute a part of his seizure, but also he may decline to voluntarily divulge bizarre sensations that he fears constitute a threat to mental integrity. Both the patient and witnesses to his attacks should provide a precise and complete chronological account of each event leading up to, comprising, and immediately following his attack.

Dementia

The syndrome of dementia is frequently the earliest and at times the only manifestation of an intracranial lesion. Dementia implies deterioration in those specific intellectual spheres dependent upon brain function in a person whose performance in these spheres was previously normal. Deterioration of (1) memory (especially that for recent events), (2) orientation in time and immediate environment, (3) ability to think abstractly, and (4) fund of general information are the cardinal manifestations to be sought. Other manifestations of altered mentation such as depression, loss of insight and judgment, visual or auditory hallucinations, delusions, personality change, and impairment of concentration may occur as components of the total syndrome; but they are not primary manifestations of dementia or necessarily indicators of organic brain disease. Nevertheless, the history of even subtle and nonspecific changes in the individual's behavior such as irritability, change in sleep habits, loss of interest and initiative at work or recreation, and unaccustomed errors in intellectual performances should alert one to the possibility of early dementia and lead one to search for loss of capacity in those specific spheres indicative of organic disease. Dementia often is a manifestation of medical diseases such as hypothyroidism, syphilis, or arteriosclerosis. Of interest in neurosurgical diagnosis, however, is the fact that the identical syndrome may herald intracranial tumor, subdural hematoma, and other neurosurgical lesions, whether it occurs alone or in company with other neurological findings. When other findings occur they may be focal and lateralized or they may be nonfocal ones such as grasp reflex or snout reflex, postural tremor or generalized seizures. Dementia of moderate or advanced degree, alone or in association with other neurological abnormalities, can usually be diagnosed by "bedside" tests of recent memory, orientation, ability to keep in mind and carry out a problem such as serial subtractions of 7 from 100, and knowledge of events expected of the patient's level of education and experience. Formal psychometric testing by a trained psychologist may be necessary to diagnose milder degrees.

Aphasia and Agnosia

Syndromes of disordered language (aphasia, agnosia) constitute a highly specific diagnostic finding. They signify a focal lesion involving the dominant cerebral hemisphere, which is the left hemisphere in virtually all right-handed and about half of left-handed persons. Language is a specialized intellectual function that is in essence the use of a system of symbols consisting of words and groups of words that convey meanings. The use of language is a dual process consisting of the reception and recognition of word symbols on the one hand and expression of them on the other. The entire process is dependent upon such a restricted mass of brain for its essential function that it may be profoundly impaired by a lesion sufficiently small to spare all other mental faculties. Aphasia is the term used to denote the selective loss of ability to comprehend or meaningfully to execute language in the absence of generalized mental impairment or motor impairment sufficient to account for the loss. Agnosia denotes the loss of ability to recognize or to appreciate the significance of stimuli although the perception of them is intact. Verbal agnosia is the specific agnosia for word symbols that pertains to language disorders. The diagnosis of aphasia and its use as a sign of a focal intracranial lesion rests primarily on evaluation of spoken language. Impairment of spoken language is usually accompanied by impairment of ability to write (agraphia) or to read (alexia), but neither of these components of written language is likely to be impaired alone as a result of an intracranial lesion. Mild degrees of aphasia (dysphasia) often manifested by only occasional misuse of a word in the course of conversation, are of equally important localizing value as more severe disturbances. Furthermore, in the individual's language armamentarium there exists a hierarchy of vulnerability that becomes manifest when speech is progressively or only partially impaired: primitive and emotional speech (e.g., exclamations, swearing) and speech that is automatic by virtue of having been learned early or repeated often (e.g., salutations, the alphabet, childhood prayers and poems, the names of the months) are least vulnerable and remain relatively intact; propositional or symbolic speech, i.e., that which conveys ideas rather than feeling, is more vulnerable and is impaired to some degree in virtually all dysphasics; polyglots lose use of recently learned tongues more readily than their native and longer-used tongue. In order to elicit milder degrees of dysphasia, therefore, it is necessary to engage the patient in sufficiently extensive conversation involving propositional speech and to maintain a keen ear for recurrent mispronunciations or tendency to stereotyped responses. This can usually be accomplished during the course of taking the patient's history. Additional testing by having the patient name objects shown him, read aloud a passage from the newspaper, write a sentence to dictation, and carry out a complicated oral command will provide confirmatory evidence of a disturbance of language in the suspected case.

Two syndromes of aphasia can be recognized clinically, one of which indicates a lesion anteriorly and the other posteriorly in the dominant cerebral hemisphere. Although neither is often seen in pure form, one or the other pattern will be predominant in individual cases frequently enough to help in localization.

1. *Expressive (motor) aphasia* is characterized by impairment of ability to say what one wishes to say, whether it be ex-
pressing oneself, reading aloud, or repeating what is said to him. The patient usually is alert and gives the appearance of being mentally clear. He is able to comprehend all or most of what is said to him and what he reads, but cannot execute spoken language normally. He usually cannot write without making errors in the formation of letters or spelling of words that were normally at his command. He may be able to identify objects by pantomime or circumlocution, but not call their names; parts of an object (e.g., heel, lace, sole) may be more difficult to name than the whole object (shoe). The mild expressive dysphasic may be able to use words or short phrases appropriately, but fail in attempts at more sustained expression. The severe aphasic may be unable to utter a word or may be reduced to emotional speech or to simple "yes" or "no" responses inappropriately used. The patient is aware of his language deficit and manifests exasperation at his inadequacy. The lesion causing this type of aphasia is almost always located in or upon the convex surface of the dominant (usually left) frontal lobe just anterior to the inferior extent of the fissure of Rolando, occasionally to the subjacent insular cortex and external capsule (Fig. 1–1). It is often accompanied by right hemiplegia (left hemiplegia in left-handed persons).

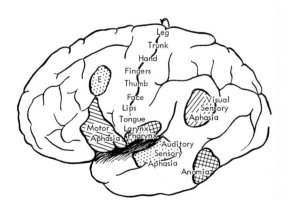

FIGURE 1–1 Convex surface of the left cerebral hemisphere showing the areas of major importance in disturbance of language. E, Exner's "writing center," injury to which causes dysgraphia. Both the auditory and visual areas of sensory aphasia must be involved to produce the total picture of sensory (Wernicke's) aphasia. Anomia depends on involvement of the inferior temporal area when it accompanies sensory aphasia.

2. *Receptive (sensory or Wernicke's) aphasia* is more variable in the details of language deficit present, but most often consists of: inability to comprehend spoken language (auditory verbal agnosia), inability to comprehend written language (visual verbal agnosia), and inability to write (agraphia).

The patient is able to speak and often talks profusely, but after the first sentence or two, what he says becomes progressively unrelated to what has been said to him. Being unable to comprehend the meaning of his own words, he tends to talk in disjointed sentences and phrases. In some cases there is an associated nominal (or amnesic) aphasia, characterized by inability to say the names of objects although able to recognize the names when they are spoken or to describe their use. Unlike the motor aphasic, the sensory aphasic is unaware of his language dysfunction; therefore he becomes annoyed at those speaking to him rather than at himself. The irrelevant voluble speech and annoyed behavior of the sensory aphasic may give the impression that he is mentally disturbed or hostile. For this reason, it is important to avoid mistaking his aphasic condition for the erratic behavior of the manic or the schizophrenic. *This type of aphasia results from a focal lesion involving the posterior superior portion of the convex surface of the dominant temporal lobe, called Wernicke's area* (Fig. 1–1).

Aphasia must be differentiated from more diffuse disorder of mental function. Deterioration of language not infrequently occurs as a part of the total picture in dementia, in which case it is of dubious localizing value. Aphasia must also be differentiated from other disorders of speech mediated at a lower level: (1) dysarthria is impairment of the articulation of words resulting from motor impairment of the muscles of the lips, tongue, and pharynx involved in speaking; (2) dysphonia is loss of voice or hoarseness due to motor impairment of laryngeal muscles; (3) mutism is a nonspecific loss of speech or refusal to speak that is usually a hysterical manifestation or part of the deaf-mute state. Akinetic mutism is the clinical state in which there is loss of power or ability to speak along with generalized severe loss of motor power.

The Frontal Lobe

The most conspicuous clinical manifestations of frontal lobe lesions are motor ones (Fig. 1–2). Contralateral "upper motor neuron paralysis" results from involvement of the motor and premotor frontal areas or the axons projecting from these areas to form the corticobulbar-corticospinal tract. When the premotor area is involved, the sucking and grasp reflexes and groping response are present contralaterally. A premotor lesion that involves the projection pathways to and from the cerebellum may produce ataxia and tremor of the contralateral limbs ("frontal lobe ataxia") simulating the lateral cerebellar syndrome. Extrapyramidal signs and, when bilateral, inability to stand or walk (astasia-abasia) may be produced. These premotor signs are more prominent in widespread bilateral involvement or with a midline interhemispheric lesion than with unilateral involvement. Interference with turning of head and eyes to the contralateral side (paralysis of conjugate gaze) results from involvement of a restricted cortical region immediately anterior to the premotor cortex. Motor (expressive) aphasia resulting from involvement of the posterior inferior area on the convex surface of the frontal cortex of the dominant hemisphere is described in the previous section.

THE FRONTAL LOBE SYNDROME. Anterior to these areas related to motor func-

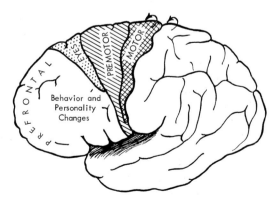

FIGURE 1–2 Lateral surface of the left cerebral hemisphere showing the areas of the frontal lobe related to the clinical signs described in the text. *Eyes,* the frontal motor eye field, associated with conjugate deviation of the eyes. The arrows at the top indicate extension of the precentral and postcentral gyri onto the medial cortical surface forming the *paracentral lobule* illustrated in Figure 1–3.

tions lies the prefrontal area, an extensive area of the frontal lobe in the human brain that distinguishes it grossly from the brain of lower animals (Fig. 1–2). Disturbance of this portion of the frontal lobes results in an array of changes in mentation and personality that have been designated collectively as the frontal lobe syndrome. Historically, this syndrome is identified with the case of Phineas Gage reported by Harlow in 1848.[4] Gage, a 25-year-old railroad worker survived for 13 years following extensive injury to both frontal lobes from a dynamite explosion that drove an iron tamping rod through his skull. Prior to the injury he had been a reverent, industrious, steady provider. Upon recovery, and thereafter for the rest of his life, he remained an irreverent, profane, impulsive vagrant.

In more recent years, study of patients following frontal lobe excision for tumors and patients subjected to prefrontal leukotomy in the treatment of mental illness has served to define the syndrome more precisely. The changes are most pronounced with bilateral prefrontal involvement; but they occur to a lesser extent with unilateral involvement, especially if it is in the dominant hemisphere. The syndrome consists in essence of loss of those traits of behavior, emotional restraint, and intelligence that characterize man's higher cultural development, including: (1) lack of emotional restraint, which may take the form of restless impulsiveness, inappropriate joking, childish excitement, outbursts of temper, facetiousness, social indiscretions, or loss of sexual inhibitions; (2) impairment of certain intellectual functions: distractibility and inability to concentrate, loss of initiative, mental torpor, impairment of recent memory (usually mild), difficulty adapting to new tasks, and impairment of abstract reasoning; and (3) dulling of certain neurotic traits such as worry, rigidity, compulsiveness, and anxiety. Concern over persistent pain is also reduced.

Since cultural development varies widely among normal people, one must take into account the individual's previous personality, educational accomplishments, and behavior patterns in diagnosing the frontal lobe syndrome. In equivocal cases, search for accompanying premotor changes such as the primitive snout or grasp reflexes will

often help in the diagnosis. These will only be found if the causative lesion extends sufficiently far back in the frontal lobe to involve those areas concerned with motor functions. The intellectual changes found in the frontal lobe syndrome are the same as some of those constituting the syndrome of dementia, but the latter encompasses additional features not found in disease limited to the frontal lobes.

The Temporal Lobe

From the standpoint of clinical diagnosis, the temporal lobes, with the exception of Wernicke's area in the dominant hemisphere, have been regarded traditionally as "silent areas" because lesions involving these areas often must reach sufficient proportion to produce increased intracranial pressure or encroachment on adjacent structures before becoming manifest clinically.

Lesions involving the deep white matter of the temporal lobe, however, will encroach on the lower fibers of the optic radiation (Meyer's loop), resulting in a contralateral homonymous upper quadrantanopsia—the so-called "pie in the sky" visual field defect. *This important finding may be the only clinical evidence of a lesion in this location,* and is one of which the patient is usually unaware.

The cortical projection areas for hearing and labyrinthine function are located on the superior surface of the temporal lobe. Although dizziness, tinnitus, and transient impairment of ability to localize sound have been reported in some instances of temporal lobe lesions, there usually is no defect in these functions because they are bilaterally represented at cortical level and, therefore, remain intact unless there is bilateral involvement.

PSYCHOMOTOR EPILEPSY. This is a clinically descriptive term introduced by Gibbs and Lennox in 1937 to denote seizures that were associated with a common electroencephalographic pattern, but with a wide variety of individual clinical patterns. The clinical patterns include: dreamy states, sensory illusions or hallucinations (olfactory, visual, auditory), automatisms (complex and purposeful but inappropriate motor acts such as smacking of lips or disrobing), emotional experiences, and amnesia for events during part or all of the attack.

Seizures of this general category have been found frequently related to abnormal electroencephalographic changes localized to one or both temporal lobes and, less frequently, to focal lesions in the same location. Accordingly, in recent years it has become common practice to use the terms "psychomotor epilepsy" and "temporal lobe epilepsy" synonymously on the assumption that such seizures are indicative of temporal lobe lesions. While the correlation is sufficiently frequent to be clinically useful, exceptions are also frequent.[9] Repeated instances are reported in which the lesion causing psychomotor attacks is found remote from the temporal lobe, usually involving components of the limbic system other than those within the temporal lobe.

In summary, aside from the signs of increased intracranial pressure when the lesion is of sufficient size, the usual clinical manifestations of a lesion in the dominant temporal lobe are: aphasia of sensory and "nominal" types; contralateral "pie in the sky" homonymous visual field defect; or certain patterns of psychomotor epileptic seizures. In the nondominant temporal lobe, the only likely localizing manifestations are the contralateral visual field defect or psychomotor type of seizures.

The Limbic System

Although functionally separable to a great extent, the limbic system and the temporal lobe should be considered together because they overlap anatomically. The limbic lobe consists of cortex and subcortical structures that form a rim (limbus = border) surrounding the opening of the lateral ventricle on the medial surface of each cerebral hemisphere (Fig. 1–3). On the surface it includes the septal region and part of the orbital cortex on the inferomedial surface of the frontal lobe, the cingulate gyrus, isthmus, hippocampal gyrus, uncus, and primary olfactory cortex. Its subjacent structures include the cingulum and septal nuclei, the hippocampal formation lying deep to the hippocampal gyrus, and the amygdala. These structures

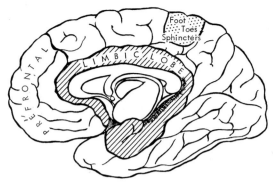

FIGURE 1–3 Medial surface of the cerebral hemisphere showing the cortical areas constituting the *limbic lobe*. The remainder of the limbic system lies subcortical to the area outlined. Also shown is the *paracentral lobule (dotted)*, the extension of the precentral and postcentral gyri onto the medial surface of the hemisphere.

are richly interconnected with one another and with the mamillary bodies, the olfactory tract, the diencephalon, and the upper reticular formation of the midbrain to form the limbic system. This system constitutes the anatomical and physiological substrate for those cerebral functions having to do with visceral activity, with emotions, and with memory.

Since the limbic lobe anatomically includes almost the entire inferomedial aspect of the temporal lobe, the question of which lobe to assign a given clinical manifestation topographically would seem optional. However, the divergence of function and of structural connections of the two probably accounts largely for discrepancies not infrequently encountered in anatomical localization of lesions manifested by visceral, emotional, or memory changes. As already suggested, psychomotor seizures in many instances signify disturbance in the limbic system rather than in the temporal lobe proper.

THE KLÜVER-BUCY SYNDROME. In 1937, Klüver and Bucy reported a striking syndrome in the monkey following bilateral removal of the limbic components of the temporal lobes. It consisted of visual agnosia, compulsive oral exploration of objects, excessive attention to and reaction to visual stimuli (hypermetamorphosis), change from aggressiveness to emotional passivity, loss of fear, increased sexual activity, and bulimia. Essentially the same syndrome has been reproduced in man, as reported by Terzian and Ore.[12]

The essential features of the syndrome in man are emotional changes (poverty of feeling and docile behavior), profound loss of memory and recognition, indiscriminate hypersexuality (self-abuse, exhibitionism, heterosexual or homosexual behavior), excessive eating (bulimia), and excessive attentiveness to visual stimuli (hypermetamorphosis). It is a profoundly disabling syndrome that renders the person permanently ineffectual socially. The accumulated evidence to date indicates that its cause is the destruction, bilaterally, of the components of the limbic system located in the inferomedial part of the temporal lobes (hippocampus, uncus, and amygdaloid nucleus). The syndrome or components of it are most likely to be encountered clinically following severe head injury, or conceivably with a midline lesion in or near the third ventricle or interpeduncular space of sufficient size to encroach upon the medial aspect of both temporal lobes. It may also be caused inadvertently by a unilateral temporal lobectomy that includes the limbic structures if the patient has pre-existing unrecognized damage to the limbic lobe on the opposite side.

Current knowledge permits only limited and fragmentary correlation of clinical signs and symptoms with the highly complex limbic system otherwise. One should suspect disease involving it when disturbance of visceral functions, emotions, or memory is encountered as a part of any cerebral syndrome. Malamud has summarized the manifestations of tumors involving the system.[8]

The Parietal Lobe

The cortex of the parietal lobes, in addition to being the end-station for sensory impulses from the homolateral thalamus, is essential to the individual's orientation and awareness of the parts of his own body, his orientation in space, and his awareness of the spatial relationship of objects in his immediate environment. Lesions that irritate the parietal cortex are manifested clinically by focal sensory epileptic

seizures. These may consist of primitive sensations such as tingling, or of more elaborate sensory experiences such as a feeling that a limb is disproportionate to the rest of the body in size, shape, or position. Such sensory phenomena may constitute the entire seizure or may be the aura for a generalized seizure.

THE PARIETAL LOBE SYNDROME. Destructive lesions limited to parietal cortex cause selective impairment of sensory discrimination rather than the primitive cutaneous sensations of pain, temperature, and touch. These discriminatory sensations, collectively referred to as cortical sensation, include: sense of position of body parts, ability to correctly localize a cutaneous stimulus without the aid of vision, ability to identify objects by feel (stereognosis), and two-point tactile discrimination. Along with deficit in these there may be the phenomenon of sensory extinction in which, when bilateral simultaneous cutaneous stimuli are presented, the patient fails to appreciate the stimulus applied to the affected side. In addition to cortical sensory deficit, there may be motor weakness in the same parts. The patient may have one or more of the following manifestations of body disorientation or neglect contralateral to the lesion: inability to recognize or locate a part (autotopagnosia), unawareness or denial of the motor or sensory defect in the involved part (anosognosia), or neglect of the involved side of the body in dressing and grooming himself. He may also manifest disorientation in external space by neglect of that part of the environment contralateral to his lesion. When asked to describe the details of a composite picture shown him or draw a symmetrical diagram such as a clock face, he is likely to neglect that side of the picture or drawing contralateral to his lesion while attending adequately to the half homolateral to the lesion. When the lesion extends to involve the white matter deep to parietal cortex, there may be an associated contralateral homonymous visual field defect due to encroachment on the optic radiations passing through this area en route to the calcarine cortex. In summary, the parietal lobe syndrome includes sensory deficit of cortical type contralateral to the lesion, contralateral hemiparesis (sometimes), neglect of body parts contralateral to the lesion, neglect of external space contralateral to the lesion, and, sometimes, contralateral homonymous visual field defect.

It is characteristic of this syndrome that its component manifestations tend to fluctuate from one examination to the next and from day to day; therefore, more than one examination of sensory functions is often necessary to demonstrate fully its manifestations in the individual patient. When the lesion is on the dominant side, all or a part of the Gerstmann syndrome may also be present. This and the accompaniment of sensory aphasia make demonstration of many of the parietal manifestations difficult or impossible in dominant hemisphere lesions.

GERSTMANN'S SYNDROME.[3] This is a symptom-complex somewhat related to sensory aphasia in that it includes impairment in the use of mathematical symbols, the inability to calculate (acalculia). Impairment of ability to perform mathematical calculations is likely to be encountered as a relatively early manifestation of mental deterioration from any cause, and is thus of less value as a localizing sign than aphasia. It occurs in the absence of general deterioration of mental function, however, as a component of the Gerstmann syndrome, which consists also of finger-agnosia (inability to identify, name, or select the individual fingers of either of his own hands or those of others), right-left disorientation, and agraphia. *This syndrome signifies a focal lesion localized to the junctional area of cortex between the parietal and occipital lobes of the dominant cerebral hemisphere.*

The syndrome varies in its components in individual cases and is rarely encountered in pure and complete form. It may be accompanied by components of parietal lobe syndrome, by components of sensory aphasia in addition to agraphia, by homonymous hemianopia and other occipital lobe manifestations. In the presence of severe aphasia it is often impossible to demonstrate because of inability to communicate with the patient. Because of the rarity of the syndrome and its variability from case to case, some have questioned its validity and usefulness in clinical diagnosis.[2]

Other Syndromes of the Intracranial Cavity

There are several syndromes of importance in diagnosis of intracranial lesions that do not lend themselves to classification with the lobes of the cerebral hemispheres or with specific cerebral functions. They may indicate a lesion involving multiple cerebral areas or one located within a restricted area but manifesting itself by encroachment upon contiguous but functionally separate structures in the intracranial cavity. Some permit no more precise localization than to indicate that the causative lesion is somewhere within the cranial vault. Other syndromes are quite precise in pointing to the site of the lesion even though they signify involvement of multiple structures.

THE SYNDROME OF INCREASED INTRACRANIAL PRESSURE. Headache, mental torpor, vomiting, bilateral papilledema, and sometimes unilateral or bilateral sixth (abducens) cranial nerve palsy constitute a syndrome resulting from crowding of the structures within the bony confines of the cranial cavity. They may result from a diffuse intracranial disorder such as meningitis or bilateral subdural hematomas or may be due to a focal intracranial lesion at or anywhere above the foramen magnum. Nevertheless, this syndrome is a very reliable indicator of disease within these confines, whether it occurs alone or in company with other neurological findings.

THE FOSTER KENNEDY SYNDROME. This syndrome, as originally defined, consisted of "true retrobulbar neuritis with the formation of a central scotoma and primary optic atrophy on the side of the lesion, together with concomitant papilledema in the opposite eye."[6] These findings, along with anosmia on the same side as the optic atrophy, were described in cases proved to have a mass lesion of the inferior part of the frontal lobe on that side. Optic atrophy with more variable involvement of the visual field in the eye homolateral to the lesion is more likely than central scotoma alone. Subsequent experience has related this syndrome to tumors of the sphenoidal ridge or olfactory groove in the floor of the anterior cranial fossa as well as lesions within the frontal lobe. Homolateral exophthalmos may accompany the ocular findings of the syndrome when the causative lesion encroaches on the bony orbit. Anosmia may be absent when the lesion is more laterally placed, or it may be present bilaterally if the lesion extends across the midline of the floor of the anterior fossa. Lesions other than tumor or abscess may cause the syndrome, including vascular abnormalities and local arachnoiditis. It is a rare syndrome, occurring in only a small percentage (1.5 per cent in one reported survey) of cases of mass lesion in the anterior cranial fossa.[13] Nevertheless, when encountered, it is of value in defining the locus of disease in an otherwise often "silent area" of brain.

PARASAGITTAL LESIONS. Lesions situated in the interhemispheric fissure may be manifest clinically by signs implicating the paracentral lobule unilaterally or bilaterally (Figs. 1–3 and 1–4). These signs include (1) paresis in the lower extremities (paraplegia), usually beginning in one foot and progressively spreading in that limb and then to the opposite member, (2) focal motor or sensory seizures beginning in the foot, (3) incontinence of urine or feces, and (4) mental changes of the frontal lobe syndrome.

The tendon reflexes may be normal, hypoactive, or hyperactive, and the Babinski sign may or may not be present early in the course. In the early stages, weakness limited to the distal parts of one lower extremity may simulate peroneal nerve palsy. Babinski's sign or hyperactive ankle jerk, if present, will permit easy differentiation. When both lower extremities are involved, and especially when this is accompanied by sphincter incontinence, the syndrome may simulate spinal cord disease. However, the paraplegia with parasagittal lesions is almost always asymmetrical and almost never as pronounced, even in advanced stages, as with cord lesions. Furthermore, accompanying focal seizures and mental changes, when present, will define the correct regional level of the causative lesion. The most common parasagittal lesion causing this syndrome is meningioma arising on one side of the falx cerebri and producing its earliest signs in the contralateral lower extremity. Thrombosis of the superior sagittal sinus may cause a similar clinical pattern, but is of more abrupt onset with more rapid development of the total deficit.

PERISELLAR LESIONS. Lesions arising in or around the sella turcica manifest themselves by (1) endocrine dysfunctions, (2) visual loss due to involvement of the optic nerves and chiasm, (3) hypothalamic signs, and (4) increased intracranial pressure due to protrusion of the lesion into the floor of the third ventricle.

The most readily recognized endocrinop-

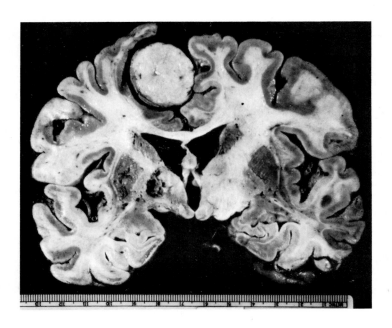

FIGURE 1–4 Parasagittal meningioma compressing both cerebral hemispheres.

athy is diabetes insipidus resulting from involvement of the pituitary stalk and posterior hypothalamus. Other alterations of endocrine function are more subtle and depend upon the degree to which the pituitary is involved and the age of the patient. They may be those of either hypofunction or hyperfunction, depending upon the nature of the lesion, and they usually require ancillary laboratory studies for their diagnosis and identification. The neurosurgeon will be more likely to encounter patients with lesions of this region because of the neurological manifestations.

The earliest neurological abnormality usually is bitemporal visual field defect due to encroachment on the midportion of the optic chiasm. At this stage it is usually asymptomatic and will be found only by special attempt on the part of the examiner. Later, progression to more extensive encroachment on optic chiasm or optic nerves results in subjective impairment of vision. The patterns of visual loss from lesions in this location are discussed in Chapter 14.

The disturbances of hypothalamic function may include alterations of sleep pattern, eating habits (with resultant cachexia or adiposity), temperature regulation and other autonomic functions, and metabolism.

The signs and symptoms of increased intracranial pressure are likely to occur early in the clinical course of suprasellar lesions with headache and papilledema as the initial findings in some instances. However, even in these instances careful testing will often reveal the characteristic abnormality in the visual fields. Anosmia, unilateral or bilateral, may be found if the lesion extends forward along the base of the brain. "Uncinate fits," focal seizures initiated by hallucinations of smell or taste, may occur when the lesion encroaches on posterior orbital surface of the frontal lobe or medial temporal lobe cortex.

SYNDROMES OF THE INTRACRANIAL VENOUS SINUSES. The venous sinuses within the cranial cavity are channels formed between layers of the dura mater. The veins draining the brain and other structures in and around the cranial cavity empty into them; thus they constitute the main avenue for venous drainage from the contents of the cranial cavity. They may become occluded by thrombosis from cachexia or blood dys-

crasias, trauma, or spread of nearby inflammatory or neoplastic disease. Those in which occlusion is most likely to produce a recognizable intracranial syndrome are the superior sagittal, the cavernous, and the lateral sinuses. Isolated occlusion of the smaller dural sinuses is rare and their manifestations are usually obscured by those implicating these three major sinuses.

Superior sagittal sinus. The superior sagittal sinus is situated in the midsagittal plane of the intracranial cavity along the superior border of the falx cerebri. It receives the veins that drain most of the convexity of both cerebral hemispheres. It also receives the cerebrospinal fluid through the arachnoidal villi located in recesses along its walls. Occlusion causes symptoms and signs of increased intracranial pressure, seizures (generalized or jacksonian), edema of forehead and scalp (especially in children), engorgement of scalp veins (especially in children), and spastic paralysis that is most marked in the lower extremities. When the clot begins in or extends into tributary veins over the cortical surface of the brain, various focal signs may appear, depending on the area of brain drained by the occluded veins. Thus there may result hemiplegia rather than paraplegia, parietal lobe signs, aphasia, homonymous hemianopsia, and the like.

Cavernous sinuses. The cavernous sinuses are situated on each lateral wall of the sella turcica. The lateral wall of each sinus is formed by a layer of dura mater extending posteriorly from the superior orbital fissure to the anterior surface of the petrous bone. The two sinuses are connected by narrow channels across the anterior and posterior margins of the sella turcica. Each cavernous sinus receives venous drainage from the upper face as well as intracranially. Through each sinus pass: the internal carotid artery on its medial wall; and, from above downward, the third, fourth, and sixth cranial nerves, and the first (ophthalmic) and second (maxillary) divisions of the fifth cranial nerve on its lateral wall. The syndrome of the cavernous sinus varies in its details, depending on which of these structures are involved. The complete syndrome consists of homolateral proptosis, chemosis, and papilledema; dilated retinal veins and retinal hemorrhage; paralysis of the homolateral third, fourth, and sixth, and the ophthalmic division of the fifth cranial nerves; pain in the eye and upper face; and normal or slightly impaired vision homolaterally. Even with unilateral lesions the syndrome may be bilateral, owing to communication between the two sinuses. Infection spreading along draining veins from the face is a common cause, in which case the signs of general septicemia are often superimposed. Aneurysm of the intracavernous portion of the carotid artery or traumatic carotid-cavernous fistula may cause the syndrome in part, accompanied by bruit and visible pulsations of the homolateral eye. Tumor in or adjacent to the sinus may produce a part or all of the syndrome, usually more gradual in its development than with the other causes.

Lateral sinuses. The lateral sinuses pass laterally and forward on either side along the line of attachment of the tentorium cerebelli to the wall of the cranial vault from the torcular Herophili near the internal occipital protuberance to the internal jugular foramen on each side. Anteriorly the sinus assumes a tortuous course on the inner wall of the mastoid bone just before emptying into the internal jugular vein. This recurring mastoid portion is designated separately by some as the *sigmoid sinus*. The lateral sinuses are usually asymmetrically developed, one (usually the right) being a large direct continuation of all the sinuses that converge at the torcular Herophili and thus the channel through which most venous drainage from the brain ultimately leaves the cranial vault. The most common cause of lateral sinus occlusion is spread of inflammation from otitis or mastoiditis. In addition to the local signs of ear infection and systemic signs of septicemia (chills, fever, and malaise), the most constant neurological manifestations are those of increased intracranial pressure. Focal brain signs are rare, but seizures of generalized or jacksonian type sometimes occur. There may be tenderness and swelling in the mastoid region, the superficial mastoid veins, and along the course of the internal jugular vein in the neck.

The syndromes of the individual cerebral arteries are not discussed here. They rarely are of concern in neurosurgical diagnosis. Their detailed description can be found in most textbooks of clinical neurology.

Manifestations of Posterior Cranial Fossa Lesions

The posterior cranial fossa contains the brain stem, through which traverse the sensory and motor "long tracts"; cranial nerves III through XII from their nuclear origins within the brain stem to their points of exit through their respective foramina in the base of the skull; the cerebellum and its peduncles; and the caudal termination of the ventricular system, including its communication with the subarachnoid space. The cardinal manifestations of lesions localized to this region result from involvement of these structures singly or in combinations. They are: "crossed paralysis"; multiple cranial nerve palsies alone (III through XII); cerebellar signs alone; or any combination of cranial nerve palsies (III through XII), cerebellar signs, and long tract signs.

"Crossed paralysis," also called alternating hemiplegia, is the term used to designate sensory or motor paralysis that involves one or more cranial nerves on one side (homolateral to the lesion) and the limbs on the opposite side. *This finding is pathognomonic of posterior fossa localization.* In crossed motor paralysis, the cranial nerve palsy will be of the lower motor neuron type, while the limb paralysis will be of the upper motor neuron type owing to involvement of the motor tracts coursing through the brain stem. In addition to crossed hemiplegia, paralysis of one or more cranial nerves also occurs in association with disturbances of other motor functions. The following syndromes will permit precise localization of the level of the lesion within the posterior fossa.

THIRD (OCULOMOTOR) NERVE PALSY ASSOCIATED WITH DISTURBANCE OF MOTOR TRACTS. The signs of third cranial nerve palsy are described in Chapter 14. Unilateral palsy of this nerve combined with crossed hemiplegia results from involvement of the basis pedunculi and third nerve on the ventral surface of the midbrain (Weber-Leyden syndrome). *However, this combination is more often encountered as a complication of an expanding lesion of one cerebral hemisphere when the expansion causes the medial aspect of the temporal lobe to herniate through the tentorial notch and compress the third nerve.* Dilation of the pupil or ptosis of the eyelid ipsilateral to the herniation is the earliest, and sometimes only, sign of third nerve involvement in this critical situation in which only slight increase in the herniation may result in compression of the midbrain with serious threat to life.

Unilateral involvement of third nerve and red nucleus, when the lesion encroaches on the tegmentum of the midbrain, results in homolateral third nerve palsy and contralateral choreiform movements, tremor, and sometimes ataxia (Benedikt's syndrome). The lesion may also involve the sensory tracts in the midbrain tegmentum, adding contralateral hemianesthesia to the findings.

Unilateral involvement of third nerve and superior cerebellar peduncle by a dorsal tegmental lesion of midbrain results in the combination of third nerve palsy and cerebellar ataxia, both homolateral to the lesion (Nothnagel's syndrome).

Unilateral involvement of the third, fourth, and sixth cranial nerves and the ophthalmic division of the fifth nerve (syndrome of Foix) by a lesion in or near the cavernous sinus has already been described.

SIXTH (ABDUCENS) AND SEVENTH (FACIAL) NERVE PALSY ASSOCIATED WITH DISTURBANCE OF MOTOR TRACTS. Unilateral involvement of these two cranial nerves and the corticospinal tract in one side of the pons causes the combination of paralysis of abduction of the eye and facial paralysis homolateral to the lesion and contralateral hemiplegia (Millard-Gubler syndrome). Sometimes the facial nerve is spared, resulting in paralysis of abduction of the eye and hemiplegia alone (Raymond-Céstan syndrome). A lesion in the vicinity of the sixth nerve may extend far enough laterally to involve the para-abducens area, resulting in paralysis of conjugate gaze toward the side of the lesion in addition to the other signs (Foville's syndrome). In such a case, not only will the eye on the side of the lesion be medially rotated and unable to abduct, but the opposite eye also will not rotate medially on

attempting gaze to the side of the lesion. It will rotate medially on convergence.

It is well to remember that unilateral or bilateral sixth nerve palsy may occur as a part of the syndrome of increased intracranial pressure; therefore when papilledema accompanies sixth nerve palsy it does not necessarily signify brain stem or posterior fossa involvement.

Paralysis of the facial nerve alone (Bell's palsy) may be due to a lesion within the posterior fossa or along the course of the nerve through the facial canal within the petrous bone. If the lesion is within the posterior fossa it is likely to involve also the acoustic (tinnitus and hearing loss) and vestibular (vertigo and nystagmus) functions of the eighth cranial nerve and some dysfunction of the fifth (trigeminal) cranial nerve (e.g., unilateral loss of the corneal reflex or hemifacial numbness along with the facial paralysis). This combination is characteristic of tumors in the cerebellopontine angle. Homolateral cerebellar ataxia and horizontal nystagmus usually accompany the cranial nerve involvements in this situation. As the lesion enlarges to encroach further on posterior fossa structures there will be involvement of additional cranial nerves and long tracts and ultimately increased intracranial pressure.

Occasionally an inflammatory or neoplastic process involving the facial nerve or its nucleus will irritate rather than paralyze it, resulting in unilateral facial spasms or contraction. This finding, when combined with contralateral hemiplegia (Brissaud's syndrome), signifies a lesion of the posterior fossa homolateral to the facial involvement.

The syndrome of the lateral medulla oblongata (Wallenberg's syndrome) results from involvement of the nucleus ambiguus of the tenth (vagus) cranial nerve, descending root and tract of trigeminal nerve, vestibular nuclei, inferior cerebellar peduncle and cerebellar hemisphere, and spinothalamic tract. The resulting signs are: homolateral palatal paralysis causing dysphagia and dysarthria, loss of pain and thermal sensation on the face, and cerebellar signs; and contralateral loss of pain and thermal sensation of trunk and limbs. Horizontal nystagmus and homolateral Horner's syndrome (due to involvement of the descending sympathetic fibers coursing through the tegmentum of the brain stem) are also found with the complete syndrome.

The syndrome of the lateral pontine tegmentum is similar to the lateral medulla oblongata syndrome except that the main sensory nucleus of the trigeminal nerve and the nuclei of the seventh and eighth nerves are involved, while the descending trigeminal root and tract and nucleus ambiguus are spared. The resulting signs are: deafness, facial paralysis, loss of facial tactile sensation, Horner's syndrome, and cerebellar signs, all homolateral to the lesion, and contralateral hemianesthesia to pain and temperature, which may involve the face as well as the trunk and limbs. Horizontal nystagmus occurs also.

Also closely resembling the syndrome of the lateral medulla is that in which the lesion extends more medially and ventrally to involve the medial lemniscus, the nucleus of the twelfth (hypoglossal) cranial nerve, and the pyramid. In addition to, or instead of, loss of pain and temperature sensation, there will be loss of proprioceptive and tactile sensation and hemiplegia contralateral to the lesion. Homolateral atrophy and paralysis of the tongue and sometimes of the upper part of the trapezius muscle (eleventh nerve) will also occur (syndromes of Céstan-Chenais and of Babinski-Nageotte). These various syndromes of the caudal part of the posterior fossa, including those described later implicating the bulbar (lower) cranial nerves, vary from case to case and by eponymic designation owing to slight variations in the extent of the lesion in this compact and neurologically critical region.

SYNDROMES OF THE LOWER (BULBAR) CRANIAL NERVES. The ninth (glossopharyngeal), tenth (vagus), and eleventh (spinal accessory) cranial nerves exit from the cranial cavity through the jugular foramen. The twelfth (hypoglossal) nerve exits through the immediately adjacent hypoglossal foramen situated at the lip of the foramen magnum. As would be expected, therefore, a lesion in this vicinity of the posterior fossa or retropharyngeal space will produce varying combinations of involvement of these nerves. In the syndrome of the jugular foramen (Vernet's syndrome), there is paralysis of the ninth, tenth, and eleventh cranial nerves. These, along with

paralysis of the twelfth nerve (syndrome of Villaret), occur with a retropharyngeal lesion invading the posterior fossa. In some instances, involvement of two or more of these nerves in other combinations is encountered (Jackson's vagoaccessory hypoglossal paralysis, Schmidt's vagoaccessory syndrome, Tapia's vagohypoglossal palsy).

Cerebellar Signs

Although not solely a motor structure, the cerebellum is important in diagnosis for its effect on motor function. It is discussed here because the clinical manifestations of its dysfunction usually indicate disease in the posterior fossa. There are two fairly distinct syndromes of cerebellar dysfunction, based on the difference in the major connections of its component parts.

1. The flocculonodular or midline syndrome occurs when the lesion affects chiefly the flocculus, the nodulus, and the posterior vermis. These structures receive their afferent stimuli primarily from the vestibular apparatus in the brain stem. The primary clinical sign is disturbance of equilibrium manifested mostly in the axial musculature of the trunk and lower extremities (truncal ataxia). The patient stands or walks with feet apart, thus broadening his base to compensate for the loss of equilibrium. He reels or staggers on attempting to walk. When he sits without support to his body, he often assumes the "tripod" position of propping on his hands to prevent wavering of his trunk and head (titubation). Use of the individual limbs is affected little if any in performing volitional movements, and there is no lateralization. Speech is dysarthric. Horizontal nystagmus is often present. The entire syndrome resembles vestibular disturbance in many respects.

2. The cerebellar hemisphere (lateral cerebellar) syndrome occurs when there is a laterally placed lesion affecting one cerebellar hemisphere. It is characterized predominantly by disturbance of coordination of the limbs homolateral to the lesion in executing volitional movements and consists of (1) decomposition of volitional movements, (2) tremor during performance of movements (intention tremor), (3) hypo-

tonia of the involved limbs, and (4) instability of the limb on attempting to maintain a posture against gravity.

Decomposition of movement consists of loss of proper integration of contraction of agonist and synergist muscles with relaxation of antagonists. As a result, a movement such as touching the nose with the fingertip is broken down ("decomposed") into the various components of movement at the individual joints rather than occurring as smoothly integrated parts of the whole movement. Furthermore, each individual component may be ill-timed or ill-measured so as to cause overshooting or undershooting of its goal.

Hypotonia is a kind of mild flaccidity of the limb so that it is hyperextendible or hyperflexible to passive movement at the joints.

The characteristic *cerebellar tremor* is that which occurs only when the limb is brought into action to perform a movement. It often has a tendency to increase in a crescendo manner as the target is approached, therefore is sometimes referred to as terminal tremor. A postural tremor is sometimes present in addition when an attempt is made to maintain an antigravity posture with the limb.

It is well to remember that, due to the major efferent connections from each cerebellar hemisphere via the superior cerebellar peduncle to the premotor cortex of the opposite cerebral hemisphere, the lateral cerebellar syndrome may be closely simulated by a lesion in the frontal lobe (frontal lobe ataxia). The signs are homolateral to lesions of cerebellar hemisphere or superior cerebellar peduncle and contralateral to lesions in the frontal lobe. Furthermore, in the latter there are likely to be other manifestations of frontal lobe disturbance associated with the cerebellar signs.

The reflex postural changes that characterize posterior fossa lesions involving the brain stem are almost always associated with impaired consciousness. These reflex changes are discussed in Chapter 3. Increased intracranial pressure may accompany any of the foregoing manifestations of posterior fossa disease when the lesion encroaches upon the aqueduct of Sylvius or fourth ventricle or interferes with egress of cerebrospinal fluid via the foramina of Luschka and Magendie.

Manifestations of Lesions of the Spinal Canal

Lesions within the spinal canal, whether intramedullary or extramedullary, may produce clinical findings indicative of involvement of the spinal cord or the spinal roots and nerves or their neurons of origin in the spinal cord or ganglia. Precise localization depends upon knowledge of the details of cross-sectional and longitudinal anatomy of the spinal cord. This is found in any of the textbooks of neuroanatomy. The primary purposes here are to define those syndromes that are of help to the examiner in localizing disease within the spinal canal and to point out some limitations of the clinical method of examination alone in regional diagnosis at this level of the nervous system. Only those anatomical features of special usefulness in clinical diagnosis are reviewed.

The spinal cord extends from the foramen magnum of the skull, where it is continuous with the medulla oblongata, to the interspace between the first and second lumbar vertebrae, where it ends. Lesions of the spinal canal caudal to the first lumbar vertebra, therefore, will produce only signs of involvement of the spinal roots constituting the cauda equina and not signs of spinal cord involvement. (The cauda equina syndrome is discussed later.)

There are usually 31 pairs of spinal nerves (8 cervical, 12 thoracic, 5 lumbar, 5 sacral, and 1 coccygeal), each formed by a dorsal root entering and a ventral root leaving the spinal cord at as many segments. The first cervical (C1) pair of spinal nerves leaves the spinal canal above the first cervical vertebra (atlas); the others leave through the intervertebral foramina between the vertebrae. There being eight pairs of cervical nerves and only seven cervical vertebrae, the nerves C2 through C7 leave via the foramina above their corresponding vertebrae, and the C8 nerves leave via the foramina below the C7 vertebra. From the first thoracic (T1) pair down, the remaining spinal nerves leave the canal through the foramina immediately below their corresponding vertebrae.

Owing to the discrepancy between the length of the spinal cord and that of the spinal canal, the segments of the spinal cord (each represented by a pair of spinal nerves) do not coincide in horizontal plane with their corresponding vertebrae (Fig. 1–5). Therefore care must be taken in describing the location of a lesion in the spinal canal to specify whether one is designating the spinal cord segment or the vertebral level of the lesion.

Each segment of spinal cord has its topographical zone of representation on the skin (dermatome) from which it receives the cutaneous sensations of pain, temperature, and touch. Figures 1–6 to 1–8 show the two dermatomal maps most widely accepted. Because of overlap of nerve supply between adjacent dermatomes, no demonstrable sensory deficit can be found unless two or more adjacent posterior roots or spinal nerves are interrupted; however, irritation of a single root or nerve will cause pain or paresthesias in that dermatome.

Within the spinal cord the structural and functional components of greatest diagnostic usefulness are: (1) the descending motor tracts in the posterior part of each lateral white column, chiefly the lateral corticospinal tract, (2) the ascending fasciculus gracilis and fasciculus cuneatus in each posterior white column, conveying proprioceptive (position and vibratory) sensation to higher centers, (3) the ascending lateral spinothalamic tract in the anterior part of each lateral white column, conveying cutaneous pain and temperature sensation to higher centers, (4) the autonomic suprasegmental descending fibers in each lateral white column and autonomic cell groups of the intermediate gray column in the thoracic segments, which give rise to preganglionic sympathetic fibers, and (5) the cervical and lumbar enlargements of the spinal cord in which the innervation and reflex arcs of the upper and lower extremities respectively are concentrated.

The Long Tracts

In addition to the corticospinal (pyramidal) fiber tract, which arises from axons in the cerebral cortex, the lateral white columns carry other descending crossed

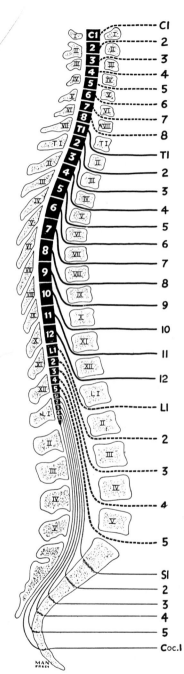

FIGURE 1–5 Illustration of the relationship of the spinal cord and spinal nerve segments to the vertebrae. The bodies and spinous processes of the vertebrae are indicated by Roman numerals and the spinal segments and nerves by Arabic numbers. (From Haymaker, W., and Woodhall, B.: Peripheral Nerve Injuries. 2nd Ed. Philadelphia, W. B. Saunders Co., 1953, p. 32.)

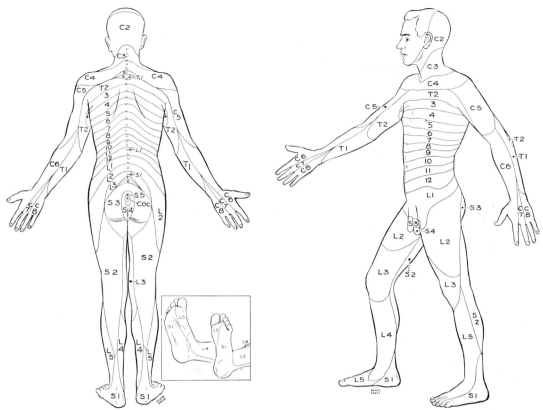

FIGURE 1–6 Posterior view of the dermatome patterns. (From Haymaker, W., and Woodhall, B.: Peripheral Nerve Injuries. 2nd Ed. Philadelphia, W. B. Saunders Co., 1953, p. 26—after Foerster, 1933.)

FIGURE 1–7 Lateral view of dermatome patterns. (From Haymaker, W., and Woodhall, B.: Peripheral Nerve Injuries. 2nd Ed. Philadelphia, W. B. Saunders Co., 1953, p. 27—after Foerster, 1933.)

axons arising at subcortical and brain stem levels and collectively referred to as extrapyramidal pathways. All these descending pyramidal and extrapyramidal axons exert influence on the lower motor neurons of the anterior gray columns. Interruption of the lateral corticospinal tract produces the syndrome of "upper motor neuron" paralysis below the level of the lesion. Involvement of the extrapyramidal axons, which travel nearby, is usual, producing varying degrees of rigidity in addition to the upper motor neuron signs.

Both the lateral corticospinal tract (descending) and the fasciculi gracilis and cuneatus (ascending) undergo decussation approximately at the level of the foramen magnum of the skull in the caudal end of the medulla oblongata; therefore lesions within the spinal canal that unilaterally impair the functions mediated by these tracts will pro-

duce signs homolaterally, whereas those above the foramen magnum produce the same signs contralaterally. The lateral spinothalamic tract, on the other hand, arises as a crossed tract within the spinal cord; therefore a lesion involving it on one side either within the spinal canal or above the foramen magnum will produce deficit of pain and temperature sensation contralaterally below the level of the lesion.

The fibers of the lateral spinothalamic tract conveying impulses from the sacral segments run most laterally (i.e., peripherally) in the tract, and those joining it at successively higher levels are added on medially. Thus, it is laminated in terms of topographical cutaneous representation with the sacral dermatomes represented nearest the periphery of the spinal cord, the cervical dermatomes represented nearest the center, and the lumbar and thoracic in

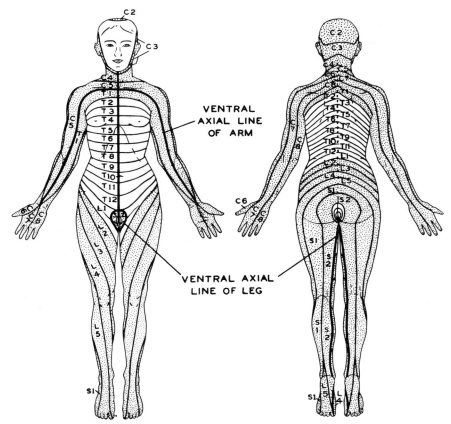

FIGURE 1-8 Anterior and posterior views of the dermatome patterns. (From Keegan, J. J., and Garett, F. D.: Anat. Rec., *102*:411, 1948.)

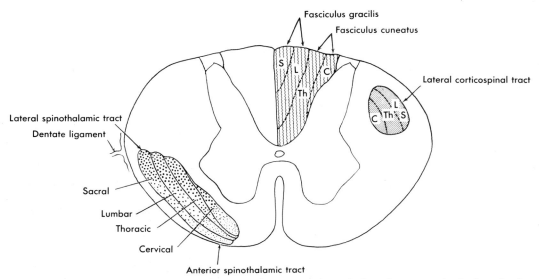

FIGURE 1-9 Laminar arrangement of the axons from successive spinal cord segments in the lateral spinothalamic tract (*left*). Laminar separation of the fibers mediating temperature (*large dots*), pain (*medium dots*), and light touch (*small dots*) within the tract is also illustrated. Similar laminations for the ascending proprioceptive (posterior column) and descending lateral corticospinal tract are shown on the right. (From Haymaker, W.: Bing's Local Diagnosis in Neurological Diseases. 15th Ed. St. Louis, C. V. Mosby Co., 1969, p. 8.)

between (Fig. 1–9). A lesion located laterally in the spinal canal anywhere above the level of entry of the sacral segments to the tract (approximately the first lumbar vertebra) may encroach upon the spinal cord in such a way as to interfere with pain and temperature sensation of the sacral region only. For this reason in the early stages of a progressing lesion, a "sensory level" on the trunk is not reliable in indicating the level of the lesion, although it is a reliable indication that the lesion is in the spinal canal. An intramedullary spinal cord lesion, on the other hand, may encroach on only the most medial fibers of the tract to produce loss of pain and temperature sensation limited to a few segments with sparing of these sensations both above and below. This finding, referred to as a suspended sensory level or segmental sensory loss, constitutes a helpful diagnostic sign indicating that the causative lesion is most likely within the parenchyma of the spinal cord. Similar laminar arrangements of fibers in the other tracts and in the cell groups within the gray matter of the cord also exist, but they are less useful diagnostically.

Disturbance of Autonomic Function

The entirety of the paravertebral sympathetic chains receive their preganglionic nerve supply from cells in the intermediate gray columns from the T1 through L2 segments of the spinal cord whose axons leave the canal via the spinal nerves corresponding to these cord segments. These preganglionic neurons are under the control of the higher centers (cerebral cortex, hypothalamus, and brain stem reticular formation) via axons passing through the brain stem and into the spinal cord in the lateral white columns on the same side, where they form a diffuse pathway extending down to the upper lumbar cord segments. Lesions at the cervical and upper thoracic levels of the canal are likely to affect these structures, producing alterations of vasomotor activity, sweating, and respiration. Orthostatic hypotension, resulting from interruption of the descending central axons controlling vasopressor and cardiac reflexes may occur with lesions above the T7 segment. Respiratory disturbances may occur with lesions at the upper cervical levels because of disturbance of innervation of intercostal and bronchial muscles as well as phrenic nerve paralysis. Alterations of sweating may occur with lesions that involve either the descending central axons or the preganglionic cell column down to the L2 cord segment. Horner's syndrome may occur homolateral to a lesion at or above the T1 segment.

Disturbance of the urethral and rectal sphincters, when of neurogenic origin, is usually indicative of a lesion in the spinal canal. The urethral sphincter receives its motor supply from neurons in the S2, S3, and S4 segments of the spinal cord. These neurons are under suprasegmental control of axons from the paracentral lobule of the frontal lobe, descending in the lateral white columns in close proximity to the lateral corticospinal tract. Different patterns of urinary dysfunction may occur, depending on the level at which the lesion occurs. The uninhibited neurogenic bladder, characterized by urinary frequency and urgency progressing to automatic micturition with a contracted bladder, is the type usually seen in parasagittal lesions of the frontal lobes. The automatic (reflex) bladder, characterized initially by urinary retention that progresses to overflow incontinence and then to automatic intermittent emptying, occurs with bilateral interruption of the suprasegmental axons traveling with the lateral corticospinal tracts at any level above the S1 spinal cord segment. Incomplete or early lesions may produce the uninhibited bladder pattern instead. The autonomous neurogenic bladder, characterized by dribbling incontinence without automatic emptying contractions of the detrusor muscle, results from lesions at the sacral segments of the spinal cord or involving the spinal roots from them that supply the bladder and its sphincters.

Disturbances of sexual function often accompany or precede impaired bladder function with lesions in the spinal canal. Priapism and frequent reflex ejaculation are the usual disturbances with lesions involving the spinal cord above the sacral segments, and especially those above the lower thoracic segments. Ability for normal erection may be retained. Lesions involving the lower sacral (S3, S4, and S5) segments of the cord or the nerve roots therefrom in the cauda equina usually cause total impotence with loss of ability for erection and ejaculation.

The suprasegmental *control of the rectal sphincter* is mediated by the same pathways as that for the external urethral sphincter. Its peripheral innervation is via the S3, S4, and S5 spinal cord segments. Lesions above these segments, involving the suprasegmental pathways, cause constipation associated with a spastic sphincter. Lesions of the sacral segments of spinal cord or the nerve roots from them result in loss of sphincter tone with fecal incontinence.

The Cervical and Lumbar Enlargements

Lesions at the level of the spinal canal corresponding to the cervical enlargement of the spinal cord (C4 through T1) are likely to involve the peripheral sensory, motor, and autonomic nerve supply of one or both upper extremities and, in addition, the tracts to and from higher centers influencing the spinal segments below. Therefore, it is characteristic of lesions here to produce: "lower motor neuron" (flaccid) paralysis and segmental sensory loss in upper extremities associated with "upper motor neuron" (spastic) paralysis in one or both lower extremities, sensory loss over the trunk and lower extremities that follows one or another pattern of sensory tract involvement, and sphincter disturbance. When the lesion is limited to the middle or lower levels of the enlargement, sparing the descending motor tracts and peripheral innervation of the upper cervical segments, it is not unusual to find components of both upper motor neuron and lower motor neuron types of motor impairment (e.g., atrophy and fasciculations accompanied by hyperactive tendon reflexes) in the upper extremities, resembling the clinical picture of amyotrophic lateral sclerosis. The anterior horn cells in the cervical enlargement that give rise to the peripheral motor innervation of each upper extremity are grouped in a laminar arrangement from medial to lateral so that functionally related muscle groups may be selectively involved while other motor supply to the extremity is spared. The cells located most laterally give motor supply to the muscles of the hands and fingers; those

most medial supply the shoulder girdle muscles. It is possible, therefore, for a lesion at the cervical enlargement to encroach on the anterior horn in such a way as to involve, for example, only those motor neurons to the hand and fingers, giving a distribution of motor loss that resembles ulnar nerve paralysis. In some instances, these patterns of loss make it extremely difficult to determine by clinical examination alone whether the lesion involves the spinal cord, the spinal roots from the cervical segments, the brachial plexus, or the individual peripheral nerves of the upper extremity.

Lesions involving the lumbar enlargement (L1 through S2 segments) of the spinal cord are likely to impair the peripheral motor, sensory, and autonomic innervation to the lower extremities. The motor loss will be of the lower motor neuron type and may be difficult to differentiate from that resulting from involvement of spinal nerves of the cauda equina or the peripheral nerves. Loss of cutaneous sensation to pain and temperature in the saddle area of the trunk with varying extension of the loss onto the lower extremities may occur. Disturbance of sphincter function is also likely. Examination for sensory loss in the saddle area and sphincter disturbance is important in the correct localization of lesions at this level.

The Cauda Equina Syndrome

Lesions within the spinal canal below the level of the first lumbar vertebra will not produce findings referable to the spinal cord tracts, since the spinal cord ends here. The findings will be limited to those of involvement of the lumbar and sacral spinal nerve roots making up the cauda equina. Motor loss will be of the lower motor neuron type limited to one or both lower extremities. Sensory loss is limited to the lower extremities and the saddle area. Impairment of sphincter control is likely and will be of the sacral segmental type (i.e., fecal incontinence with loss of tone of the anal sphincter and urinary incontinence indicative of the autonomous bladder). Loss of sensation of the urge to void or to defecate is also likely. As already noted, it may be impossible to differentiate between lesions in this level of the spinal canal and those of the lower segments of the spinal cord on the basis of the clinical findings alone. Myelography and other ancillary techniques are usually required. Since the cauda equina is constituted of nerve roots that are peripheral nerves, both structurally and functionally, the prognosis for return of function following removal of the lesion is good in contradistinction to the poor prognosis when the lesion involves the spinal cord.

The foregoing discussion of manifestations of spinal canal disease has dealt mostly with the localization of lesions in terms of the longitudinal plane of the structures within the spinal cord. Localization in terms of the transverse (cross-sectional) plane is of equal importance. The following syndromes indicate the transverse extent to lesions at the particular level of their maximum encroachment upon the spinal cord whether they are of considerable longitudinal extent (e.g., tumor) or sharply localized (e.g., knife wounds). Etiologically, they may be produced by operatively remediable lesions, but frequently they result from inoperable neurological diseases such as multiple sclerosis, amyotrophic lateral sclerosis, and syringomyelia.

Transection of the Spinal Cord ("Transverse Myelitis")

The manifestations of interruption of the continuity of the spinal cord in its cross-sectional plane will vary depending on several factors: the speed with which the interruption occurs; the length of time elapsed between the occurrence of the insult and the examination of the patient; whether the transection is complete or incomplete; the level of the spinal cord involved; and the etiology. Sudden complete transection results immediately in spinal shock: flaccid total paralysis of all skeletal musculature and loss of all spinal reflexes below the segmental level of the lesion, loss of all cutaneous and propioceptive sensation at and below the segmental level of the lesion, and transient urinary and fecal retention. Transection within the upper three cervical segments is usually incompatible with life because of the accompanying loss of vital functions (respiratory and vasomotor control, regulation of body temperature). Transection below the T2 spinal segment will spare the upper extremities, but vasomotor instability, especially orthostatic hypotension, is likely with transection at any level above the midthoracic segments. The latter is important to remember when transporting such patients. Bilateral Horner's syndrome will be produced by lesions at or above the T1 segment.

Spinal shock persists for one to six weeks in those who survive. Spinal reflexes then begin to return and become increasingly active over the ensuing weeks. Reflex bladder emptying develops. Clonus develops. The Babinski sign appears bilaterally. Flexor spasms begin to appear in response to cutaneous stimulation and become increasingly active on the slightest stimulation. A mass reflex response, consisting of bouts of profuse sweating and flushing, wide fluctuations in blood pressure, reflex voiding, and massive reflex contraction of the trunk and limbs below the lesion may develop in response to cutaneous stimulation. Within 6 to 12 months after the insult, extensor spasms in the limbs begin to occur, and for an indefinite period of time thereafter, reflex movements of alternating flexor spasms and extensor spasms may appear, sometimes resembling stepping movements of the lower limbs. Extensor spasms usually predominate as time passes, and ultimately sustained extensor rigidity of the lower extremities (paraplegia-in-extension) prevails. In some cases, the increased tone in flexor muscle groups rather than extensors predominates, resulting in sustained flexion posture of the lower limbs (paraplegia-in-flexion). Earlier reports based on study of paraplegics in World War I suggested that paraplegia-in-extension resulted with complete transections, and paraplegia-in-flexion resulted when the transection was incomplete; however, subsequent studies since the advent of antibiotics and other improvements in the care of such patients have led to modification of this concept. The indications are that the difference is more likely due to the *level* of the transection: transection at the cervical levels is more likely to result in paraplegia-in-extension, whereas that at midthoracic levels is more likely to result in paraplegia-in-flexion.

When the transection occurs suddenly, but is incomplete, there may be a transient period of spinal shock due to the concussive effects of the causative lesion on the spinal cord. This state will soon become clinically evident, sometimes within hours or several days, by the finding of some degree of return of the motor and sensory function originally lost. The prognosis for recovery in such cases is improved, although it may take weeks or months to assess it.

When gradual transverse encroachment on the spinal cord occurs, as in compression by tumor, the clinical manifestations of spinal shock usually do not appear. Instead, there develop a gradual upper motor neuron type of paralysis and progressing sensory loss below the lesion.

The Brown-Séquard Syndrome

Transverse hemisection of the spinal cord, interruption of the lateral half of the spinal cord on either side above the lumbar segments, results in homolateral upper motor neuron paralysis, vasomotor paralysis and loss of position and vibratory sensation below the level of the lesion, and contralateral loss of pain and temperature sensation below the level of the lesion. At times there may be a narrow band of hyperesthesia just above the level of analgesia bilaterally or homolateral to the lesion, presumably owing to irritation of the dorsal root at the site of the lesion.

This syndrome rarely occurs in pure form clinically. Acute lesions (e.g., stab wound or fracture of the spine) will usually involve less or more than this precise transverse area. Slower lesions (e.g., encroaching tumor) will present clinical signs of the incomplete syndrome before the entire syndrome develops. The essential feature of greatest diagnostic usefulness is the homolateral spastic weakness in association with a contralateral cutaneous sensory level on the trunk. As has been pointed out already, the level on the trunk below which cutaneous sensation is lost is not a reliable indication of the level of the lesion; therefore precise localization usually requires myelography unless the site is evident on inspection (e.g., stab wound).

The Anterior Spinal Artery Syndrome

The arterial supply to the spinal cord is via the single anterior spinal artery, which runs in the anterior median fissure and supplies approximately the anterior two thirds of the cord bilaterally, and the paired posterior spinal arteries, each supplying half of the posterior one third. These arteries receive reinforcing blood supply at multiple segments along the canal by anastomoses from the intercostal and lumbar arteries. Anastomoses at the cervical and upper thoracic level with the thyroid artery, at the lower thoracic level, and at the upper lumbar level are especially large and are essential to maintenance of adequate supply of blood to the spinal cord throughout its length. Infarction of the spinal cord may result not only from thrombosis of its nutrient arteries, but also from lesions that occlude any of these crucial reinforcing arteries outside the spinal canal or along the nerve roots with which they enter the canal. The blood supply to any level of the cord may also be interrupted by compression on the artery by an expanding lesion such as tumor in the spinal canal. The arterial syndrome most readily recognizable clinically is that of the anterior spinal artery. Compromise of blood flow through it results in infarction or ischemia of motor cells in the anterior gray horns, the lateral spinothalamic tracts in the anterior portion of the lateral white columns, and the descending motor tracts more posteriorly in the lateral white columns (Fig. 1–10). In the thoracic and cervical segments, the autonomic pathways will also be involved. The posterior white columns are spared. Thus there results bilateral motor paralysis and cutaneous sensory loss below the level of infarction and bilateral sparing of proprioceptive (position and vibratory) sensation. Infarction involving the segments carrying the autonomic suprasegmental tracts and the preganglionic sympathetic fibers will produce autonomic signs in addition.

Central Lesions of Spinal Cord

Just anterior to the central canal in the anterior commissure, the axons from the second-order neurons of the dorsal gray

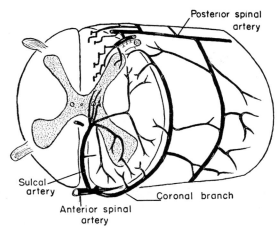

Posterior spinal artery

Sulcal artery

Coronal branch

Anterior spinal artery

FIGURE 1–10 Diagram showing blood supply to spinal cord in cross-sectional plane. The illustration is that of one side of the cord illustrating that the major supply to the areas of the lateral spinothalamic and lateral corticospinal tracts as well as the anterior two thirds of gray matter receive their major supply from the anterior spinal artery. (From Peele, T. L.: The Neuroanatomic Basis for Clinical Neurology. 2nd Ed. New York, McGraw-Hill Book Co., Inc., 1961, p. 112—after Herren and Alexander.)

horns conveying pain and temperature entering each segment of the cord cross to the opposite side to form the lateral spinothalamic tract. As has already been noted, these fibers form the most centrally (medially) placed axons within the tract as they join at successively higher levels. A lesion in the vicinity of the central canal will involve these crossing sensory fibers and may also encroach upon the medial aspect of the tract on one or both sides. The result will be a segmental sensory loss (suspended sensory level) over both sides, the extent of which will depend on the longitudinal extent of the lesion along the cord and the transverse extent of its encroachment on the lateral spinothalamic tracts. A dissociation of pain and temperature perception may also occur, since the fibers conveying thermal sensation are grouped dorsolaterally in the lateral spinothalamic tract while pain fibers are grouped anteromedially (see Fig. 1–9). The extent of the segment of sensory loss will likely differ on the two sides, especially when the lesion is asymmetrical in its transverse encroachment on the tracts. A syrinx of the cord is the lesion with which this sensory pattern is most often associated, but it may also occur with hematomyelia or with intramedullary tumors.

Manifestations of Peripheral Nerve Lesions

In terms of its gross anatomy, the peripheral nervous system consists of all the mixed nerves located outside the bony enclosures housing the central nervous system and carrying the motor, sensory, and autonomic innervation of all the deep and superficial somatic structures of the head, trunk, and limbs. From the standpoint of histological structure and potential disturbance of function, however, it should be considered as extending from the point at which the segmental nerve roots enter and leave the spinal cord to the distal terminations of its constituent axons. The clinical manifestations of its involvement by disease or injury are fundamentally the same, regardless of the point along this extent at which the involvement occurs; only the pattern of distribution of the disturbed function differs, depending on the changes in distribution of the constituent axons in their course from the spinal cord to the structures that they innervate. These axons vary in size and thickness of their myelin sheaths in relation to the type of impulse that they transmit and the speed of transmission. Their susceptibility to some noxious agents also differs in relation to these same structural factors. *Unlike the axons within the central nervous system, those constituting the peripheral nervous system are capable of regeneration after destruction.*

The paired spinal nerves representing each spinal cord segment are formed by junction of their respective dorsal (posterior) and ventral (anterior) nerve roots at the intervertebral foramen from which they exit from the spinal canal. The axons constituting the ventral roots arise from parent motor neurons in the anterior gray column of the spinal cord; at the T1 through L3 segments they are accompanied by the axons of the preganglionic sympathetic neurons situated in the intermediate gray column bound for the paravertebral chain of sympathetic ganglia (white rami communicantes). Just distal to each paravertebral ganglion, the gray rami communicantes—the axons arising from postganglionic neurons within the ganglion — rejoin the nerve to reach their peripheral distribution. The axons constituting the dorsal spinal roots arise from parent sensory neurons located in the dorsal root ganglion at each segment. It will be remembered that the dorsal and ventral roots arising from the lower thoracic, the lumbar, and the sacral segments and forming the cauda equina travel for a considerable distance down the spinal canal before reaching their respective intervertebral foramina where they join. The meninges (dura and arachnoid) covering the spinal cord form a root sleeve around each pair of nerve roots extending to the intervertebral foramen where they end by fusing with the periosteum of the foramen and the connective tissue sheath of each spinal nerve.

The spinal nerves of the T2 through T12 segments continue peripherally as the intercostal nerves. Those from the C1 through C4 segments form the cervical plexus. Those of the segments C5 through T1 undergo redistribution of their constituent axons to form the brachial plexus, from which arise the peripheral nerves innervating the upper extremity and shoulder girdle. Those of the L1 through L4 segments form the lumbar plexus, and those from the L4 through S4 segments form the sacral plexus. (Because of the variation in overlap between the two, it is clinically useful to consider these together as the lumbosacral plexus, from which arise the peripheral nerves innervating the lower extremity and pelvic girdle). In this process of redistribution of axons from spinal nerves to plexus to peripheral nerves, an individual peripheral nerve ends up with axons arising from several spinal cord segments, and the axons constituting a single spinal nerve root may be distributed in more than one peripheral nerve.

Each peripheral nerve has its territory of cutaneous sensory supply and its somatic motor supply, just as each spinal segment has. As a result of the redistribution of the sensory axons from spinal segmental roots to peripheral nerves, the peripheral nerve territories differ substantially from the dermatome pattern shown in Figures 1–6 to 1–8. Figures 1–11, 1–12 and 1–13 map the cutaneous territories of the individual peripheral nerves. Since there is considerable overlap between adjacent peripheral nerve

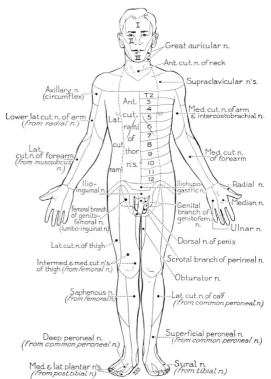

FIGURE 1–11 The cutaneous territories of the individual peripheral nerves viewed anteriorly. This and Figures 1–12 and 1–13 can be compared with Figures 1–6, 1–7, and 1–8, which show the *dermatomes of the spinal cord segments* to differentiate between central and peripheral lesions. The numbers on the trunk indicate the zones supplied by each of the intercostal nerves. The asterisk beneath the scrotum indicates the territory of the posterior cutaneous nerve of the thigh as viewed anteriorly. (From Haymaker, W., and Woodhall, B.: Peripheral Nerve Injuries. 2nd Ed. Philadelphia, W. B. Saunders Co., 1953, p. 43.)

territories, the actual area of sensory deficit on the skin is usually less extensive when a single peripheral nerve is interrupted than that shown. It is useful, therefore, especially in the cutaneous nerve supply to the extremities, to define those zones of autonomous supply characteristic of each peripheral nerve. In examining the patient with a cutaneous sensory deficit, a helpful technique is to begin testing within the area of definite sensory loss and work out radially from this focus in mapping the entire area of deficit.

The peripheral nerves are mixed nerves in that they include axons conveying

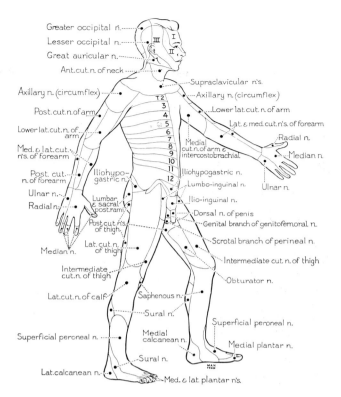

FIGURE 1–12 Lateral view of the cutaneous territories of the peripheral nerves. (From Haymaker, W., and Woodhall, B.: Peripheral Nerve Injuries. 2nd Ed. Philadelphia, W. B. Saunders Co., 1953, p. 42.)

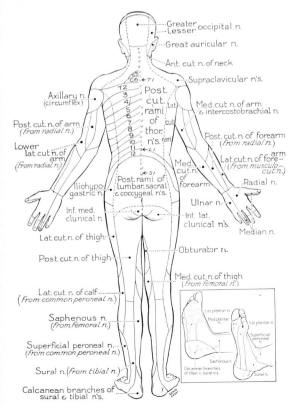

FIGURE 1–13 Posterior view of the cutaneous territory of the peripheral nerves. (From Haymaker, W., and Woodhall, B.: Peripheral Nerve Injuries. 2nd Ed. Philadelphia, W. B. Saunders Co.)

motor, sensory, and autonomic impulses. Therefore, lesions that affect them might produce disturbance of any or all of these functions, depending on the level at which they are affected. As a nerve courses peripherally, its component axons separate off into more specialized branches; therefore, the more proximally it is affected, the more likely one is to find disturbance of all three functions in its territory of supply. The general manifestations of peripheral nerve lesions are (1) motor paralysis of lower motor neuron type only; (2) sensory changes, which may consist of deficit of pain, temperature, touch, position, or vibratory sensations alone or in combinations, and subjective sensations of numbness, dysesthesias, paresthesias, or pain; (3) decrease or absence of tendon reflexes, but sparing of cutaneous reflexes and absence of pathological reflexes (e.g., Babinski sign, flexor spasms); and (4) autonomic and trophic changes consisting of edema, peripheral vasomotor instability (flushing or pallor), thick or shiny skin with regional loss of cutaneous hair, and trophic ulcers.

The patterns of distribution that these manifestations may take are (1) individual spinal root syndromes, (2) plexus syndromes, (3) mononeuropathy, in which an isolated peripheral nerve is paralyzed in part or in its entirety, (4) polyneuropathy, in which multiple adjacent peripheral nerves are involved simultaneously in a bilaterally symmetrical pattern, and (5) mononeuropathy multiplex (rare), in which two or more individual peripheral nerves are paralyzed simultaneously.

Those that are of primary concern in neurosurgical diagnosis are the syndromes of the spinal roots and plexuses and the mononeuropathies.

Polyneuropathy is invariably due to medical diseases of toxic, metabolic, or inflammatory etiology and is only of concern to the neurosurgeon in that its manifestations may sometimes simulate certain neurosurgical lesions. It consists of bilaterally symmetrical distribution of flaccid weakness (diplegia), diminution or loss of tendon reflexes, sensory deficit, and autonomic changes that involve the extremities earliest and often exclusively. It may involve the lower extremities alone, the upper extremities alone, or occasionally the face alone (facial diplegia). The motor

and sensory manifestations generally begin in the distal parts of the involved extremities; they may remain limited to this distal distribution or progressively ascend the extremities. The trunk musculature becomes involved only late in the course of the disease if at all, even when all four extremities are severely involved. One never finds a sensory level on the trunk. There rarely is any impairment of sphincter function, although the occasional patient may void in bed if too weak to get out of bed. This syndrome may on occasion be difficult to diagnose because it simulates transverse myelitis or a lesion of the cauda equina. Table 1–1 lists the features that distinguish the two. In rapidly progressive cases of either, the distinction may be clouded, but rarely should it be necessary to subject the patient with rapidly advancing polyneuropathy to the hazard of myelography or other technical procedures to establish the correct diagnosis.

The syndromes of the individual nerves are described in Chapters 81, 82, and 83. The manifestations of disorders involving the major nerve plexuses and the individual peripheral nerves are also described in detail in the excellent monograph *Peripheral Nerve Injuries,* by Haymaker and Woodhall.[5]

Manifestations of Disorders of Skeletal Musculature

These disorders are rarely of concern in neurosurgical diagnosis. They are manifested clinically by muscular wasting and weakness, impairment of tendon reflexes, and sometimes muscular pains. They may in some instances simulate lesions of the peripheral nervous system or the spinal canal in which only motor function is disturbed. Usually they can be readily distinguished from such lesions by the following cardinal features that characterize the primary myopathies:

1. Motor loss is of the flaccid type. It is generally of bilaterally symmetrical distribution and may be generalized or restricted to certain muscle groups. It tends to predominate in the muscles of the trunk, the limb girdles, and the proximal parts of the limbs. Pseudohypertrophy of involved muscles, i.e., hypertrophy in which the muscles appear larger than nor-

TABLE 1-1 *CLINICAL MANIFESTATIONS OF SPINAL CORD, PERIPHERAL NERVE, AND SKELETAL MUSCLE DISEASES*

CLINICAL MANIFESTATIONS	SPINAL CORD LESIONS (Myelopathies)	PERIPHERAL NERVE LESIONS (Neuropathies)	MUSCLE DISEASES (Myopathies)
Motor	Upper or lower motor neuron type weakness, depending on acuity and "age" of the lesion and its location in relation to cord segments *Trunk and limb(s) below the lesion affected* Atrophy from disuse only	Lower motor neuron (flaccid) weakness only Predominantly in extremities; tends to involve distal limb segments more than proximal Atrophy early	Flaccid weakness only Tends to involve trunk and proximal limb segments earliest
Sensory	Cutaneous "sensory level" or "suspended sensory level" on trunk Sensory dissociation, if present, usually in terms of cord tracts	Rarely involves trunk; tends to begin distally in limbs and ascend limbs or follows distribution of a peripheral nerve supply Dissociation, if present, may be of any combination of modalities	None
Reflexes	Hyperactive tendon reflexes below lesion except during "spinal shock" with acute lesions At level of lesion, if limb segments are involved, hyporeflexia or areflexia persists or both hyper- and hyporeflexia occurs in same limb(s) *Pathological reflexes* (Babinski sign, spontaneous flexor or extensor spasms) below lesion likely Cutaneous reflexes lost below lesion	Hyporeflexia or areflexia found early and persists No pathological reflexes Cutaneous reflexes spared unless their effector muscles are completely paralyzed	Tendon reflexes normal early, become progressively hypoactive as disease advances Cutaneous reflexes spared No pathological reflexes
Sphincters	External urethral and anal sphincters often impaired	Sphincters very rarely involved	No sphincter disturbance

mal but are markedly weakened, is sometimes seen.

2. The tendon reflexes are diminished or occasionally absent as in lower motor neuron paralysis, but they tend to be preserved longer than in lower motor neuron involvement with comparable degrees of weakness and wasting. The cutaneous reflexes are preserved, and pathological reflexes do not appear.

3. Sensation is preserved in all modalities.

4. The sphincters are spared.

Table 1-1 lists the clinical findings that differentiate primary diseases of somatic musculature from polyneuropathy and spinal cord lesions.

THE ETIOLOGICAL DIAGNOSIS

The final step in neurosurgical diagnosis by the clinical method is determination of the etiology of the lesion. Sometimes this will have already been accomplished in the process of localizing the lesion and simultaneously considering salient items of information obtained in the process. Nevertheless, it is advisable as a conscious step in the diagnostic process to consider all the causes that are reasonably possible; the most likely is not always the correct one. Ancillary techniques are frequently required for refinement of diagnosis and planning management; the more thoroughly one has considered the etiological possibilities, the more judicious will be his choice of procedures and their priority.

The etiology of the neurosurgical diseases is considered in detail in subsequent chapters. The purpose here is not to preview these, but to provide the neurosurgeon with a "vest pocket" mental picture of the spectrum of diseases of the nervous system and their temporal profiles that he may find useful in the examining room with his patient. Of course, not all of them are generally considered "surgical diseases," whatever the implications of such a classification; but the neurosurgeon as a diagnostician is required to have a working knowledge of all categories of disease that may affect the nervous system if he is to fulfill his role as a physician and diagnostician as well as a surgical technician.

The following is an outline of the categories of nervous system diseases and a capsule condensation of their salient distinguishing features. It will be seen readily that *the determination of etiology depends primarily on adequate and accurate history* from the patient and relatives or other witnesses to his illness, whereas *anatomical localization depends primarily on the abnormal findings elicited by examination* of the patient.

Developmental Defects

Developmental defects are usually present from birth or become recognized very early in life. The clinical course of deficits in function produced by most of them is usually static (i.e., nonprogressive) or very slowly progressive over a period of years with modifications imposed by overall development of the nervous system in early life and its deterioration in later life. An exception to this general rule is that group of developmental anomalies in which rapid progression of deficit results from increasing pressure on neural structures (e.g., craniostenosis or congenital hydrocephalus).

Neoplasms

Neoplasms vary in age of onset depending on the type of tumor. Their onset is generally insidious (except when heralded by a sudden event such as an epileptic seizure), and the course of the symptoms produced is usually cumulative and progressive over a period of months or very few years. The rate of progression of symptoms within this range will vary depending on the location of the lesion and its degree of malignancy. Metastatic lesions to the nervous system not infrequently produce symptoms antecedent to those in the primary site.

Vascular Diseases

Vascular diseases predominantly occur in middle and late adult life with the exception of congenital vascular anomalies and the (rare) inflammatory vascular diseases, which may become clinically manifest at any age. The clinical onset of vascular diseases is nearly always sudden with progression to maximal deficit in minutes to hours (occasionally a few days), followed by a plateau of static (nonprogressive) deficit, then improvement in function if the patient survives the earlier phases. Within this general time range the onset and course vary in details depending on whether the lesion is a hemorrhage or an occlusion. In some instances the symptoms will occur intermittently over a period of days, weeks, or months, simulating demyelinative disease or occasionally a neoplastic growth. Differentiation from demyelinative disease can usually be made on the basis of the age of the patient at the time of initial symptoms and the recurrence of essentially the same manifestations with each episode. The occasional slowly progressing course seen in patients with occlusive arterial disease in the sixth decade or later can be very difficult to differentiate from the course of intracranial neoplasm; such cases usually require ancillary techniques for clarification of the diagnosis.

Demyelinative Disease

Demyelinative disease is a pathological category peculiar to the nervous system, resulting from the destruction of the myelin sheaths of axons in the central nervous system (brain, brain stem, cerebellum, and spinal cord). *Multiple sclerosis* is the most common disease in this group. The onset of its symptoms usually takes place during adolescence or early adult life, rarely after the third decade. It tends to occur in one or more acute or subacute episodes, each of which evolves to maximal deficit over a period of from 12 hours to several days, followed by a plateau of deficit, then gradual complete or partial subsidence. Successive attacks may be spaced weeks, months, or years apart, each differing in signs of localization but similar in temporal profile. Often an individual episode will subside only partially, leaving a background of permanent residual deficit upon which the deficits of subsequent attacks are superimposed. *Thus, the long-term clinical course is usually one of progressive accumulation of permanent deficit upon which are superimposed acute transient exacerbations of variable abnormal signs* indicative of involvement, successively, of different motor and sensory tracts up and down the neuraxis. Mental and emotional changes become a prominent part of the picture, usually in the later stages, because of the predilection of the cerebral lesions to cluster around the ventricular walls. Optic or retrobulbar neuritis, acute cerebellar or brain stem syndromes (or both), and acute partial or complete transverse syndromes of the spinal cord are the common forms that individual attacks tend to take. In an individual case the course may be fulminant to total disability or death within a few months, whereas in another case the attacks may be years apart and disabling residua minimal.

Acute postinfectious or postvaccinal encephalomyelitis, another fairly common demyelinative syndrome, differs from multiple sclerosis in that it usually occurs as a single acute episode with simultaneous involvement of multiple levels of the neuraxis. It most often occurs in children following immunization with certain vaccines or during the early convalescent phase of an acute exanthematous infection, usually heralded by a secondary rise in temperature, impairment of consciousness, and seizures. Its course varies from a few days to several weeks with gradual recovery to varying degrees of normalcy.

The diffuse cerebral scleroses are the other likely form that demyelinative disease takes. The onset and course vary widely depending on which of the two major types —inflammatory (exogenous, myelinoclastic) or degenerative (leukodystrophic) —occurs. The former is exemplified by Schilder's disease, which runs a rapid course of a few weeks to three years from onset to death. It is characterized by successive episodes of deficit corresponding to lesions in varying areas of white matter of the cerebral hemispheres (hallucinations and mental changes, motor or sensory hemiplegias, loss of vision, and convulsive seizures). It occurs most often in childhood or adolescence, but may begin in the third and fourth decades. The degenerative forms of cerebral sclerosis are more insidious in onset and progress over a period of several years with the development of a combination of corticospinal, extrapyramidal, mental, and cerebellar manifestations. Some types begin in early childhood and are familial; others begin in the later decades of life. *Both the inflammatory and degenerative forms of diffuse cerebral sclerosis are of importance to the neurosurgeon in that their clinical manifestations and course may closely simulate brain tumor, including the development of papilledema and other signs of increased intracranial pressure.*

Infections

Infections of the nervous system have some important differences in clinical manifestations from infections elsewhere in the body. They may take any one or a combination of three forms:

Abscess, focal infection, behaves as an expanding intracranial lesion just as a tumor does and often runs a similar course in time. It frequently is not accompanied by the usual systemic symptoms of abscess elsewhere (fever, leukocytosis). A history or findings of a source of infection (e.g., paranasal sinuses, ear, lung, preceding head trauma) is the most helpful information in differentiating it from neoplasm.

Meningitis, a diffuse infection of meninges, may run an acute or chronic course, depending on the infectious agent. In addition to initial signs of meningeal irritation (headache, stiff neck), the chronic forms or the more prolonged acute cases may produce "neighborhood reaction" in the cortical surfaces of brain (meningoencephalitis) and surface blood vessels or multiple cranial nerve palsies. The diagnosis usually rests on examination of the cerebrospinal fluid.

Encephalitis, a direct infection of brain parenchyma, is most often of viral etiology. Its course is acute or subacute with signs indicative of diffuse cerebral or brain stem involvement.

Degenerative Disease

Degenerative diseases of the nervous system usually occur in adult life, have an insidious onset and run a progressive course of several to many years. Some may simulate neoplasm in time course and in their early manifestations. They differ from neoplasm in clinical manifestations in that they are generally systems diseases — i.e., limited to one or a combination of two neuronal systems subserving a specific function — throughout their course, whereas neoplasm is a regional lesion. Familial incidence is not uncommon, a point of some help in the early differential diagnosis when present. The degenerative diseases often are manifest unilaterally at their outset, but eventually develop a bilaterally symmetrical distribution as they progress.

Trauma

Traumatic lesions are usually self-evident by the history, but the delayed effects of trauma may present a diagnostic problem when the onset of their symptoms is remote, when the trauma may have been too trivial for the patient to mention, or when the history is inadequate.

Metabolic and Toxic Diseases

Metabolic and toxic diseases are mostly secondary to systemic diseases such as diabetes, thyroid dysfunction, or poisoning. Some are limited to the nervous system; several of those diseases previously classified as degenerative are now regarded as metabolic with the discovery of a causative metabolic defect, and others are likely to be so reclassified in the future. The onset of metabolic or toxic syndromes of the nervous system may occur at any age, and their course may be episodic, progressive, or one of a single acute and self-limited episode, depending on the causative disturbance. The manifestations are generally diffuse and bilateral, but sometimes (e.g., in diabetic neuropathy) are localized or limited in distribution. The diagnosis usually rests on a history of precedent systemic metabolic disorder and laboratory studies.

Recurrent Episodic Syndromes

Recurrent episodic syndromes of the nervous system may be encountered as part of many diseases, or some may occur in the absence of known underlying cause. They are more properly regarded as syndromes than diseases. Even when their underlying causative disease is known, they often must be managed per se when the cause cannot be removed. The more common of these are: epilepsy, narcolepsy-cataplexy syndromes, headaches of certain categories (migraine, muscle-contraction, or tension headaches), recurrent syncope, and Ménière's syndrome.

It is emphasized that these are general characteristics of each of the categories of disease to which many exceptions may be found. They are intended only as "handles" that one may find helpful in attempting to arrive quickly at a working diagnosis, or more likely a differential diagnosis, in the individual case — a most important step for the mature diagnostician in planning the subsequent diagnostic and therapeutic management of his patient.

REFERENCES

1. Adams, R. D.: The clinical method of neurology: Comments and suggestions. Med. Clin. N. Amer., 36:1393, 1952.
2. Benton, A. L.: The fiction of the "Gerstmann syndrome." J. Neurol. Neurosurg. Psychiat., 24:176–181, 1961.
3. Gerstmann, J.: Syndrome of finger agnosia, disorientation for right and left, agraphia and acalculia. Local diagnostic value. Arch. Neurol. Psychiat., 44:398–408, 1940.
4. Harlow, J. M.: Passage of an iron rod through the head. Boston Med. Surg. J., 39:389, 1848.
5. Haymaker, W., and Woodhall, B.: Peripheral Nerve Injuries. 2nd Ed. Philadelphia, W. B. Saunders Co., 1953.
6. Kennedy, F.: Retrobulbar neuritis as an exact diagnostic sign of certain tumors and abscesses in the frontal lobes. Amer. J. Med. Sci., 142: 355–368, 1911.
7. Kuhn, R. A.: Functional capacity of the isolated human spinal cord. Brain, 73:1–51, 1950.
8. Malamud, N.: Psychiatric disorder with intracranial tumors of the limbic system. Arch. Neurol., 17:113–123, 1967.

9. Schneider, R. C., Crosby, E. C., and Farhat, S. M.: Extratemporal lesions triggering the temporal lobe syndrome. The role of association bundles. J. Neurosurg., *22*:246–263, 1965.

10. Talbert, O. R., and Clark, R. M.: Clinical manifestations of focal epilepsy. Southern Med. J., *61*:363–369, 1968.

11. Tarlov, I. M., and Herz, E.: Spinal cord compression studies. IV. Outlook with complete paralysis in man. Arch. Neurol. Psychiat., *72*:43–59, 1954.

12. Terzian, H., and Ore, G. D.: Syndrome of Klüver and Bucy reproduced in man by bilateral removal of the temporal lobes. Neurology, *5*:373–380, 1955.

13. von Wowern, F.: Foster Kennedy syndrome: Evaluation of its diagnostic value. Acta Neurol. Scand., *43*:205–214, 1967.

14. Williams, D.: The structure of emotions reflected in epileptic experiences. Brain, *79*:29–67, 1956.

2 ✓

CLINICAL EXAMINATION IN INFANCY AND CHILDHOOD

Adequate neurological diagnosis, at any age, is based on full and accurate clinical data. Findings on examination are expected to provide information as to the locus of the disease; the historical data provide information pertinent to its etiology. Neurological diagnosis in the child is more complex than in the adult. The child's nervous system grows in mass, and its physiology changes with age. His behavioral repertoire expands and reflects the nervous system's growth and development. The examiner must have knowledge of the child's behavioral development and function, in longitudinal and cross-sectional perspective, in order to make an accurate neurological diagnosis. With this one important exception, the principles and objectives of clinical neurological diagnosis in childhood are identical to those in adulthood.

BEHAVIORAL MANIFESTATIONS OF CEREBRAL MATURATION

The cerebral hemispheres (telencephalon) and the cerebellum have only slight influence over the behavioral repertoire of the newborn infant. Intelligence and sensory-motor coordination progressively increase with age as cerebellar and cerebral physiological maturation occurs.[1]

The newborn infant possesses a remarkable efficiency for maintaining homeostasis of vital functions. When hungry he roots, sucks, and swallows effectively. Movement of limbs appears fitful and variable. Responses to stimuli are gross, generalized, and poorly discriminating. Postural sets are largely dominated by tonic reflex automatism. The most important afferent forces for this reflex behavior are through the vestibular division of the eighth cranial nerve, proprioceptive mechanisms from the neck and trunk, and sensory elements originating in the skin and mucous membranes. The neonate is capable of almost no volitional behavior. The telencephalon influences neurophysiological behavioral functions to such a slight extent that lesions of the cerebral hemispheres may be difficult to detect at this stage in development.

Volitional control over body postures and adaptive motor performance begins early and proceeds rapidly according to predictable patterns. The normative behavior of infants and children has been well documented by Gesell and colleagues.[1] During the first three months of life, the infant gains control over his eye movements. He fixes gaze and follows bright objects with conjugate eye movements. By age 6 months, he has gained useful control over neck and arm muscles. He supports his head, he reaches for and grasps objects, and he manipulates objects crudely, using the whole hand. A bright object brought into the periphery of his field of vision is seen, and he turns his eyes toward that object. He also turns his head in the direction of sound stimuli. He maintains some of his weight when supported in standing. The infant at 10 months of age sits indefinitely, steadily, with almost straight back and re-

G. F. YOUNG

laxed postures of limbs. On volition he can go to the prone position, creep on hands and knees, pull himself to standing, and make stepping movements while holding on. Sensory-motor coordination of finger movements has developed so that he can prehend a pellet with a pincer maneuver involving the thumb and index finger. By age 15 months, the infant says words, indicates some of his needs for food and toilet, and walks unaided. He is beginning to have some control over the sphincters of bowel and bladder. His knowledge and understanding have grown to encompass concepts of multiple objects, container and contained, and larger and smaller magnitudes. He can place a cube into a cup, remove it, and construct a tower of two or three cubes. During the first year of life, the automatisms that were determined by spinal and brain stem reflex mechanisms have been superseded by improved sensory-motor coordination of adaptive acts, which is controlled by the cerebral cortex and subject to the child's will.

A 2-year-old child walks steadily and well, and he runs. He talks in words, phrases, and short sentences. He has gained control over the sphincters. He quickly puts several objects into a container and he can construct a tower of some six or eight cubes. By age 3, the child is very sociable. He carries on a meaningful conversation and he can dress and undress himself with some supervision and assistance. He walks up and down steps with little difficulty and jumps from the bottom step. By age 4, he knows the primary colors and rudimentary number concepts and he argues by analogy. He does a standing broad jump, stands momentarily on one foot, and tries to hop. The 5-year-old hops and skips, is largely independent in performing self care, and can describe some of his personal experiences. He counts to 12, he copies a triangle, and he can draw an unmistakable human figure.

The 5-year-old can cooperate and participate in the neurological examination with almost the same degree of competence as the adult patient except for tests that require academic skills (such as reading, writing, and mathematical calculations) that have not yet come into his learning experience. Examination of cranial nerves I through XII, primary sensory modalities, motor performance, and reflex activity are all tested by techniques similar to those applicable to the adult. The major difference between the neurological examination of adults and of young children relates to tests of the higher cerebral functions.

THE HISTORY AND EXAMINATION

The neurological surgeon who deals with children must include in his historical survey pertinent information that begins with the health of the mother prior to conception and any complications or difficulties during pregnancy, labor, and parturition. He should know the physical and functional status of the infant at birth, and he should trace systematically the progress of somatic growth and behavioral development from birth to the time of the examination. Special cognizance should be taken of any structural defects of the bony skeleton and other somatic malformations. If the patient is age 4 years or older, it is wise to question him about the nature of his illness. The examiner is often gratified by the candid recitation of pertinent symptoms that can sometimes be elicited from small children. However, youngsters, and even teenagers, have an imperfect concept of dates and times. They are not often reliable in this respect.

It is of primary importance to determine whether a child's neurological abnormalities are due to a static and unchanging lesion or to a progressing one. In this connection, examinations repeated after an interval of time can be of immeasurable help. However, if the results of the examination are to be relied upon, it must be conducted in a standardized and reproducible manner. The record of the results of these examinations should be precise. In order to achieve these objectives quickly, efficiently, and reliably, it is profitable to engage the young child in constructive play activities using standard test objects and procedures (such as the items — some of them taken from the Gesell developmental examination — shown in Figure 2–1).[1,2,4] Use of such standardized tests allows the

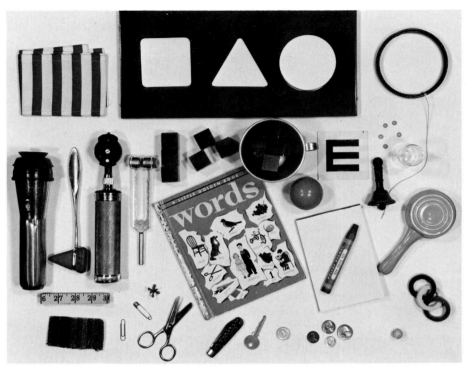

FIGURE 2–1 Neurological examination materials appropriate for infants and children.

examiner to profit by the wealth of normative data that have been accumulated. He will then be able to compare his findings with the norm as he documents changes in the individual child's performance from one examination to another. Regardless of the techniques of examination, the examiner will have to be flexible and sometimes inventive in order to elicit behavior that will allow him to correctly infer whether a given neuronal system or region of the nervous system is functioning properly. The order of performance of the numerous parts of the examination must be adapted to the circumstances. However, regardless of the manner in which the observational data are obtained, the results should be recorded in a standardized manner that makes it easy to ascertain whether there is derangement in "a system of physiologically related neuronal assemblies," or in a particular "region of the nervous system." The six customary subdivisions are recommended: cerebral function, cranial nerve functions, sensory sys-

tem, motor system, cerebellar function, and reflex status.

COMMENTS ON THE ANATOMICAL AND ETIOLOGICAL DIAGNOSES

Systems Syndromes

The syndromes of upper motor neuron paralysis, cortically derived extrapyramidal motor symptoms, and cerebellar dysfunction are as readily discerned in the child of 4 or 5 years of age as in the adult. Even in some younger children, the syndromes may have classic manifestations. However, during early infancy, even severe and extensive lesions in cerebrum or cerebellum may be manifested in ways that are different from those in the adult. Not infrequently, suprasegmental lesions in the young infant will be manifested by hypotonia and delayed development of gross motor capabilities. The more classic signs of spasticity, rigidity, dyskinesia, or ataxia may become manifest later, as growth and maturation of the nervous system occur.

Regional Diagnosis

For the most part, the classic manifestations of peripheral nerve, spinal cord, and brain stem lesions are similar at all ages. Diagnostic difficulties arise, however, when one undertakes localization within the supratentorial compartment. It is rare that one can identify a classic "frontal lobe syndrome," or "parietal lobe syndrome" in a preschool child. The concepts inherent in these terms indicate loss of or qualitative changes in neurological function that had previously been acquired by the patient. The developmental language disorders, specific learning disabilities, and some childhood behavior disorders related to brain disease appear to have a more complex and less well-understood localization.[3]

A special problem in regional diagnosis is often encountered when the young patient has a tumor situated in the midsagittal plane. The manifestations may be those of increased intracranial pressure, dulling of cognitive functions, slowness of reactions, a tendency to somnolence, and general lack of precision in sensory-motor performance. Ascertaining whether the lesion is a tumor, whether the tumor is in the infratentorial or supratentorial compartment, or whether the syndrome is due to diffuse brain swelling is usually not possible on the basis of the clinical examination alone. These patients must have the thoughtful application of special technical procedures such as electroencephalography, echoencephalography, radioisotopic brain scanning, cerebral angiography, and pneumography. Some patients require special metabolic and endocrine studies.

Etiological Diagnosis

The prevalence and importance of dysgenetic, encephaloclastic, traumatic, and neoplastic disease of congenital origin cannot be overemphasized. It is in the differentiation of these from other childhood neurological illnesses that the longitudinal health and developmental histories of the patient assume prime importance. Careful inspection for skeletal, integumental, and other developmental malformations often contributes evidence of overriding diagnostic importance. Differentiating the syndromes of mental retardation, developmental language and learning disorders, and most cases of childhood epilepsy from the nervous system diseases that require a more concerted neurosurgical effort can usually be achieved on the basis of clinical evidence alone.

A frequently recurring diagnostic dilemma is encountered in children who have poorly controlled epilepsy. Such children may appear to have dementia or another progressive brain disorder. In many such cases, the syndrome can be shown to be caused by uncontrolled epilepsy and a toxic encephalopathy produced by overdosage of ineffective antiepileptic medications. All such children will require an extensive inpatient diagnostic and therapeutic effort. The electroencephalogram provides very useful diagnostic information. Skillful adjustment of antiepileptic medicines will also help to clarify the diagnosis. Nevertheless, some of these patients will require special neuroradiological and metabolic studies in order to prove what is wrong.

REFERENCES

1. Gesell, A., and Amatruda, C. S.: Developmental Diagnosis. 2nd Ed. New York, Paul B. Hoeber, 1947.
2. Harrison, T. R., et al.: Principles of Internal Medicine. 5th Ed. New York, McGraw-Hill Book Co., 1966, pp. 1249–1266.
3. Orton, S. T.: Reading, Writing, and Speech Problems in Children. New York, W. W. Norton & Co., Inc., 1961.
4. Paine, R. S., and Oppe, T. E.: Neurological Examination of Children. Surrey, England, William Heinemann Medical Books Ltd., 1966.

3 ✓

DIFFERENTIAL DIAGNOSIS OF ALTERED STATES OF CONSCIOUSNESS

Consciousness is the highest function of the brain, and its subtlest impairment in disease provides a cardinal clinical sign. The preservation of sentient existence stands equal with the relief of suffering as the physician's first responsibility.

Consciousness ranges in degree from *alert wakefulness* to *deep coma*. The former is characterized by full and appropriate responses to both internal and external stimuli, and the latter by apparently complete unresponsiveness to even the most compelling stimuli. The gradations between these extremes are also important, for even subtle changes can influence diagnosis, management, and prognosis. The following states may be defined:

Lethargy means drowsiness, inaction, and indifference in which responses are delayed and incomplete, and an increased stimulus may be required to evoke a response. *Obtundation* refers to duller indifference in which little more than wakefulness is maintained. *Stupor* is the state from which the subject can only be aroused by vigorous and continuous external stimulation. *Coma* means that psychological and motor responses to stimulation are either completely lost (*deep coma*) or reduced to only rudimentary or reflex motor responses (*moderately deep coma*). In some closely allied states, e.g., *delirium* and *organic confusion*, consciousness is deranged as much as it is depressed, often by the same processes that may progress to cause coma.

Examples of stupor and coma as urgent problems in diagnosis and care are common in any busy emergency room. Table 3–1 itemizes the final diagnosis in 386 patients presenting with "coma of unknown etiology," and reflects the diverse diseases that can cause severe brain dysfunction and coma. That a large proportion are reversible if given appropriate medical or surgical treatment underlines the importance of rapid and accurate diagnosis.

TABLE 3–1 *FINAL DIAGNOSIS IN 386 PATIENTS WITH "COMA OF UNKNOWN ETIOLOGY"**

Supratentorial mass lesions		69
Epidural hematoma	2	
Subdural hematoma	21	
Intracerebral hematoma	33	
Cerebral infarct	5	
Brain tumor	5	
Brain abscess	3	
Subtentorial lesions		52
Brain stem infarct	37	
Brain stem hemorrhage	7	
Brain stem tumor	2	
Cerebellar hemorrhage	4	
Cerebellar abscess	2	
Metabolic and diffuse cerebral disorders		261
Anoxia and ischemia	51	
Concussion and postictal states	9	
Infection (meningitis and encephalitis)	11	
Subarachnoid hemorrhage	10	
Exogenous toxins	99	
Endogenous toxins and deficiencies	81	
Psychiatric disorders		4

*Reprinted from Plum, F., and Posner, J. B.: Diagnosis of Stupor and Coma. 2nd Ed. Contemporary Neurology Series, Vol. 10, 1972, with permission of F. A. Davis Co.

F. PLUM

R. W. BRENNAN

44

CLINICAL EXAMINATION OF THE UNCONSCIOUS PATIENT

The emergency care of the less than fully conscious patient must combine treatment and diagnosis. The patient must be protected from further insult by insuring a patent airway and adequate ventilation, mechanical if necessary. In every case of unexplained stupor or coma, glucose (50 ml. of a 50 per cent solution) should be given intravenously immediately *after* blood has been drawn for glucose determination. The treatment is innocuous, and in hypoglycemia it gives prompt protection against further and sometimes irreversible neuronal injury. Diagnosis properly begins with a careful history, but often the sum of available information from the patient, his friends, his family, or the ambulance or police personnel is either incomplete or conflicting. Hence the need for an orderly, selective physical examination that may give findings with specific diagnostic value.

The observations listed in Table 3–2 give important clues, but diagnosis depends upon the total findings. The first question is anatomical, i.e., where does the lesion causing unconsciousness lie? Can the signs be due to a single lesion? Or, do they point to multifocal or diffuse disease? Finally, and most important for management, in what direction is the process evolving?

A plan for evaluating the nervous system in the unconscious patient follows, based on changes observed in five physiological functions: the state of consciousness, the pattern of breathing, the size and reactivity of the pupils, the eye movements, and the skeletal muscle responses.

The Physiology and Pathology of Consciousness

Consciousness may be thought of as having two components, one being its crude "off-on" quality, and the other its content. In general, crude "all or none" consciousness depends upon the integrity of specific areas of the upper brain stem, while the content of consciousness depends more upon the functions of the cerebral hemispheres.

Studies of patients with disease restricted to the cerebral hemispheres led

TABLE 3–2 *IMPORTANT PHYSICAL SIGNS IN COMA*

Vital signs
Hypertension	Hypertensive encephalopathy; cerebral hemorrhage; subarachnoid hemorrhage
Hypotension	Inadequate cerebral perfusion secondary to myocardial infarction, hemorrhagic shock, or pulmonary infarction
Hyperthermia	CNS infection; subarachnoid hemorrhage; bacterial endocarditis; pneumonitis with hypoxia; heat stroke
Hypothermia	Metabolic or toxic coma of any cause, particularly barbiturate or phenothiazine intoxication, other depressants, or insulin coma; destructive brain stem lesions; myxedema

Skin changes
Multiple petechiae or purpura	Thrombotic thrombocytopenic purpura; meningococcemia; bacterial endocarditis; fat embolism
Cherry pink skin	Carbon monoxide poisoning
Multiple healed venipunctures	Drug addiction
Evidence of head trauma; scalp contusion, edema; blood or CSF in nares or behind tympanic membrane; subgaleal or subperiosteal blood ("raccoon eyes," Battle's sign)	Skull fractures; cerebral concussion, contusion; acute epidural or subdural hemorrhage
Nuchal rigidity	Meningitis; cerebellar tonsillar herniation; rarely, acute subarachnoid hemorrhage. (in which stiff neck takes several hours to develop)

Wolff to conclude that man's highest integrative abilities are lost in proportion to the amount of involved cortex.[8] Patients with moderately advanced but selective cortical disease, e.g., Alzheimer's disease, typically show a profound decline in the content of consciousness but fully retain wakefulness. More extensive or rapid losses of the functioning cortical mass blunt responsiveness, and in functional or anatomical decorticate states, only rudiments of behavioral responsiveness remain. Even then such features as intact chewing and swallowing, food preferences, and sleep-awake cycles are preserved. However, such global but selective cortical lesions are rare, and the great bulk of unconsciousness has other causes.

Evidence that the crude element of consciousness depends heavily on brain stem structures goes as far back as clinico-pathological analyses published in the late nineteenth century.[21] Many examples are now known of discrete lesions, including tumors, infarcts, and hemorrhages restricted to paramedian areas of the pons, midbrain, and hypothalamus, that abolish or reduce consciousness.[7, 14, 19, 20]

Experimental studies of the brain stem reticular core have further defined much of its normal function. Magoun and Moruzzi identified an ascending reticular activating system (ARAS) within the paramedian tegmentum of the midbrain and extending to the hypothalamus and thalamus.[29] This system diffusely projects to the cerebral cortex and profoundly influences both arousal and the electroencephalographic (EEG) pattern. In experimental animals, stimulation leads to alert behavior and an activated, desynchronized electroencephalogram, while destruction causes behavioral unresponsiveness and a slow electroencephalogram. Depressant and anesthetic drugs act selectively on the ARAS, presumably because of its highly polysynaptic organization.[1]

An earlier view held that both sleep and coma arose passively when the tonic activating influence of the ascending reticular activating system decreased, but this concept has been disproved. Recent evidence reveals that sleep is an active process, regulated by functional subunits of the reticular core. Cerebral blood flow and metabolism remain normal even in the deepest stages of sleep, or may actually increase. In coma, on the other hand, cerebral metabolism is consistently subnormal. Sleep is a highly physiological state and coma is a most unphysiological one, and there is no basis for equating the two.

Respiration

Many of the metabolic abnormalities that cause coma increase or decrease the chemical stimuli to pulmonary ventilation. Also, because damage or depression of the brain at nearly every level affects the act of breathing, appraisal of this function becomes useful in anatomical localization. Table 3–3 lists some of the metabolic influences that can cause coma and at the

TABLE 3–3 METABOLIC DISORDERS CAUSING COMA AND AFFECTING RESPIRATION

Hyperventilation
  Acute metabolic acidosis
    Uremia
    Diabetic ketoacidosis
    Exogenous poisoning (paraldehyde, methyl alcohol, ethylene glycol)
    Anoxic lactic acidosis
  Respiratory alkalosis
    Hepatic encephalopathy
    Salicylate intoxication
    Cardiopulmonary disease
    Central neurogenic hyperventilation
Hypoventilation
  Respiratory acidosis
    Depressant drug poisoning
    Pulmonary disease with CO_2 retention
  Metabolic alkalosis
    Rarely causes stupor or coma except perhaps with severe hyperadrenocorticism

same time will alter an anatomically intact respiratory system. The remainder of this section describes neuroanatomical influences on breathing that aid the clinician in reaching a localizing diagnosis.

In normal awake subjects, a significant portion of the resting stimulus to pulmonary ventilation comes from nonchemical neural sources. As a result, when a neurologically intact subject is asked to hyperventilate briefly, he continues to breathe rhythmically *after* the hyperventilation at a time when carbon dioxide and oxygen stimuli are in abeyance. This altogether unconscious and automatic influence is impaired with even moderate degrees of bilateral cerebral dysfunction, and such subjects demonstrate *posthyperventilation apnea,* usually lasting 10 to 25 seconds, after taking five good deep breaths. This abnormality is useful in distinguishing a dulled or confused subject with cerebral dysfunction from one with a psychologically induced behavioral alteration.

More severe bilateral hemispheric dysfunction impairs the nonchemical influences on the act of breathing even more, and in addition, in many such patients there is an increased respiratory responsiveness to chemical stimuli. As a result, many of them develop a breathing pattern with regular oscillations between hyperpnea and apnea. This is *Cheyne-Stokes* respiration. The regular waxing and waning, being dependent on stimuli reaching the respiratory system, has a period length equal to twice the lung-to-brain circulation time.

Involvement of anatomical centers in the posterior hypothalamus and midbrain produces moderate pulmonary edema in many patients, and a pattern of hyperpnea with a low arterial carbon dioxide tension combined with a below-normal oxygen tension is the result. A less common manifestation of midbrain–upper pontine lesions in man is a true *central hyperventilation*. This condition occurs in patients with destructive depression or compression of the paramedian tegmentum, and is marked by respiratory rates as high as 25 to 40 per minute, a low arterial blood carbon dioxide tension, and an above-normal blood oxygen tension.

Damage or depression to the brain stem's paramedian reticulum at or below the pons produces *irregularly irregular breathing* patterns. These may take various forms including inspiratory or expiratory apneusis, cluster breathing, gasping, or long periods of ataxic irregular breathing patterns in which the timing and depth of the next breath cannot be predicted from the past pattern. All these last-mentioned abnormalities tend to be associated with abnormal blood gases and underventilation, and thus they tend to accentuate whatever neurological injury or depression is already present.

Extensive damage or depression of the medullary reticular formation generally destroys the central control of respiration and produces severe hypoventilation or apnea.

Pupils

At rest or in reflex motion, pupil size reflects a balance between opposite tonic motor inputs. The parasympathetic system acts upon the pupilloconstrictor muscle to induce miosis, while the sympathetic system innervates the radially arranged pupillodilator fibers that produce active mydriasis.[9] The selective loss of either influence leaves the other unopposed, with corresponding changes in pupil size. The central pathways for both pupilloconstrictor and dilator effects course through the upper brain stem

and are often interrupted by lesions in this area that threaten consciousness.

Lesions above the diencephalon have little effect on pupillary size or function, although sleep and cerebral depression are associated with bilateral pupilloconstriction. Stimulation of the lateral hypothalamus produces ipsilateral pupil dilatation; destruction or functional depression of the same area results in pupilloconstriction. These effects are mediated through pupillodilator pathways that descend from the hypothalamus through all levels of the brain stem to reach second order neurons in the upper thoracic spinal cord; the pathway then travels through peripheral fibers to third order neurons in the superior cervical ganglion, and finally through postganglionic fibers passing with branches of the internal carotid artery to the orbit.

Active pupilloconstriction results from stimulation in another diencephalic structure, the pretectum. Destruction or depression of this area may result in bilateral pupillary dilatation. The light reflex is typically impaired as well, from involvement of the afferent limb or the pretectal relay nuclei. This and perhaps other pupilloconstrictor influences play upon the Edinger-Westphal nucleus, which is interposed between the oculomotor nuclei of the paramedian midbrain. Preganglionic parasympathetic fibers pass in the peripheral parts of the oculomotor nerve, to synapse in the ciliary ganglion in the orbit.

Localizing Value of Pupillary Abnormalities in Coma

The size of the normal pupil varies widely. Miosis is common in drowsiness or sleep, while mydriasis accompanies arousal, intense emotion, or the perception of pain. Patients with bilateral cerebral dysfunction commonly exhibit small pupils (2 to 3 mm) that are reactive to light and fluctuate with the state of spontaneous and reflex arousal. The pupils may undergo cyclic changes with Cheyne-Stokes respiration, dilating in hyperpnea and constricting in apnea. In such patients, the mobility and symmetry of the pupils exclude structural injury to the brain stem proper.

Miosis on the same side as a large hemispheric lesion may indicate encroachment on the more specific pupillodilator center in the ipsilateral hypothalamus, and thus herald impending transtentorial herniation.

Midbrain damage produces clear-cut pupillary signs. Tectal or pretectal lesions interrupt the light reflex, producing mid-position or slightly dilated pupils (5 to 6 mm) that are round, regular, but sometimes asymmetrical and relatively fixed to light. Such "tectal pupils" commonly have the spontaneous movements of hippus and retain reflex dilatation to noxious body stimuli. Discrete lesions that involve the oculomotor nerve in the ventral midbrain, or in the interpeduncular fossa, produce widely dilated (8 to 9 mm) and immobile pupils. Major injury to the midbrain, as in central infarction or hemorrhage or in the compression and distortion wrought by transtentorial herniation, nearly always interrupts both sympathetic and para-sympathetic pathways. The resulting pupils are in midposition (4 to 5 mm), fixed to light, and sometimes irregular and slightly asymmetrical; such pupils may still dilate slightly in response to noxious stimuli de-livered to neck or trunk (the ciliospinal reflex).[2]

Several patterns of pupillary response may occur in combination; supratentorial mass lesions, such as epidural hematomas situated laterally, may compress the ipsilateral oculomotor nerve and produce a dilated fixed pupil as a prelude to the more typical changes of transtentorial hernia-tion.[33, 37]

Pontine lesions involving the tegmentum may interrupt descending sympathetic pathways and produce small pupils on one or both sides. The acute and extensive damage of pontine hemorrhage produces pinpoint pupils (1 to 2 mm), which at least briefly may lose their light reaction.[36]

Laterally, medullary lesions cause a mild Horner's syndrome, with slight ptosis and pupillary constriction, on the homo-lateral side, but consciousness is not impaired.

In most metabolic encephalopathies, in-cluding sedative poisoning, the pupils are small but symmetrical, regular, and fully reactive to light. In extreme cases, as with unremitting anoxia or very severe meta-bolic or drug depressions, the pupillary light reflex may be lost terminally. The ex-ception to this rule is glutethimide poison-ing, in which the anticholinergic effect of the drug can result in fixed wide pupils (5 to 8 mm) with only moderately severe cen-tral nervous system depression. In narcotic intoxication, pupils are intensely miotic (1 to 2 mm), but reactive, and dilate in response to topical nalorphine solution.

Ocular Movements

Both voluntary and reflex conjugate movements of the eyes depend on mechan-isms represented at several levels of the neuraxis. Oculomotor abnormalities in stuporous or comatose patients give clinically useful information concerning the site of the lesion that is depressing con-sciousness.

Supranuclear fibers from voluntary or reflex conjugate gaze centers in the cere-bral hemispheres descend through or medial to the internal capsule into the brain stem, decussate, and pass down the contra-lateral pontine paramedial tegmentum to synapse near the abducens nucleus in the low pons.[3, 10] Fibers controlling conjugate vertical gaze and originating in the cere-brum travel through the regions of the pre-tectal and posterior commissural nuclei to reach the oculomotor nuclei bilaterally. *Internuclear fibers* connecting the oculo-motor, trochlear, and abducens nuclei course in the median longitudinal fasci-culus (MLF) just ventral to the periaque-ductal gray matter of the midbrain and pons. This pathway decussates in the pons just rostral to the abducens nucleus. It serves to coordinate ipsilateral lateral rectus and contralateral medial rectus muscle action initiated through supranu-clear conjugate gaze mechanisms. The *labyrinthine-vestibular system* also in-fluences conjugate eye movements. Fibers from the semicircular canals, otoliths, and the fastigial nucleus of the cerebellum synapse in the vestibular nuclei, from which second order fibers traverse the median longitudinal fasciculus to the ocular motor nuclei. Fibers conveying proprioception from the upper cervical segments probably reach the ocular motor nuclei through the caudal continuation of the MLF, which descends into the spinal cord as far as C2 or C3.

In stuporous or comatose patients, reflex eye movements may be elicited to test the integrity of many of the foregoing pathways.[32] The *oculocephalic reflex* or "doll's eyes" phenomenon is demonstrated by observing the eyes as the head is briefly rotated and held at the extreme position. A positive response to side-to-side movement is transient conjugate deviation of the eyes opposite to the direction of head movement (e.g., if the head is rotated to the right, the eyes deviate to the left). Vertical reflex movements may be sought by brisk flexion and extension of the head and the neck. A positive response is deviation of the eyes upward on flexion, downward on extension. The stimulus for the oculocephalic reflex involves either the labyrinthine vestibular system or proprioceptive afferents from the neck, or possibly both.[18] The *oculovestibular reflex* refers to reflex conjugate eye movements or nystagmus or both induced by caloric stimulation of the labyrinth. The head is elevated 30 degrees above the horizontal so that the lateral semicircular canal is vertical, a position in which stimulation can provoke a maximal response. A soft catheter is placed in the external canal near the tympanic membrane, and a small volume of ice water is slowly syringed into the canal of the unresponsive patient until either horizontal nystagmus or tonic ocular deviation occurs; 1 ml is usually sufficient, and volumes of more than 20 ml are rarely necessary. To test for vertical eye movements, one can irrigate both auditory canals simultaneously with ice water. In a comatose patient with intact brain stem vestibular-oculomotor connections, the eyes deviate downward. With the lateral canal inverted (head 60 degrees below horizontal), the same maneuver elicits upward eye movement.

In most patients in coma, the reflex eye movements in response to caloric stimulation and to passive head turning relate to each other as if the two stimuli differed only in degree, the first being the stronger. In the oculovestibular reflex, an induced convection current in the labyrinthine endolymph of the lateral canal alters the balance in the paired vestibular systems to produce tonic conjugate eye deviation toward the same side with cold stimuli, or to the opposite side with warm stimuli.[39] In the oculocephalic reflex, the relative currents generated by inertia of the endolymph as the head is moved stimulate the receptors of both lateral canals to produce similar but less pronounced effects. In addition, stimuli from proprioceptors in the upper cervical segments also play a role, so that some patients with pontine lesions may lose the caloric response but retain the oculocephalic response.

In awake alert patients the eyes are directed straight ahead at rest. Oculocephalic responses cannot normally be elicited, and caloric stimulation yields nystagmus rather than sustained deviation.

In coma due to bilateral hemispheral depression, the eyes are directed straight ahead. For the first 24 hours or so after onset of asymmetrical or unilateral cerebral dysfunction the eyes typically deviate to the side of the lesion, occasionally with some nystagmus to that side. In patients with moderate bilateral cerebral depression, as in metabolic stupor or coma, labyrinthine stimuli cause tonic eye movements rather than nystagmus, since the quick or eye-centering phase depends on interaction between the oculovestibular system and the cerebrum and disappears as cerebral influences are reduced. In such patients, oculocephalic reflexes may be of large amplitude and easily elicited, and caloric responses may be sustained for several minutes, as if released from suprasegmental inhibition. Such hyperactive responses are characteristic of patients who have diffuse cortical dysfunction from anoxia, hypoglycemia, or hepatic coma.

With coma from brain stem lesions, reflex eye movements are depressed, or otherwise abnormal. With midbrain or pontine lesions involving the median longitudinal fasciculus, the eye on the side of the lesion fails to adduct on reflex movements. Lateral pontine lesions cause the eyes to deviate conjugately away from the side of the lesion, and reflex movements toward that side are often blocked at the midline. Skew deviation, or vertical strabismus, appears with dorsolateral pontine lesions or with lesions in the median longitudinal fasciculus. It may be brought out with reflex lateral eye movements to one or both sides. Extensive pontine lesions may block reflex eye movements in all planes, while midbrain-pretectal lesions may selectively impair vertical movements alone. "Ocular bobbing" is intermittent brisk downward eye movement followed by a slower return to the primary position. It is a reliable sign of extensive pontine destruction.[16]

Motor Function

Motor abnormalities in patients with depressed consciousness or coma give further evidence as to the side involved and the nature of the lesion.

Paratonic rigidity is a nonspecific but early sign of subcortical hemispheric motor dysfunction. It represents an abnormal increase in resistance to passive movement, but, unlike spasticity or plasticity, it is intermittent; when present, it is independent of the initial position of the extremity. The resistance often has a reactive or overactive quality suggesting that the patient is voluntarily opposing every effort of the examiner to move him. Ranging in degree from slight failure to relax to intense rigidity of the entire body, paratonia is common in states of diffuse cerebral dysfunction, i.e., widespread vascular disease or metabolic disturbances.

Motor and sensory function in patients with depressed consciousness can be estimated by applying noxious stimuli to different parts of the body and observing the response. *Appropriate responses* in a patient with acute brain dysfunction imply that both motor and sensory pathways are at least partly intact. *Inappropriate responses* are stereotypes of movement and posture in response to noxious stimuli whose pattern depends on the level of injury. *Decorticate response* consists of flexion of the arm, wrist, and fingers with adduction in the upper extremity, and extension, internal rotation, and plantar flexion in the lower extremity. The response is typically due to lesions of the frontal hemisphere, internal capsule, or rostral cerebral peduncle. *Decerebrate responses* when fully developed consist of opisthotonus, adduction and extension and hyperpronation of the arms, and extension and plantar flexion of the lower extremities. The response requires at least partial and bilateral separation of midbrain and pontine structures from hemispheral influence,

and is elicited commonly in conditions that destroy or depress the upper brain stem.

SUPRATENTORIAL LESIONS CAUSING COMA

Two main types of supratentorial processes can depress or abolish consciousness: localized hemispheral lesions that produce a deep destructive or mass effect because they either extend directly into deeper midline diencephalic structures, or secondarily compress them; and lesions that produce diffuse bilateral impairment of either the cortical mantle or its underlying white matter, but spare the brain stem. These latter usually have a metabolic origin and are discussed separately.

Anatomical Considerations

Because its confines are inelastic, the intracranial volume is essentially fixed. A progressive mass lesion must enlarge at the expense of one or more of the normal intracranial components—brain, blood, or cerebrospinal fluid. Accommodative mechanisms are limited and cannot indefinitely make room for a continually expanding process. At some point, the contents of the supratentorial space will herniate through the tentorial notch, molding and distorting the involved tissues and eventually producing hemorrhage and necrosis of the impacted area.[15, 25] The dividing line between survival and death with supratentorial masses is drawn at the point at which irreversible tentorial herniation can be prevented.

Pathogenesis

As a hemispheral mass lesion enlarges and induces brain swelling, there is a compensatory shift in the medial and deep structures of the hemisphere. One of two main syndromes of transtentorial herniation evolves, depending on the location of the lesion and, hence, on the direction of the displacing force. Central diencephalic compression produces signs reflecting bilateral and generally symmetrical failure of the diencephalon, then the midbrain, pons, and finally the medulla in progressive rostrocaudal fashion (Syndrome I, Table 3–4). In laterally placed lesions, the earliest signs may reflect herniation of the uncus and other structures of the medial temporal lobe over the adjacent lip of the tentorial notch and onto the ipsilateral third nerve (Syndrome II). If herniation continues, signs of progressive descending brain stem failure appear soon after.[30]

The course of the transtentorial herniation syndrome is usually measured in hours or even days, but very rapidly evolving masses, e.g., epidural hematoma, may cause coma from irreversible brain stem injury within an hour. More indolent lesions may cause gradual, stepwise, or even fluctuating signs of incipient herniation. Cerebral hemorrhage with intraventricular rupture produces exceptionally rapid brain stem dysfunction, and frequently there are signs of medullary failure while higher functions are still preserved.

SUBTENTORIAL LESIONS CAUSING COMA

Patients with destructive subtentorial lesions, e.g., primary hemorrhage or infarction of the midbrain or pons, often lose consciousness immediately, or as soon as the activating systems in the median tegmentum are involved.[26] Such lesions always give unequivocal localizing signs, and the anatomical diagnosis is not often in doubt. In further contrast to the brain stem injury caused by supratentorial masses, functions rostral to the lesion are preserved. Metabolic depression may mimic structural lesions of the brain stem, but pupillary light reflexes are spared, and ocular and motor signs are symmetrical in metabolic brain disease.

Expanding lesions in the posterior fossa influence consciousness as they directly compress the brain stem; in certain cases, upward transtentorial herniation may also play a role.[13] Herniation of the cerebellar tonsils through the foramen magnum distorts the medulla, and respiratory failure is the terminal event. In diagnosis, the history is crucial; with acute lesions (e.g., cerebellar hemorrhage), the sudden occipital headache, vertigo, and vomiting followed by progressive neurological impairment from pontine compression strongly suggests the correct one.[17]

TABLE 3–4 *SYNDROMES OF TRANSTENTORIAL HERNIATION*

Level	Consciousness	Respiration	Pupils	Oculocephalic Reflex	Motor Response
SYNDROME I (Central Compression and Herniation)					
Early diencephalic	Dull	Eupnea, yawns, sighs	Small, reactive	Intermittent or hyperactive	Hemiplegia, bilateral Babinski, moderate bilateral paratonia
Late diencephalic	Stupor	CSR*	Small, reactive	Hyperactive	Hemiplegia, bilateral, Babinski, decorticate pain response
Midbrain	Coma	CSR → CNH†	Midposition, fixed	Disconjugate or sluggish	Decerebrate responses
Upper pontine	Coma	CNH	Midposition, fixed	Sluggish	Less decerebrate
Lower pontine	Coma	Eupneic or ataxic	Midposition, fixed	0	Flaccid, bilateral Babinski
SYNDROME II (Lateral Compression and Herniation)					
Early diencephalic	Drowsy	Eupnea	One dilated or normal	Intact if obtainable	Developing unilateral changes
Late diencephalic	Stupor	Eupnea → CSR or CNH	One dilated → fixed	III Nerve Palsy	Decorticate → decerebrate
Midbrain	Coma	CNH	Dilated, fixed	Disconjugate	Decerebrate
Upper pontine	Coma	CNH	Midposition, fixed	Sluggish	Less decerebrate
Lower pontine	Coma	Eupneic or ataxic	Midposition, fixed	0	Flaccid, bilateral Babinski

*CSR, Cheyne-Stokes respiration.
†CNH, Central neurogenic hyperventilation.

METABOLIC CAUSES OF STUPOR AND COMA

Metabolic encephalopathy occurs when noncerebral diseases secondarily interfere with brain metabolism in any of several ways. Some examples may be given. In hypoxia and in hypoglycemia, extrinsic brain energy sources are insufficient, and rapid irreversible catabolic changes occur.[35, 41] In electrolyte imbalances, e.g., hyponatremia or water intoxication, neuronal excitability is altered.[38] Changes in the brain's acid-base or osmotic milieu may also depress function. Uremia and hepatic failure are complex states in which cerebral function often suffers; presumably, some endogenous toxin is at fault.[4, 28] Depressant drugs or other exogenous toxins are common causes of metabolic depression, sometimes to the point of profound coma.

Patients with mild metabolic encephalopathy are confused and disoriented, have mild blunting of alertness, and may show perceptual disturbances in the form of illusions or visual hallucinations. Tremor, asterixis ("flap"), or myoclonic movements are common. Diffuse and symmetrical motor abnormalities are seen, including paratonia and snouting and grasp reflexes. As the disease progresses, stupor and finally coma ensue. The pattern of respiration and motor responses varies with the stage of progression. The pupils are small, but symmetrical, and light reflexes are preserved. Oculocephalic and oculovestibular reflexes remain brisk and conjugate, except in sedative intoxication, when they are depressed or absent even in light coma.

The findings in metabolic encephalopathy bespeak widespread but selective action on brain functions, with cerebral functions being involved before those of lower structures. In certain cases, the findings suggest partial dysfunction affecting many levels of the neuraxis simultaneously, while the integrity of other functions originating at the same level is spared. Another point of difference from coma based on structural lesions is the rarity of asymmetrical or focal signs in metabolic encephalopathy. Finally, the electroencephalogram shows generalized symmetrical slowing without focal abnormality.

In certain other diseases, coma may arise from a combination of structural and metabolic effects. Coma in subarachnoid hemorrhage may come from mechanical effects, e.g., an associated hematoma acting as a supratentorial or subtentorial mass, or from some toxic metabolic action of blood products. In severe bacterial meningitis or in viral meningoencephalitis, cerebral edema is often found and may be of itself a cause of diffuse cerebral dysfunction and coma. In these several conditions, careful examination of the cerebrospinal fluid almost always gives unequivocal diagnostic information.

EPISODIC UNCONSCIOUSNESS

Some common and important neurological problems present as brief and fully reversible episodes of altered consciousness. According to the classification proposed by Lee and Plum, the causes may be assigned to five major groups: failure of systemic circulation, as in vasodepressor syncope or cardiac arrhythmia; systemic disorders impairing cerebral metabolism, as in hypoglycemia; cerebral arterial insufficiency due to structural or functional changes in the brain vasculature; primary neurological disorders, e.g., epilepsy or concussion; and other causes, e.g., psychogenic unresponsiveness.[27] Unless the episode has been witnessed by the physician, the etiological diagnosis must depend heavily on a detailed history centered on what the circumstances were, what the patient felt, and what observers, if any, may have noted.

This group of disorders is peripheral to neurosurgical practice, but recurrent episodes of unconsciousness warrant close attention, for their causes can sometimes produce irreversible neurological injury as well.

REFERENCES

1. Arduini, A., and Arduini, M. G.: Effects of drugs and metabolic alterations on brain stem arousal mechanisms. J. Pharmacol. Exp. Ther., *110*:76–85, 1954.
2. Arieff, A. J., and Pyzik, S. W.: The ciliospinal reflex in injuries of the cervical spinal cord in

man. A.M.A. Arch. Neurol. Psychiat., 70: 621–629, 1953.

3. Bender, M., ed.: The Oculomotor System, New York, Harper and Row, 1964.

4. Bessman, S. P., and Bessman, A. N.: The cerebral and peripheral uptake of ammonia in liver disease with an hypothesis of hepatic coma. J. Clin. Invest., 34:622–628, 1955.

5. Blegvad, B.: Caloric vestibular reaction in unconscious patients. Arch. Otolaryng., 75:506–514, 1962.

6. Brain, R.: The physiological basis of consciousness. Brain, 81:426–455, 1958.

7. Cairns, H.: Disturbances of consciousness with lesions of the brain stem and diencephalon. Brain, 75:109–146, 1952.

8. Chapman, L. F., and Wolff, H. G.: The cerebral hemispheres and the highest integrative functions of man. Arch. Neurol., 1:357–424, 1959.

9. Cogan, D. G.: Neurology of the Ocular Muscles. Ed. 2. Springfield, Ill., Charles C Thomas, 1956.

10. Crosby, E. C.: Relations of brain centers to normal and abnormal eye movements in the horizontal plane. J. Comp. Neurol., 99:437–479, 1953.

11. Cushing, H.: Concerning a definite regulatory mechanism of the vaso-motor centre which controls blood pressure during cerebral compression. Bull. Hopkins Hosp., 12:290–292, 1901.

12. Dodge, P. R., and Swartz, M. N.: Bacterial meningitis: II. Special neurologic problems, postmeningitic complications and clinico-pathological correlations. New Eng. J. Med., 272:954–960, 1965.

13. Ecker, A.: Upward transtentorial herniation of the brainstem and cerebellum due to tumor of the posterior fossa. J. Neurosurg., 5:51–61, 1948.

14. von Economo, C.: Sleep as a problem of localization. J. Nerv. Ment. Dis., 71:249–259, 1930.

15. Finney, L. A., and Walker, A. E.: Transtentorial Herniation. Springfield, Ill., Charles C Thomas, 1962.

16. Fisher, C. M.: Ocular bobbing. Arch. Neurol., 11:543–546, 1964.

17. Fisher, C. M.: The neurologic examination of the comatose patient. Acta Neurol. Scand., 45: suppl. 36, 1969.

18. Ford, F. R., and Walsh, F. B.: Tonic deviations of the eyes produced by movements of the head. Arch. Ophthal., 23:1274–1284, 1940.

19. French, J. D.: Brain lesions with prolonged unconsciousness. A.M.A. Arch. Neurol. Psychiat., 68:727–740, 1952.

20. Fulton, J. F., and Bailey, P.: Tumors in the region of the third ventricle: Their diagnosis and relation to pathological sleep, J. Nerv. Ment. Dis., 69:1–25, 145–164, 261–277, 1929.

21. Gayet, M.: Affection encephalique (encephalite diffuse probable). Arch. Physiol. Norm. Path. 2ᵉ ser. 2:341–351, 1875.

22. Harris, A. J., Hodes, R., and Magoun, H. W.: The afferent path of the pupillodilator reflex in the cat. J. Neurophysiol., 7:231–243, 1944.

23. Holcomb, B.: Causes and diagnosis of various forms of coma. J.A.M.A., 77:2112–2114, 1921.

24. Holmes, G.: The cerebral integration of the ocular movements. Brit. Med. J., 2:107–112, 1938.

25. Jefferson, G.: The tentorial pressure cone. Arch. Neurol. Psychiat., 40:857–876, 1938.

26. Kubik, C. S., and Adams, R. D.: Occlusion of the basilar artery—a clinical and pathological study. Brain, 69:73–121, 1946.

27. Lee, J. E., Killip, T., III, and Plum, F.: Episodic unconsciousness. In Barondess, J., ed.: Baltimore, Md., Williams & Wilkins Co., 1971, pp. 133–166.

28. Locke, S., Merrill, J. P., and Tyler, H. R.: Neurologic complications of acute uremia. Arch. Int. Med., 108:519–530, 1961.

29. Magoun, H. W.: The Waking Brain. Ed. 2. Springfield, Ill., Charles C Thomas, 1963.

30. McNealy, D. E., and Plum, F.: Brainstem dysfunction with supratentorial mass lesions. Arch. Neurol., 7:10–32, 1962.

31. Meyers, R.: Systemic, vascular and respiratory effects of experimentally induced alterations in intraventricular pressure. J. Neuropath. Exp. Neurol., 1:241–264, 1942.

32. Nathanson, M., and Bergman, P. S.: Newer methods of evaluation of patients with altered states of consciousness. Med. Clin. N. Amer., 42:701–710, 1958.

33. Pevehouse, B. C., Bloom, W. H., and McKissock, W.: Ophthalmologic aspects of diagnosis and localization of subdural hematomas. Neurology, 10:1037–1041, 1960.

34. Plum, F., and Posner, J. B.: Diagnosis of Stupor and Coma. 2nd Ed. Contemporary Neurology Series, Vol. 10. Philadelphia, F. A. Davis Co., 1972.

35. Richardson, J. C., Chambers, R. A., and Heywood, P. M.: Encephalopathies of anoxia and hypoglycemia. Arch. Neurol., 1:178–190, 1959.

36. Steegman, A. T.: Primary pontile hemorrhage. J. Nerv. Ment. Dis., 114:35–65, 1951.

37. Sunderland, S., and Bradley, K. C.: Disturbances of oculomotor function accompanying extradural haemorrhage. J. Neurol. Neurosurg. Psychiat., 16:35–46, 1953.

38. Swanson, A. G., and Iseri, O. A.: Acute encephalopathy due to water intoxication. New Eng. J. Med., 258:831–834, 1958.

39. Szentagothai, J.: The elementary vestibulo-ocular reflex arc. J. Neurophysiol., 13:395–407, 1950.

40. Walsh, F. B.: Clinical Neuro-ophthalmology. Ed. 2. Baltimore, Williams & Wilkins Co., 1957.

41. Weinberger, L. M., Gibbon, M. H., and Gibbon, J. H., Jr.: Temporary arrest of the circulation to the central nervous system: I. Physiologic effects. Arch. Neurol. Psychiat., 43:615–634, 1940.

II

Diagnostic Procedures

4

RADIOLOGY OF THE SKULL

A vast amount of radiological information relating to the skull has accumulated over the past 70 years.[1, 8, 11, 14, 15] In this chapter the approach to the skull is within the context of the present-day diagnostic armamentarium available for the neurological work-up of patients.

Prior to the availability of radioactive brain scanning and at a time when angiography carried a high rate of morbidity, extreme efforts were made to extract every possible clue from examination of the plain skull film. Many radiological features of the skull that were once considered to be diagnostic of general or specific problems have since been found to have no practical value in the management of the patient. No longer is it necessary, however, as in the past, to agonize over the meaning of certain findings in the plain skull film. Today brain scanning, low-risk angiography, and pneumography will resolve the questionable findings in the plain film studies. Thus, a more objective interpretation of the plain skull roentgenogram is possible.

The following work plan for the evaluation of a radiological finding stresses the relative value of various skull features and lists certain structures that should be looked for in the various skull projections.

The questions that should be asked in the evaluation of skull roentgenograms are:

Is the finding an artifact?

Is it a normal variation or a pathological finding?

Is the pathological finding a manifestation of systemic disease, a primary skull condition, or a manifestation of intracranial disease?

A sequential exploration of these questions will avoid many pitfalls.

EXTRACALVARIAL STRUCTURES SIMULATING LESIONS

It is imperative to consider the possibility of extracalvarial structures or objects simulating intracranial lesions. A dense external occipital protuberance, electroencephalogram paste, sebaceous cyst, hair braids, a glass eye, and gravel or sand in the hair or scalp are some structures or objects that will simulate intracranial densities (Fig. 4–1). An ulcerated scalp neoplasm may simulate a lytic skull lesion. Air in a gaping scalp wound may simulate a fracture (Fig. 4–1 E).

PSEUDOLESIONS

The following features are occasionally misinterpreted as abnormal.

Apparent Suprasellar and Sellar Calcification

Normal calvarial densities, carotid siphon calcifications, or ligamentous calcifications may simulate sellar and suprasellar calcified masses (Fig. 4–2). Stereoscopic lateral radiograms are of great help, and multiple projections or laminagraphy may establish the true situation.

Dural plaques of calcification may be diagnosed by demonstrating that the calcification is adjacent to the inner surface of

M. M. SCHECHTER

E. L. KIER

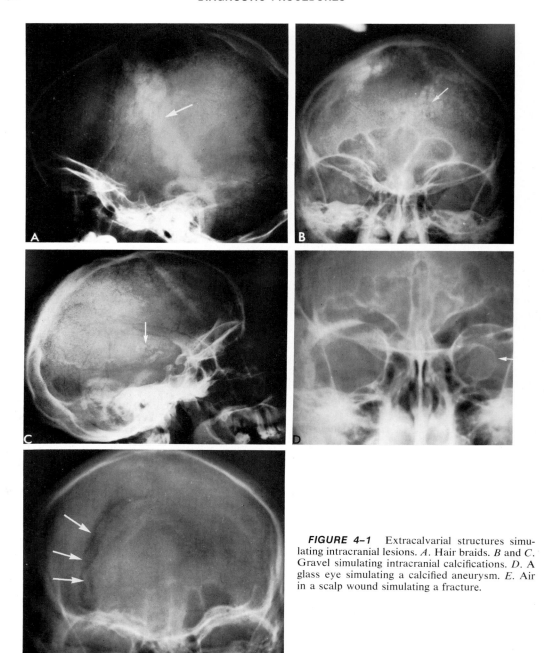

FIGURE 4–1   Extracalvarial structures simulating intracranial lesions. *A*. Hair braids. *B* and *C*. Gravel simulating intracranial calcifications. *D*. A glass eye simulating a calcified aneurysm. *E*. Air in a scalp wound simulating a fracture.

the vault or in the falx. Calcification of the carotid siphon is manifested by curved linear streaks of calcification parallel to one another, superimposed on the sella, and they usually occupy the cavernous portion of the carotid siphon. The superior wall of

the carotid siphon is usually more densely calcified (Fig. 4–2). This calcification may be recognized in the anteroposterior projection, in which it shows through the ethmoid air sinus, but tomography in the coronal plane will usually demonstrate it to better advantage. Even after most extensive and meticulous studies one may have to resort to angiography to make a final diagnosis.

Absence of Greater and Lesser Sphenoidal Wings

There may be great variation in the bony density and configuration of these structures. Asymmetry is more the rule than the exception.

The bone of the wings of the sphenoid is at times so thin that routine radiograms may suggest their absence (Fig. 4–3). This presents a problem that becomes more difficult in cases of asymmetry in which there is an apparent unilateral absence of the sphenoidal wings. When there is a clinical suspicion of a lesion related to this area, the problem is further compounded and the result may be unnecessary specialized

radiological work-ups. Rischbieth and Bull illustrated the normal asymmetry of the superior orbital fissure.[12] Because of its extreme variability, a diagnosis of abnormality should not be based on a single projection. The greater sphenoidal wing frequently is not seen in the Caldwell projection. If the structures are not recognized in the base projection, stereoscopic and laminagraphic examinations may be critical. Extension of the sphenoidal sinus into the greater sphenoidal wing should not be mistaken for erosion or dysplasia (Fig. 4–3).[9]

"Eroded" Foramen Ovale and Foramen Spinosum

In spite of their notoriety, the diagnostic value of these two foramina is extremely limited and they should be evaluated with much caution.

Developmental variations are frequent.

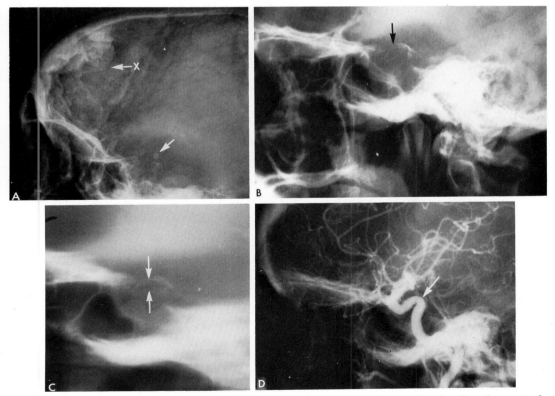

FIGURE 4–2   *A.* Calvarial densities (*arrows*) simulating sellar and suprasellar calcification. Note hyperostosis frontalis interna (**X**). *B.* Carotid siphon calcification (*arrow*) in lateral view. *C.* Carotid siphon calcification laminagram. Note the two parallel lines of calcification. *D.* Carotid siphon calcification confirmed by angiography.

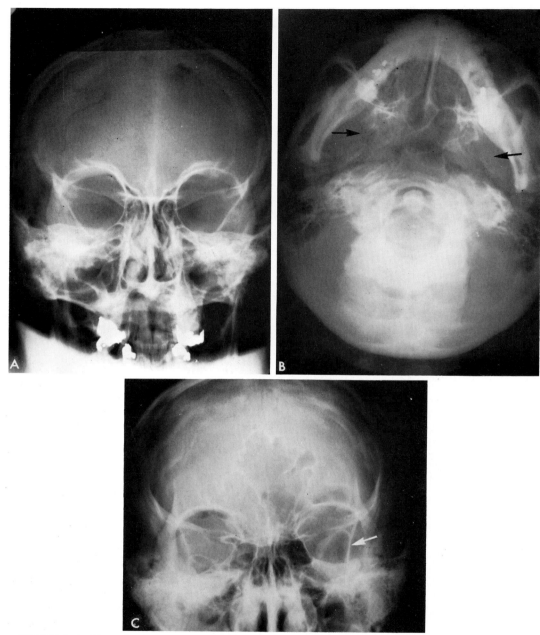

FIGURE 4–3 Normal structures suggesting abnormalities. *A*. Thin greater sphenoidal wing suggesting its absence. *B*. Indistinct foramen ovale and foramen spinosum. *C*. Huge sphenoid sinus simulating an eroded greater sphenoidal wing.

The posterior wall of the foramen spinosum is the last to ossify and frequently remains unossified. The foramina spinosum and ovale may ossify as a single structure. The walls of the foramina may slant. The overlying nasopharyngeal soft tissue structures may obscure the anatomy. All these factors plus the direction of the radiographic beam may contribute to the appearance of indistinct canals (Fig. 4–3 *B*). There is poor correlation between the caliber of the middle meningeal artery and the size of the foramen spinosum. Lesions involving these foramina are usually related to fifth nerve and nasopharyngeal tumors (see Fig. 4–35). The diagnostic value of these foramina in meningiomas is limited.

"Widened" Coronal Suture

The diagnosis of early changes of sutural diastasis is difficult, particularly in the very young in whom ossification is incomplete. The coronal suture is more difficult to evaluate than the others. The superior segment of the coronal suture may remain open during childhood. Frequently this presents a problem in children who are being evaluated for a possible intracranial lesion. The suture will be interpreted as widened or normal, depending upon the clinical convictions of the physician who is making the evaluation. Because of the normal variations in closure of the coronal suture, care should be taken not to base a diagnosis of increased intracranial pressure solely on the appearance of this structure (Fig. 4–3).

The "J" Sella

The terms "J sella" and "omega sella" are widely used in the literature and in the everyday evaluation of infant skull roentgenograms. Although these terms are frequently used by radiologists and neurosurgeons, there has always been considerable disagreement as to the diagnostic value of the findings. This unsatisfactory situation resulted from the previous lack of basic correlative anatomical-radiological information about the sphenoid during infancy, information that is now available from studies correlating the developmental anatomy of the sella with its radiological manifestations.[5, 6] With this information pathological changes can be differentiated from normal growth patterns. A review of the normal adult sphenoid anatomy is necessary to understand the developmental changes (Fig. 4–4). An important feature of the developing sphenoid is that the planum sphenoidale is not present at birth. Prior to the formation of the planum, an elongated sulcus chiasmatis should not be mistaken for an abnormal feature.

The normally prominent roof of the optic canal during early infancy should not be mistaken for the planum sphenoidale (Fig. 4–5). This mistake accounts for many of the normal infants who have been presented in the literature as showing "abnormal excavation" of the sulcus chiasmatis. In effect, very few pathological conditions represent true abnormalities of the tuberculum sellae, sulcus chiasmatis, planum sphenoidale, and optic canal roof. Craniopharyngiomas in infancy are almost invariably associated with sellar abnormalities. Sellar abnormalities in optic gliomas are inconstant and depend upon whether the optic nerve is involved and whether the chiasm is pre-fixed or post-fixed. Sellar changes due to posterior fossa masses are very rare. The terms "J sella" and "omega sella" and the like are diagnostically meaningless, harmful to the objective assessment of the sphenoid in infancy, and should be discarded.

The "Enlarged" Optic Canal

The radiological evaluation of the optic canal is difficult because of the direction of its axis and its complex three-dimensional architecture. A review of the normal anatomy is appropriate at this time. The term "foramen" should not be used, as it is actually a canal with two openings (Fig. 4–6). An obviously enlarged canal presents no diagnostic difficulty (Fig. 4–7). Figures for its normal dimensions are available.[14] A difference between the transverse diameters of the two canals of over 25 to 30 per cent as an indicator of disease is an easy figure to remember.[3]

Mistaking a normal variation for a pathological condition has not been infrequent in the past. This resulted from the previous lack of information about the changing features of the infantile optic canal, information that has now been provided by study of the development of the canal, correlating its radiological and anatomical features.[6] The optic canal roof was found to be a very prominent structure during early infancy. The optic canal floor develops slowly and demonstrates many developmental variations. Normal variations such as vertical optic canal, asymmetry, absence of the

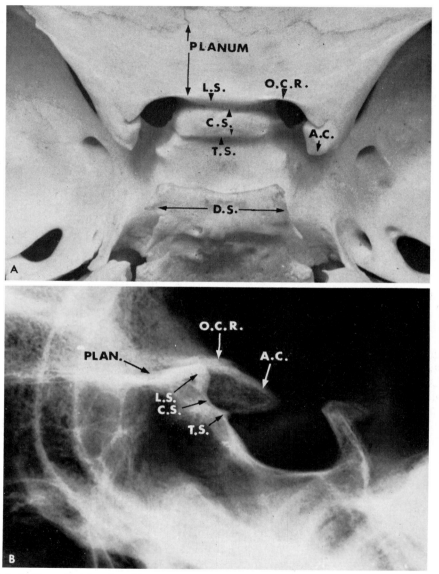

FIGURE 4–4 Normal adult sphenoid. *A.* Superior aspect of sphenoid bone specimen. *B.* Lateral skull roentgenogram. Note that the optic canal roof (O.C.R.) is not a prominent structure in the lateral skull roentgenogram. A.C., anterior clinoid process; C.S., chiasmatic sulcus; D.S., dorsum sellae; L.S., limbus sphenoidale; PLAN., planum sphenoidale; T.S., tuberculum sellae. (From Kier, E. L.: Amer. J. Roentgen., *102*:747–767, 1968. Reproduced by permission of the publisher.)

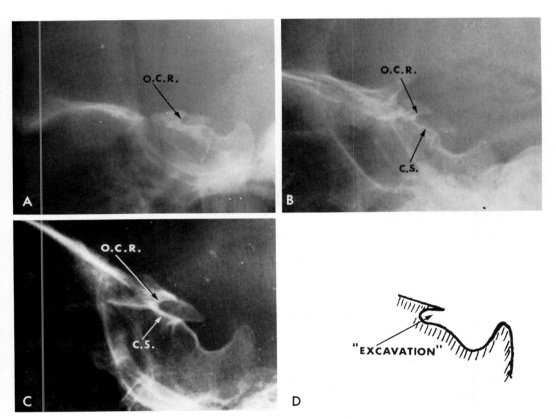

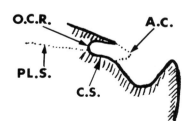

FIGURE 4–5 Elucidation of the mythical "excavation." *B* and *C*. Children with normal presellar sphenoids. These are similar to the cases presented in the literature as showing "excavation under the anterior clinoid process." *D*. Tracing similar to the ones presented in the literature to illustrate the "abnormal excavation." Note that the so-called excavation is a roentgenological illusion resulting from the prominence of the optic canal roof (O.C.R.) during infancy. The laterally positioned optic canal roof forms the superior component of the so-called excavation and projects as a dense white line that appears to be continuous with the normal and midline chiasmatic sulcus (C.S.). *E*. Tracing demonstrating the correct anatomical components of the "excavation." A.C., anterior clinoid process; PL.S., planum sphenoidale. Cases such as these have resulted in the loss of the diagnostic value of this term. (From Kier, E. L.: Amer. J. Roentgen., *102*: 747–767, 1968. Reproduced by permission of the publisher.)

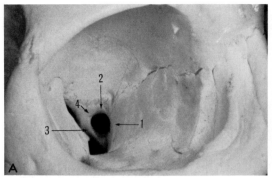

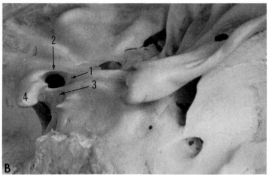

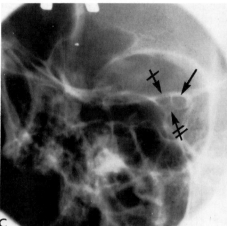

FIGURE 4-6 Normal adult optic canal. *A.* View of apex of orbit showing the orbital opening. *B.* View of the cranial opening within the skull. Note that cranial opening has its long diameter in the horizontal plane and the orbital opening has its long diameter in the vertical plane. The canal walls are formed by the lateral wall of the sphenoid sinus (1), the lesser sphenoid wing (2), the optic strut (3), and the anterior clinoid processes (4). The optic strut separates the superior orbital fissure from the optic canal. *C.* A pneumatized anterior clinoid process (*arrow*) should not be mistaken for the optic canal (*arrow with single crossed shaft*). Note the optic strut (*arrow with double crossed shaft*) separating the superior orbital fissure from the optic canal. (From Invest. Radiol., *1*:346–362, 1966. *A* and *B* reproduced by permission of the publisher.)

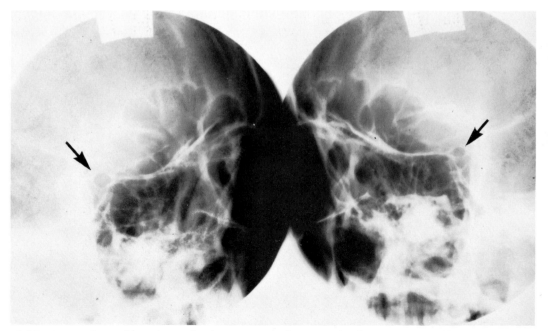

FIGURE 4-7 Case with optic canal enlargment secondary to optic glioma. Note the difference in size between the two sides.

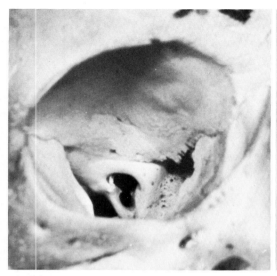
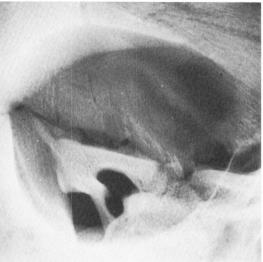

FIGURE 4–8 Optic canal anomalies. The fetal "keyhole" configuration of the optic canal may persist through childhood. The configuration in childhood should not be mistaken for erosion of the floor or an enlarged canal in the vertical diameter. (From Kier, E. L.: Invest. Radiol., *1*:346–362, 1966. Reproduced by permission of the publisher.)

floor of the cranial opening of the canal, and the vertically large orbital opening of the canal in childhood should not be mistaken for pathological features (Figs. 4–8 and 4–9). The transverse diameter of the canal is a more reliable index of abnormality than the vertical diameter. The roof of the optic canal may be normally so thin as to not be demonstrated radiographically.

Sphenoid "Meningioma"

Normal densities at the junction of the greater and lesser sphenoidal wings should not be mistaken for hyperostosis resulting from a sphenoid meningioma (Fig. 4–10).

"Fractures"

Among the structures that should not be mistaken for fractures are: the metopic suture of the frontal bone, the vascular grooves on the cranial bones, and the inner table suture lines.

The frontal bone ossifies from two centers. Usually ossification is complete at birth; occasionally the two ossification centers do not unite at all or unite late in child-

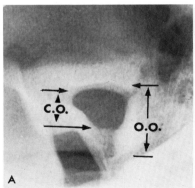
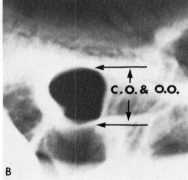

FIGURE 4–9 The difference between infantile and adult optic canals. *A.* In the child the vertical diameter of the orbital opening (O.O.) is much larger than the vertical diameter of the cranial opening (C.O.). *B.* In the adult the two openings are about equal. This should be considered in the stereoscopic and laminagraphic evaluation of the infantile optic canal. (From Kier, E. L.: Invest. Radiol., *1*:346–362, 1966. Reproduced by permission of the publisher.)

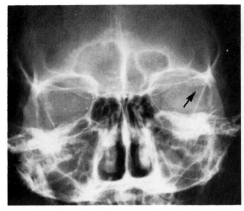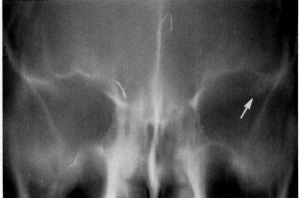

FIGURE 4-10   Normal sphenoidal densities (*arrows*) at the junction of the greater and lesser sphenoidal wings.

hood. The nonunion will result in a transitory or permanent frontal (metopic) suture (Fig. 4-11 *A*). Vertical midline fractures of the frontal bone are rare. Furthermore, digitations will be recognized in a careful perusal of the area in question, and perisutural densities are present. Caffey has documented other infantile sutures and synchondroses that should not be mistaken for fractures. These include wormian bones, the mendosal suture, and other occipital bone changes (Fig. 4-11 *C*).[2]

A recurrent problem in trauma to the back of the head in childhood is the presence of a linear lucency extending through the occipital bone to the foramen magnum. Embryological studies show no suture formation simulating this lucency. These lines, therefore, usually constitute fractures.

Grooving of the external surface of the frontal bone and the external surface of the temporal squama is produced by the supraorbital artery (a branch of the ophthalmic artery) and by the middle temporal artery (a branch of the superficial temporal artery) respectively. When the markings are bilateral they tend to be symmetrical, and the question of a fracture should hardly arise.

The inner table of a suture line has a linear appearance and might be mistaken for a fracture. The outer table, however, has interdigitations and if these are recognized a mistaken diagnosis will not be made (Fig. 4-11 *B*).

The grooves for the middle meningeal artery are slightly tortuous, taper gradually, and have branches. Middle meningeal vascular grooves do not cross one another. Occasionally the two borders of the groove have slightly sclerotic margins. The shadow they cast is usually not as dense as that of a fracture since they do not involve the entire thickness of the skull.

Calcified "Lesions"

The following structures may be calcified and should not be interpreted as pathological: the dura including the falx and the tentorium, the petroclinoid and interclinoid ligaments, the carotid siphon, the pineal gland, the choroid plexus, the habenular commissure, and pacchionian granulations (Fig. 4-12).

Reference already has been made to dural calcification and calcification in the carotid siphon. The most characteristic changes of dural calcification relate to the region where it encompasses the sagittal sinus and where it joins the tentorium. The Y-shaped streaks of calcification in the region of the sinus are characteristic (Fig. 4-12). In the anteroposterior projection, calcification of the point where the falx meets the tentorium may be mistaken for pineal calcification. When the streak of calcification exhibits an inverted V shape, the situation is obvious, but when the calcification is more marked in one lateral leaf of the tentorium it may be mistaken for a displaced pineal gland.

The frequently calcified petroclinoid ligament should not be mistaken for a retrosellar or clivus lesion. The calcification is distinguished by its attachment to the posterior clinoid processes and by the way it extends obliquely downward toward the apices of the petrous pyramids (Fig. 4–12 B).

The most common site of calcification in the choroid plexus is the glomus, which is situated in the trigone of the lateral ventricle. When both are symmetrically calcified there is usually no problem of mistaken diagnosis. When one calcifies or one calcifies asymmetrically it may be mistaken for a tumor or for a displaced pineal gland. Calcification of the glomus is usually more extensive than that of the pineal and is usually situated behind and below the pineal calcification (Fig. 4–12 D).

Pacchionian granulations, when calcified, may be recognized as small densities lying just to the side of the sagittal sinus (Fig. 4–12 E).

The calcified pineal is discussed later in this chapter.

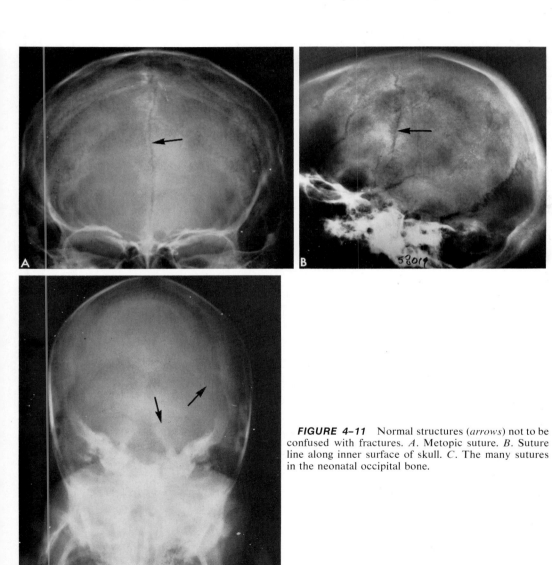

FIGURE 4–11 Normal structures (*arrows*) not to be confused with fractures. *A*. Metopic suture. *B*. Suture line along inner surface of skull. *C*. The many sutures in the neonatal occipital bone.

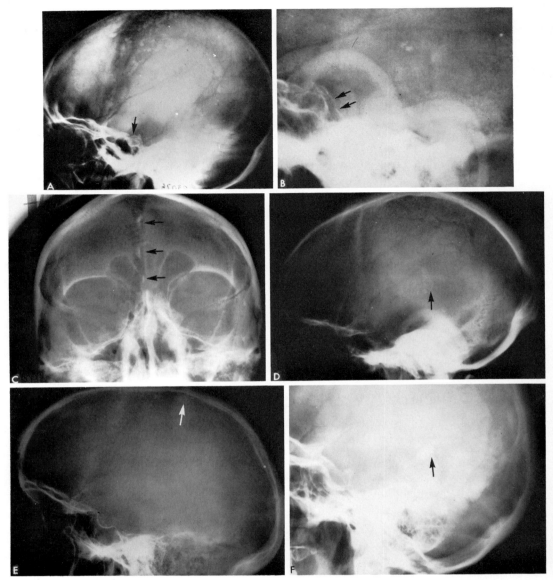

FIGURE 4–12   Normal intracranial calcification. *A*. Bridged sella. *B*. Petroclinoid ligament. *C*. Falx. *D*. Glomus of choroid plexus. *E*. Pacchionian granulations. *F*. Calcification in tentorium.

PROBLEM STRUCTURES

The following questions present an almost daily radiological dilemma. Are the vascular markings abnormally increased? Are the convolutional markings abnormal? Is the skull lucency abnormal? Can the pineal body be evaluated in a rotated skull film?

Vascular Markings

There are numerous vascular markings on the inner and outer tables of the skull and also between the two tables. These include dural sinuses, dural veins, diploic veins, and arterial grooves. The extremely wide range of normal venous vascular markings limits the diagnostic value of these structures. The recognition, if possible, of a hypertrophied arterial channel may suggest the presence of a meningioma or a tumor that has invaded the dura, or an arteriovenous malformation. The meningeal vascular grooves accommodate arteries and veins. The channels transmitting mainly arteries may be distinguished from those transmitting veins because the margins are straighter and more regular than those of the veins. A large groove with regular margins that transports an artery and that enlarges as it courses distally is usually associated with a meningioma (Fig. 4–13). Other grooves may be seen to converge toward the area where the meningioma has its attachment. Thus the problem is: (1) to distinguish between an arterial groove and a venous groove; and (2) to decide if the arterial groove is normal or abnormal. Fortunately the availability of brain scanning greatly helps to resolve this problem. The majority of lesions producing increased vascular markings will also produce positive brain scans.

Convolutional Markings

Experience confirms the statement that convolutional markings as a single finding are of no significance.[15] In the presence of long-standing raised intracranial pressure, digital markings are usually accompanied by other more diagnostic changes such as an eroded sella.

Skull Lucencies

Benign-appearing skull lucencies are an extremely frequent radiological diagnostic dilemma. A large number of undiagnosable cases remains even after the exclusion of obvious lesions such as pacchionian granulations, venous lakes, emissary veins, parietal foramina, epidermoids, and hemangiomas. These problem cases are extremely vexing and cannot be resolved except by periodic follow-up to determine if they change in appearance, and by specialized contrast studies.

The Pineal in Rotated Films

An experimental study with a pineal model has demonstrated that the normal pineal body in the rotated skull films stays within its range of normal variation (2 to 3 mm) in both anteroposterior and posteroanterior projections.[7] This is related to the center of rotation of the skull on the spine. The pineal is located near the axis of rotation of the skull on the spinal column.

The pineal is also at the center of an imaginary circle formed by the middle and posterior fossae. As a result of these relationships, it remains in the midline in rotated skull films. In extremely rotated skull films the pineal should be correlated with the occipital bone and greater sphenoidal wing, which respectively form the posterior and anterior margins of the imaginary circle.

THE PATHOLOGICAL SKULL

Once an artifact is excluded and it is determined that the finding is of pathological significance, the sequential exploration continues. Then the question must be asked: Is the pathological finding a mani-

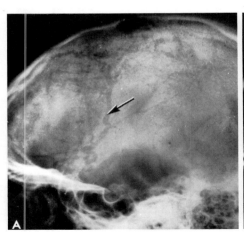
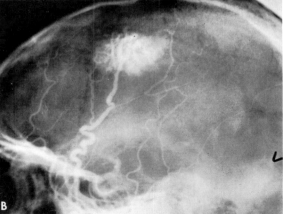

FIGURE 4–13 *A*. Unilaterally enlarged meningeal groove (*arrow*). *B*. External carotid angiogram demonstrates an enlarged middle meningeal artery within the groove and supplying a meningioma.

festation of systemic disease, a primary skull condition, or a manifestation of intracranial disease?

In an evaluation of the pathological changes, certain features are of importance, and usually one or more of these will be present.

The Sella Turcica

Changes in the sella may be due to raised intracranial pressure, lesions in adjacent structures, or intrasellar lesions. Definite signs of sellar abnormality are a complete or partial absence of the dorsum sellae and posterior clinoid processes, the floor of the sella, the tuberculum sellae, and the anterior clinoids. A single structure may be involved or the complete sella may be destroyed. In the senile skull these structures may be indistinct, and caution should be exercised in not overinterpreting their absence (Fig. 4–14). A large pituitary adenoma, craniopharyngioma, carotid aneu-

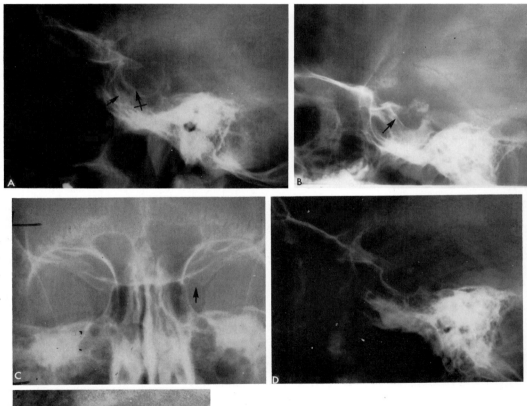

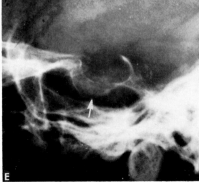

FIGURE 4–14 Sellae. *A.* Absence of floor. Anterior part of floor of sella is destroyed. The line (*crossed arrow*) is in the lateral skull wall. *B.* Erosion of tuberculum sellae by craniopharyngioma. *C.* Absence of anterior clinoid processes secondary to chromophobe adenoma. *D.* Senile sella showing demineralized dorsum. *E.* Double sella floor secondary to chromophobe adenoma.

rysm, chordoma, metastatic deposit, and nasopharyngeal tumor may cause total destruction of the sella.

Intrasellar and suprasellar calcifications, craniopharyngiomas, chordomas, meningiomas, aneurysms, and teratomas may show intracranial calcification (see discussion of calcification later in this chapter).

Hyperostosis definitely indicates sellar abnormality. Meningiomas may arise from the clinoid processes, planum sphenoidale, diaphragma sellae, or tuberculum sellae (Figs. 4–15 to 4–19). The area of tumor attachment may show marked bone thickening. A particular type of hyperostosis, the blistering effect of the planum sphenoidale is considered almost pathognomonic for this condition.

Various estimations of the size of the sella in the lateral projection have been described. Any sella with a depth of over 15 mm and an anteroposterior diameter of over 20 mm is definitely abnormal.

Certain changes in the sella have been referred to in the past as definite signs of abnormality. The signs listed as follows are now considered questionable since they have not proved to have consistent diagnostic value. They are: (1) sloping floor (double floor), (2) depth of 13 to 15 mm and anteroposterior diameter of 17 to 20 mm, (3) pointed anterior clinoids, and (4) a demineralized dorsum and floor. The J-shaped sella has been covered earlier in this chapter.

The distinction between an intrasellar

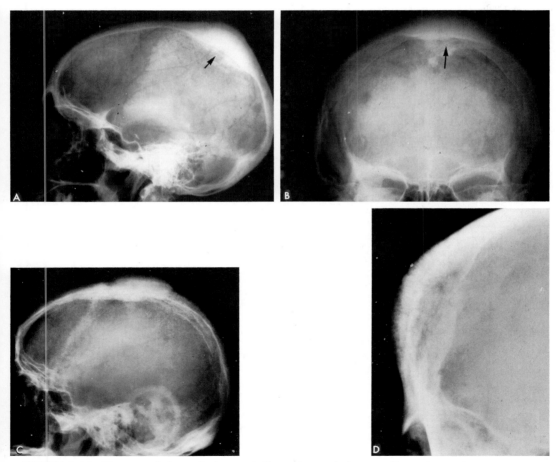

FIGURE 4–15 Hyperostosis in meningiomas. *A.* Convexity meningioma. *B.* Convexity meningioma. *C.* Parasagittal meningioma. *D.* Frontal meningioma with sunburst appearance, widening of diploë, and extension through the inner table.

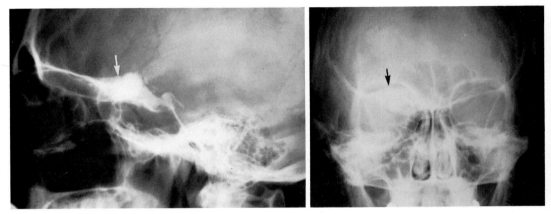

FIGURE 4–16   Meningioma of lesser sphenoid wing.

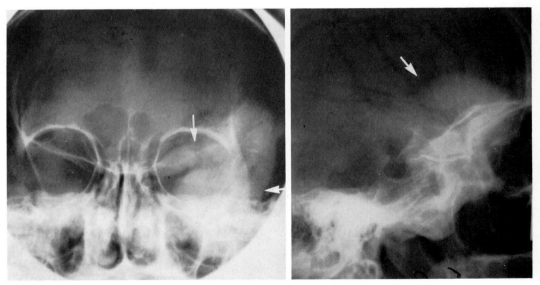

FIGURE 4–17   Meningioma of greater and lesser wing of the sphenoid bone.

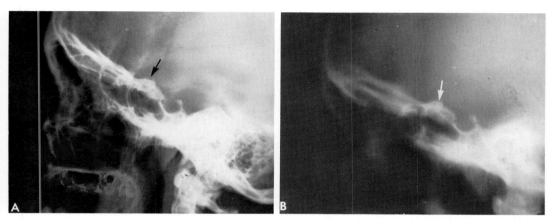

FIGURE 4-18 Meningioma of planum sphenoidale. *A*. Lateral view. *B*. Tomogram.

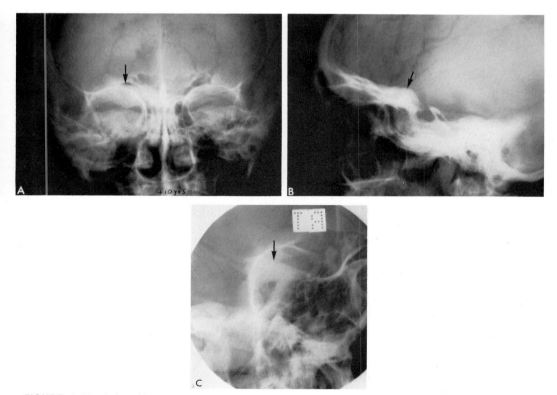

FIGURE 4-19 Sphenoid meningioma surrounding optic canal. *A*. Anteroposterior view. *B*. Lateral view. *C*. Optic canal view.

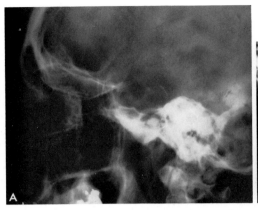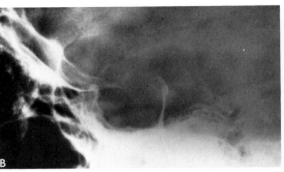

FIGURE 4–20 *A.* Chromophobe adenoma demonstrating an enlarged sella, absence of floor of sella, anterior clinoid processes tipped up, destruction of tuberculum sellae, displaced dorsum sellae, and "floating" posterior clinoid processes. *B.* Chromophobe adenoma. Note large sella, destruction of floor, pointed anterior clinoid process, and thinning of posteriorly displaced dorsum sellae.

lesion and an extrasellar lesion may be assessed as shown in Table 4–1.

DISPLACED PHYSIOLOGICAL CALCIFICATIONS

The best known method for evaluating pineal position in the lateral projection is the Vastine-Kinney method.[16] The method described by Oon is simple, reliable, and easy to master.[10] Pineal displacements are usually to the side and downward. Upward displacements are unusual (Fig. 4–21).

The calcified glomus has been discussed earlier in this chapter.

TRAUMA

The vault may be fractured and there may be a tear in the membranous coverings of the brain. When the fracture line passes through a nasal sinus or through the mastoid air cells, cerebrospinal fluid may es-

cape into the sinuses and mastoid spaces with rhinorrhea and otorrhea resulting. Air may pass from these structures into the subarachnoid spaces and into the ventricles. Blood may also enter the sinuses, which then become radiopaque. A fluid level may be present in the sinuses (Fig. 4–22).

Fractures may be linear, depressed, diastatic, and comminuted (Fig. 4–23). The fracture line may further involve an air sinus or may traverse a middle meningeal artery or a dural sinus. The indriven spicule may tear a dural sinus or damage brain cortex. The foramina of the skull have an area of thick bone surrounding them, and it can be readily understood how fracture lines take a zig-zag course following the lines of least resistance.

The radiological evidence of a skull fracture is the fracture line and displacement of bone. Infants may, however, have fractures without evidence of a fracture line, since the soft skull may indent like a ping-pong ball. Loose skin folds in the neonate should not

TABLE 4–1 *DISTINCTION BETWEEN INTRASELLAR AND EXTRASELLAR LESIONS*

INTRASELLAR LESIONS	EXTRASELLAR LESIONS
Sella ballooned	Sella enlarged, not ballooned
Anterior clinoids undermined	No undermining
Double floor	Usually single floor
Posterior clinoids preserved	Posterior clinoids usually destroyed
Posterior clinoids floating	No sloping of dorsum sellae
Dorsum sellae sloping backward	

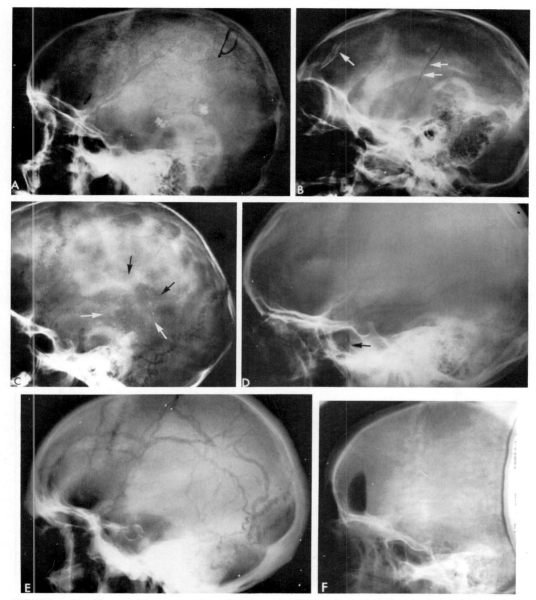

FIGURE 4–21 Abnormal features on lateral studies. *A*. Displaced calcified glomus of choroid secondary to a mass lesion. *B*. Depressed fracture (*single arrow*). Linear fracture (*double arrow*). *C*. Fine calcifications secondary to ependymoma. *D*. Fluid level in sphenoid sinus secondary to trauma. *E*. Opaque sphenoid secondary to nasopharyngeal carcinoma. Note vascularity of skull. *F*. Unsuspected air-fluid level in frontal brain abscess. Gas-forming organism.

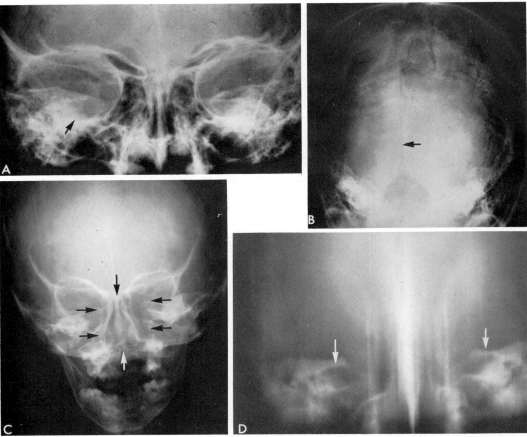

FIGURE 4–22 Abnormal features on anteroposterior, posteroanterior, and Towne's projections. *A.* Widened internal auditory meatus secondary to acoustic tumor. *B.* Occipital fracture. *C.* Absence of body of sphenoid secondary to nasopharyngeal tumor. Note the bony void in the center of the face in the region of the nose. *D.* Laminagram of petrous bones of a patient with von Recklinghausen's disease with widening of both auditory canals.

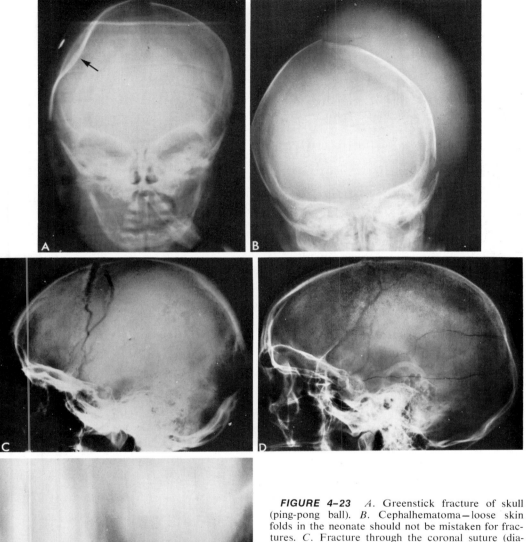

FIGURE 4-23 *A.* Greenstick fracture of skull (ping-pong ball). *B.* Cephalhematoma—loose skin folds in the neonate should not be mistaken for fractures. *C.* Fracture through the coronal suture (diastatic fracture). *D.* Fracture extending from one side to the other (horseshoe). Note that the longer fracture line extends to the middle meningeal groove and its sharper margins suggest that that side was closest to the film. *E.* Fracture at base of skull seen only with laminagraphy.

be mistaken for fracture lines. Fracture lines appear as dark radiolucent shadows when the x-ray beam passes directly through the plane of the fracture. If the ray passes a little obliquely to the fracture plane, the margins of the fracture will be less sharp and may even appear wider apart. The fracture may not be recognized at all if the x-ray beam meets the fracture plane at right angles. The fracture line is usually sharper on the side closest to the film. This may be an important lateralizing sign when the fracture cannot be recognized in other projections. In depressed fractures the fragments may overlap. Overlapping of the margins will cause them to appear more dense radiologically. Without overlap of the margins or turning of a fragment so as to increase its density, depression of a fracture may be missed unless tangential views are taken (Fig. 4–24).

A cephalhematoma, in the chronic stage, may calcify and appear as a dense mass attached to the outer table of the skull. The sutures limit its extent (Fig. 4–25).

The dura may tear during skull trauma, and gradually the edges of the fracture may become scalloped while the gap grows larger (Fig. 4–25). These changes result in the so-called growth fracture or leptomeningeal fracture and may present as a lytic lesion.

CALCIFICATION

Physiological calcification has already been discussed. There are also many conditions that may produce pathological intracranial calcification (Fig. 4–26). Because of the large number of conditions that may produce it and the difficulty of establishing the nature of the intracranial calcification

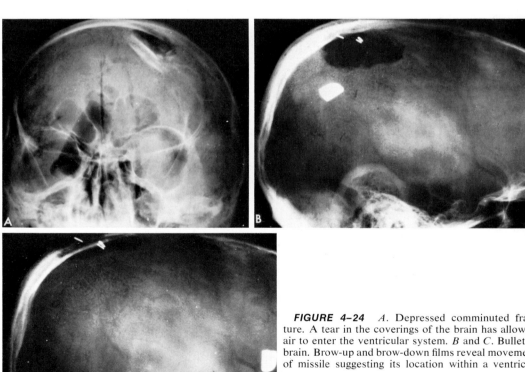

FIGURE 4–24 *A.* Depressed comminuted fracture. A tear in the coverings of the brain has allowed air to enter the ventricular system. *B* and *C.* Bullet in brain. Brow-up and brow-down films reveal movement of missile suggesting its location within a ventricle.

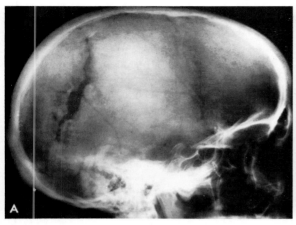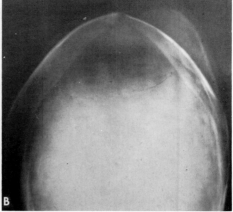

FIGURE 4-25 *A*. Growth fracture in an adult. Note scalloped margins. *B*. Calcified cephalhematoma.

TABLE 4-2   *CAUSES OF INTRACRANIAL CALCIFICATION*

FOCAL CALCIFICATION	DIFFUSE CALCIFICATION
Arteriovenous malformation	Tuberous sclerosis
Aneurysm	Encephalitedes
Tumor	Viral
Sturge-Weber syndrome	Parasitic
Chronic subdural hematoma	Endocrine disorder
Teratoma	Tuberculoma
	Tuberculous meningitis

the causes are divided into focal and diffuse as shown in Table 4-2.

Curvilinear calcification at the base of the skull usually suggests an aneurysm, and multiple linear shadows in parallel pairs may suggest an arteriovenous malformation. Sturge-Weber calcification is usually related to the occipital area and has a classic appearance (Fig. 4-27).

The calcification of tumors is usually not characteristic except for lipomas of the corpus callosum, in which two large vertical curvilinear streaks outline the tumor. Teratomas are usually in the midline and may have teeth in them. Other calcifications may be topographically related to particular structures such as the pineal gland, the choroid plexus, the great vein of Galen, the wall of the ventricle, and the basal ganglia, in which case their location is suggestive of their etiology (Fig. 4-28).

LYTIC AND HYPEROSTOTIC LESIONS

The lesions may be single or multiple (Table 4-3). A few of these conditions have characteristic changes such as those in Paget's disease, in which a diffuse area of lysis occurs and basilar invagination is marked. The epidermoid has a sclerotic margin and the eosinophilic granuloma has sharp, punched-out margins without sclerosis. The hemangioma expands the tables of bone and has a soap-bubble appearance (Fig. 4-30).

The hyperostotic lesions are usually meningiomas (shown in Figs. 4-15, 4-16, 4-17, 4-18, and 4-19) and fibrous dysplasia (Fig. 4-32). Fibrous dysplasia is usually associated with a young age group and may be confined to the base of the skull. Meningiomas tend to occur at a later *Text continued on page 86.*

TABLE 4-3   *LYTIC AND HYPEROSTOTIC LESIONS*

SINGLE LESIONS	MULTIPLE LESIONS
Surgical defect	Pacchionian granulations
Osteoporosis circumscripta	Paget's disease
Meningioma	Persistent parietal foramina
Osteomyelitis	Radiation necrosis
Metastatic disease	Osteomyelitis
Solitary myeloma	Metastatic disease
Epidermoid	Multiple myeloma
Eosinophilic granuloma	
Hemangioma	

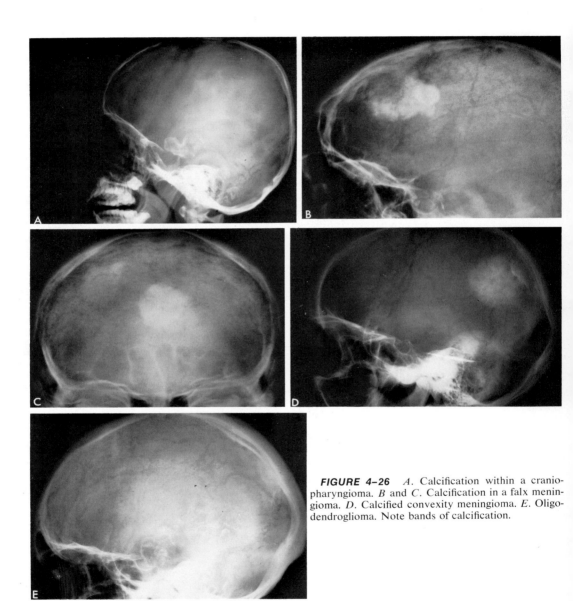

FIGURE 4–26 *A.* Calcification within a cranio-pharyngioma. *B* and *C.* Calcification in a falx meningioma. *D.* Calcified convexity meningioma. *E.* Oligodendroglioma. Note bands of calcification.

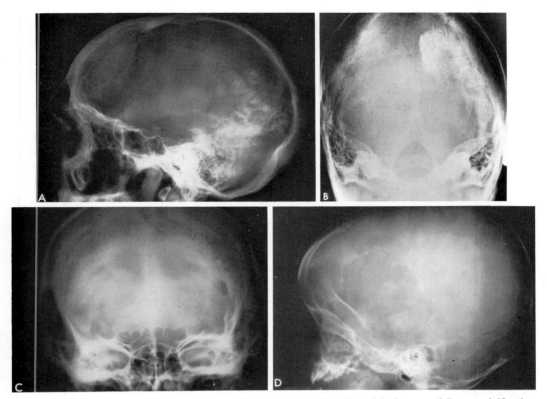

FIGURE 4–27 *A.* Sturge-Weber syndrome. Note classic unilateral occipital areas of linear calcifications paralleling one another. *B.* Sturge-Weber calcification in the anteroposterior projection. *C.* Calcification in the wall of an aneurysm. *D.* A large lucent lesion representing the fatty tissue of an intracerebral teratoma. The margins are calcified. The presence of a tooth was confirmed at operation.

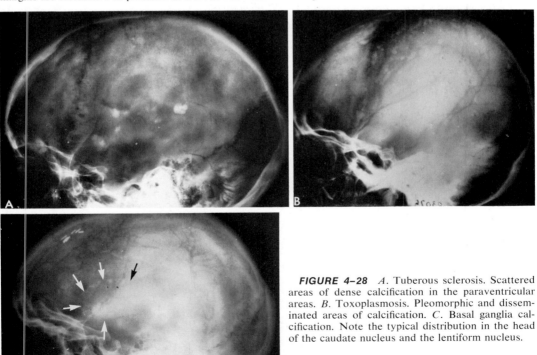

FIGURE 4–28 *A.* Tuberous sclerosis. Scattered areas of dense calcification in the paraventricular areas. *B.* Toxoplasmosis. Pleomorphic and disseminated areas of calcification. *C.* Basal ganglia calcification. Note the typical distribution in the head of the caudate nucleus and the lentiform nucleus.

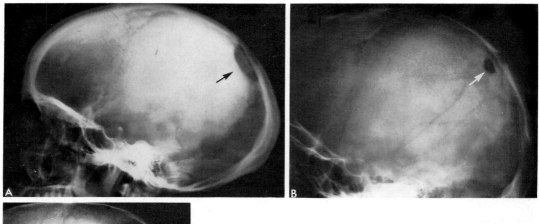

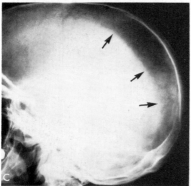

FIGURE 4–29 *A* and *B*. Parietal foramina are usually situated in upper part of parietal bone, 1 to 2 inches above the lambda, and are bilateral. Similar but more extensive changes are seen in parietal thinning, *C*.

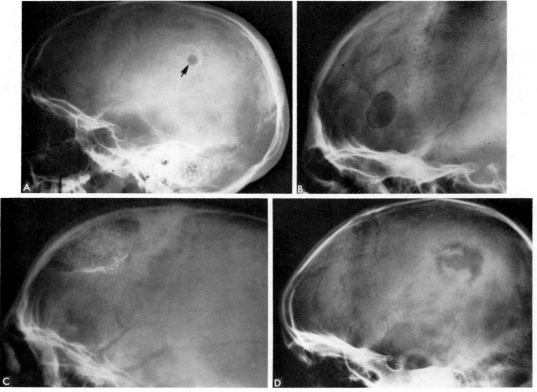

FIGURE 4–30 *A*. Epidermoid. There is a smooth sclerotic margin around the translucency. *B*. Eosinophilic granuloma. Note the sharp punched-out appearance without a sclerotic margin. *C*. Hemangioma. This expands the table of the skull and has a soap-bubble appearance. *D*. Osteomyelitis has an irregular lytic area with a "moth-eaten" appearance. A similar appearance may be seen in syphilis, tuberculosis, and focal radiation necrosis.

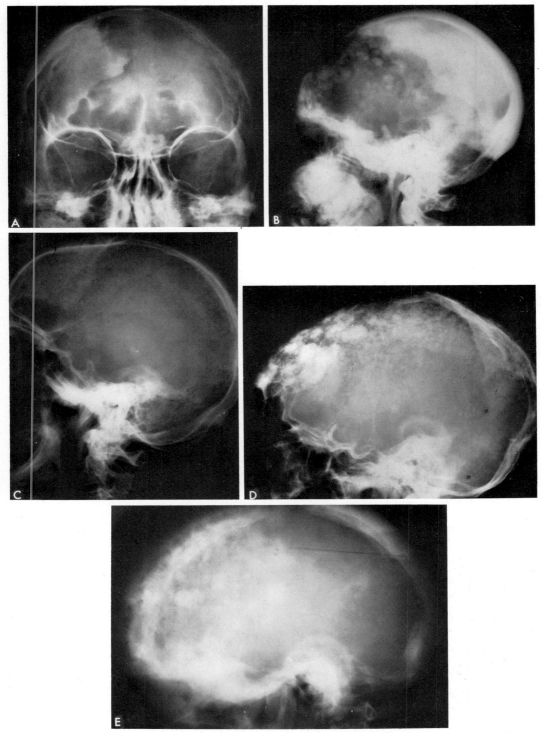

FIGURE 4–31 *A*. Osteoporosis circumscripta involving mainly frontal bone; *B*, involving multiple bones; and *C*, involving frontal and temporal area. *D*. Paget's disease with widened separation of tables of the skull and a mixture of translucent and dense paths. Note the basilar invagination. *E*. Paget's disease with extreme basilar invagination.

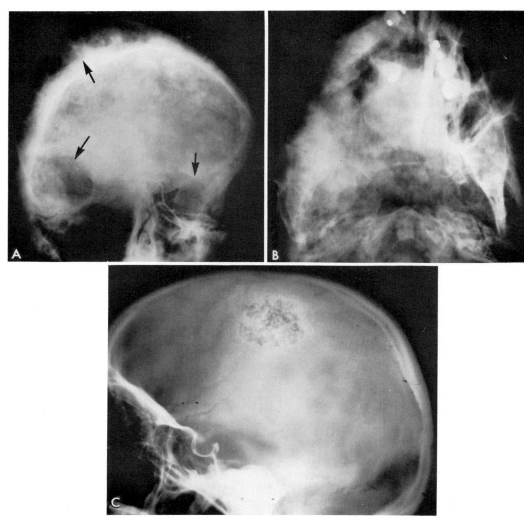

FIGURE 4–32 *A.* Fibrous dysplasia. Mixture of lucencies and sclerosis resembling Paget's disease, but areas of sclerosis are better defined and more homogenous. The blister type of expansion of the vertex is typical of this condition. Arrows point to "blistering" and to orbits. *B.* In base view note that the disease is more extensive on the right side. *C.* Localized form of fibrous dysplasia.

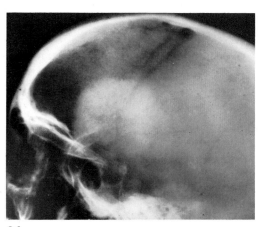

FIGURE 4–33 Osteoma of parietal region. This affects the outer table. Specialized views differentiate this from a meningioma, which usually affects the inner table.

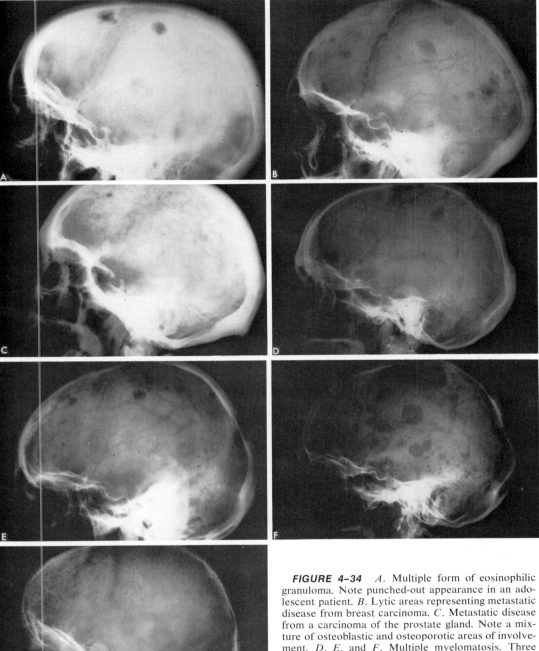

FIGURE 4–34 *A.* Multiple form of eosinophilic granuloma. Note punched-out appearance in an adolescent patient. *B.* Lytic areas representing metastatic disease from breast carcinoma. *C.* Metastatic disease from a carcinoma of the prostate gland. Note a mixture of osteoblastic and osteoporotic areas of involvement. *D, E,* and *F.* Multiple myelomatosis. Three progressive stages of the disease. *G.* Neuroblastoma. Note the widened suture. The tumor involves the skull and meninges and infiltrates the suture lines.

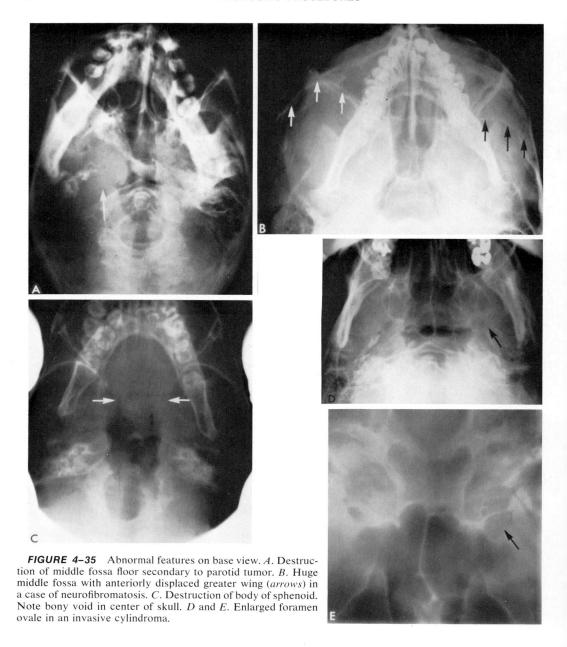

FIGURE 4–35 Abnormal features on base view. *A.* Destruction of middle fossa floor secondary to parotid tumor. *B.* Huge middle fossa with anteriorly displaced greater wing (*arrows*) in a case of neurofibromatosis. *C.* Destruction of body of sphenoid. Note bony void in center of skull. *D* and *E.* Enlarged foramen ovale in an invasive cylindroma.

age and favor females. Various bone changes are described in meningiomas, ranging from diffuse hyperostosis of bone to the sunburst appearance of spicules laid down vertically to the skull surface. Meningiomas occasionally produce lytic lesions of bone.

Certain basic projections are taken in the evaluation of the skull. Each projection may show particular structures to better advantage. Occasionally specialized projections may be taken to outline areas such as the petrous pyramid, the optic canals, and the foramina at the base of the skull. Certain features are best seen in the various projections. The frontal view is most useful to study the position of the pineal gland. If the pineal gland is not recognized in the lateral projection it will not be visible in the anterior projection. The sphenoid wings,

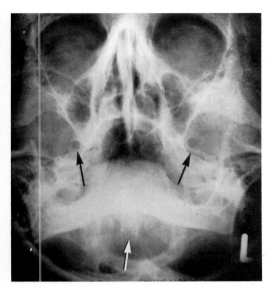

FIGURE 4–36 Special view for foramen ovale. This is an extended Water's view, useful for visualization of the odontoid through the foramen magnum.

the orbital fissures, the internal auditory meatuses, and the anterior clinoids, however, are seen to better advantage in this projection.

Special oblique views are necessary for visualization of the optic canals. Laminagraphy is essential for the evaluation of the components of the optic canal such as the cranial and orbital openings, roof, floor, and optic strut. Because of marked normal variability in its vertical diameter, the horizontal diameter of the canal should be used for assessment of pathological enlargement. A difference of at least 25 per cent of this measurement between the two sides is an indication of an expanding lesion in this area. A pneumatized anterior clinoid should not be mistaken for the optic canal (see Fig. 4–6).

Laminagraphy is also essential for the evaluation of the internal auditory canal and its components such as the posterior wall of the meatus and the crista falciformis. Because of frequent asymmetry between the two sides, the height of the canal is not a reliable indicator of pathological change. Because of earlier diagnosis today, the percentage of abnormalities of the petrous bone recognized in the routine x-ray studies is diminishing.

The base view is useful for study of the basal foramina, the greater sphenoidal wing, the pterygoid plates, and the body of the sphenoid. (The evaluation of the foramen ovale and foramen spinosum was dealt with earlier in the chapter.) This projection is particularly useful for visualization of the jugular foramen when lesions of this region such as glomus jugulare tumors are suspected.

REFERENCES

1. duBoulay, G. H.: Principles of X-Ray Diagnosis of the Skull. London, Butterworth and Co., 1965.
2. Caffey, J.: Pediatric X-Ray Diagnosis. 5th Ed. Chicago, Year Book Medical Pub., 1967.
3. Farberov, B. J.: Roentgenological diagnostics of the foramen opticum. Acta Radiol., *18*:594, 1937.
4. Kier, E. L.: Embryology of the normal optic canal and its anomalies; an anatomic and roentgenographic study. Invest. Radiol., *1*:346, 1966.
5. Kier, E. L.: The infantile sella turcica; new radiologic and anatomic concepts based on a developmental study of the sphenoid bone. Amer. J. Roentgen., *102*:747, 1968.
6. Kier, E. L.: 'J' and 'omega' shape of sella turcica; anatomic clarification of radiologic misconceptions. Acta Radiol., *9*:91, 1969.
7. Kier, E. L., and Schechter, M. M.: Criteria for Interpreting Rotated Neuroradiologic Studies. Submitted for publication.
8. Kohler, A.: Borderlands of the Normal and Early Pathologic in Skeletal Roentgenology. 10th Ed. New York, Grune and Stratton, 1956.
9. Morley, T. P., and Wortzman, G.: The importance of the lateral extensions of the sphenoidal sinus in post-traumatic cerebrospinal rhinorrhea and meningitis. Clinical and radiologic aspects. J. Neurosurg., *22*:326, 1965.
10. Oon, C. L.: New method of pineal localization. Amer. J. Roentgen., *92*:1242–1248, 1964.
11. Pendergrass, E. P., Schaeffer, J. P., and Hodes, P. J.: The Head and Neck in Roentgen Diagnosis. 2nd Ed. Springfield, Ill., Charles C Thomas, 1956.
12. Rischbieth, R. H. C., and Bull, J. W. D.: The significance of enlargement of the superior orbital (sphenoidal) fissure. Brit. J. Radiol., *31*:125–135, 1958.
13. Schechter, M. M., and Elkin, M.: The role of radiology in the management of head trauma. *In* Brock, S., ed.: Injuries of the Brain and Spinal Cord. 5th Ed. New York, Springer Pub., In publication.
14. Schinz, H. R., ed.: Roentgen Diagnosis. Vol. III. New York and London, Grune & Stratton, 1969.
15. Taveras, J. M., and Wood, E. H.: Diagnostic Neuroradiology. Baltimore, Md., Williams & Wilkins Co., 1964.
16. Vastine, J. A., and Kinney, K. K.: The pineal shadow as an aid in the localization of brain tumors. Amer. J. Roentgen., *17*:320, 1927.

5

CEREBRAL ANGIOGRAPHY

The discovery of the x-ray beam by Röntgen in 1895 was rapidly followed by its diagnostic application to the nervous system. Walter Dandy's ingenious discovery of pneumography was inspired by Luckett's report of air within the ventricular system of a patient who had sustained serious head trauma.[30, 120] It was not long before Dandy introduced air into the lumbar subarachnoid space, and so encephalography was born.[31] In 1927, Egas Moniz published a report of his first attempts at cerebral angiography in human patients.[129] The first attempt at carotid angiography, performed on a patient suffering from general paralysis of the insane, was by means of a percutaneous carotid injection of 7 cc of a 70 per cent solution of strontium bromide. The patient did not complain of any unpleasant sensations, and so it was assumed that this had been injected into the jugular vein. The radiograms showed no filling of the vessels. With the second and third cases (parkinsonism), he was also unsuccessful. In the fourth case, the needle was dislodged and 10 cc of solution was extravasated into the tissues of the neck. Moniz therefore decided to modify his technique and inject into the carotid artery after operative exposure. In the fifth case, therefore, the right internal carotid artery was exposed and ligated. The artery was punctured twice and 4 cc of 70 per cent strontium bromide was injected. The patient complained of a painful sensation and became agitated. He had difficulty with speech and later stopped speaking (the first neurological complications of cerebral angiography), but was well on the third day.

The radiographic exposures were made a little late and no angiogram was obtained.

In the sixth case, a 48-year-old patient with Parkinson's disease, a temporary ligature was placed on the internal carotid artery for two minutes and 13 to 14 cc of 70 per cent solution of strontium bromide was injected. The first film showed contrast filling of the middle and posterior cerebral arteries. This was the first carotid angiogram in a living patient. Unfortunately, the patient died eight hours later from thrombophlebitis. This prompted Moniz to abandon the bromides for the iodides. In 1933, Moniz and Aleves reviewed 600 carotid angiograms from their archives and also described the radiological anatomy of the carotid tree.[130]

Engeset popularized the percutaneous technique of carotid angiography, and Shimidzu also described his percutaneous technique for carotid angiography and his technique for vertebral angiography.[44, 193] The older toxic contrast media have today been modified or replaced by safer solutions.

Thus angiography, a one-time hazardous technique, has passed through phases of development and has today become a simple and safe procedure. In recent years the pendulum has swung away from pneumographic studies toward angiography, and with further refinements and improvements it is anticipated that fewer air studies will be undertaken as the primary contrast diagnostic technique of choice.

ANGIOGRAPHIC TECHNIQUE

Many techniques are used today to visualize the major vessels leading to the

M. M. SCHECHTER

head and their intracranial course. The choice of technique depends, in part, on the particular problem and also upon personal preference.

The diagnostic quality of radiograms and the amount of information obtained from a cerebral angiogram are greatly enhanced if the techniques are controlled by a radiologist competent in the field and fully conversant with the problem. Joint consultations between the neurology, neurosurgery, and neuroradiology services are mandatory in deciding upon the information required and the choice of procedure.

Approaches

Carotid Angiography

To opacify the carotid tree, the following approaches may be used.

1. Direct puncture (usually performed percutaneously) of the internal carotid artery, the external carotid artery, or the common carotid artery.

2. Direct puncture of the carotid artery with catheterization of the internal carotid artery, the external carotid artery, or the common carotid artery (either anterograde or retrograde).

3. Retrograde catheterization of the carotid artery via the superficial temporal artery.

4. Selective catheterization via the femoral artery (with catheter tip in the common carotid artery on either side).

5. Segmentally selective opacification via the femoral artery (catheter tip in innominate artery), the brachial artery (with or without catheterization), or the axillary artery.

6. Nonselective opacification (aortic arch opacification) via the femoral artery (catheterization), the brachial artery (with or without catheterization), the common carotid artery (retrograde catheterization) or the axillary artery.

7. Intravenous technique.

Vertebral Angiography

To opacify the vertebral tree, the following approaches may be considered.

1. Direct vertebral artery puncture, either high cervical and occipital or mid and low cervical with Sheldon needle and modifications with needle opening directed up or down, short-beveled needles, Cournand needle, Touhy needle, or by catheterization.

2. Selective catheterization via another vessel (accomplished either percutaneously or through open exposure) via the brachial, the femoral, the radial, or the subclavian artery.

3. Segmentally selective opacification by means of brachial artery puncture (with or without catheterization); subclavian artery puncture, either supraclavicular (with or without catheterization) or infraclavicular; axillary artery puncture with or without catheterization; radial artery puncture with open exposure and catheterization; femoral artery puncture with catheter tip in innominate or subclavian artery; retrograde carotid artery opacification with or without catheterization; or retrograde superficial temporal artery catheterization.

4. Nonselective opacification (aortic arch opacification) via the femoral artery (catheterization), the brachial artery (with or without catheterization), the common carotid artery (with catheterization) or the axillary or subclavian artery.

5. Intravenous techniques.

A few of the foregoing techniques are seldom used; only the more popular are considered here.

Equipment

Skull Unit

This is a matter of personal taste. There are quite a few skull units on the market, some of which have facilities for rotating the patient through 360 degrees.

Film Changing Equipment

A single-exposure technique should not be acceptable today. The use of biplane rapid serial angiography should be routine practice because of the advantages it affords, such as a comparison of the anterior projection and lateral projection viewed simultaneously, the early angiographic changes, and sequential changes. Simultaneous biplane angiography also eliminates one injection.

Image Intensifier

This facilitates the placement of catheters and, of course, must be available when cinematography is used.

Automatic Injectors

Most injections are made by hand unless high pressures are required. Some centers routinely use an automatic injector. The author reserves the automatic injector for catheterization techniques in which the rapid introduction of a bolus of contrast medium is necessary or chronologically comparable phase studies are to be made.

All percutaneous vertebral artery injections should be made by hand. When a needle becomes dislodged, the increased resistance to the introduction of saline or contrast medium will immediately become obvious and the injection can be terminated.

Syringes

The routine use of the following syringes will help to obviate the chance of a mistake: (1) 20-ml conventional for irrigating with saline, (2) 10-ml conventional for contrast medium, (3) special long narrow (20-ml BD X2003) syringe for pressure injections of contrast media, and (4) 4-ml for local anesthetic agent.

Head Binder

A binder should be used for immobilization. This might consist of a muslin band, which is attached to two rollers on the side of the skull table, and adhesive tape passing over the forehead and over the chin to the sides of the table. Even with a cooperative patient, a head binder may help to give him an extra sense of stability.

Protection

Various types of protection have been designed. Detailed descriptions can be found in radiological texts.

Preparation and Positioning of Patient

The patient has usually fasted for six hours before the examination. Sensitivity tests to iodine compounds may be used, but are not very reliable.

The neck should be shaved before the procedure is started and surgically prepared by applying pHisoHex or Betadine. A waterproof sheet is placed over the patient's chest and abdomen, and sterile towels are draped about the operative field. After being removed from their solutions, all catheters, guides, needles, connecting tubes, and adapters are rinsed carefully in saline before use. The procedure should have already been explained to the patient and the risks discussed. The patient is warned of a possible burning sensation behind the eyes or in the jaw, teeth, tongue, and lips that may last for a few seconds. He is told not to move during the injection and is assured that the burning sensation is only momentary.

In apprehensive patients and in young children and in hospitals where excellent anesthesiology is obtainable, it may be desirable to conduct the procedures under a general anesthetic. If local anesthesia is used, pentobarbital sodium (Nembutal, 100 mg) may be given a half hour prior to the examination. All cases should receive atropine alkaloids (atropine sulfate, 0.4 mg) intramuscularly, for protection against carotid sinus effects, and a barbiturate (Luminal, 30 mg) in an effort to avoid reactions to the local anesthetic. Patients with head injuries should receive a minimum of premedication for fear of masking signs and symptoms.

It is necessary that the patient have an adequate airway, and apparatus for suctioning should be present in the room. Resuscitation apparatus should be immediately available, and the angiographer should be familiar with its use.

The patient usually lies in the supine position, but under very exceptional circumstances, the study may be performed with the patient in other positions. It is important that no packing be placed under the shoulders to extend the neck. Neck extension stretches muscles, ligaments, and fascial planes, rendering the vessels less palpable. The neck should be flexed with the chin brought in toward the chest. In this position the vessels will be much more easily palpable.

Projections Used

The three most useful views are the lateral, the 20-degree anteroposterior or

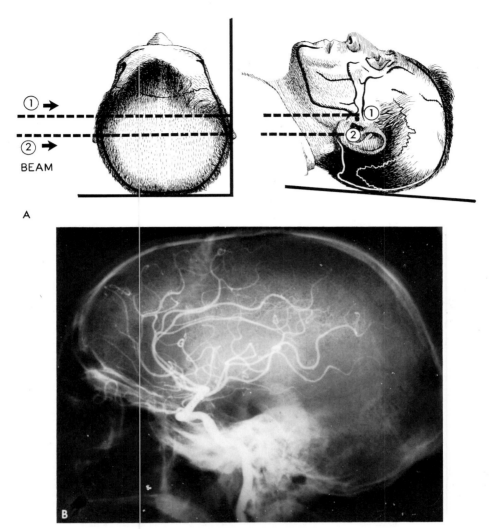

FIGURE 5-1 Lateral projection. *A*. The orbitomeatal line may be at right angles to the table top, and the central beam is directed 2.5 cm above and 2.5 cm in front of the external auditory meatus for carotid angiography (1). For vertebral angiography (2), the beam should be directed 2.5 cm behind the auditory meatus. *B*. Angiogram produced by this technique.

fronto-occipital, and the half-axial or Towne's view.

For the lateral projection the film is arranged vertical to the table top, and the direction of the x-ray beam is horizontal to the table top. It is not satisfactory to turn the head to the side and use a vertical beam, as it is difficult to obtain a true lateral projection in this position. For carotid angiography the central beam is directed 2.5 cm above and 2.5 cm anterior to the external auditory meatus. For vertebral angiography the beam should be directed 2.5 cm behind the external auditory meatus (Fig. 5–1).

The 20-degree anteroposterior or fronto-occipital projection is obtained by tilting the tube (Fig. 5–2).

The half-axial or Towne's view is particularly useful in vertebral angiography because it projects the posterior cerebral arteries and superior cerebellar arteries above the petrous bone (Fig. 5–3).

Other useful projections are the 15- or 20-degree anteroposterior oblique, the true anteroposterior, the periorbital, the full axial, and the tangential views.

A 15- or 20-degree anteroposterior oblique projection with the head turned

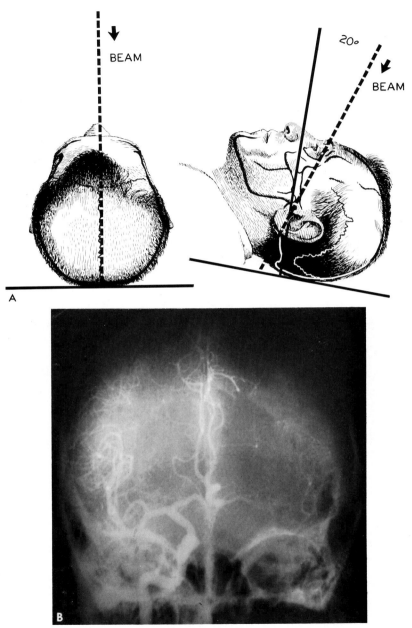

FIGURE 5–2. Twenty-degree fronto-occipital or anteroposterior projection. *A*. The baseline is at right angles to the table top. The central beam passes through the frontal bone and through the external auditory meatus. The central beam makes an angle of 20 degrees with the baseline. *B*. Carotid angiogram made using this technique.

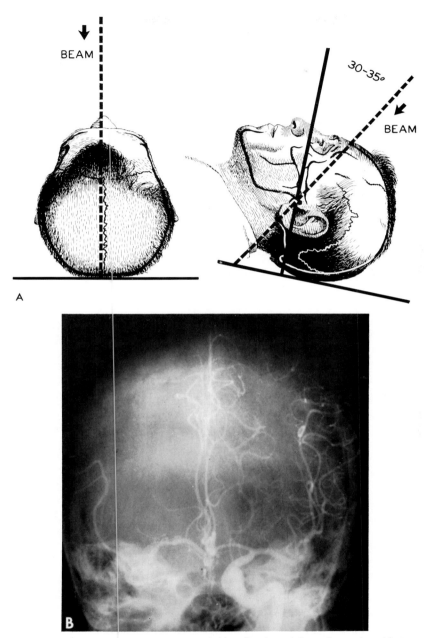

FIGURE 5–3 Towne's or half-axial projection. *A*. The baseline is at right angles to the table top, and the central beam passes through the external auditory meatus and makes an angle of 30 to 35 degrees with the baseline. *B*. Carotid angiogram made in this position—contralateral carotid compression has resulted in filling of branches of opposite carotid artery.

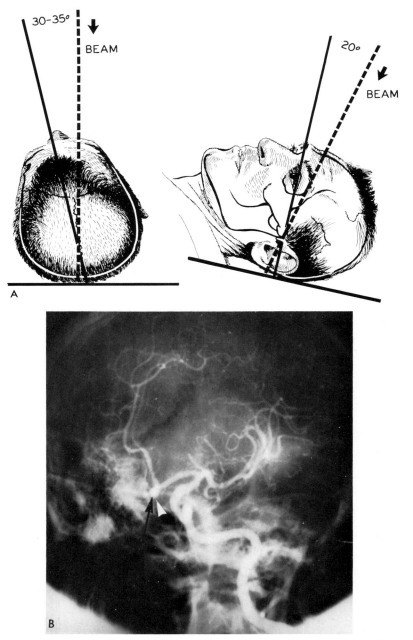

FIGURE 5–4   Fronto-occipital oblique or anteroposterior oblique projection. *A*. The orbitomeatal line is at right angles to the film. The head is rotated 30 to 35 degrees away from the injected side. The central beam passes through the frontal bone toward the feet and is centered 4 cm lateral to the glabella and 2 cm above the superior margin of the orbit. The central beam makes an angle of 20 degrees with the orbitomeatal line. *B*. Carotid angiogram made in this position. Note aneurysm of anterior communicating artery (*arrows*) shown in this projection.

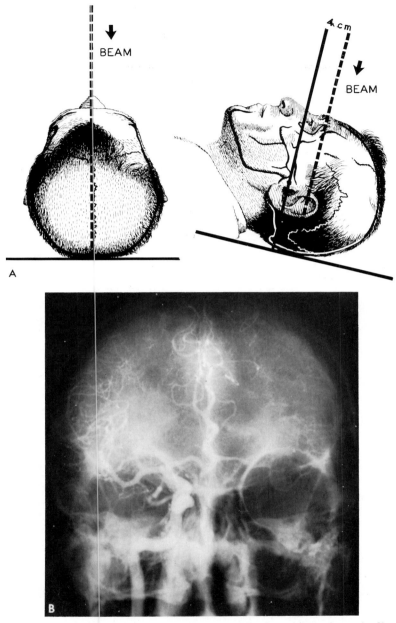

FIGURE 5–5 Anteroposterior projection. *A*. The orbitomeatal line is at right angles to the film, and the central beam is directed 4 cm above the superior margin of the orbit and parallel to the orbitomeatal line. *B*. Carotid angiogram made in this position.

away from the side of the puncture is particularly useful for the region of the anterior communicating artery and also to outline the deep dural sinuses and veins during the venous phase of the study (Fig. 5–4). The beam is directed 20 degrees, caudally, and the head is turned through 30 to 35 degrees.

The opposite oblique view may also be used.

A true anteroposterior view is shown in Figure 5–5.

The perorbital view for the trifurcation of the middle cerebral artery is particularly useful in examining the first part of the

middle cerebral artery. Here the head is
turned 10 degrees toward the side injected.
The x-ray beam is vertical and is directed
through the center of the orbit (Fig. 5–6).

The full axial (submentovertical) view
is useful in investigating aneurysms in the
region of the anterior communicating artery
and the middle cerebral artery (Fig. 5–7).

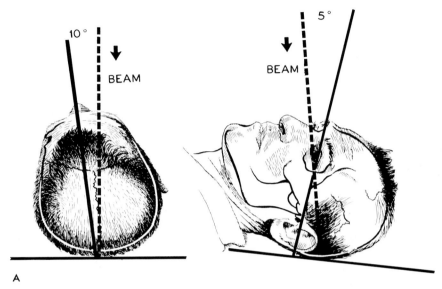

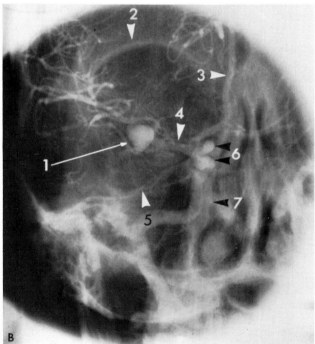

FIGURE 5–6   Perorbital projection. *A*. The orbitomeatal line is at right angles to the table top. The head is
displaced and rotated 10 degrees toward the injected side. The central beam is tilted upward 5 degrees through
the center of the orbit. *B*. Carotid angiogram made in this position: (1) aneurysm of middle cerebral artery, (2)
superior margin of orbit, (3) anterior cerebral artery, (4) middle cerebral artery, (5) inferior margin of orbit,
(6) carotid siphon, (7) intracavernous portion of carotid artery.

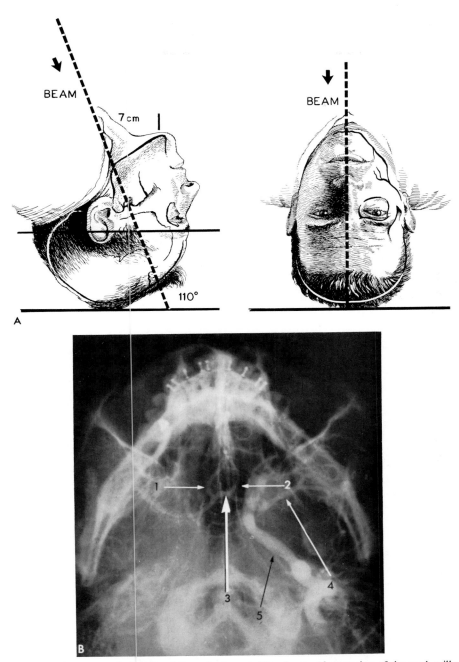

FIGURE 5-7 Submentovertical (full axial) projection. *A*. The degree of extension of the neck will vary with each patient. The central beam is directed midway between the angles of the jaw and about 7 cm behind the symphysis mentis. The angle between the baseline and the central beam should be 110 degrees. *B*. Carotid angiogram made in this position. Although other projections suggested aneurysm in the region of the anterior communicating artery, this projection cleared this region. (1 and 2) Anterior cerebral arteries, (3) anterior communicating artery, (4) middle cerebral artery, (5) internal carotid artery.

The tangential view, with the head turned about 20 degrees away from or toward the side injected, may sometimes show a subdural hematoma to better advantage (Fig. 5–8).

Time Interval Between Films

This will vary from case to case. Usually two films per second for a total of six seconds is recommended, but with a rapid

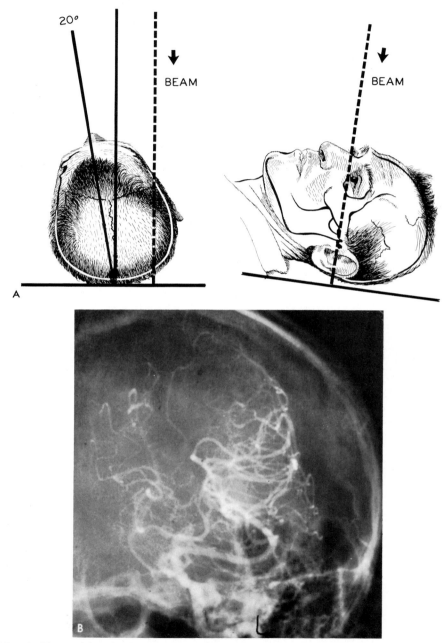

FIGURE 5–8 Tangential projection. The head is displaced so that the involved side is over the center of the film. *A.* The head is turned away 20 degrees from the injected side, and the central beam is directed at a tangent to the parietal region and at right angles to the film. *B.* For subdural hematomas situated in the frontal region, the head is rotated 10 degrees toward the injected side.

circulation or with fistulae, it might be desirable to have films taken at shorter intervals. In certain circumstances it might be advisable to prolong the interval between films. The venous phase is usually obtained about six seconds after the start of the injection.

Contrast Media

Most medical centers use 60 per cent methylglucamine diatrizoate (Renografin) or 50 per cent sodium diatrizoate (Hypaque). The amount and concentration will depend upon the site of introduction and the timing of the radiographic exposures. With a catheter or needle in the common carotid artery, 6 to 8 ml of contrast medium is usually sufficient. When the catheter is in the internal carotid artery, 6 ml is sufficient. Six milliliters is usually sufficient for the vertebral artery, and when a catheter in the subclavian artery is near the origin of the vertebral artery, 10 to 15 ml is sufficient. When the arch of the aorta is opacified to outline the major vessels in the neck, 40 ml of a more concentrated solution is used with a pressure apparatus so that the bolus of contrast medium is introduced within about 1.3 seconds.

Catheter Preparation

For simple percutaneous carotid catheterization, a PE 160 catheter is usually used. Either a 30-cm length of sterile catheter is obtained in a separate packet or a 30-cm length is cut from a reel of tubing. One end of the catheter is tapered by stretching it over a flexible guide wire (Fig. 5-9 A), and the other end is attached to a connector (Fig. 5-10), which is then attached to a syringe. When thicker catheters are used, such as the radiopaque catheters for segmental opacification via the axillary or femoral route, the stretching of

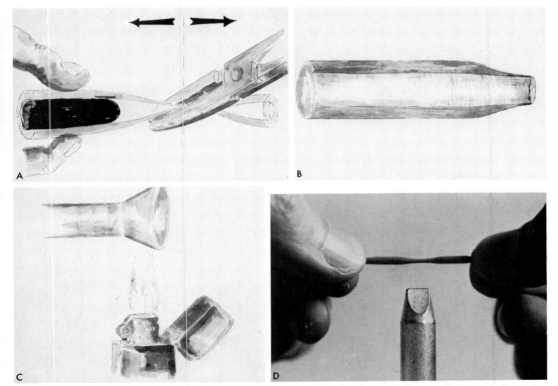

FIGURE 5–9 *A*. Preparation of catheter for angiography. *B*. Tip of catheter. *C*. Heat applied to end of catheter for flaring aperture. *D*. Note heating element in the center. Guide wire is in lumen of catheter.

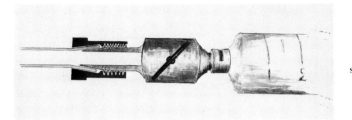

FIGURE 5–10 Connector between syringe and catheter.

the catheter and tapering of its end is facilitated by heating it over an open flame or radiant heat (Fig. 5–9 *C* and *D*).

Every detail in the preparation of the catheters must be carefully followed since omitting an apparently trivial step may result not only in an unsuccessful examination, but in most undesirable complications.

The vinyl and polyethylene catheters are prepared as follows. Having selected a suitable thickness and length of catheter, the rigid end of the guide is introduced into the catheter to within 1 cm of the end of the catheter. The tip of the catheter is now held in a pair of forceps and, while the catheter and guide are held in the other hand, this is stretched (Fig. 5–9 *A*). The guide is now removed, and the catheter tip is cut with a sharp scalpel or pair of scissors just distal to its narrowing (Fig. 5–9*B*). In this way a tapered leading tip of catheter is obtained that will fit snugly over the guide and will pass easily through the skin and arterial wall. The more rigid catheters are prepared in a similar fashion, by applying heat (from an open flame or a source of dry heat) over the region to be tapered (Fig. 5–9 *C* and *D*). A few rapid passages through a spirit flame is usually all that is required. Should side openings be desired (with the larger bores), these may be drilled in the sides with either an ordinary sawed off No. 18 (standard wire gauge) needle or a special instrument. The holes should be drilled with the channel directed backward so that the jets will leave the catheter retrogradely. These retrojets will counteract the recoil effect of the forward stream at the tip of the catheter. Three or four holes are usually sufficient and should be drilled in a spiral fashion around the catheter so as not to weaken it (Fig. 5–11). The opposite end of the catheter may be flared by holding it over

a flame or a heating element, or using a flanged instrument, to accept the special connector (Fig. 5–10). When pressure injections are not used the introduction of a closely fitting needle into this end will be quite satisfactory. Other radiopaque polyethylene and vinyl tubings are prepared in a similar manner. Some catheters are commercially available, preshaped and with a syringe adaptor attached.

Special connectors may, however, be used at this end. Figure 5–10 demonstrates their application. These are manufactured in various sizes and may be provided with a tap or a nonreturn valve. When the end of the catheter is too short to reach the pressure injector, a length of connector tubing must be used. This may be made of heavy duty tubing that will withstand high pressures. This tubing should have an internal diameter at least three times that of the catheter used. High-pressure connecting tubing sets are available in lengths of 25 cm (10 inches), 50 cm (20 inches), and 75 cm (30 inches) and will withstand pressures up to 100 lb per square inch or 7 kg per square centimeter. Luer-Lok connectors should be used when high pressures are anticipated.

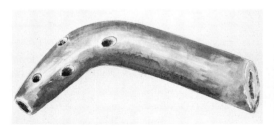

FIGURE 5–11 Note that the side openings in the catheter are directed backward so that the jet stream is directed backward.

To preshape the ends of the catheters, a thin rigid wire about 10 inches long may be inserted into the tapered end. The catheter end accommodating the wire may now be shaped (the stiff wire will retain the shape), and the end placed in boiling water for about five seconds. Next, the catheter is plunged into cold water, and the wire is removed. The "elastic memory" of the catheter ensures that it will spring back into its shape after being straightened during the manipulations during passage of the spring guide and passage along the femoral or axillary artery. A variety of thicknesses and shapes should be available for use in each particular situation.

Carotid Angiography

Direct Puncture Techniques

Direct carotid artery puncture may be made into the common carotid artery, the internal carotid artery, or the external carotid artery. The site of puncture depends on the suspected pathological process and the information required. Denser opacification with greater intracranial definition will result from an internal carotid puncture. The external carotid circulation may be useful in demonstrating the collateral supply between the extracranial and intracranial circulation and also for the tumor circulation in meningiomas and other tumors and pathological processes supplied by the external carotid artery. If the internal carotid artery is selected for direct puncture, this should be attacked as high up in the neck as possible to avoid the carotid sinus, which is situated at the bifurcation. Furthermore, the internal carotid artery becomes progressively less mobile as it approaches the base of the skull and is therefore easier to puncture. The common carotid should be punctured as low down in the neck as possible to avoid the carotid sinus. Since most pathological conditions in the cervical carotid artery occur at the bifurcation, the injection should be made as low as possible to avoid puncturing the area and to visualize it radiographically.

About 3 ml of 2 per cent procaine hydrochloride are infiltrated into the skin and around the carotid artery. Larger amounts of local anesthetic will obscure the local anatomy and make palpation of the artery difficult. The procaine is introduced around the carotid artery, there being no necessity to infiltrate the wall of the vessel. An attempt is made to introduce the No. 18 (standard wire gauge) needle through the same opening made by the local anesthetic needle. No attempt is made to puncture the artery at this stage, but the needle is advanced with the right hand until its tip impinges on the wall of the vessel. The vessel is now anchored by placing the separated index and middle fingers of the left hand on either side of the needle, considering the operator on the right side (Fig. 5–12). The left carotid artery may be pulled over toward the vertebral bodies and trachea, and anchored, while the right carotid artery may be pushed toward the midline. Using the right hand, the needle is briskly pushed into the lumen of the vessel. For beginners, it is perhaps easier to penetrate both walls of the vessel with the needle vertical to the long axis of the vessel; it is, of course, preferable to puncture only one wall. The needle is then tilted parallel with the vessel and is withdrawn slowly, using a rotary motion. Usually a characteristic flick is felt as the needle point leaves the distal wall of the vessel and pops into the lumen. This part of the puncture is performed with the bare needle, i.e., with a stylet or a connecting tube. The advantage of omitting the stylet lies in the

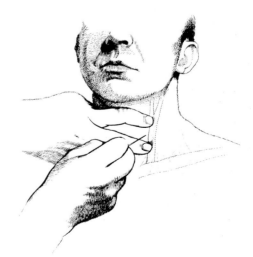

FIGURE 5–12 Technique of percutaneous carotid angiography.

recognition of the puncture of only one wall when blood under systolic pressure will spurt from the needle. This would be missed with a stylet in position. In young patients an extremely mobile vessel in the neck may resist puncture because of its elasticity and movements. A useful trick here is to embed a 2-inch 22-bore needle alongside the carotid artery and to anchor the vessel against this with the index and middle fingers.

The connecting tube, which has already been attached to a stopcock and a 20-ml syringe containing saline (stopcock is between tubing and syringe) is now attached to the needle, and saline infusion is continued until the examination is terminated; the saline may be heparinized. A continuous drip will release a pair of hands during the examination. It is not as satisfactory, however, as hand injection by a trained operator, who will immediately recognize displacement of the needle and immediately institute appropriate corrective measures. Cardiac patients should not be overloaded with saline.

To puncture the external carotid artery, the patient's neck is turned away from the side of injection. In this way the external and internal carotid arteries are separated. If a needle is introduced into the wrong vessel, it should be left in position and a puncture of the other vessel attempted. Leaving the first needle in position will aid in identifying the correct vessel.[169]

Saline is used only in 20-ml syringes and contrast medium in 10-ml syringes. This will prevent confusion. Ten milliliters of contrast medium — 50 per cent sodium diatrizoate (Hypaque) or 60 per cent methylglucamine diatrizoate (Renografin) — are drawn up into the syringe and injected into the connecting tube. The plunger of the syringe containing the contrast medium should be well lubricated with saline to obviate jamming from crystallization of the contrast medium on its surface. At a given command, about 2 ml before the end of the injection, the technician starts exposing the films. Since the connecting tubing with catheter accommodates about 3 ml, only 7 ml of contrast medium is introduced.

The number of films and the time intervals between them will depend upon such factors as the vascular circulation rate, the disease present, and the information required. When an aneurysm is suspected, the arterial phase will perhaps supply the vital information, and a film in the intermediate or venous phase may demonstrate the pooling of contrast medium in the aneurysm. In occlusive disease, delayed films may show the collateral circulation. Arteriovenous malformations will require a very short interval between films because of the rapid shunt of arterial blood through the anastomotic vessels to the venous system. The circulation time in infants and children is faster than in adults.

Automatic injectors may be used and can be coupled to the exposure mechanism. In this way the exposure is started automatically after a predetermined amount of contrast medium has been introduced. When a rapid circulation is expected (in children and in patients with arteriovenous fistulae), the exposure should be started after about 3 ml of contrast substance has been introduced. The contrast material in the connecting tube and needle may act as an anticoagulant, to prevent clotting in the tube, which may allow the stopcock to be turned off at this stage in preparation for the next injection. The author, however, prefers to allow this amount of medium to drain away by opening the top; continuous saline perfusion should be resumed.

There are valid arguments for starting the examination with the anteroposterior projection, but equally convincing reasons for beginning with the lateral projection. Where biplane angiography is used, both views are obtained simultaneously.

If the contrast medium passes into the internal carotid artery, the patient may experience a burning sensation behind the eyes, whereas this sensation may be felt in the cheek, gums, and teeth if the medium enters the external carotid. Fifteen milliliters of saline injected rapidly usually produces blanching of the conjunctiva and skin over the face if the flow has entered the external carotid artery. It must be remembered, however, that with puncture of a common carotid or even of an internal carotid artery, this subjective sensation may be an unreliable indicator, and a scout film using 2 ml of contrast medium and the Polaroid cassette will show precisely which vessel has been entered.

With the needle (or catheter, as described later) in position, the 2 ml of contrast medium is injected and an exposure of the neck is made in the lateral projection, proximal to the intracranial course of the carotid artery. Using a cassette with a Polaroid film, the position of the needle and its relation to the vessels can be obtained within 10 seconds of film exposure. Similarly, the position of the catheter tip relative to the vessels in the neck may be appreciated. If the situation is not satisfactory, the needle or catheter may be adjusted.

The anteroposterior (modified) and lateral projections (Figs. 5–1 and 5–3) are usually all that are necessary. Under certain circumstances other views may be indicated. Compression of the contralateral carotid artery will usually result in filling of the vessels of the opposite hemisphere. In the anteroposterior projection the two sides may now be compared, and asymmetry will become obvious (Fig. 5–13).

Anterior communicating aneurysms may not fill unless the contralateral carotid artery is compressed. The presence or absence of contralateral flow is an important factor in determining the operative approach to aneurysms. Contralateral compression does not give a valid assessment of the flow from the uninjected to the injected side, but only evaluates the patency of the anastomosis from the injected to the uninjected side. Saltzman claims that compression of the ipsilateral vertebral artery during carotid artery injection will fill the posterior communicating and posterior cerebral arteries.[172, 174]

If the ipsilateral anterior cerebral artery does not fill with the carotid injection, technical causes should be looked for before considering an anatomical basis. Poor filling of the carotid artery in the neck owing to spasm, hematoma, and extravascular passage of contrast medium is not infrequently associated with nonfilling of the anterior cerebral artery (Figs. 5–14 and 5–15). Partial withdrawal of the catheter may eliminate vascular spasm and permit demonstration of a normal vessel.

After removal of the needle, compression over the puncture site should be maintained for at least five minutes by "riding the carotid pulsations." The neck should then be carefully watched for an additional 15 minutes before the patient leaves the radiology department. Inspection at frequent intervals for the next 12 hours should be made.

Catheterization Techniques

The Seldinger apparatus with slight modifications can be used for carotid,

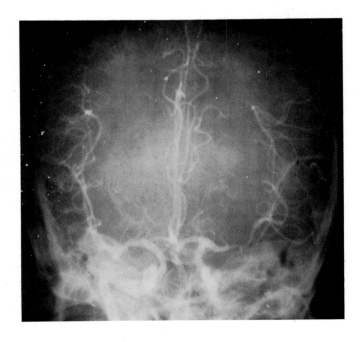

FIGURE 5–13 Right carotid angiogram with compression of the left carotid artery in the neck. Note that the contrast medium has passed from the right side to the left anterior, middle, and internal carotid arteries.

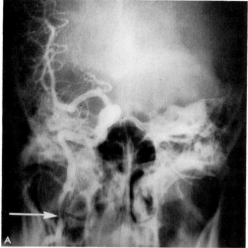

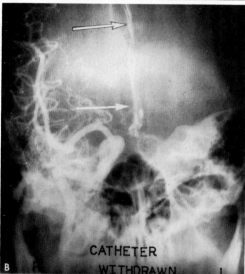

CATHETER

WITHDRAWN

FIGURE 5–14 *A*. Note area of spasm in internal carotid artery from high placement of catheter tip. There is no filling of anterior cerebral artery. *B*. When catheter was withdrawn, a little contrast medium filled the anterior cerebral artery.

brachial, and femoral catheterizations.[190] The author has dispensed with the large-size guide and uses only the small size for all angiography. The author has also found that the examination is facilitated by simply replacing the three-part special needle with the regular No. 18 (standard wire gauge) thin-walled needle. The technique for introducing the catheter into the carotid artery is the same as for the brachial and the femoral arteries.

With catheters larger than the PE 160, it is advisable to make a small nick in the skin and subcutaneous tissues using a tapered scalpel blade. This will facilitate the entry of the tip of the catheter through skin and soft tissues. A dilator may also facilitate vascular entry. Most punctures are performed percutaneously, but under certain circumstances, such as in infants, the brachial artery may have to be exposed operatively before puncture.

The Seldinger Technique

The common carotid artery is punctured as low in the neck as possible using an 18-gauge thin-walled needle and the previously described technique. A Seldinger guide, 50 cm long, is introduced (flexible end first) into the needle and advanced about 3 cm beyond the tip of the needle (Fig. 5–16). If there is any resistance at all to the passage of the guide, the needle, without being removed, should be rotated through 180 degrees, and a second attempt made. Absolutely no effort should be used to overcome any resistance to the passage of the guide. If resistance is encountered, the introduction of a few milliliters of saline into the needle may result in better placement, and another attempt may be made to introduce the guide. If an attempt is made to overcome resistance during the introduction of the guide, a thrombus or atheromatous plaque may be dislodged. Furthermore, the end of the guide may be kinked and may catch on the end of the catheter, preventing withdrawal of the guide, or may catch on the artery wall, causing considerable difficulty during withdrawal of the guide. If resistance is still encountered, the guide should be removed, and with the needle still in the artery, an ordinary conventional angiogram performed.

If no resistance is encountered, then after advancing the guide 3 cm beyond the tip of the needle, the needle is removed over the guide. A 30-cm catheter (PE 160) that has been specially prepared is then threaded over the free end of the guide to approximate the skin surface. The catheter tip should fit snugly over the guide. Catheter and guide are now advanced, using a slight rotatory movement of the catheter and guide together, for about 4 cm. The

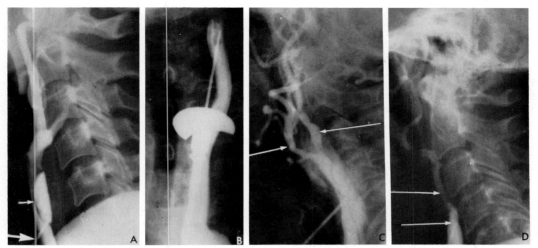

FIGURE 5-15 *A*. Subintimal injection of contrast medium. Note needle point and negative shadow (*smaller arrow*) representing an intimal flap. *B*. Injection into the carotid sheath simulating occlusive disease. *C*. Contrast medium injected partially into tissues of the neck and into the common carotid artery. There is partial filling of the internal and external carotid arteries. *D*. Second carotid injection into the same vessel. Note now no filling of internal carotid artery.

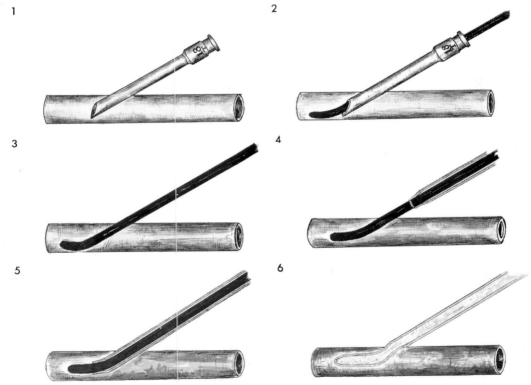

FIGURE 5-16 Schematic drawings illustrating the various steps of arterial catheterization.

guide is then withdrawn, leaving the catheter in position. Free flow of blood now issues from the end of the catheter, which is connected to an adapter and this to a syringe with saline.

If the special adapter is to be used, the catheter must be threaded through it before being threaded over the guide. Saline perfusion prevents clotting of blood in the catheter, although the tube may be heparinized before use. Saline may be introduced into the catheter and the tap closed. A little blood, however, creeps into the tip of the catheter, and it is therefore necessary to perfuse with saline every minute or two. Before introducing saline, always open the stopcock and allow the blood to reflux through the tube. This is particularly important should the catheter remain unflushed for a few minutes. In this way embolization will be prevented if a clot does form.

The advancing catheter will enter the internal carotid artery from the common carotid artery 9 times out of 10 if the neck is flexed. In this position the internal carotid artery forms a direct line with the common carotid artery.[115, 178] There is a far greater chance for external carotid cannulation if the neck is markedly extended during the passage from the common carotid artery.

The length of catheter inside the vessel lumen may be determined by measuring the length of catheter outside the vessel and subtracting this amount from 30 cm (allow 2 cm for passage through tissues in the neck). Should the catheter enter the external carotid artery, it may be withdrawn until its tip is in the common carotid artery; advancing it once again with the neck flexed will result in its entry into the internal carotid artery in most cases. Should the catheter again enter the external carotid artery, it may be withdrawn until the tip is present in the common carotid artery; the introduction of contrast medium here results in a simultaneous internal and external carotid angiogram.

With the catheter in position, 2 to 3 ml of saline rapidly injected will usually indicate whether the catheter is in the external or internal carotid artery. With the catheter in the external carotid artery, the patient usually has a slight burning or cold sensation along the distribution of the branches of the external carotid (i.e., the nose, mouth, tongue, and teeth). Slight blanching of the skin may also be observed on that side of the head. With the catheter in the internal carotid artery, there is usually no sensation or perhaps a slight burning sensation behind the eye on the side of the injection. There might be blanching of the skin over the distribution of the anastomosis of the ophthalmic artery.[91] These symptoms are markedly exaggerated when contrast medium is used.

Six to eight milliliters of medium (methylglucamine diatrizoate [Renografin] 60 per cent or sodium diatrizoate [Hypaque] 50 per cent) is now introduced, and the radiographic exposure is made 2 ml before the end of the injection. Exposures made with only 3 ml of contrast substance have resulted in perfectly adequate films. Accurate timing of exposure is necessary for success with these small amounts of contrast medium. Should subtraction techniques be contemplated, then radiographic exposure should be started a little before the injection is made so that the first film shows no contrast medium in the vasculature.

The common carotid artery may be punctured and the catheter introduced retrograde, down the carotid artery to outline the origin of this vessel. On the right, compression above the tip of the catheter will result in passage of contrast medium down the right common carotid to the innominate artery and to the subclavian artery and may outline the vertebral artery.[10, 214] Ecker described opacification of the vertebral artery by compressing the right carotid artery just distal to the needle in its lumen.[42] The advantages and disadvantages of carotid catheterization are covered in greater detail elsewhere.[178] A catheter tip lying free in the lumen of the vessel is less likely to result in subintimal extravasation than a needle. Multiple projections may be obtained without fear of dislodging a rigid needle. Should a combined right carotid and vertebral angiogram be required a catheter (PE 205 or 240) may be advanced retrograde down the common carotid artery. An injection at this stage will opacify the carotid tree. The catheter tip may then be advanced until it enters the innominate artery. Opacification will now be obtained of the vertebral artery and its branches.[10, 178, 214] A compression cuff on the right arm with distal compression of the carotid artery may give better definition of the vertebral tree. Using this technique with larger-lumen catheters, opacification of the aortic arch and its major branches has been obtained.[203]

At the completion of the examination the catheter is removed, and compression is applied to the puncture site for at least five minutes. Care must be taken to apply firm pressure and by "riding with the pulsations" not to occlude the circulation completely. Patients with atherosclerosis may require compression for longer periods, up to 20 minutes.

Weiner and associates described a technique of carotid catheterization via the exposed superficial temporal artery.[221] The superficial temporal artery is exposed under local anesthesia, and after making a nick into the vessel, a catheter (PE 160) is inserted and advanced until its tip enters the common carotid artery. Introduction of saline into the catheter during its passage along the vessel facilitates negotiating bends in the vessel by straightening the short segment of the artery immediately ahead of the advancing catheter. This technique is more time consuming, but is useful when a puncture of the carotid in the neck or a catheter study via the axillary or femoral artery is difficult or contraindicated.

Segmental Selective Catheterization

The PE 205, 240, or the more rigid catheters will give the best results. A stab wound should be made in the skin after the preliminary steps already described for carotid catheterization. The catheter may be advanced under fluoroscopic control (an image intensifier will facilitate this part of the examination); the polyvinyl or polyethylene tube may be rendered opaque with contrast medium. The right radial, brachial, or subclavian artery may be punctured and the catheter advanced until its tip lies in the innominate artery (Fig. 5-17). The brachial artery may be punctured percutaneously in the antecubital fossa. After operatively preparing the area, as described previously, about 3 ml of 2

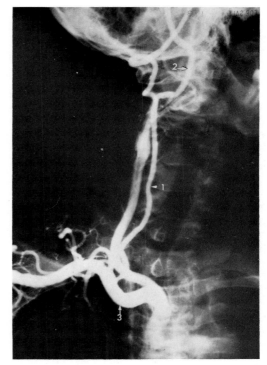

FIGURE 5–17 Brachial artery catheterization. Tip of catheter is in innominate artery. Note filling of vertebral artery (1) (origin stenosed), of common carotid and internal carotid arteries (2), and of subclavian artery (3).

per cent procaine hydrochloride is infiltrated around the brachial artery at a point where it can be readily palpated. This is usually in line with the medial and lateral epicondyles. The index and middle fingers of the left hand anchor the vessel and immobilize it. The right hand is then used to introduce the No. 18 thin-walled needle into the brachial artery, using the same technique employed for the carotid artery puncture. Care must be taken to avoid damage to the median nerve. The brachial artery may be punctured in the bicipital groove, midway along the humerus, as it passes from the posterior to the medial surface of this bone. Twelve to fifteen milliliters of 50 per cent Hypaque or 60 per cent Renografin introduced manually will result in adequate contrast of the carotid and vertebral arteries. Many workers have obtained contrast with the catheter tip in the brachial artery with or without a pressure injector. Thirty milliliters of 75 per cent Renografin introduced by pressure injector through a large cannula (No. 12) into the exposed right brachial artery may outline the carotid and vertebral arteries and their intracranial branches. Kuhn cuts down on the brachial artery and introduces a No. 8 cannula and 30 ml of 50 per cent Hypaque as rapidly as possible by hand.[103] A constricting bandage (Baumanometer cuff) around the arm, occluding the distal brachial artery during injection, may enhance the definition of the carotid and the vertebral arteries. A pilot injection of 2 ml of contrast medium is desirable to determine the precise position of the catheter in relation to the openings of the major vessels before the final bolus of medium is introduced.

In infants, Castellanos and Pereiras obtained excellent opacification of the aorta and its branches with the cannula or needle tip in the brachial artery.[23] This they have named "countercurrent aortography." Good intracranial opacification is obtained in infants using this technique, but results in adults are not as satisfactory. A recent revival of interest in it, however, has shown some promising results.[96]

Although not a catheterization technique, percutaneous injection of the right brachial artery has been used to outline the right subclavian, right vertebral, and right common carotid arteries and their branches. Percutaneous injection of the left brachial has been used to opacify the left subclavian and left vertebral arteries. The patient is premedicated as described earlier and, after the antecubital fossa is prepared, the course of the brachial artery is palpated. After infiltration with local anesthetic a No. 16 or No. 17 thin-walled short-beveled needle is introduced into the brachial artery. The needle is gently and carefully advanced up the lumen of the vessel. If difficulty is encountered in palpating the brachial artery in the antecubital fossa, it may be felt higher in the arm as it courses around the humerus (bicipital groove). A pilot dose of a few milliliters of contrast medium and an exposure with Polaroid film will quickly show the position of the needle in the vessel. One milliliter of Hypaque 50 per cent per kilogram of body weight is introduced using a pressure injector so that the bolus is in-

jected in less than 1.5 seconds. Exposures are made 2 seconds later, at the rate of two or three exposures a second. The number and rate of exposures will depend on the suspected pathological condition. Using this technique, excellent definition of the major vessels in the neck is obtained, but opacification of intracranial vessels is not consistently good with simultaneous filling of the carotid and vertebral trees. The superimposed shadows often present a confusing picture.

Odman uses preshaped catheters and has successfully catheterized the various major vessels in the neck.[140] This author has selectively catheterized the carotid vessels via the femoral artery using catheters with preshaped ends (Figs. 5–18 and 5–19). This, at times, may be a tedious procedure; if any difficulty is encountered, a nonselective catheterization technique of the aortic arch will supply the information desired.

Rossi prefers the axillary route for selec-

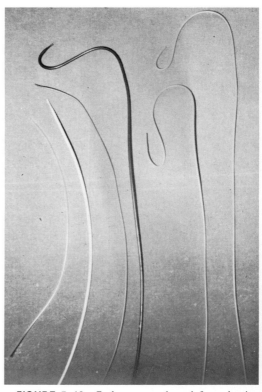

FIGURE 5–18 Catheters preshaped for selective introduction into the major vessels of the arch of the aorta.

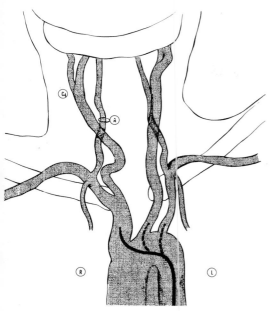

FIGURE 5-19 Drawing showing selective catheterization of major vessels in neck by a specially shaped catheter. C_4 = level of fourth cervical vertebra. A = foramen transversarium.

tive catheterization of the major vessels of the neck.[166] When tortuous vessels resist the passage of the guide, he has used the "floppy guide" technique in which a variably adjusted length of the flexible end of the guide facilitates passage around curves.

Nonselective Catheterization or Aortic Arch Studies

The four avenues of approach here are the femoral, brachial, axillary, and common carotid arteries. Since the brachial artery is so notoriously liable to spasm and there is danger of compromising its circulation with a wide-bore catheter, the femoral or the axillary artery is the vessel of choice.[224] A radiopaque catheter with side openings or the PE 240 polyethylene catheter is introduced over the Seldinger guide. The tip of the catheter is premolded so that its bend will negotiate the arch of the aorta. (Image intensification will facilitate placement of the catheter.)

The right or left thigh (the author prefers the right) is prepared for the operative procedure as described earlier, and about 4 ml of 2 per cent procaine hydrochloride is infiltrated around the femoral artery 2 to 3 cm below the inguinal ligament. Puncture

of the femoral artery above the inguinal ligament will make postpuncture compression difficult or impossible. After piercing the skin at this level with a tapered scalpel blade, the No. 18 thin-walled short-beveled needle is introduced through the opening, the femoral artery is anchored with the index and middle fingers of the left hand placed on either side of the vessel, and the needle is introduced into the lumen of the vessel as in carotid arteriography. The metal spring guide is then introduced through the needle. Either of the following two methods may be followed:

1. The guide (of suitable length) is introduced until its tip is at the level that the catheter tip will assume. The catheter with side openings is now threaded over the guide and, using a rotary movement, is advanced through the skin and artery wall along the guide until its tip approximates the desired level. The guide is now removed.

2. The guide is introduced a few centimeters, and after the catheter has been threaded over it, the two are advanced together to the desired level, when the guide is removed. The tip should be placed in the ascending aorta about 2 to 3 cm proximal to the origin of the innominate artery. This location of its tip reduces the danger of its springing into a major branch during the pressure injection. Retrojets will maintain the position during the injection.

A pilot injection of 2 ml of contrast medium with an exposure of the neck in the anteroposterior projection will demonstrate the position of the tip of the catheter relative to the major branches and will also check the radiographic technique. Forty milliliters of 60 per cent Renografin or 50 per cent Hypaque is introduced using a mechanical pressure injector that introduces the bolus of contrast medium in less than 1.3 seconds. An oblique projection (right posterior oblique) will outline the aorta and its major branches. An anteroposterior projection of the head may be useful to demonstrate the cerebral circulation (Fig. 5–19). The lateral projection is not as helpful since the vessels of the two sides are superimposed. The submentovertical position is often helpful for visualization of the intracranial circulation since it obviates the superimposition of vessels that occurs in the lateral projection. After removal of the catheter, manual pressure over the puncture site should be applied for at least 15 minutes.

A tortuous iliac vessel may render introduction of the Seldinger guide difficult. The Gensini guide may facilitate passage around these sharp bends.[38, 39] The spring metal guide (BD) also has a removable metal core that renders it much more flexible to negotiate the tortuous vessels. Rossi popularized the "floppy wire" technique.[166]

Vertebral Angiography

Contrast filling of the vertebral artery has been attempted by many maneuvers and often ingenious devices. Schechter and DeGutierrez-Mahoney demonstrated the evolution of the techniques that have been rewarding in the hands of each particular investigator.[180]

Direct Puncture Technique

The direct puncture of the vertebral artery will result in a high degree of intracranial definition, but will not always outline the origin of the vertebral artery. With the side-opening needle, however, contrast medium may be directed up or down the vertebral artery (Fig. 5–20).[177] The high cervical approach (suboccipital puncture of Maslowsky and Zielke and Weidner) has few followers.[123, 235]

The anterior cervical approach is perhaps

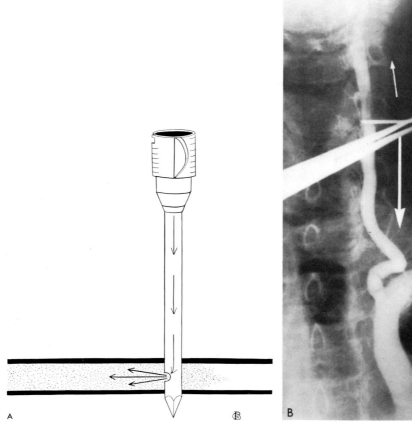
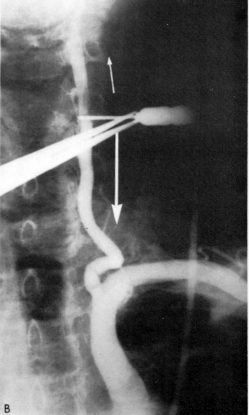

FIGURE 5–20 *A*. The vertebral artery is purposely transfixed by this needle, and by rotating the hub of the needle, the side opening at the end may be directed up or down the vessel. *B*. Vertebral angiogram produced by this technique using the anterior cervical approach and with the needle rotated so as to direct contrast medium from the side opening downward to outline the cervical course of the vertebral artery and its origin from the subclavian artery.

the simplest and the most rewarding of the direct vertebral puncture techniques.[110, 201, 207] The preparation of the patient is the same as for carotid angiography. Any level from C1 to C6 may be selected, but one should remember that when osteoarthritis is present a lower cervical approach may be more difficult. Unless there is an indication to examine the right vertebral artery (the right posterior inferior cerebellar artery arises from the vertebral artery a centimeter or two proximal to its union with the opposite vessel to become the basilar artery), the left side is usually selected. Statistically this is the larger vessel.[101, 200] A submentovertical view of the base of the skull rarely demonstrates a significant difference in the size of the foramina transversaria, but the larger opening, when found, transports the larger vessel. It would be wise to attempt puncture of the vertebral artery on this side.

After the skin and subcutaneous tissue have been infiltrated with local anesthetic, the needle is advanced and local anesthetic is infiltrated around the intervertebral foramen. The vertebral arteriogram needle is attached to a plastic tube or other convenient connector; the system is filled with saline and connected to a syringe; the needle is introduced through the skin; and the syringe is disconnected from the connecting tube, rendering the system completely patent, so that any flow from the needle will spill freely from the end of the connecting tube. The right-handed operator displaces the trachea toward the opposite side; the carotid artery is displaced lateralward (Fig. 5–21). The right hand introducing the needle directs it between the anterior tubercles of the spine; an opening in the bony resistance will become apparent. Once the intervertebral foramen is entered, the tip of the needle is directed lateralward, and a few rapid short stabs are made inside the intervertebral foramen. The withdrawal movements of the needle should be very slowly and carefully executed, since the positioning of the hole in the needle relative to the vessel is critical.

It is unusual to actually feel the passage of the needle through the vertebral artery. Once flow is established, the connecting tube is attached to the syringe for perfusion with saline. There is no need to introduce

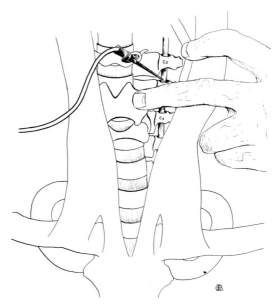

FIGURE 5–21 Technique of anterior cervical approach for vertebral angiography.

contrast substance with great force. Approximately 6 ml of 60 per cent Renografin or 50 per cent Hypaque is used. Firm pressure on the plunger of the syringe is all that is required.

The connecting tube should be transparent, so that air bubbles may be recognized; should a faulty puncture produce blood mixed with cerebrospinal fluid, this will also be recognized. If the returned blood appears very dilute, this situation must always be suspected. Introduction of contrast medium under such circumstances has been reported and may have very undesirable effects.[17, 205] To reduce this complication of the anterior approach, the vertebral needle is directed outward, i.e., away from the midline. If the needle with the side opening is used, the introduction of the needle may be vertical to the long axis of the neck. If an end-opening needle is used, the approach will differ in the sense that the hub of the needle is inclined caudally. Because of the anatomy of the parts, the side-opening needle is recommended. A notch on the hub of the needle indicates which way the opening faces (Fig. 5–20 A).

To outline the cervical course of the vertebral artery and its origin from the subclavian artery, the side-opening needle may be rotated through 180 degrees without repuncturing the vessel, directing the orifice downward. The origin of the vertebral artery will be outlined using this technique (Fig. 5–20 B).[177] The injection for opacification of the lower end of the vertebral artery should be made using a little more force than is used for the intracranial definition. It should be mentioned that even with the opening directed downward, contrast medium will eventually pass up the vessel to outline the basilar tree. Thus total vertebrobasilar opacification may be achieved with a single injection. Approximately 8 ml of 60 per cent Renografin or 50 per cent Hypaque are used with this retrograde technique.

With the end-opening needle, the vertebral artery may be catheterized. This has been attempted successfully but is not recommended. The lumen of the vertebral artery may be very small, and the removal of the guide may be difficult.

Catheterization Techniques

Catheterization of the vertebral artery from the brachial, radial, and femoral arteries employs the catheterization techniques already described.[27, 76, 112, 154, 204, 156, 157] In the hands of the experienced, a high success rate is claimed, and the examination is quite simple.

For partial segmental opacification of the vertebral artery, the brachial artery is punctured under local anesthesia, and the small-size Seldinger guide is introduced.[154] The brachial artery may be punctured where it is easily felt in front of the elbow or at a higher level where it runs in the bicipital groove. Cannulation is accomplished with a PE 205 catheter, although a PE 160 will often suffice. An appropriate length of catheter (usually 50 cm) should be introduced so that the tip lies opposite the vertebral artery. Side openings in the catheter are a distinct advantage. If a radiopaque catheter is used, fluoroscopic control for placement can be utilized. When a polyethylene tube is used, the introduction of a milliliter or two of contrast medium will show the position of the catheter. For the definitive study 12 to 15 ml of 60 per cent Renografin or 50 per cent Hypaque introduced as rapidly as possible by hand is usually sufficient. The cervical course of

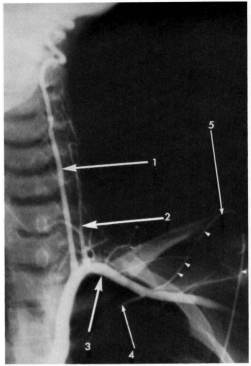

FIGURE 5–22 Catheter introduced percutaneously through a puncture of the left subclavian artery infraclavicularly. (1) Vertebral artery, (2) thyrocervical trunk, (3) subclavian artery, (4) internal mammary artery, (5) catheter, polyethylene PE 160.

the vessel is well outlined, but the intracranial definition is usually not as good as that resulting from direct vertebral artery punctures (Fig. 5–22).

For partial segmental opacification of the vertebral artery without catheterization via a brachial artery injection, the technique must be modified slightly. A No. 12 or No. 14 needle is introduced into the brachial artery in the antecubital fossa. This may be the Robb-Steinberg needle or a thin-walled short-beveled needle. Thirty milliliters of 60 per cent Renografin are introduced as rapidly as possible by hand. Serial exposures should be made. A needle of smaller caliber (No. 17 thin-walled) may also be used with a pressure injector to introduce the contrast medium.

With the femoral approach, the artery is punctured below the inguinal ligament under local anesthesia, and the catheter is advanced using the usual technique. The femoral artery should be punctured at least 2 cm below the ligament to facilitate postinjection compression, and the artery should be compressed for at least 15 minutes after the catheter or needle is withdrawn.

Roy has described another approach in which he punctures the axillary artery and introduces a catheter, using the catheterization techniques previously described.[168] The axillary artery is palpated with either arm abducted. The author claims few complications and no spasm or thrombosis. Hanafee has used the axillary approach for selective catheterization of the vertebral artery.[69] Rossi has also used this technique with very good results.[165]

Since many variables are involved in catheterization techniques, including the length of catheter, the number and size of side openings, and the viscosity of the contrast medium, the pressure recording registered on the injector in no way resembles the pressure at the tip of the catheter. For this reason individual calibrations will have to be made by workers using these pressure injectors.

THE NORMAL ANGIOGRAM

Radiological Anatomy of the Arterial System

Carotid and Vertebral Arteries

The three major vessels arising from the arch of the aorta are the innominate artery, the left carotid artery, and the left subclavian artery. The innominate artery divides into the right subclavian and right common carotid arteries, and the two vertebral arteries arise from the two subclavian arteries respectively (Fig. 5–23). Variations sometimes occur. A common trunk for the origin of the innominate and the left common carotid artery is a not uncommon variation in the Negro, and this possibility should be kept in mind and suspected when the carotid arteries on both sides fill from an injection into the right subclavian or innominate artery. The vertebral arteries may arise directly from the arch of the aorta, a situation that should be considered when a subclavian injection does not opacify the vertebral artery (Fig. 5–24). The common carotid artery usually divides

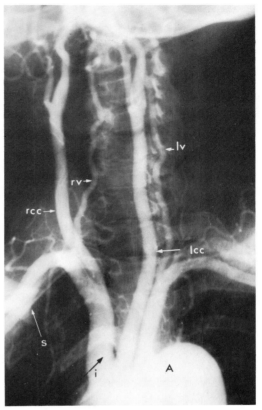

FIGURE 5–23 Aortic arch study with catheter introduced from the femoral artery with its tip in the ascending aorta. i = innominate artery. rcc = right common carotid artery. s = subclavian artery. lcc = left common carotid artery. rv = right vertebral artery. lv = left vertebral artery. A = aorta.

into the internal and external carotid arteries at the level of the superior margin of the thyroid cartilage.

The external carotid artery is anterior and medial to the internal carotid artery at its origin and, progressing cephelad, it assumes a lateral position. Branches of the external carotid artery enter the cranial cavity and assume an important role in the establishment of collateral pathways and supply to tumors.

Anatomists divide the internal carotid artery into four parts: cervical, petrous, cavernous, and cerebral (Figs. 5–25 and 5–26). The cervical internal carotid artery begins at about the level of the upper border of the thyroid cartilage and progresses vertically in the long axis of the common carotid artery to enter the skull through the

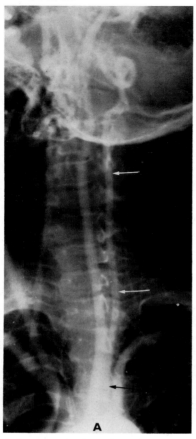

FIGURE 5-24 Aortic arch study. Note that the right vertebral artery arises from the subclavian artery, whereas the left vertebral artery indicated by three arrows arises directly from the arch of the aorta. A = aorta.

carotid canal. It is here that the petrous portion of the carotid artery begins. The petrous portion is divided anatomically into the ascending portion, the knee, and the horizontal part. This horizontal or third part is the longest and runs anteriorly, upward, and medially. The petrous portion of the artery terminates as it passes between the lingula and the petrosal process of the sphenoid bone. It is here that the cavernous portion begins. The artery is situated between layers of the dura mater forming the cavernous sinus, where it is bathed in venous blood—the only site in the body where such a situation exists. The artery ascends and then runs along the carotid sulcus, and again curves upward on the medial side of the anterior clinoid process and perforates the dura mater to enter the

subarachnoid space and assume its course as the cerebral portion. The meningohypophyseal trunk arises from the intracavernous portion of the carotid artery. The significance of hypertrophy of these vessels is discussed later.

The first branch of the cerebral carotid artery is the ophthalmic artery. Tiny vessels usually arise from the intracavernous portion of the artery to supply the wall of the cavernous sinus and its contents, but are not usually recognizable because of their tiny caliber unless they enlarge, when pathological change may be suspected. The normal radiological anatomy of the intracavernous artery has been well documented.[20] Its variations and their significance are discussed later. Having perforated the dura mater on the medial side of the anterior clinoid process, the internal carotid artery passes between the optic and oculomotor nerves and then gives off its anterior and middle cerebral artery branches. The course of the internal carotid artery including the intracavernous portion and the supraclinoid portion has been referred to as the "carotid siphon" by Moniz.[129]

The ophthalmic artery is the first intradural branch of the internal carotid artery. (Ruptured aneurysms at the site of origin of the ophthalmic artery will result in subarachnoid hemorrhage.) It passes laterally and inferiorly to enter the orbit through the optic foramen. The radiological anatomy of this vessel has been well covered by Lombardi.[119] The vessel is the major supply to the eyeball through the central retinal artery and also supplies the structures of the orbit and surrounding tissues. Occasionally the anterior meningeal artery takes origin from the ophthalmic artery (Fig. 5-27).[57] The ophthalmic artery forms the major collateral supply to the carotid siphon in occlusion of the carotid artery. In a high proportion of cases, the choroidal blush is recognized and outlines the back of the orbit. This is a useful landmark in expanding lesions of the orbit.

The posterior communicating artery is the next major branch of the internal carotid artery and arises from the dorsal aspect of the carotid siphon and courses posteriorly and medially to unite with the posterior cerebral artery; they both con-

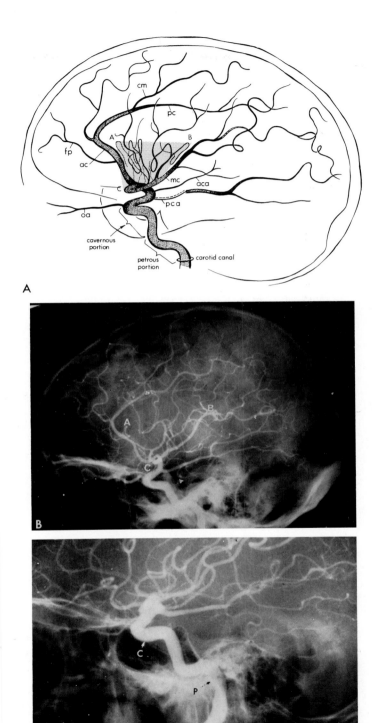

A

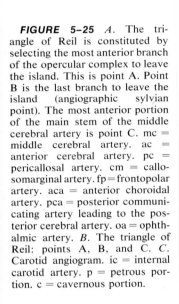

FIGURE 5–25 *A*. The triangle of Reil is constituted by selecting the most anterior branch of the opercular complex to leave the island. This is point A. Point B is the last branch to leave the island (angiographic sylvian point). The most anterior portion of the main stem of the middle cerebral artery is point C. mc = middle cerebral artery. ac = anterior cerebral artery. pc = pericallosal artery. cm = callosomarginal artery. fp=frontopolar artery. aca = anterior choroidal artery. pca = posterior communicating artery leading to the posterior cerebral artery. oa = ophthalmic artery. *B*. The triangle of Reil: points A, B, and C. *C*. Carotid angiogram. ic = internal carotid artery. p = petrous portion. c = cavernous portion.

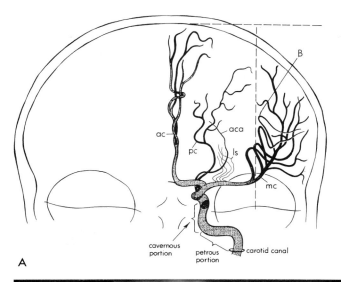

A

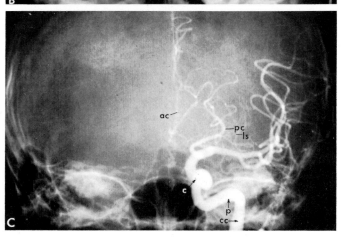

FIGURE 5–26 *A.* The angiographic sylvian point is the point at which the last branch of the middle cerebral artery leaves the island of Reil (B). In the frontal projection this should be halfway between a line drawn tangentially to the inner table of the skull and another line drawn parallel with and at the upper margin of the orbital roofs or the petrous crest, whichever is lower. ac = anterior cerebral artery. pc = posterior cerebral artery. aca = anterior choroidal artery. ls = lenticulostriate arteries. mc = middle cerebral artery. *B.* Construction of lines to evaluate the position of the angiographic sylvian point. *C.* Carotid angiogram. cc = carotid canal. p = petrous portion. c = cavernous portion. pc = posterior cerebral artery. ac = anterior cerebral artery. ls = lenticulostriate artery.

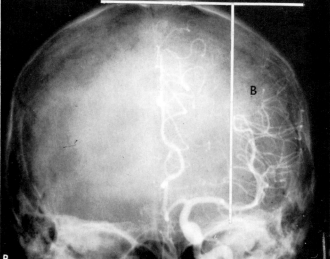

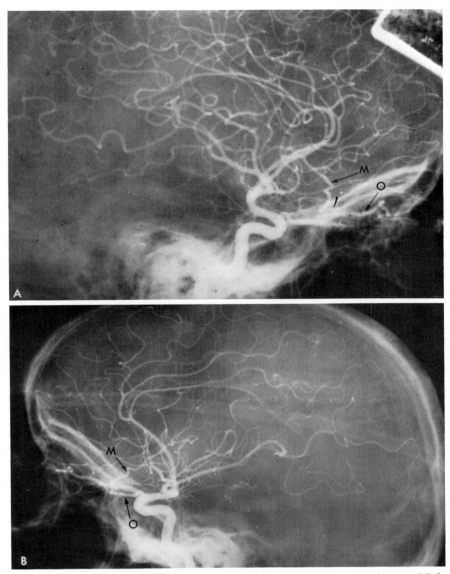

FIGURE 5–27 *A.* Right carotid angiogram showing the origin of the right meningeal artery (M) from the left ophthalmic artery (O). *B.* Left carotid angiogram in the same patient. Note origin of the left meningeal artery (M) from the left ophthalmic artery (O).

stitute part of the circle of Willis. This vessel, because of its tiny lumen, may not be opacified in the cerebral angiogram. When opacified, however, it may be seen as a fine shadow; occasionally it is well developed. Occasionally the posterior cerebral artery appears to arise directly from the internal carotid artery. The posterior communicating artery or posterior cerebral artery fills in a high proportion of cases. Saltzman found that it did so in almost 50 per cent of internal carotid angiograms and in 30 per cent of common carotid angiograms.[172] Filling of this vessel depends upon various factors that alter hemodynamic flow. Vertebral artery compression during carotid angiography is one. At the origin of the posterior communicating artery, one sometimes sees infundibular widening of the carotid artery (Fig. 5–28).[173]

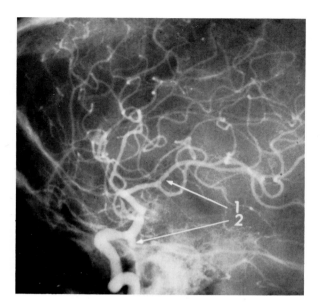

FIGURE 5-28 Carotid angiogram. The head has been purposely rotated into an oblique position to throw the branches of the middle cerebral artery (1) clear of the posterior cerebral artery. There is infundibular widening at the origin of the posterior cerebral artery from the internal carotid artery (2).

It has not been conclusively established whether this represents an aneurysm or a preaneurysmal state. Hassler and Saltzman found anatomical defects in the wall of this widening in a few cases.[74, 75] The significance of this finding becomes important when one is looking for a cause of subarachnoid hemorrhage.

Anterior Choroidal Artery

This is the next branch of the internal carotid artery, arising just distal to the posterior communicating artery, and can be identified in over 90 per cent of cases (Fig. 5-29). From its origin, which may show infundibular widening similar to that

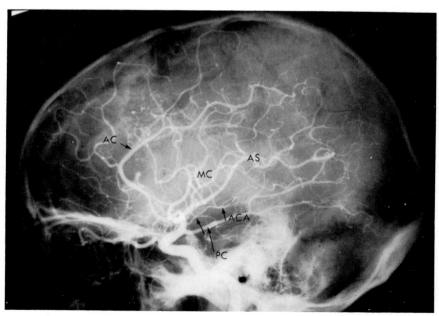

FIGURE 5-29 Normal carotid angiogram. AC = anterior cerebral artery. MC = middle cerebral group. PC = posterior cerebral artery. AS = angiographic sylvian point. ACA = anterior choroidal artery. (Also see Figure 5-66 A for anterior choroidal artery.)

seen in the posterior cerebral artery, the anterior choroidal artery passes posteriorly and laterally and usually has a convex upward course. It finally enters the temporal horn and supplies the internal capsule and the choroid plexus of the inferior horn of the lateral ventricle. Occasionally a blush can be recognized angiographically that represents the choroid plexus. Sjögren refers to the cisternal and plexal course of the anterior choroidal artery, representing the length of artery from its origin through the cisternal space of the parasellar region and the length from its entry into the temporal horn to its supply to the choroid plexus.[196]

Anterior Cerebral Artery

This arises at the division of the internal carotid artery into its two major branches. It passes forward and medialward across the anterior perforated substance, above the optic nerve, to the commencement of the longitudinal fissure. The anterior communicating artery usually connects the anterior cerebral artery to the anterior cerebral artery of the opposite side. From this point the two vessels run alongside each other in the longitudinal fissure, curving over the genu of the corpus callosum as the pericallosal artery, and finally anastamosing with the branches of the posterior cerebral artery. The frontopolar branch of the anterior cerebral artery usually arises from the anterior cerebral artery just before the parent vessel takes a turn over the corpus callosum and passes toward the frontal lobe. The callosomarginal branch of the anterior cerebral artery distal to the frontopolar branch usually runs in the callosomarginal sulcus, but may emerge and return to the sulcus. This undulating course may be recognized in the frontal projection; the vessel wanders away from the midline and its fellow of the opposite side returns to the midline. In the lateral projection the vessel often runs a course roughly parallel to that of the pericallosal artery.

Middle Cerebral Artery

This is the largest branch of the internal carotid artery and often appears to be a continuation of this vessel. It, at first, passes lateralward in the sylvian fissure and then passes upward and backward over the island of Reil to distribute over the surface of the brain. The proximal portion of the middle cerebral artery is directed forward and lateralward and, if not horizontal, then usually a little downward; in the lateral projection it is therefore normally foreshortened. When the course of this portion of the middle cerebral artery is displayed in a well-centered, lateral radiogram, then abnormal displacement of the vessel should be suspected. The middle cerebral artery then trifurcates and continues between the island of Reil and the temporal lobe and, passing backward, divides into numerous branches before leaving the sylvian fissure (Fig. 5–30). Two groups of small branches arise from the horizontal segment of the middle cerebral artery, the medial and lateral lenticulostriate arteries. About two to six in number, these vessels pass directly upward to enter the anterior perforating substance (Fig. 5–31). The medial group supplies the medial ganglia (thalamus, caudate, and lentiform) and the internal capsule, while the lateral group supplies the more laterally situated structures such as the putamen. In the anterior projection, the lenticulostriate arteries describe an S-shaped curve (Fig. 5–32). They are not always easy to recognize in the lateral projection, being superimposed on the other branches of the middle cerebral artery. The anterior temporal branch of the middle cerebral artery passes downward near the tip of the temporal lobe, and the orbitofrontal artery along the under surface of the frontal lobe. The ascending branches or the candelabra group (so called because it sometimes resembles a candelabra) is probably the most conspicuous group of the middle cerebral artery branches. The island of Reil is roughly triangular in shape and is covered in part by the operculum of the frontal, parietal, and temporal lobes.

The insular branches of the middle cerebral artery course over the island of Reil. As the branches that are directed upward meet the upper border of the island they enter a cul-de-sac and turn on themselves to run downward and then leave the sylvian fissure and are directed upward over the surface of the brain. Most of the branches pass upward and outward. Where the vessels turn on themselves or reverse direction,

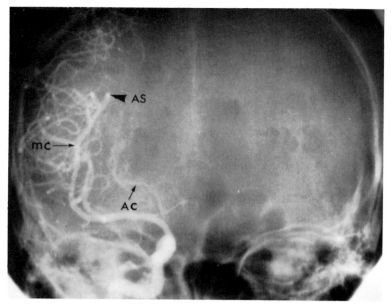

FIGURE 5–30 Carotid angiogram showing anterior choroidal artery (AC), middle cerebral artery (MC), and angiographic sylvian point (AS).

one may recognize a dense dot, the contrast-filled artery foreshortened. If these dots are joined by an imaginary line, we have the upper margin of the island of Reil. This is usually horizontal and constitutes the hypotenuse of the triangle of Reil (Figs. 5–25 and 5–33).

The course of the artery as it emerges from the sylvian fissure is usually recognizable, and one can predict the course of the sylvian fissure from this. The point of exit of the last of the insular branches to leave from the sylvian fissure is usually recognizable and has been termed the

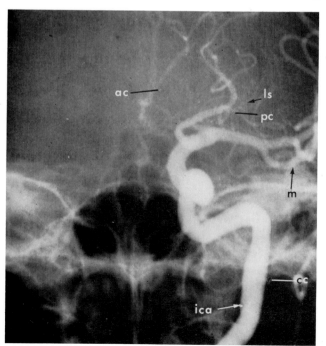

FIGURE 5–31 Carotid angiogram showing the fine lenticulostriate arteries (ls). m = middle cerebral arteries. ica = internal carotid artery. pc = posterior carotid artery. cc = carotid canal. ac = anterior cerebral artery.

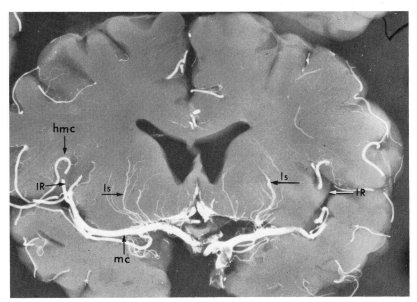

FIGURE 5–32   Postmortem angiogram using a barium and gelatin mixture. Note the course of the middle cerebral artery (mc) and the lenticulostriate arteries (ls) on both sides. The island of Reil (IR) is shown on both sides. Note the "hairpin bend" (hmc) of the middle cerebral artery.

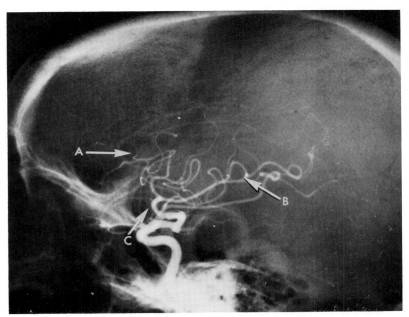

FIGURE 5–33   Carotid angiogram with only faint opacification of the anterior cerebral artery but with excellent filling of the middle cerebral artery group. Points A, B, and C constitute the triangle of Reil (see also Figure 5–25 *A* and *B*).

angiographic sylvian point (Figs. 5–25 and 5–26). In the anterior projection the loops of the middle cerebral artery as they leave the sylvian fissure are readily recognizable. The lower loops are the anterior vessels and the superior loops the posterior branches. The height of the angiographic sylvian point in the frontal projection is midway between the highest point of the skull and the upper margin of the orbit.[212] The distance between the angiographic sylvian point and the inner table of the skull varies from 30 to 43 mm.[212] The terminal branches of the middle cerebral artery pass backward and have been called, after Moniz, the posterior parietal, the angular, and the posterior temporal arteries. In infants and children the middle cerebral artery runs a more vertical course than in adults; this should not be misinterpreted as abnormal (Fig. 5–34).[211]

Vertebral Artery

For purposes of description the normal roentgenological anatomy of the vertebral artery is divided into four segments: the origin of the vertebral artery from the subclavian artery to C6 (its usual site of entering the foramen transversarium); the course from C6 to C1; from C1 to its entry into the skull; and from its entry into the skull to its union with the opposite vertebral artery to become the basilar artery (Fig. 5–35).

Many variations of the origin of the vertebral artery have been described.[32, 76, 101, 110] Of practical importance is absence of the vertebral artery in caroticobasilar anastomosis. Here the vertebral artery may arise from the carotid artery.[131] This situation may be misinterpreted as occlusive disease. The origin of the vertebral artery from the arch is of practical importance when vertebral angiography from the subclavian artery is attempted.

Variations of the second part are rare. Only a few anomalies have been described. Rivaglia, quoted by Krayenbühl and Yasargil, described the vertebral artery leaving the canal between C2 and C3.[161] An incidental finding during angiography has been noted in which the vertebral artery entered the foramen transversarium at C3 (Fig. 5–36).

Multiple variations are seen in the third part. In some persons there may be differences between the two sides. In one case described by Krayenbühl and Yasargil, there was no foramen in C1, so the artery went below C1.[101]

In the intracranial segment or the fourth

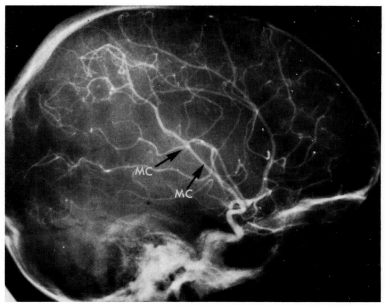

FIGURE 5–34 Carotid angiogram showing the middle cerebral artery running a more vertical course than usual. mc = middle cerebral artery.

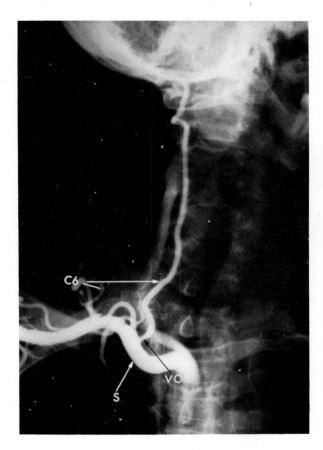

FIGURE 5-35 Subclavian opacification. The origin of the vertebral artery (VO) from the subclavian artery (S) is outlined. C6 is the level at which the vertebral artery usually enters the foramen transversarium. The origin of the vertebral artery to C6 is the first part. C6 to C1 is the second part.

part, there are variations in the course of the vessels as they enter the basilar artery. Anatomical anomalies are rare. In Krayenbühl and Yasargil's series, the vertebral artery in the lateral projection appeared to be parallel to the clivus in 47 per cent of cases (Fig. 5-37; see also Fig. 5-47) and slightly bent posteriorly in 39 per cent of cases or markedly bent posteriorly in 14 per cent of cases (Fig. 5-38).[101]

The displacement may be as much as 1 cm according to Lindgren.[110] Sergent reports displacements in normal subjects of 0.8 to 1.2 cm, and Krayenbühl and Yasargil noted a displacement of 1.6 cm in a normal vertebral angiogram.[101,191] The junction of the vertebral arteries may be projected approximately in the midline of the foramen magnum or definitely lateral to this (Figs. 5-39 and 5-40). The point of juncture of the two vertebral arteries varies considerably in the normal angiogram and may be quite laterally placed (compare with

the tip of the basilar artery, which is usually midline). It is important to recognize a laterally placed origin of the basilar artery and not interpret these findings as abnormal.[67]

Caliber of the Vertebral Artery

Stopford, examining these vessels in 150 cadavers, found a wider vertebral artery on the left in 51 per cent of cases, a wider vertebral artery on the right in 41 per cent of cases, and vertebral arteries of equal width in 8 per cent of cases.[200] Thus, in 92 per cent of cases, the vertebral arteries were of unequal width. Stopford also found an abnormally small vertebral artery on the right side in 9 per cent of cases (Fig. 5-41), abnormally small vertebral arteries on the left side in 5 per cent of cases, and abnormally small vertebral arteries on both sides in 1 per cent of cases.[200]

In a series of postmortem studies by

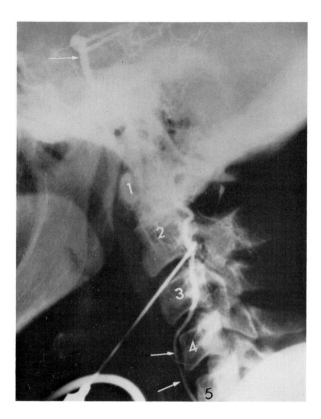

FIGURE 5–36 Vertebral angiogram. Note course of vertebral artery (*arrows*) in the lower cervical region where it enters foramen transversarium between C3 and C4.

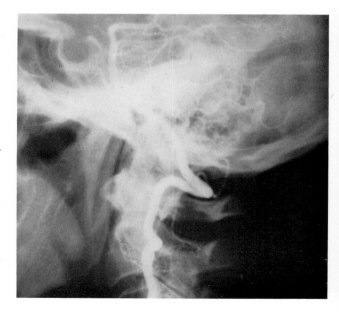

FIGURE 5–37 Note that the basilar artery is parallel to the clivus.

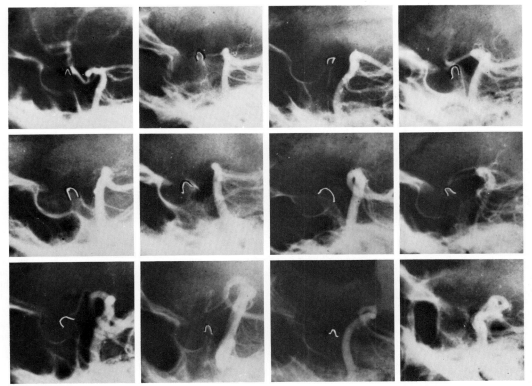

FIGURE 5-38 Twelve normal vertebral angiograms. The posterior clinoid has been retouched for identification. Note the variations in the height of the basilar artery and its distance (horizontal) from the tip of the posterior clinoid.

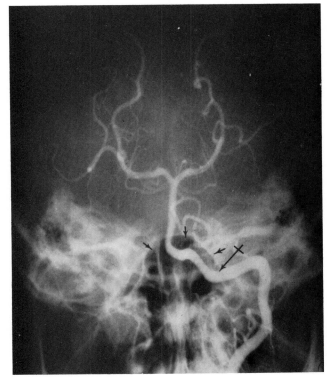

FIGURE 5-39 The junction of the two vertebral arteries is projected in the midline of the foramen magnum (*foramen magnum identified by arrows*); ⊢→ represents the point of entry of the vertebral artery into the subarachnoid space.

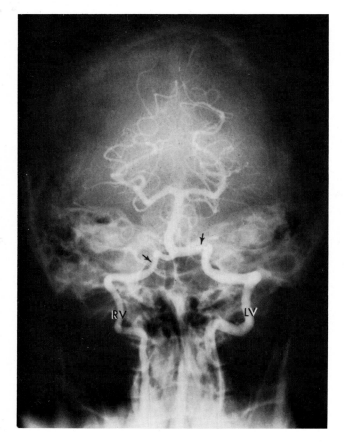

FIGURE 5–40 Vertebral angiogram. Note that the caliber of the left vertebral artery (LV) is larger than that on the right side (RV). The junction of the two vertebral arteries is projected to the right of the midline. Note that the basilar artery is concave toward the vertebral artery of the larger caliber.

Krayenbühl and Yasargil, 42 per cent had wider vertebral arteries on the left side, 32 per cent had wider vertebral arteries on the right side, and 26 per cent had vertebral arteries of equal width. In 72 per cent the difference in caliber was clearly visible; in 20 per cent the caliber was minimal. They also found abnormally small vertebral arteries on the right side in 6.2 per cent, abnormally small vertebral arteries on the left side in 4.5 per cent, and abnormally small vertebral arteries on both sides in 0.75 per cent; in two cases, one vertebral artery was as thin as a string.[101] Of interest here is that when the foramina transversaria are of unequal size (this can be recognized in the basal view) the larger foramen transmits the larger vertebral artery.

The most dorsal point of the artery seen in the lateral angiogram corresponds with its entry into the subarachnoid space, and this is roughly the middle of the foramen magnum. In the fronto-occipital projection, the entrance into the subarachnoid space corresponds with the lateral margin of the foramen magnum (Fig. 5–39).

Height at Which Vertebral Arteries Join

In the Stopford series, 72 per cent joined below the inferior margin of the pons, 8 per cent joined above the inferior margin of the pons, and 19 per cent joined at the level of the olivary nucleus of the medulla. In the Krayenbühl and Yasargil series, 66 per cent joined at the inferior margin of the pons, 12 per cent above this point, and 22 per cent below this point; one case joined at the middle of the pons.[101]

Reflux Down Contralateral Side

Visualization of the contralateral vertebral artery depends on many factors. One important factor is the rate of injection. Compression of the ipsilateral vertebral artery over the supraclavicular region might

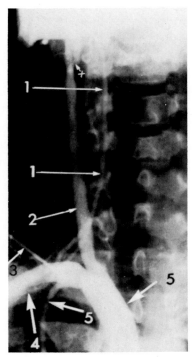

FIGURE 5–41 Supraclavicular puncture of the subclavian artery. Note needle (3), subclavian artery (4), innominate artery (5), common carotid artery (2), with marked narrowing at origin of internal carotid artery (x). Vertebral artery has a narrow and hypoplastic lumen (1).

promote reflux. Twenty to thirty per cent of cases show filling of the contralateral vertebral artery during percutaneous vertebral angiography.[157, 206] Since there is no reflux in over 70 per cent of cases, the opposite vertebral artery must be opacified if pathological change such as an aneurysm at the origin of the posterior inferior cerebellar artery is suspected. Scatliff et al. investigated the factors involved in vertebral artery reflux.[175] Hypotension, turning of the head, and variations in the caliber of the vertebral artery are considered.

Posterior Inferior Cerebellar Artery

The first large artery arising from the vertebral is the posterior inferior cerebellar artery. The vessel usually arises from the vertebral artery 1 to 2 cm proximal to the origin of the basilar. The medial extension of the cerebellar hemisphere, which presents at or just above the foramen magnum, is called the cerebellar tonsil. A portion of

the posterior inferior cerebellar artery is intimately associated with this part. The posterior inferior cerebellar artery arises from the vertebral artery and passes dorsolaterally with a caudal loop around the medulla, and then divides into a medial and a lateral branch. The lateral branch passes over the inferior surface of the cerebellum while the medial branch runs along the medial aspect of the tonsil. The medial branch has a caudal loop and a cranial loop. The caudal loop passes under the cerebellar tonsil, and the cranial loop passes close to the caudal and lateral limits of the fourth ventricle. The vessel then distributes to the medial part of the cerebellar hemisphere. Thus, viewed at right angles to the median plane, a caudal loop is formed defining the approximate outline of the caudal part of the tonsil, and a cranial arterial loop indicating the cranial border of the tonsil.

By outlining this vessel with contrast medium it is possible to judge the position of the cerebellar tonsil and the caudolateral part of the fourth ventricle. Herniations of the tonsils may therefore be demonstrated by showing the hairpin bend of the posterior inferior cerebellar artery below the foramen magnum (Figs. 5–42 and 5–43).

Cases have been reported in which the origin of the posterior inferior cerebellar artery was from the basilar artery and in which one vertebral artery became the posterior inferior cerebellar artery, while the one on the other side continued to become the basilar artery; that is, there was nonfusion of the vertebral artery.[101, 157]

The posterior inferior cerebellar artery is unfortunately sometimes absent or too small to be clearly visualized during vertebral angiography. Krayenbühl and Yasargil state that it is identified in the lateral projection in 88 per cent of cases, and not visualized in 12 per cent of cases.[101] In four cases, the loop of the posterior inferior cerebellar extended markedly below the foramen magnum. In 9 per cent of demonstrable posterior inferior cerebellar arteries, the loop was just below the foramen magnum in a narrow coil, while in 8 per cent the coil entered the foramen magnum in a broad sweep. Lindgren identified this vessel in the lateral projection in 90 per cent of cases.[111, 112]

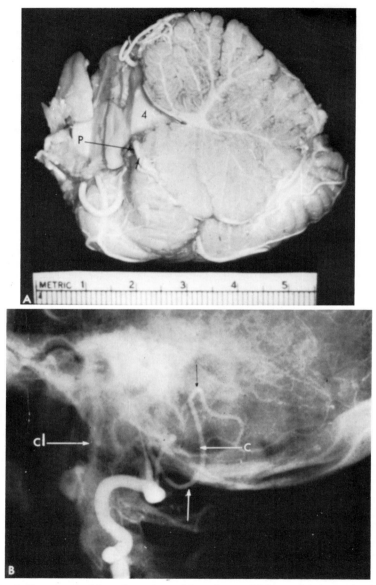

FIGURE 5-42 *A*. Postmortem injected specimen. Note the cranial loop of the posterior inferior cerebellar artery and its proximity to the fourth ventricle (↑). (Specimen by courtesy of Dr. Wollschlaeger.) *B*. Vertebral angiogram outlining the posterior inferior cerebellar artery. The caudal loop of the posterior inferior cerebellar artery outlines the inferior pole of the cerebellar tonsil (c), and the cranial loop (cl) is related to the caudolateral portion of the fourth ventricle.

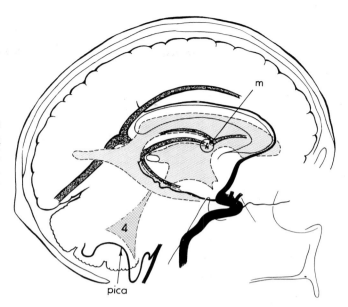

FIGURE 5-43 Diagram of relationship of ventricular system, arteries and veins. M = foramen of Monro. A = junction of thalamostriate vein, septal vein, and internal cerebral vein. 4 = fourth ventricle. pica = posterior inferior cerebellar artery.

The posterior meningeal branches arising from the vertebral artery are sometimes recognized during angiography. These course along the inner table of the occipital bone. The anterior spinal artery can be identified in 50 per cent of vertebral angiograms. It may outline the anterior margin of the spinal cord, may act as a collateral pathway in occlusive disease, and may feed pathological processes, e.g., angiomas.[183,184]

Basilar Artery

The first part of the basilar artery, as seen in the lateral angiogram, is overlapped by the dense petrous bones. The artery then shows a curve with a ventral convexity. The variations in distance from the tip of the basilar to the dorsum sellae, according to Krayenbühl and Yasargil, are as follows: in 39 per cent of cases 0.1 to 0.5 cm; in 48 per cent of cases 0.5 to 0.9 cm; in 13 per cent of cases 1.0 cm or more. The average is 0.6 cm; the minimum is 0.1 cm; the maximum is 1.4 cm.[101]

The point of basilar bifurcation also varies longitudinally. As a landmark, a line was projected backward from the anterior clinoids parallel to the baseline of the skull. In 51 per cent of cases the tip of the basilar was the same height; in 19 per cent of cases the tip of the basilar was less than half the height of the dorsum sellae; and in 30 per cent of cases the tip of the basilar was more than half the height of the dorsum sellae above. The maximum height above this line was 1.3 cm (Fig. 5–38). When the tip is projected above the posterior clinoids, the usual appearance in the lateral and anteroposterior projection is a W, like the handlebar mustache, but when projected below the posterior clinoids, the appearance in the lateral and anteroposterior projection is like a V or Y (Fig. 5–44). The W and V forms were described by Lindgren.[113]

Anterior Inferior Cerebellar Arteries

These are not seen in the lateral projection as they are covered by the dense petrous bone. These vessels run laterally toward the auditory meatus. Some authors have described changes in the course of the vessel produced by acoustic neuromas.

Pontine Perforating Branches

These are sometimes seen in the lateral projection. They are five vessels running parallel to one another and posteriorly from the basilar artery to the pons.

Superior Cerebellar Arteries

These, in their most ventral part, follow the course of the posterior cerebral arteries

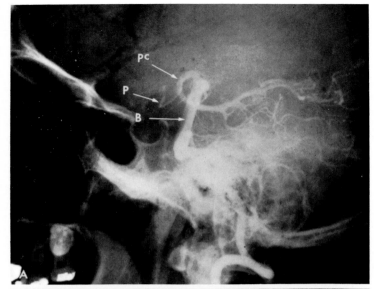

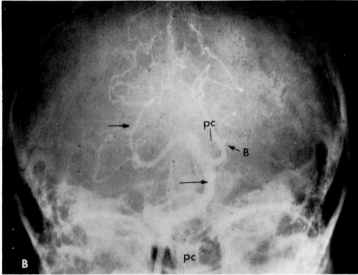

FIGURE 5–44 *A*. Lateral projection of a vertebral angiogram showing an elongated basilar artery extending for a considerable distance above the posterior clinoids. B = basilar artery. pc = posterior cerebral artery. p = posterior communicating artery. *B*. Anterior projection of the same vertebral angiogram. With the vertical extension of the basilar artery the configuration in the anterior projection is the **W** type.

and curve around the midbrain. This part of the artery may arch caudally in a single curve or show irregular loops. The majority of the branches of this artery are projected in a region that corresponds with the lateral projection of the tentorium. The superior cerebellar arteries divide into medial and lateral branches, which pass over the superior aspect of the cerebellum. Congenital anomalies are not common. The superior cerebellar arteries may arise from the posterior cerebrals, and two superior cerebellar arteries have been seen on the left

and one on the right. Wollschlaeger and Wollschlaeger have shown numerous variations of the vessels arising from the basilar artery.[227]

Posterior Cerebral Arteries

The two posterior cerebral arteries course over the tentorium and, proximal to their bifurcation, pass straight back, or may even show a marked curve with a caudal convexity.[222] Usually, in most of their course, the two arteries run approximately the same course. The occipital branch of the posterior cerebral artery arches superiorly, and the branches are distributed in a wedge-shaped area in the occipital fossa. The calcarine branch of the posterior cerebral artery is more or less a straight continuation of the artery. The temporal branch of the posterior cerebral artery crosses the first part of the posterior cerebral artery and passes caudally. The lateral branches are projected in a triangular region, which in the lateral projection corresponds with the tentorium. In the anteroposterior projection there is no constant bilateral symmetry of the branches of the posterior cerebral artery. The vessel gives off its temporal branch and then continues, forming a "Grecian vase" when viewed in the anterior projection, to divide into the occipital and calcarine branches (Fig. 5–45). Fetterman and Moran drew attention to the fact that with advancing age the posterior communicating arteries become reduced to filamentous strands, and this may explain the flow dynamics in which there may be filling of the posterior cerebral artery from both the carotid artery and the basilar artery or only from one of them.[50]

When one posterior cerebral artery fills from the carotid and one from the basilar artery, the resulting asymmetry may simulate a disease process (Fig. 5–46). Both posterior cerebral arteries may arise from the carotid artery while both superior cerebellar arteries arise from the basilar artery (Fig. 5–47). Saltzman reported an increased incidence of filling of the posterior cerebral artery and posterior communicating artery when the ipsilateral vertebral artery was compressed low in the neck.[172, 174]

Posterior Choroidal Arteries

Lateral to the cerebral peduncle, the posterior cerebral artery gives off two posterior choroidal arteries — the medial branch, which supplies the choroid plexus in the third ventricle, and the lateral branch, which supplies the choroid plexus in the lateral ventricle. Branches also pass to the neighboring structures. The arteries first run parallel to the posterior cerebral and then, in the choroid fissure, swing around the medial posterior part of the thalamus to proceed upward in a concave curve forward. They extend at the same time in a medial direction and run laterally to and over the pineal body up into the tela choroidea of the third ventricle. Here, near the midline, they meet the internal cerebral

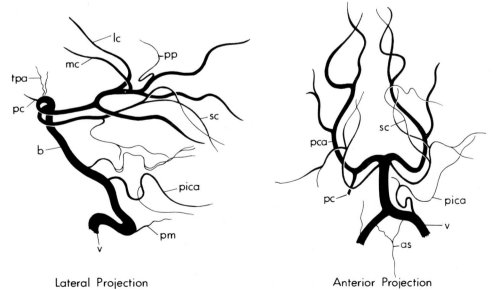

Lateral Projection   Anterior Projection

FIGURE 5–45 Vertebral arteriogram. v = vertebral artery. pm = posterior meningeal artery. pica = posterior inferior cerebellar artery. b = basilar artery. pc = posterior communicating artery. tpa = thalamoperforating arteries. sc = superior cerebellar artery. pp = posterior pericallosal artery. mc = medial posterior choroidal artery. lc = lateral posterior choroidal artery. as = anterior spinal artery. pca = posterior cerebral artery.

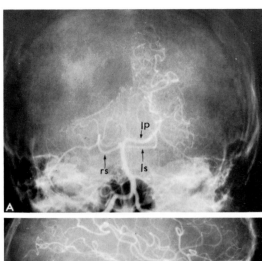
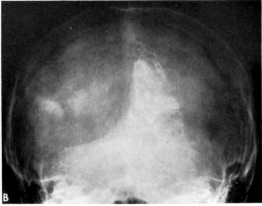
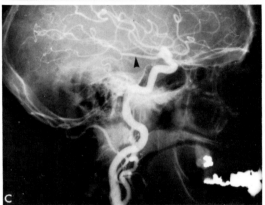

FIGURE 5–46 *A*. Vertebral angiogram showing filling of the right superior cerebellar artery (rs), the left superior cerebellar artery (ls) and the left posterior cerebellar artery (lp). *B*. Later phase in the same angiogram shows opacification of cerebellar vessels on the right side and of the cerebellar vessels and the territory of the posterior cerebral artery. The asymmetry here is accounted for by the lack of filling of the right posterior cerebral artery, which arose from the carotid artery. *C*. Right carotid angiogram. The posterior cerebral artery (*arrow*) is filling from the carotid artery and not from the basilar artery.

vein, which they follow anteriorly in the roof of the third ventricle. The lateral posterior choroidal artery passes through the intraventricular foramen and supplies the choroid plexus in the upper part of the lateral ventricles. Only rarely can these vessels be identified in the anteroposterior projection. In the lateral view, two main arteries are usually distinguished, one on either side, each running a convex curve backward and upward from the posterior cerebral artery toward the interventricular foramen (Figs. 5–45 and 5–48). Except for deviations of a few millimeters, the pathways of these two main vessels usually coincide. A number of finer vessels are also seen along their course, but sometimes the branches are more distinct. The lateral posterior choroidal arteries form the largest curve, and situated anterior to them are the medial posterior choroidal arteries forming more narrow curves.

The main branch of the posterior choroidal artery arises from the posterior

cerebral artery 1 to 2 mm posterior to the basilar artery. It usually runs backward together with the posterior cerebral artery, but in 15 per cent of cases, it courses 2 to 5 mm above and parallel to the posterior cerebral artery, which it then leaves in an upward curve. As a rule, the posterior choroidal arteries on either side differ from one another by only a few millimeters. There is no difference in the adult and in the child.[116]

Posterior Communicating Arteries

The posterior communicating and the anterior portion of the posterior cerebral artery give off some small branches—the thalamoperforating arteries — extending backward and upward. In 71 per cent of cases, according to Krayenbühl and Yasargil, one or both posterior communicating arteries filled.[101] The posterior communicating arteries were not seen in 29 per cent of cases (Figs. 5–38 and 5–49). The poste-

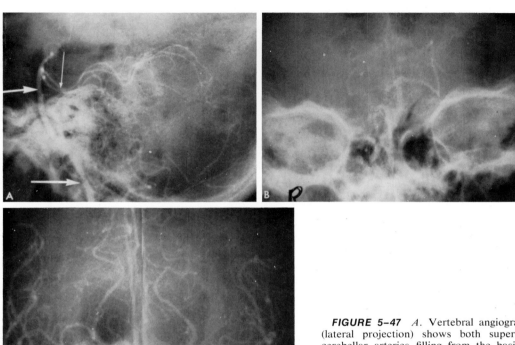

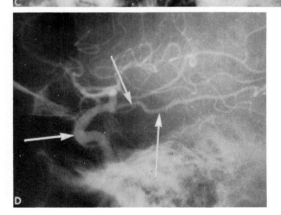

FIGURE 5–47 *A*. Vertebral angiogram (lateral projection) shows both superior cerebellar arteries filling from the basilar artery. *B*. Anteroposterior projection also shows both superior cerebellar arteries filling from the basilar artery. *C*. Both posterior cerebral arteries arise from the carotid arteries. *D*. Origin of the left posterior cerebral artery in the lateral projection.

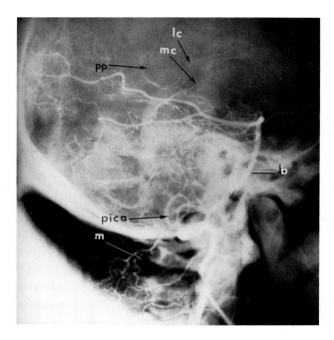

FIGURE 5-48 Vertebral angiogram. The lateral posterior choroidal arteries (lc) and the medial posterior choroidal arteries (mc) are outlined arising from the posterior cerebral artery. Note the course of the posterior pericallosal artery (pp) passing around the splenium of the corpus callosum. The posterior inferior cerebellar artery (pica) and the muscular branches (m) of the vertebral artery are identified. Note the basilar artery (b) parallel to the clivus.

rior pericallosal artery (artery of the splenium of the corpus callosum) is sometimes seen arising from the posterior cerebral artery. It passes forward beneath the splenium to double back on itself and pass over the splenium of the corpus callosum (Fig. 5-48). The significance of this vessel is discussed in the section on the abnormal angiogram.[58]

Anastomoses of Vertebral-Basilar Tree with Carotid Tree

The vertebral and basilar tree anastomoses with the carotid tree in the following sites: (1) the posterior communicating artery and (2) the occipital branch of the external carotid artery and the vertebral artery in the neck (Fig. 5-49), (3) the

FIGURE 5-49 Vertebral angiogram. Both posterior communicating (PC) have filled and the anterior and middle cerebral arteries (MC) are outlined. The muscular branches of the vertebral artery are anastamosing with the occipital branch (M and O) of the external carotid artery and other branches of the external carotid artery (EC) have filled.

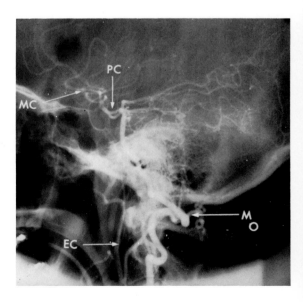

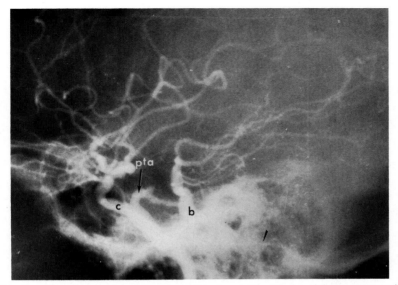

FIGURE 5-50 Carotid angiogram. The internal carotid artery (c) has filled, and the contrast medium has passed via a persistent trigeminal artery (pta) to the basilar artery (b). The vertebral artery on the same side of the trigeminal artery is usually absent.

anterior and posterior choroidal arteries, (4) the parieto-occipital and callosomarginal branches, and (5) the posterior pericallosal artery and the pericallosal artery (Fig. 5-48), and (6) the persistent trigeminal artery (Fig. 5-50).

Radiological Anatomy of the Venous System

The venous system may be conveniently described under the dural sinuses and superficial cortical veins, and the deep cerebral veins.

Dural Sinuses and Superficial Cortical Veins

The superficial sagittal or longitudinal sinus usually originates just above the nasion, and as it extends backward it increases in caliber to pass to the torcular Herophili and thence to the transverse or lateral sinuses to the jugular vein. The right lateral sinus is larger than the left, and not infrequently the superior sagittal sinus drains directly into the right transverse sinus. The cortical veins usually pass upward and enter the sagittal sinus against the stream (except the most anterior two or three tributaries). Streaming is often present where opacified and unopacified blood mix. This accounts for thinning of the stream of contrast medium, which should not be mistaken for an organic defect (Fig. 5-51).

The inferior sagittal sinus courses in the free margin of the falx. The great vein of Galen passes into the straight sinus at the level of the junction of the free margin of the falx and the tentorial opening, and is directed backward and downward to enter the torcular. The petrosal sinuses are frequently identified and may provide a clue to the presence of angle tumors. The vein of Trolard is the largest superficial draining vein that enters the sinus. The vein of Labbé anastomoses with the vein of Trolard and usually enters the transverse sinus. The superficial middle cerebral vein runs in the sylvian fissure downward, outlining the temporal lobe, to enter the cavernous sinus. The dural sinuses are usually undisplaced by acquired cerebral disease. The deep cerebral veins may be displaced and are much more constant in position in the normal phlebogram.

Deep Cerebral Veins

The internal cerebral vein begins at the foramen of Monro by the union of the

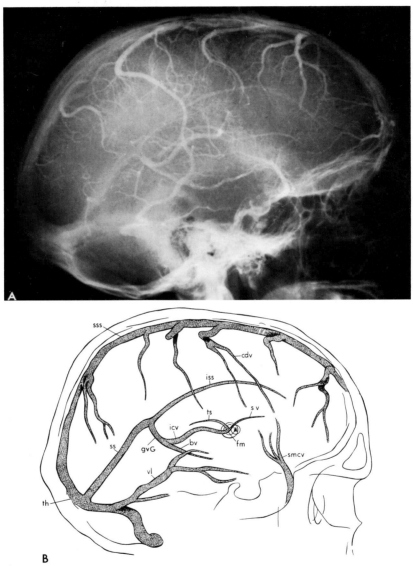

B

FIGURE 5–51   *A*. Venous phase of a carotid angiogram. *B*. Identification of structures shown in *A*. sss = superior sagittal sinus. ss = straight sinus. th = torcular Herophili. gvG = great vein of Galen. bv = basilar vein. icv = internal cerebral vein. ts = thalamostriate vein. fm = region of <u>foramen magnum</u> (i.e., junction of thalamostriate and septal and internal cerebral vein). sv = septal vein. smcv = superficial middle cerebral vein. cdv = cortical draining vein. iss = inferior sagittal sinus.

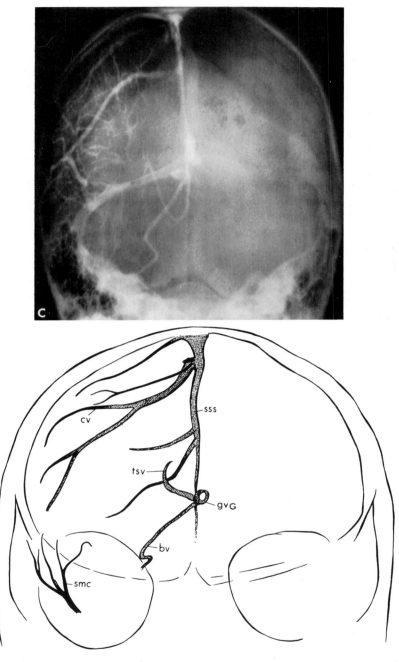

FIGURE 5–51 *(Continued)* *C.* Venous phase of a carotid angiogram. There is some slight ventricular dilatation present. *D.* Identification of structures shown in *C.* sss = superior sagittal sinus. gvG = great vein of Galen. bv = basilar vein. tsv = thalamostriate vein. cv = cortical vein. smc = superficial middle cerebral vein.

thalamostriate vein and the septal vein. The vessel is paired and runs in the roof of the third ventricle in the midline. The veins are arched upward and unite at the level of the quadrigeminal cistern to become the great vein of Galen. The thalamostriate vein is formed by veins from the walls of the lateral ventricle and the choroid plexus (Fig. 5–51 A and B). The ependymal veins, if well opacified, will outline the lateral ventricles (Fig. 5–52). The thalamostriate vein, traced backward from the internal cerebral vein, extends backward and slightly upward in the groove between the caudate nucleus and the thalamus. In this portion it outlines the inferolateral aspect of the lateral ventricle. In the lateral projection the thalamostriate vein runs parallel to the internal cerebral vein. In the frontal projection, the vein has the shape of the horns of an African cow (Fig. 5–53). With ventricular dilatation, the arc becomes much wider, resembling a pair of short horns.[189] This is a much more reliable sign of ventricular dilatation than the shape of the anterior cerebral artery. The point where the thalamostriate vein enters the internal cerebral vein usually relates to the foramen of Monro. This has, therefore, been called

the venous angle by Krayenbühl and Richter (Fig. 5–43).[100] Occasionally the thalamostriate vein enters the internal cerebral vein posterior to the foramen of Monro; here it forms a false venous angle and apparent shortening of the internal cerebral vein (Fig. 5–54).

The basilar vein or the vein of Rosenthal originates at the level of the temporal horn and anterior perforating substance in a group of small veins resembling a fine web. The vein passes backward around the brain stem to join the internal cerebral immediately before the origin of the great cerebral vein. The course of the basilar vein is similar to that of the posterior cerebral artery.

The veins of the posterior fossa may be divided into three groups: a superior group draining superiorly or deeply into the galenic system; an anterior group draining anteriorly into the petrosal sinuses; and a posterior group draining posteriorly or laterally into the torcular and neighboring straight and lateral sinuses.[81]

The anterior pontomesencephalic vein lies in front of the pons and extends into the depth of the interpeduncular fossa. The precentral cerebellar vein lies in the depth

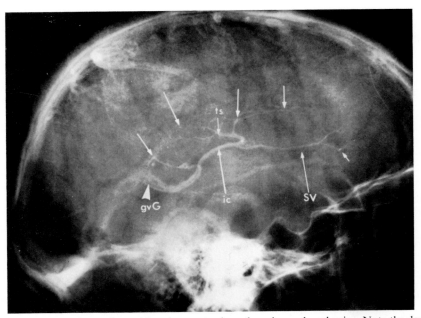

FIGURE 5–52   Venous phase of carotid angiogram to show the subependymal veins. Note the dense shadows created by the veins as they reverse direction. The shape and size of the ventricle can be determined from these shadows. ic = internal cerebral vein. ts = thalamostriate veins. gvG = great vein of Galen. Arrows point to subependymal veins (SV).

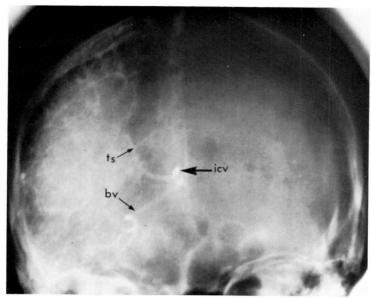

FIGURE 5–53 Venous phase of a carotid angiogram. ts = thalamostriate vein. bv = basilar vein. icv = internal cerebral vein. Note that there is some ventricular dilatation present.

of the precentral cerebellar fissure. A detailed account of this venous drainage system is outside the scope of this text. The reader, if interested in more detail, is referred to the excellent work of Wolf, Huang, and Newman.[226]

THE ABNORMAL ANGIOGRAM

Extracranial Lesions

Vascular Occlusive Disease

Ischemic lesions of the brain may result from occlusive disease anywhere along the arterial tree leading to the brain. The common occurrence of infarction of the brain without demonstrable vascular occlusion confirms the observations of many previous workers. Recent publications have stressed the high incidence of extracranial vascular disease as a localized entity.[55] Fields and co-workers claim that over 25 per cent of strokes have their causative lesions situated extracranially.[51] In some centers the operative correction of these lesions has been emphasized.[33, 41, 162]

The clinical picture produced by carotid occlusion is variable and may mimic other conditions such as neoplasms and space-occupying lesions. Even the most astute neurologists will, in some cases, admit to difficulty in distinguishing clinically between an internal carotid occlusion in the neck and one in the branches of the vessel in the head. Silverstein and associates examined 30 patients with proved occlusion of the common and internal carotid arteries in an attempt to evaluate certain procedures considered diagnostic for carotid occlusion.[195] Diminished carotid pulsations were present in only 17 per cent of these patients. An increase in carotid pulsations was reported, in two cases, on the occluded side. Carotid or intracranial bruits were not very helpful. Response to manual compression of the carotid artery was positive in 70 per cent of these cases, but many false positives do occur. Ophthalmodynamometric differences in retinal artery pressure were a fairly good diagnostic test. These clinical diagnostic modalities would sometimes, therefore, appear to be misleading, but a positive reaction would justify further investigation with angiography. Angiography plays a major role in the investigation and evaluation of patients with strokes. Many centers still limit their radiological examinations to the intracranial vasculature despite publications that emphasize the high incidence of an extracranial lesion being responsible for the patient's condition.[51]

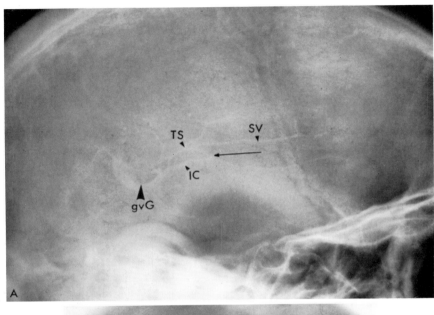

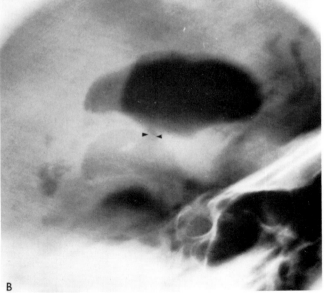

FIGURE 5-54 *A.* Venous phase of a carotid angiogram. The arrow directed towards the white dot is a false venous angle and does not represent the position of the foramen of Monro, which is identified in *B.* SV = septal vein. TS = thalamostriate vein. gvG = great vein of Galen. IC = internal cerebral vein. *B.* Air study showing the dilated ventricular system. The two arrows are directed to the foramen of Monro. Note that this does not correspond with the false venous angle.

Recent investigations have shown occlusive arterial disease in the cervical vessels in up to 80 per cent of patients with "stroke." Stenosis of the internal carotid artery at the bifurcation and stenosis of the vertebral artery at its origin are the most frequent findings. In 16 patients, all with severe neurological deficits, examined with aortocervical angiography as well as with selective angiography of the carotid and vertebral arteries, occlusive disease was found in 88 per cent. In 35 patients, many with intermittent strokes, examination with aortocervical angiography alone revealed disease in only 63 per cent. Aortocervical angiography alone revealed changes in the clinically relevant vessel in only 39 per cent, but selective angiography of the relevant vessel disclosed occlusive disease in 68 per cent of cases. These figures would indicate the value of a very careful investigation of the vascular tree, including selective vessel opacification. The validity of published reports of the incidence of disease may indeed be questioned when such a work-up is not undertaken. The incidence of carotid narrowing or occlusion in routine unselected autopsies is as high as 9.5 per cent.[55] By far the most common cause is atherosclerosis. The most common site of involvement is the carotid bifurcation.[8] Hutchinson and Yates reviewed 100 patients who came to necropsy as the result of a cerebrovascular lesion or whose clinical history suggested such an event in the past.[85, 86] In these 100 cases, the complete lengths of the vertebral and the carotid arteries were examined both radiologically and by dissection. Their findings indicate that unless the arch of the aorta is opacified with contrast medium during angiography, the origin of the major vessels leading from it will not be seen. Thus, occlusive disease of the origin of the common carotid and vertebral arteries will be missed. Significant stenosis or occlusion of the carotid artery was more common than of the vertebral artery. In 5 per cent of cases a carotid and a vertebral artery were involved, the same incidence as for bilateral carotid involvement. The pathological basis was always atheroma with an occasional addition of either old or recent thrombosis. A not uncommon finding was hemorrhage into the base of the plaques of atheroma.

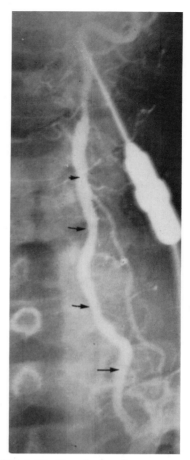

FIGURE 5-55 Vertebral angiogram. Note that at each level of cervical spondylosis there is narrowing of the caliber of the vertebral artery.

Recently the ulcerated atheroma appearing in the extracranial carotid circulation has been incriminated as a source of intracranial emboli. The most common sites of involvement were the internal carotid artery just beyond its origin near the bifurcation of the common carotid artery and the origin of the vertebral artery. Yates stressed the importance of cervical spondylosis and its effects on the cervical portion of the vertebral arteries (Fig. 5-55).[233] Bony outgrowths may displace the vessel, which, if already narrowed by atheroma, may undergo complete occlusion with movements of the neck. DeKleyn, Sheehan et al., and Maslowski have shown the effect of extension and rotation of the neck on the vertebral artery.[35, 124, 192]

Of 646 patients examined angiographically by Fields and co-workers for symptoms suggesting cerebral insufficiency, 16 were found to have complete occlusions bilaterally.[52] The lesion usually involves the internal carotid artery just at and beyond its origin from the common carotid artery, but may extend to involve the external and common carotid arteries (Fig. 5–56). Little or no neurological deficit may occur even with complete occlusion, providing that adequate collateral channels are functioning. These channels may be via the circle of Willis or via the collaterals of the external carotid circulation.

Sites of anastomosis between the internal cerebral circulation and the extracranial circulation occur between the middle meningeal artery and the ophthalmic artery and between the superficial temporal artery, external maxillary artery, and the ophthalmic artery (Fig. 5–57). The occipital branch of the external carotid artery frequently anastomoses with the muscular branches of the vertebral artery in the upper cervical region (Fig. 5–58). Intracranial anastomoses between the major vessels and their branches occur at the circle of Willis between the two anterior cerebral arteries through the anterior communicating artery, and the two posterior communicating arteries. The cortical branches of the anterior, middle, and posterior cerebral arteries anastomose over the surface of the cortex (Fig. 5–59), and there is an anastomosis between the anterior and posterior choroidal arteries. The collateral circulation has been most adequately covered in the literature.[3, 48, 132, 182, 210, 213, 218]

Occlusive disease of the subclavian artery proximal to the origin of the vertebral artery may result in a reversal of blood flow in the ipsilateral vertebral artery from the basilar artery and thence to the subclavian artery beyond its point of occlusion. Contorni first described this interesting phenomenon, later named the "subclavian steal" by Reivich et al.[25, 158] This reverse flow in the vertebral artery may deprive the brain of blood and result in cerebral ischemia. It may occur also in occlusion of the innominate artery when blood will reach the right vertebral, right subclavian, and right common carotid arteries via the basilar artery and the opposite vertebral artery. Other neck vessels may take part in establishing the flow to the occluded vessel.

Reports have appeared of kinks in the carotid and vertebral arteries that have resulted in ischemic attacks.[9, 62, 71, 84, 155, 160] Hurwitt and co-workers state that kinked and buckled internal carotid arteries may be

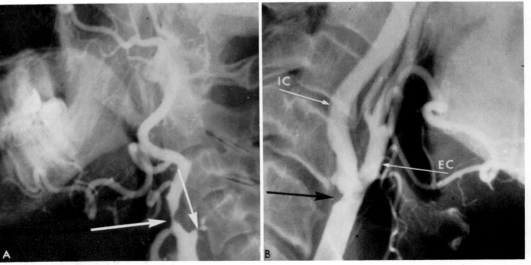

FIGURE 5–56 *A.* A carotid angiogram demonstrating complete occlusion of the internal carotid artery at its origin and a severe degree of narrowing of the external carotid artery. *B.* A defect in the lumen of the internal carotid artery at its origin (*black arrow*). IC = internal carotid artery. EC = external carotid artery.

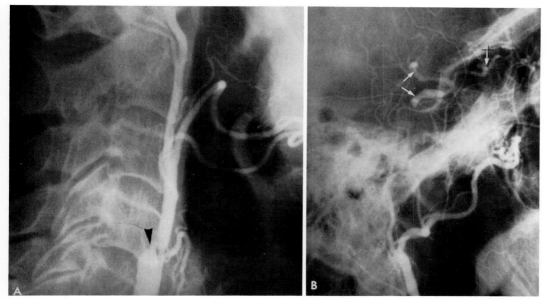

FIGURE 5-57 *A*. Carotid occlusion just beyond the origin of the internal carotid artery. There is also some narrowing of the lumen of the external carotid artery. *B*. Filling of the carotid siphon (→) via extracranial anastomoses such as the ophthalmic artery (↦).

FIGURE 5-58 A vertebral angiogram in a patient with occlusion of the common carotid artery. Note filling of the vertebral artery (1), the basilar artery (2), the posterior communicating artery (3), the anterior and middle cerebral arteries (4), and filling of the occipital branch of the external carotid (5) and other branches (6) of the external carotid artery via the anastomosis in the neck between the muscular branches of the vertebral artery and the occipital artery. Note that the flow in the external carotid artery has reversed itself. On occasions the reverse flow continues from the external carotid artery to the bifurcation and then becomes anterograde up the internal carotid artery.

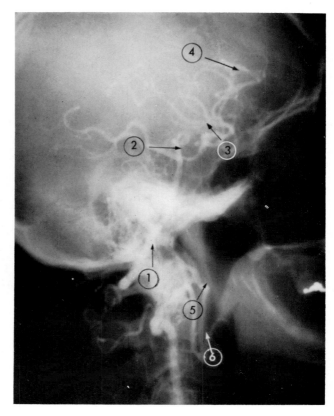

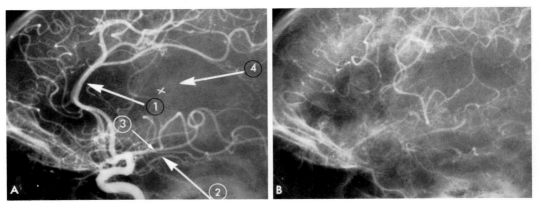

FIGURE 5–59 *A.* A carotid angiogram with filling of both anterior cerebral arteries (1), the anterior choroidal (2), and the posterior branches of the middle cerebral artery (3). The major branches of the island of Reil are missing; their absence results in a bare area (x and 4). *B.* Branches of the island of Reil filling retrogradely via the anterior cerebral artery branches.

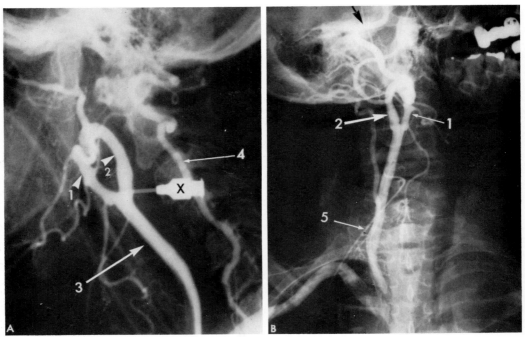

FIGURE 5–60 Right common carotid angiogram. *A.* Note that there is a kink in the internal carotid artery (2) without the passage of contrast medium beyond this point. The external carotid artery and its branches (1) have filled, and contrast has passed retrogradely down the common carotid artery (3) to the subclavian artery and anterogradely up the vertebral artery (4). Note the irregularities in the lumen of the vertebral artery. The needle (X) is artefactitious and is not related to the angiographic study. *B.* With the neck rotated, the kink no longer obstructs the flow of contrast into the internal carotid artery (*black arrow*). The polyethylene catheter (5) is in the common carotid artery.

obstructed just as effectively as those with internal blocking lesions (Fig. 5–60).[84] Rarely do kinking and tortuosity of cerebral arteries alone give rise to symptoms of cerebral ischemia.[9] This is usually an incidental finding. However, in cases of diffuse atherosclerotic disease, stenosis and vertebral artery compression by osteophytes (Fig. 5–55), loops, or kinks in a vessel may further embarrass the cerebral circulation and result in ischemic attacks. In 241 patients with cerebrovascular disease, Harrison and Davalos operatively corrected buckling or tortuosity of carotid arteries in 39 of 46 cases demonstrating this phenomenon.[71] The curves in the vessel varied from S or V shapes to complete loops.

Aneurysms and Arterial Buckling

Dissecting aneurysms of the carotid artery are usually caused by trauma, the result of a subintimal injection of contrast medium or blunt injury to the neck. A rare spontaneous dissecting aneurysm of the internal carotid artery was reported by Anderson and Schechter.[4]

Aneurysms in the neck are rare. A pulsatile swelling in the neck is not infrequently misdiagnosed as an aneurysm. Tortuous and kinked vessels may be mistaken for aneurysms. Buckling or kinking of the major vessels in the neck occurs when the atherosclerotic aorta elongates and unfolds, and shadows of the tortuous vessels in the neck may be mistaken for aneurysms (Fig. 5–61).[187] In a case recently investigated by the author, the patient had received antimalarial, arsenical, and penicillin medications over a period of 20 years for a swelling in the neck diagnosed 20 years ago as an aneurysm of the carotid artery. A bruit and thrill in the neck were elicited. An angiogram demonstrated a large carotid body tumor (see Fig. 5–66). Sutton reported a pulsatile mass in the tonsillar fossa that at angiography proved to be a large carotid aneurysm in the cavernous sinus that had eroded through the base of the skull and had presented in the tonsillar fossa.[205] One pulsatile mass in the tonsillar fossa examined angiographically by the author was a kink in the internal carotid artery; a second patient with a

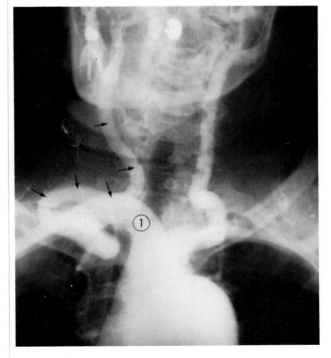

FIGURE 5–61 Elongation of the major vessels in the neck has led to tortuous vessels. The innominate artery is particularly prominent (1) and was mistaken for an aneurysm. Note the tortuous elongated course of the right carotid artery (*arrows*).

similar clinical presentation had an aneurysm of the internal carotid artery, which was resected with an end-to-end anastamosis of the carotid artery stumps.[24] Ullrich and Sugar reported a case of a carotid aneurysm in the neck with four other aneurysms in the head of the same patient.[217] Alexander et al. reported a case of bilateral extracranial aneurysms of the carotid arteries.[2] Other reports of extracranial aneurysms have appeared in the literature.[102,171] The internal carotid artery is almost invariably the vessel involved (Fig. 5–62).

Arteriovenous Fistulae

Most arteriovenous fistulae in the neck result from trauma, although there have

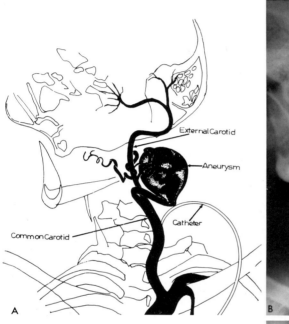

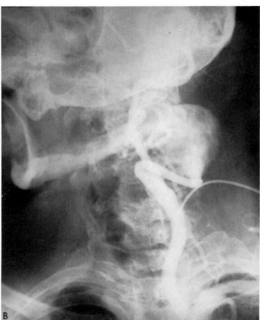

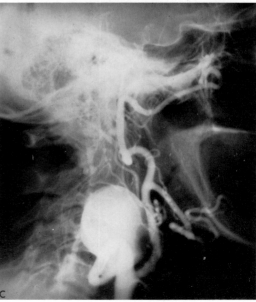

FIGURE 5–62 Aneurysm of the internal carotid artery. *A* and *B*. Note that the external carotid artery is unaffected. The tortuous internal carotid artery enters directly into the aneurysm. *C*. The lateral projection of the angiogram shows this to best advantage.

been reports in the literature of their spontaneous occurrence. In a case reported elsewhere, this appeared to develop spontaneously in a patient at rest, while listening to the radio.[65] Four weeks before hospitalization, the patient noted the sudden onset of occipital pain followed two hours later by a swishing noise in the head. On examination a to and fro murmur was heard over the posterior triangle of the neck. A vertebral angiogram demonstrated the fistula. Aronson reported a case of an arteriovenous fistula of the vertebral artery that followed trauma in a 23-year-old patient who, falling from a truck, struck his neck on the sharp corner of a box.[5] Arteriovenous fistulae of the vertebral artery have been described following percutaneous vertebral arteriography. Stab wounds (Fig. 5–63) and missile injuries are the most

common cause.[236] Arteriovenous fistulae of the common carotid artery and jugular vein are rare and are usually associated with trauma. The author has demonstrated a fistula between the occipital artery and an adjacent vein that was caused by a gunshot wound. Tori and Garusi reported a case of a carotid-jugular fistula in which preoperative and postoperative angiography were performed in a 5-year-old child.[216] When the communication is large, the rapid shunting of blood from the arterial to the venous side may result in poor filling of the intracranial vessels. The carotid artery will also hypertrophy, and the arterialized large dilated jugular vein will be outlined almost immediately after the carotid opacification. Cardiomegaly follows large fistulae of some duration, as may heart failure. We recently had the opportunity to investigate

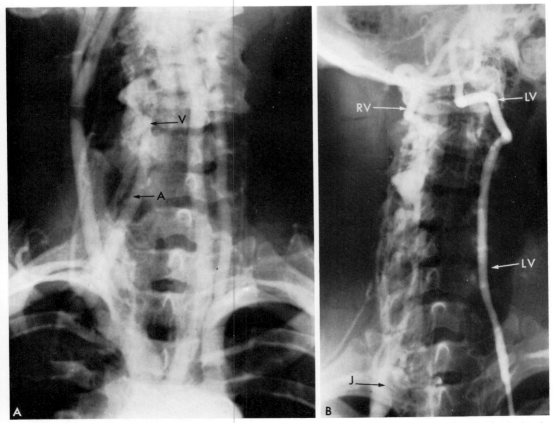

FIGURE 5–63 This patient was stabbed in the neck and developed a marked "whooshing" sound in the head. The weapon penetrated the vertebral artery and the surrounding venous plexus. *A.* An aortic arch study shows the fistula between (A) the right vertebral artery and (V) the dilated veins. *B.* A left vertebral angiogram via the femoral artery shows the catheter in the left vertebral artery with opacification of the left (LV) and right (RV) vertebral artery. Large veins can be seen transporting the contrast medium to the jugular veins (J).

a 23-year-old man, retarded since birth, who was admitted for revision of an operatively induced right carotid-jugular fistula. This had been performed in 1949 to enhance cerebral blood flow and improve the patient's mental condition. The patient now presented with incipient cardiac failure. The large arterialized aneurysm of the jugular vein was resected (Fig. 5–64).

Congenital Lesions

The common carotid artery usually bifurcates opposite the third and fourth cervical vertebral bodies. It may, however, bifurcate at a much lower level. Anomalous origins of the carotid and vertebral arteries have been described. The incidence of these congenital anomalies has been placed as high as 52.3 per cent in the Negro adult male and 22.6 per cent in the Caucasian adult male. DeGaris and associates in postmortem examinations of 203 adult Negro males found 16 different patterns of

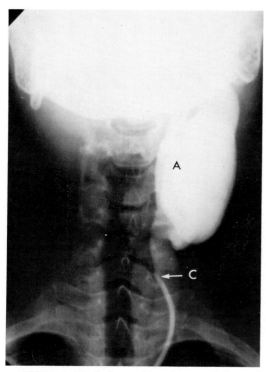

FIGURE 5–64 Left carotid angiogram via femoral catheterization with the catheter in the carotid artery (C). The large arterialized aneurysm of the jugular vein is well outlined (A).

branches of the aortic arch.[34] Some variation of the origin of the major vessels from the aorta was found in 75 per cent of stillborn fetuses studied by barium injection and dissection of the aortic arch.[238] Fisher reported a case of complete absence of both carotid arteries.[54] Many such congenital anomalies may be missed in a carotid angiogram unless the origin of these vessels is examined with particular attention.

Congenital anomalies of the origin of the vertebral artery appear to be more common than those of the carotid artery. The one vertebral artery may be absent in caroticobasilar anastomoses, and the vertebral artery may arise from the carotid artery.[131, 202] Lindgren cited four cases in which the vertebral artery arose from the carotid artery in the neck, and Hauge also reported two cases in which the vertebral artery arose from sites other than the subclavian artery.[76, 110] Krayenbühl and Yasargil have noted quite a few variations of origin of the vertebral arteries in their postmortem studies.[101] Figure 5–65 shows the origin of the left vertebral artery from the arch of the aorta.

Variations in the second part of the course of the vertebral artery are rare. The vertebral artery may enter the foramen transversarium at a level above C6, but entry at C3 has been described by Silvan.[194] The present author has encountered a similar case (Fig. 5–36). Rivaglia has seen a vertebral artery leave the canal between C2 and C3 to enter the foramen magnum.[161]

Carotid Body Tumors

These are usually benign tumors that may invade locally. They are usually single, although Engstrom and Hamberger reported a case of bilateral carotid body tumors studied angiographically.[45] The present author has recently examined such a case. These tumors have a very characteristic appearance and, as previously stated, are often mistaken clinically for carotid aneurysms. Their extreme vascularity renders them pulsatile. The radiological appearances reported in 13 cases examined by the author were quite characteristic. Because of the extreme vascularity of the lesion, contrast medium introduced into the common carotid artery is soaked up

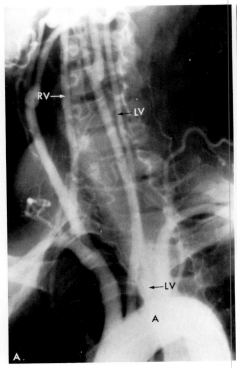

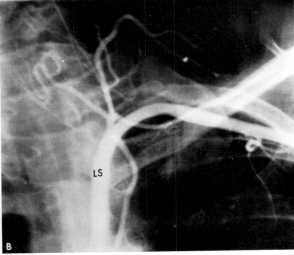

FIGURE 5–65 *A*. Arch study with tip of the catheter in ascending aorta. Note that the left vertebral artery (LV) arises directly from the arch of the aorta (A). RV = right vertebral artery. *B*. Left subclavian artery (LS) shows no origin of the left vertebral artery. (Case by kind permission of Dr. P. Rossi.)

like a sponge by the tumor that arises over the carotid body at the bifurcation of the common carotid artery and usually engulfs the vessel, narrowing its lumen.[179] One of the most characteristic changes observed was the separation of the internal and external carotid arteries by the tumor mass (Fig. 5–66).[24]

False Occlusive Patterns of the Vessels in the Neck

The false passage of the needle with the introduction of contrast medium subintimally sometimes mimics the radiological appearances of occlusive and stenotic disease.[59, 133, 136, 181] An injection beneath the intima of the artery may occlude the vessel temporarily and produce a pattern not unlike that of organic disease (Fig. 5–15). The flow distal to this point may be very slow and may simulate a narrowed lumen of the vessel, and sometimes the flow may be slowed to such an extent that streaming and layering of the heavier contrast medium may take place (Fig. 5–67). A needle or catheter in the external carotid artery may

result in filling of only the external carotid artery and suggest internal carotid occlusion. This may not be recognized by the novice, but a film of the neck including the tip of the needle and the bifurcation of the carotid artery would clarify the position.

Spasm

It is sometimes difficult to distinguish radiologically between spasm and occlusive disease. Vessels in spasm usually show gradual tapering. Factors exciting spasm are, for example, contrast in the vessel wall or in the tissues outside the vessel, or a catheter threaded high up the carotid artery. A frequent site of spasm in vertebral angiography is the point where the vertebral artery crosses over the arch of C1. The change in the caliber of vessels during angiography has been demonstrated and supports the diagnosis of spasm.

The significance of internal carotid artery occlusion at its origin has already been discussed. Rarely is the disease process situated further along the course of the vessel in the neck, although propagation of the

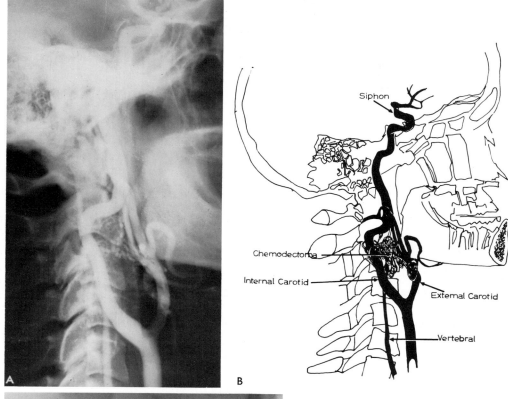

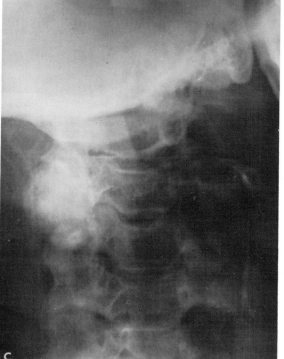

FIGURE 5–66 Carotid body tumor, mistaken clinically for an aneurysm of the carotid artery. *A* and *B*. Note the characteristic separation of the internal and external carotid arteries and the highly vascular tumor supplied by the external carotid artery and the vertebral artery. *C*. The marked vascularity of the tumor with an irregular margin is demonstrated.

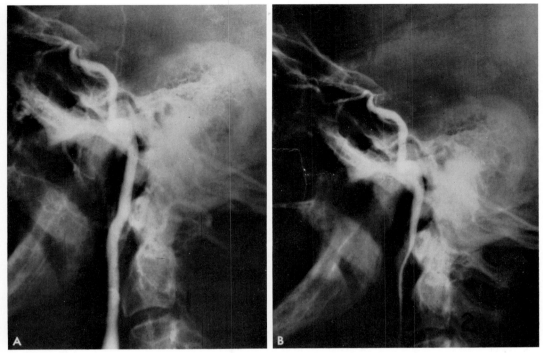

FIGURE 5-67 Internal carotid artery occlusion just distal to the origin of the ophthalmic artery. Because of slow flow, there is poor mixing of blood and contrast medium. The contrast medium with a higher specific gravity hugs the most dependent parts, in this case the posterior wall of the cervical internal carotid artery (the patient was in the supine position during this angiogram). The "streaming phenomenon" must be kept in mind when evaluating occlusive disease. *A.* The ophthalmic artery allows a runoff of the blood–contrast agent mixture, but it is slow enough to prevent through and through mixing. *B.* Further runoff through the ophthalmic artery has occurred, and unopacified blood is now passing along the carotid artery, above the attenuated layer of contrast medium.

thrombus distally from this point usually occurs. The region of the carotid siphon is not uncommonly involved, and linear streaks of calcification in this region seen on the plain film may direct one's attention to this area.

Intracranial Lesions

Occlusive Disease

Although angiography has proved to be a most valuable diagnostic test in revealing vascular occlusive disease in the neck, it has perhaps been less rewarding in the evaluation of patients who have suffered an occlusion of a vessel in the head. Various authors have indicated how erroneous the clinical diagnosis of stroke may be. The clinical diagnosis is often upset by the angiographic findings, and even the most astute physicians often find themselves unable to distinguish between middle cerebral occlusion and internal carotid artery occlusion before angiography. Various factors may be responsible for the so-called negative angiogram in the presence of a stroke. Autopsy casts of the cerebral arterial tree reveal an abundance of vessels. Even after the cast of the arterial tree is pruned, it is obvious and not surprising that only the larger branches of the part that remains will be represented and recognized in an angiogram during life. It is not surprising, therefore, that occlusion of a branch might remain unrecognized. Occlusion of a vessel may not be recognized when collateral vessels take over to irrigate the area deprived of its blood supply. Retrograde flow with a delay in local filling would confirm the presence of an occluded vessel, an observation that may only be made if serial films are taken.

Angiography may occasionally reveal a contrast stain in the presence of an infarct. Although most authors deny that there is anatomical evidence for the existence of direct connections between arteries and veins in the human brain, Hasegawa claims their presence.[72] Feindel and Perot have observed at operation cerebral veins partly or wholly filled with a stream of arterial blood.[49] These authors have outlined two major groups of cases showing this phenomenon: those in which there are structural changes, such as arteriovenous malformations, and those in which a local region of brain such as an infarct, uses oxygen inadequately. Cronqvist demonstrated a very specific angiographic pattern, which is characterized by regional rapid passage of the contrast medium.[28] Hence, early filling of veins may, on occasion, occur with a contrast blush. The regional hyperemia is due to the vasodilatory effects of the hypoxic tissue. Lassen refers to this as a state of "luxury perfusion," an unfortunate term since the tissue has an impaired oxygen consumption.[107] Poverty perfusion might perhaps be a more appropriate term. The presence of early-filling veins is not restricted to infarcts. When an early-draining vein is questioned in an angiogram, it is often helpful to examine the venous phase and trace the vessels backward to the arterial phase. I have found this useful in distinguishing between an early-draining vein and an artery.

Middle cerebral artery occlusion is more readily recognized in the lateral projection than in the anteroposterior, since the branches of the middle cerebral artery are superimposed in the latter and occlusion of a single branch of the middle cerebral artery may not be so obvious. When the main stem of the middle cerebral artery is occluded, the stump of the vessel may be seen (Fig. 5–68A). Occlusion of the ascending frontoparietal artery is readily recognized, but nonfilling of the other branches is not as easily appreciated. With serial films, vessels irrigating the middle cerebral territory may be seen to fill in the late arterial stage from collateral supply from the anterior and posterior cerebral arteries (Fig. 5–68B and C).

The diagnosis of occlusion of the anterior cerebral artery on the basis of angiographic appearances must be made with caution, since anatomical variations of the circle of Willis are so frequent. Filling of an anterior cerebral artery after contralateral compression or injection of the other side may occur.

The radiological diagnosis of posterior cerebral artery occlusion must also be made with caution. In about one third of cases the posterior cerebral artery is of the fetal type and arises from the carotid artery. On occasion, vertebral angiography will show filling of only the superior cerebellar arteries, because both posterior cerebral arteries fill from the carotid artery (Fig. 5–47). Anatomical studies of the circle of Willis explain the frequency of variation in the posterior circulation.[3, 102, 144, 227] In all cases of nonfilling of a posterior cerebral artery, ipsilateral injection of the carotid artery must be done before the significance of this lack of opacification can be fully appreciated.

Factors apart from the anatomy may also be involved in the nonfilling of vessels. The differential in heads of pressure of the two vertebral arteries, spasm in the vessels, and the rate of injection may all influence the filling of individual branches of the circle of Willis. Saltzman has shown that by compressing the ipsilateral vertebral artery during carotid artery injection, filling of the posterior cerebral was frequently achieved when a previous injection had been unsuccessful.[172] Mones reported nonfilling of the posterior cerebral artery from either the basilar or ipsilateral carotid artery in four patients.[128] All these patients had homonymous field defects contralateral to the nonfilled artery. No postmortem confirmation was obtained.

The neuroradiologist is not frequently asked to undertake angiography on a patient who presents with the "classic" symptoms and signs of basilar thrombosis. This is a disease that usually does not respond to treatment currently available. It is more common for basilar thrombosis to be demonstrated radiologically in a situation of clinical uncertainty. Various angiographic factors must be seriously considered and their effects evaluated before the diagnosis may be made. Factors such as streaming, spasm, washout from the opposite vertebral artery, temporary occlusion of the vertebral

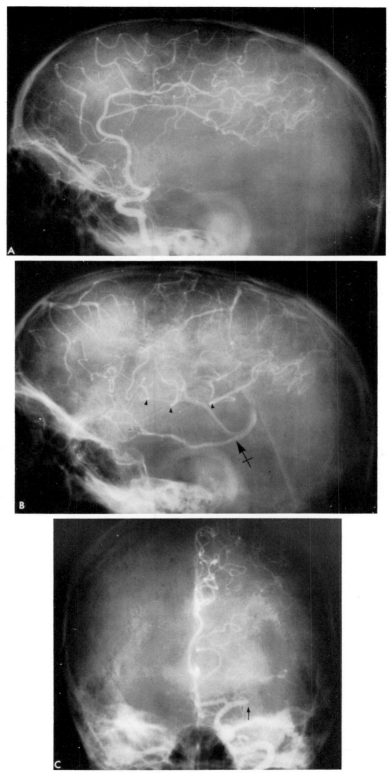

FIGURE 5-68 *A*. Lateral carotid angiogram showing nonfilling of branches of the middle cerebral artery. Only a stump (a few millimeters) has filled (cf. *C*). *B*. A later phase of the carotid angiogram. This now shows retrograde filling of branches of the middle cerebral artery (→). Note that these have eventually filled at a stage when the cortical veins and deep veins and dural sinus are filling (⊢→).

artery by the tip of the catheter or the needle end must be excluded, and strict angiographic criteria must be adhered to. There should be reflux down the opposite vertebral artery. Rapid washout would suggest mechanical effects rather than organic disease. Collateral flow would also support the diagnosis (Fig. 5–69). A carotid angiogram might show filling of the tip of the basilar artery via the posterior communicating arteries.

It is usually not possible to distinguish radiologically between thrombosis or embolism purely on angiographic evidence. The shape of the defect in the vessel may, however, be suggestive; embolism appears as a defect concave toward the column of contrast medium. Migration of the point of obstruction also suggests embolism rather than thrombosis, although emboli may arise from an area of thrombus (Fig. 5–70).

Thrombosis of the longitudinal and transverse sinuses is rarely diagnosed in life and, even when suspected clinically, is rarely confirmed in the postmortem room. Krayenbühl has shown the characteristic changes in the venous phase of the cerebral angiogram.[98] Askenasy and associates illustrated the characteristic changes in three cases of venous sinus thrombosis.[6] All three cases had postmortem verification. In two cases cerebral angiography showed absence of filling of the superior sagittal sinus during the venous phase, with prominent deep veins draining the contrast medium.

Aneurysms

Intracranial aneurysms are not infrequently encountered at postmortem (0.5 to 3.7 per cent) according to various path-

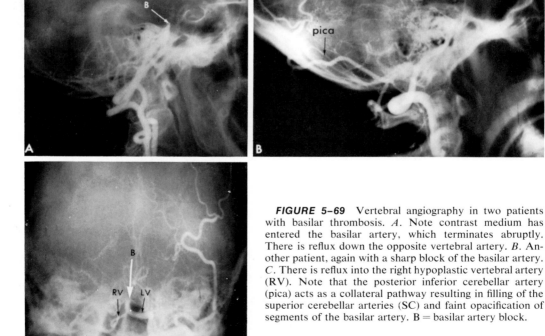

FIGURE 5–69 Vertebral angiography in two patients with basilar thrombosis. *A.* Note contrast medium has entered the basilar artery, which terminates abruptly. There is reflux down the opposite vertebral artery. *B.* Another patient, again with a sharp block of the basilar artery. *C.* There is reflux into the right hypoplastic vertebral artery (RV). Note that the posterior inferior cerebellar artery (pica) acts as a collateral pathway resulting in filling of the superior cerebellar arteries (SC) and faint opacification of segments of the basilar artery. B = basilar artery block.

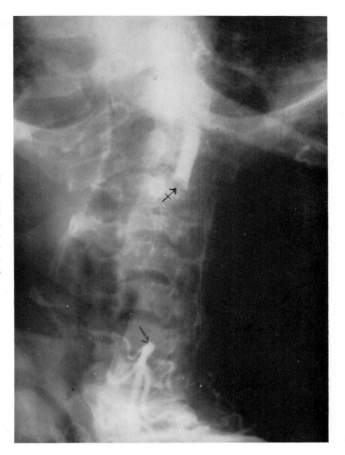

FIGURE 5-70 Carotid angiogram in a patient with a cardiac arrhythmia. An embolus has lodged in the common carotid artery. Note the concave inward defect in the carotid artery (⊢→), which is characteristic for embolism. Branches of the external carotid artery have filled via collateral channels (see Figure 5-58). The embolus, removed surgically, extended like a long sausage to the carotid bifurcation.

ologists and are the most common cause of spontaneous subarachnoid hemorrhage.[199] They are usually situated on the circle of Willis. Figure 5-71 shows the incidence of their location according to Bull.[19] Norlen and Paly claim that 15 per cent of intracranial aneurysms are situated in the posterior fossa and that 5 per cent of intracranial aneurysms arise from the vertebral artery.[137]

Aneurysms may produce their effect by gradual expansion, acting as a mass lesion, and may compress adjacent structures. The great majority of aneurysms present clinically when they rupture into the subarachnoid space, into the cerebral tissue, or into the ventricles. Contrast medium may fill the lumen of the aneurysm depending upon the position of the sac during angiography, the presence of spasm around its neck, the presence of clot within its lumen and the phase of the angiographic series. An anterior communicating artery aneurysm may be clearly demonstrated in one film of the

series and may no longer be seen in a film taken one second later. Multiple views may be required to establish the presence of an aneurysm and the anatomy of its attachment, i.e., whether a neck is present (Figs. 5-1 to 5-8 and 5-72).

In an analysis of McKissock's series of 1769 aneurysms, Bull found 14 per cent to be multiple.[18] Although Crawford claims that 12 per cent of aneurysms are multiple, a more recent large series claims that over 25 per cent are multiple.[26, 147]

Although most aneurysms appear to be of congenital origin, at the point of bifurcation of the branches of the circle of Willis where the muscular layer of the wall is deficient, other factors involved in the production of these aneurysms are high blood pressure and atheromatous lesions in these vessels.[64] The congenital aneurysms are usually saccular; atherosclerotic aneurysms are fusiform and may be dissecting.[229]

Radiological evidence of rupture of an

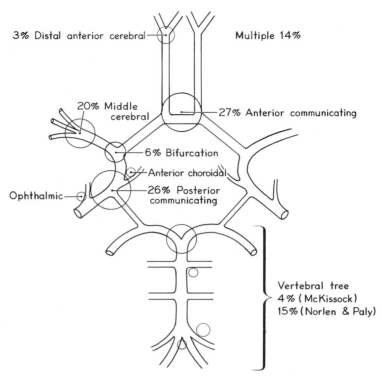

3% Distal anterior cerebral

Multiple 14%

20% Middle cerebral

27% Anterior communicating

6% Bifurcation

Anterior choroidal

26% Posterior communicating

Ophthalmic

Vertebral tree
4% (McKissock)
15% (Norlen & Paly)

FIGURE 5–71 Analysis of the 1769 intracranial aneurysms collected by McKissock (from 1950 to 1960) by Bull. (From Schobinger, R. A., and Ruzicka, F. F., eds.: Vascular Roentgenology. New York, Macmillan Co., 1964.)

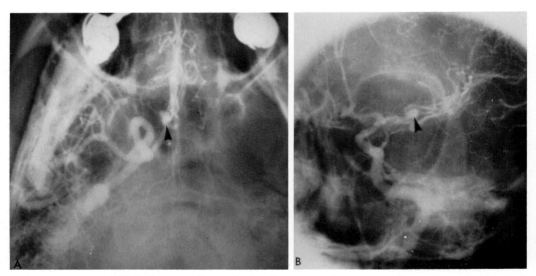

FIGURE 5–72 *A*. Multiple views may be required to demonstrate the presence of an aneurysm and its precise site of attachment. Submentovertical projection shows an aneurysm of the anterior communicating region. This was difficult to recognize in other projections. The submentovertical projection is also useful for aneurysms of the trifurcation of the middle cerebral artery. *B*. Perorbital view for an aneurysm arising at the trifurcation of the middle cerebral artery. The posterior inferior cerebellar artery is readily recognized in oblique views with the aneurysm projected through the open mouth. For other useful projections see Figures 5–1 to 5–8.

aneurysm may be displacement of other vessels by the presence of a hematoma, and spasm of vessels associated with the aneurysm. A few case reports have appeared of rupture during angiography.[89]

When multiple aneurysms are present and subarachnoid hemorrhage has occurred without localizing signs, it may be difficult to designate the offending aneurysm. Wood has offered criteria to determine the site of rupture when multiple aneurysms are present.[231] In order of decreasing dependability he lists the following angiographic signs: evidence of a mass (denoting hematoma or edematous infarct) (Fig. 5–73); the size of the aneurysm (the greater it is, the more likely it was responsible for the subarachnoid hemorrhage); and the presence of spasm (not very valuable) (Fig. 5–74). Applying these criteria, he states that it should be possible to identify the ruptured aneurysm among multiple lesions in more than 95 per cent of cases. DuBoulay has reported on the natural history of intracranial aneurysms, and his contribution is well worth referring to in this respect.[40]

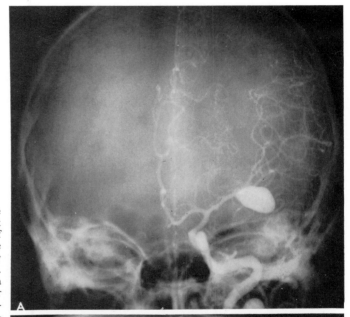

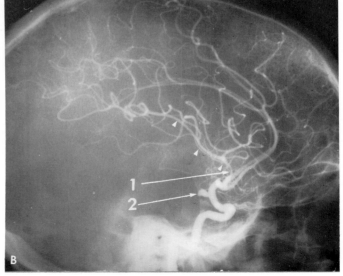

FIGURE 5–73 *A*. A large middle cerebral artery aneurysm. Note that there is a considerable displacement of the anterior cerebral artery across the midline and the middle cerebral artery has been displaced inward and upward. The aneurysm has bled and there is a surrounding hematoma. *B*. Posterior communicating aneurysm (2). The upward displacement of the middle cerebral artery and its branches (*white arrow heads*) and the narrowing of the main stem of the middle cerebral artery (1) suggest recent hemorrhage. Operation confirmed the presence of a temporal lobe hematoma.

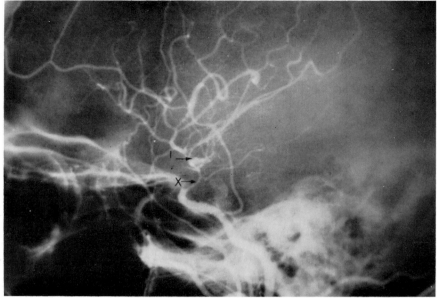

FIGURE 5–74   Anterior communicating aneurysm in a patient with subarachnoid hemorrhage. Aneurysm (1), which appears lobulated; spasm of carotid siphon (X).

Of 403 consecutive cases of subarachnoid hemorrhage reported by Sutton, 77 per cent had lesions demonstrated by bilateral carotid angiography; the findings were negative in 23 per cent. Fifty-one of the ninety-one negative cases were further investigated by vertebral angiography. Unilateral vertebral angiography showed a lesion in 40 per cent of them. In 17 cases in which the findings of bilateral carotid and unilateral vertebral angiography were negative, a second vertebral angiogram on the contralateral side showed a lesion in 7 cases (Fig. 5–75).[205]

The importance of the posterior inferior cerebellar artery origin as a site for aneu-

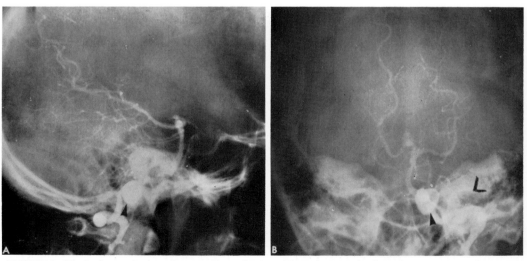

FIGURE 5–75   Left vertebral angiogram. Frontal (*A*) and lateral (*B*) projections demonstrate a left posterior inferior cerebellar artery aneurysm. Note that there is no reflux down the opposite vertebral artery (see text for explanation.)

rysm formation is stressed here; it is the second most common site by far on the posterior circulation, the most common being the tip of the basilar artery (Fig. 5–76). Sixty per cent of aneurysms on the posterior circulation arise from the tip of the basilar artery and 20 per cent arise from the origin of the posterior inferior cerebellar artery.

Spatz and Bull reviewed 60 cases of spontaneous subarachnoid hemorrhage in which bilateral carotid angiography failed to reveal a source of bleeding.[198] In 16 cases, vertebral arteriography demonstrated the lesion responsible for the bleeding. Eight of these were aneurysms and eight were angiomas. The diagnostic accuracy is considerably enhanced by a meticulous examination of the arterial tree in cases of subarachnoid hemorrhage.

Angiomas

Cushing and Bailey divided these into three groups: telangiectases, venous angiomas, and arterial (arteriovenous) angiomas.[29] Most angiomas appear to have arterial and venous components, and the terms "angioma" and "arteriovenous malformation" are here used synonymously.

These malformations vary in size and shape and may be superficially or deeply seated. They may be found supratentorially and in the posterior fossa and occasionally are situated both above and below the tentorium. Unless bleeding has occurred, these lesions are usually not space-occupying, but on occasions may be, and may even result in atrophy of surrounding cerebral structures.

Angiomas are not infrequently the cause of subarachnoid hemorrhage. The arteries supplying the angiomas are usually hypertrophied, but less so than the draining veins (Fig. 5–77). The venous return from these lesions to the deep or superficial system of veins depends on their size and situation. They are frequently supplied by the carotid and vertebral circulation, and an assessment of their extent and supply usually requires both vertebral and carotid angiography (Fig. 5–78).[6]

Large vascular glioblastomas may on occasion resemble an angioma radiographically, but the large tangle of vessels of more uniform size with an arterial supply

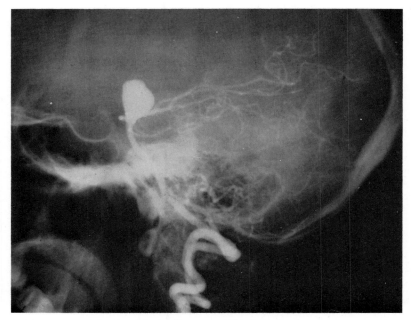

FIGURE 5–76   Aneurysm of the tip of the basilar artery. This is by far the most common site on the posterior circulation. This patient was admitted to hospital with spontaneous subarachnoid hemorrhage without localizing signs. Carotid angiography revealed an aneurysm arising from the right middle cerebral artery. During hospital stay bilateral third nerve palsy developed. A vertebral angiogram revealed a large terminal basilar aneurysm.

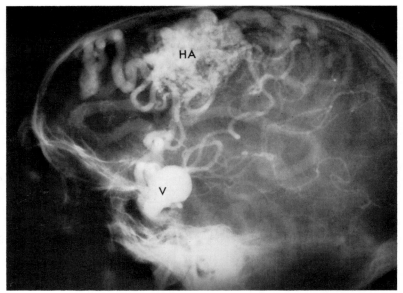

FIGURE 5-77 Carotid angiogram demonstrating a large arteriovenous malformation supplied by a tangle of hypertrophied arteries (HA). Large veins drain the malformation (V). There is also an aneurysm present arising from the region of the anterior communicating artery.

and venous return typical for angioma will usually distinguish them. These large angiomas act like sponges and attract all the contrast medium, which passes rapidly from the arterial to the venous system. Definition and detail may be enhanced by the introduction of a larger bolus of contrast medium within a shorter time interval than usual; by using an automatic serialograph both the maximum arterial and venous phases of the circulation will be obtained.

Aneurysms of the great vein of Galen are really arteriovenous malformations with secondary enlargement of the vein of Galen (Fig. 5-79). Reports of these have been published by Boldry and Miller, Hirano and Terry, Poppen and Avman, and Litvak and Ransohoff.[13, 79, 114, 150] The basic

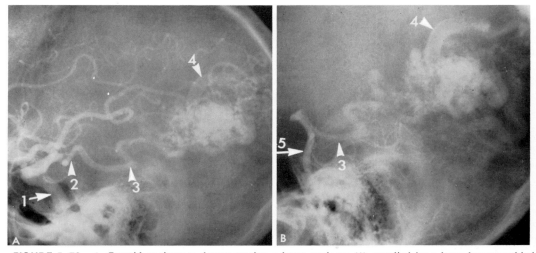

FIGURE 5-78 *A.* Carotid angiogram demonstrating a large angioma (1) supplied by a large hypertrophied posterior cerebral artery (2, 3). Note draining vein (4) during arterial phase. *B.* Vertebral angiogram in same patient showing angioma filled from basilar artery (5) via the posterior cerebral artery.

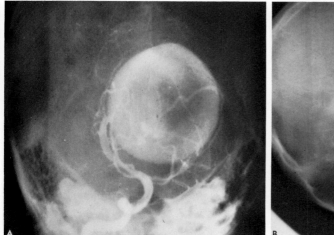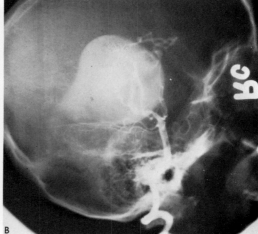

FIGURE 5–79   *A.* Right vertebral angiogram, anteroposterior Towne view. Here the aneurysm of the vein of Galen is filling from the right posterior cerebral artery. *B.* Lateral vertebral angiogram of same patient. Not only are the main stems of the posterior cerebral arteries filling the aneurysm of the vein of Galen, but enlarged choroidal arterial branches participate as well.

embryological defect is a fistula between primitive choroidal arteries and veins with the resulting malformation related to the shifting of the vascular system with brain growth. This is discussed by O'Brien and Schechter.[139]

Although the combination of aneurysm and angioma is rare, they are associated more frequently than is accounted for by mere chance (Fig. 5–77).[15, 147] Many suggestions have been made as to the nature of the association. Its significance becomes obvious when the point of bleeding in intracranial hemorrhage must be determined. Spasm of vessels and the other radiological signs of a bleeding aneurysm may be helpful in this regard, as described earlier.

Tumor

Angiography may help not only in determining the presence and site of an expanding neoplasm, but also in elucidating the nature of the mass. This information depends on two factors: the displacement of arteries and veins from their normal course, and the angioarchitecture of the tumor. The displacement of vessels depends on the size and situation of the tumor and on whether the growth is displacing or infiltrating. Displacements may also reflect such secondary changes as edema or swelling around the tumor and obstruction of

cerebrospinal pathways with ventricular dilatation.

Some tumors are highly vascular, much more than normal brain, while others may have a poor blood supply. Tumor vessels differ from normal vessels in that they have irregular lumina and shapes. They are more tortuous than normal vessels, and connections may be present between arteries and veins. Malignant tumors may have numerous arteriovenous shunts within their substance. The latter may undergo necrosis, cystic changes, and even hemorrhage, causing areas of avascularity that may be recognized in the angiogram.

The circulation rate through a tumor may suggest the pathological condition present. Glioblastomas containing numerous arteriovenous shunts may show filling of the tumor vessels during the arterial phase only and early disappearance of the contrast medium, so that very little of the tumor may retain medium during the venous phase (Fig. 5–80). Meningiomas with a more homogeneous angioarchitecture consisting of numerous capillaries usually retain the contrast medium for a longer period, and the tumor opacification will still be present during the venous phase (Fig. 5–81). Metastatic deposits have a circulation rate that usually lies between those of glioblastomas and meningiomas (Fig. 5–82). Swelling of brain tissue may

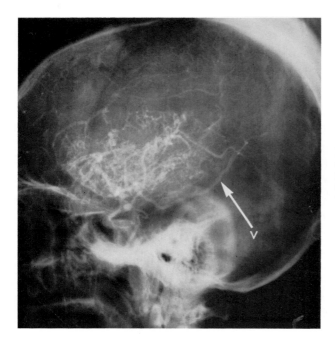

FIGURE 5–80 Glioblastoma multiforme. Note the abnormal vessels with multiple arteriovenous shunts. Also note that the draining veins have filled early in the series (v). This lesion was space-taking (compare with an arteriovenous malformation).

delay circulation time, and this will become manifest when the opacification of the tumor occurs later than that of the normal brain tissue.

Large avascular space-occupying masses such as cysts and abscesses may displace and crowd vascular channels on the periphery of a mass. These crowded normal cerebral vessels must be distinguished from the tumor vessels that form a halo or ring shadow on the surface of a glioblastoma (Fig. 5–83).

Displacement of Vessels

SUPRATENTORIAL LESIONS. The anterior cerebral artery will be displaced to the contralateral side by an expanding mass (Fig. 5–84). Masses deep in the temporal fossa, however, may not displace the artery (Fig. 5–85). The type of displacement

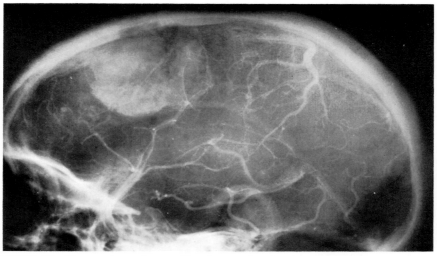

FIGURE 5–81 Venous phase of a carotid angiogram showing the tumor blush of a meningioma.

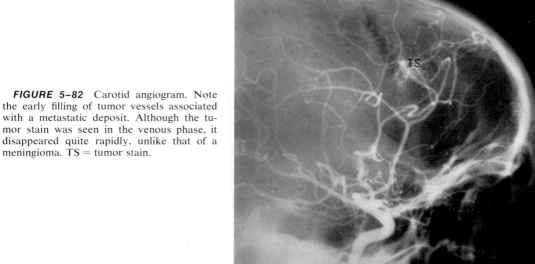

FIGURE 5–82 Carotid angiogram. Note the early filling of tumor vessels associated with a metastatic deposit. Although the tumor stain was seen in the venous phase, it disappeared quite rapidly, unlike that of a meningioma. TS = tumor stain.

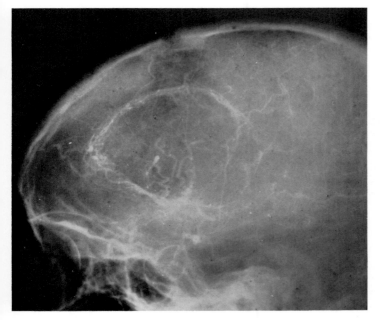

FIGURE 5–83 Carotid angiogram showing a halo of abnormal vessels surrounding a relatively avascular mass (this was a malignant glioma, astrocytoma Grade III).

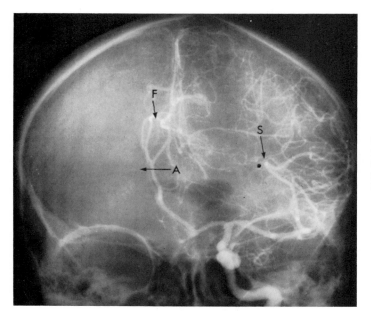

FIGURE 5–84 Displacement of the anterior cerebral artery (A) with falcine herniation (F) and downward displacement of the angiographic sylvian point (S) by a posterior frontal meningioma.

varies with the situation of the mass. Anterior frontal masses cause maximum bowing of the vessel with minor displacements of the internal cerebral vein. With lesions situated further back, there will be more displacement of the internal cerebral vein than of the anterior cerebral artery (Fig. 5–86).

Displacement of vessels in certain situations may provide evidence not only of a tumor mass, but of the specific nature of the tumor. Falx meningiomas may displace the pericallosal artery to the contralateral side and the callosomarginal artery to the ipsilateral side (Fig. 5–87). This sign is fairly specific, but may be mimicked by inter-

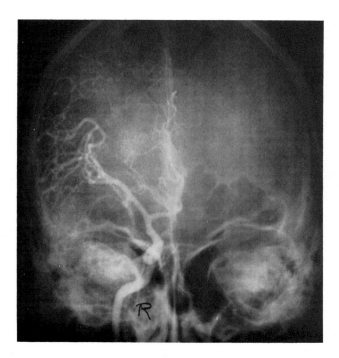

FIGURE 5–85 Upward and inward displacement of the middle cerebral artery by a temporal fossa meningioma. Note the stretched branches of the middle cerebral artery. There is little displacement across the midline of the anterior cerebral artery.

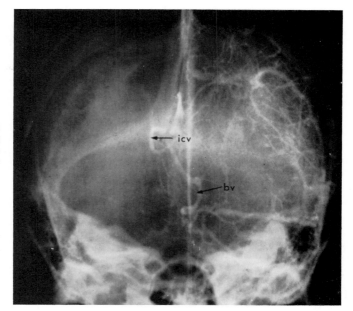

FIGURE 5–86 The internal cerebral vein (icv) is displaced more than the anterior cerebral artery when lesions are close to the midline. bv = basilar vein.

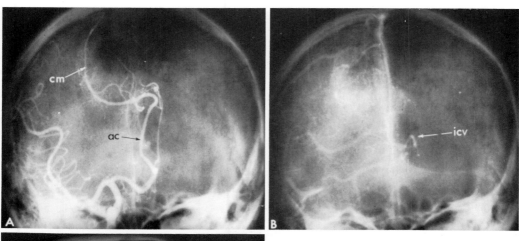

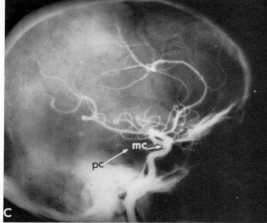

FIGURE 5–87 *A*. Falx meningioma. The displacement of vessels here is highly suggestive, almost pathognomonic for a falx meningioma. This shows the right anterior cerebral artery (ac) displaced toward the left, but the course of the callosomarginal artery (cm) is such that it cannot negotiate the falx. Since the tumor arises from the falx, this portion of the artery is displaced toward the right, i.e., the ipsilateral side. *B*. This shows the tumor stain and the displaced internal cerebral vein (icv). *C*. The callosomarginal artery is displaced laterally, the pericallosal artery (pc) depressed, and the roof of the triangle of Reil depressed (mc).

hemispheric falx hematomas and inter-hemispheric empyemas.[22] We recently en-countered an exhibition of this sign that was caused by a glioblastoma that had grown out of the hemisphere and had insinuated itself between the anterior cere-bral artery and the falx. Tentorial meningio-mas may displace the posterior end of the lateral ventricle, or the posterior cerebral artery upward, while at the same time dis-placing the superior cerebellar artery down-ward (cf. Fig. 5–104). This is a fairly specific sign for tentorial meningiomas.[185]

Venous displacements and changes in the relative rate of filling of the superficial draining veins may be present with a com-paratively normal arterial phase of the cerebral angiogram. The internal cerebral vein shows its maximum displacements with mass lesions approaching the midline (Fig. 5–86). The disproportionate dis-placement between the internal cerebral vein and the arterial tree may supply valuable diagnostic information. For in-stance, disproportionate displacement of the internal cerebral vein relative to the anterior cerebral artery would suggest a deep-seated lesion near the midline or a lesion situated more posteriorly.

The striothalamic vein and the septal vein are usually recognized in a lateral projection of the venous phase of a carotid angiogram (Fig. 5–88). The point of junc-ture usually represents the location of the foramen of Monro. Ring and Laine and co-workers have devised topograms of this point of juncture.[106, 159] Although displace-ments of the "venous angle" may be appre-ciated by applying these topograms, cau-tion must be exercised, since a false venous angle may be produced by a perforating vein entering behind the foramen of Monro (Fig. 5–54). Johansson has illus-trated the normal and the displaced internal cerebral veins in a comprehensive mono-graph.[93]

When the major displacement of the anterior cerebral artery occurs along its distal course, falcine herniation will be more pronounced (Fig. 5–84). Subfrontal masses will displace the anterior cerebral artery upward and backward and will de-press the carotid siphon (Fig. 5–89). The internal cerebral vein may be displaced backward, upward, and across the midline. Suprasellar masses may depress the carotid siphon, but elevate the anterior cerebral artery and the internal cerebral vein (Fig. 5–90).

Parasagittal tumors may simply depress

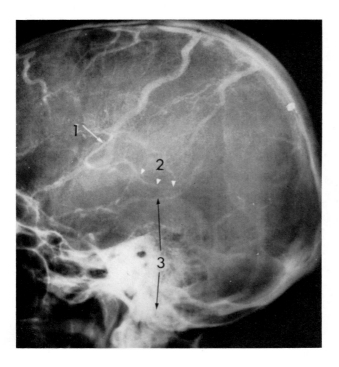

FIGURE 5–88 Venous phase of carotid angiogram. A large posterior parietal glio-blastoma resulted in depression of the in-ternal cerebral vein (2) and unfolding of the venous angle, manifested by a displaced thalamostriate vein (1). Note basal vein (3).

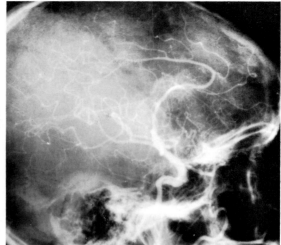

FIGURE 5-89 The typical upward and backward displacement of the anterior cerebral artery by an olfactory groove meningioma.

the pericallosal and callosomarginal branches of the anterior cerebral arteries. The internal cerebral vein may also be depressed (Fig. 5-87C). When the tumor grows more to one side, the anterior cerebral branches will be displaced across the midline (Fig. 5-87).

The branches of the middle cerebral artery in the sylvian fissure are displaced upward in expanding lesions in the temporal lobe (Fig. 5-91). Usually some displacement of the anterior cerebral artery accompanies these middle cerebral artery displacements. (Although deep temporal lesions may not displace the anterior cerebral artery, they will usually displace the internal cerebral vein.) A parietal mass will displace the sylvian group downward (Figs. 5-84 and 5-90). Lesions in the occipital lobe, if large enough, may displace the sylvian group upward and cause ruching of the vessel. This may actually appear to be a displacement of the middle cerebral artery (Fig. 5-92).

The anterior choroidal artery, which enters the temporal horn, may also show

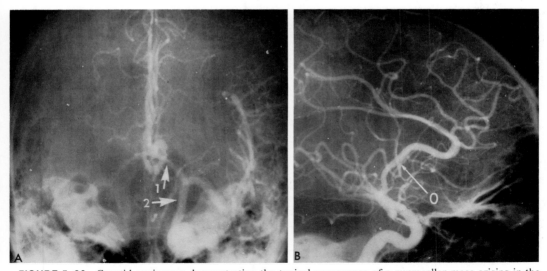

FIGURE 5-90 Carotid angiogram demonstrating the typical appearance of a suprasellar mass arising in the sella (chromophobe adenoma). Note that the carotid siphon (the intracavernous carotid artery and the supraclinoid internal carotid artery, 2) is displaced away from the midline, the anterior cerebral artery is arched upward (1 and 0), and the carotid siphon is depressed.

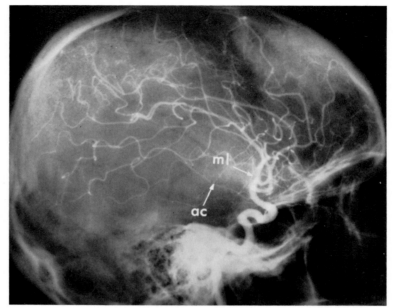

FIGURE 5–91   An avascular temporal lobe mass. The middle cerebral artery group is displaced upward, and the first portion of the middle cerebral artery (ml) is no longer foreshortened. The anterior choroidal artery (ac) is elevated and stretched.

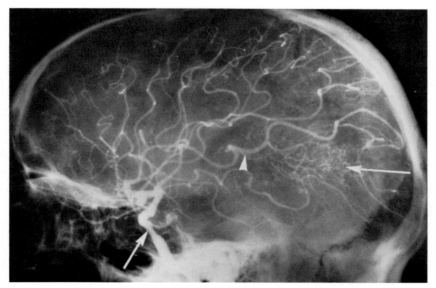

FIGURE 5–92   Carotid angiogram in a posterior parieto-occipital glioblastoma. Note the tumor vessels (*arrows*) and the apparent elevation of branches of the middle cerebral artery with ruching of the vessels (*white arrowhead*). Note atherosclerotic narrowing of the carotid siphon.

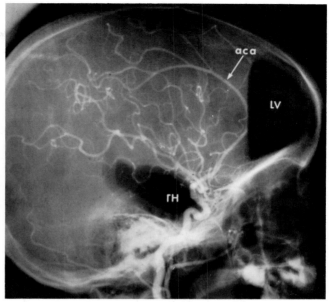

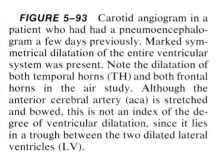

FIGURE 5-93 Carotid angiogram in a patient who had had a pneumoencephalogram a few days previously. Marked symmetrical dilatation of the entire ventricular system was present. Note the dilatation of both temporal horns (TH) and both frontal horns in the air study. Although the anterior cerebral artery (aca) is stretched and bowed, this is not an index of the degree of ventricular dilatation, since it lies in a trough between the two dilated lateral ventricles (LV).

displacements. Temporal lobe lesions stretch this artery and may displace it upward (Fig. 5-91).

Dilatation of the lateral ventricles may be reflected in the stretched course of the anterior cerebral artery. A marked degree of ventricular dilatation, however, must be present before these changes occur (Fig. 5-93). The thalamostriate vein, which runs along the lateral wall of the ventricle, will supply a much more sensitive indication of ventricular dilatation. Sears and associates have compared the appearance of these veins seen in the anteroposterior projection of the carotid phlebogram to a pair of bull's horns.[189] With dilatation of the ventricular system, they resemble a set of short horns, whereas normally they are convex inward (Fig. 5-94).

Although central expanding lesions dis-

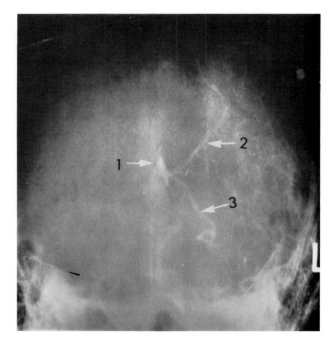

FIGURE 5-94 Venous phase of carotid angiogram. Note internal cerebral vein (1) is in midline. Thalamostriate vein (2) is separated abnormally from midline owing to ventricular dilatation. Basilar vein (3).

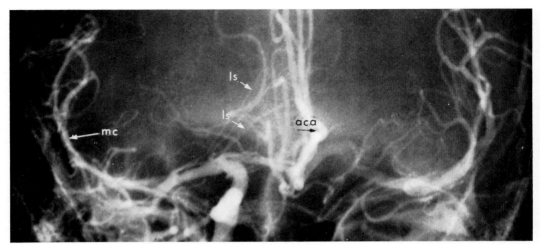

FIGURE 5–95   Carotid angiogram. Note the increased separation between the right middle cerebral artery (mc) and the anterior cerebral artery (aca). The right middle cerebral artery is stretched and displaced outward, and the lenticulostriate vessels (ls) are markedly displaced toward the midline. Compare with the left side.

play their maximum effect on the deep veins rather than on the larger arteries, angiographic magnification techniques that offer great detail and definition will allow displacement of the lenticulostriate arteries to be readily recognized (Fig. 5–95).[66]

POSTERIOR FOSSA LESIONS. Carotid angiography may supply indirect signs of a posterior fossa expanding lesion. A midline anterior cerebral artery stretched and wide-swept due to dilatation of the lateral ventricles would suggest disease in the posterior fossa obstructing the cerebro-spinal fluid pathway through the aqueduct of Sylvius. Air studies of the posterior fossa supply a more sensitive test of minor displacements of structures than does vertebral angiography, since minor changes and normal variations in the position of vessels in the posterior fossa may overlap. Vertebral angiography, however, may be more helpful in assessing the nature of the lesion rather than its precise localization.

Upward herniation through the tentorial opening may result in superior displacement of the superior cerebellar arteries and

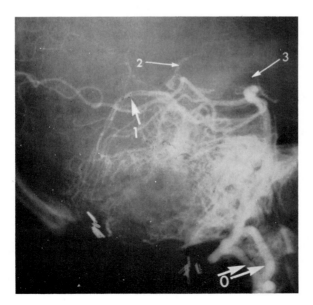

FIGURE 5–96   Posterior fossa metastatic deposit. A postoperative vertebral angiogram shows up herniation of the superior cerebellar arteries through the tentorial opening (1). The basilar artery is flat against the clivus. This latter sign has a little more significance in the infant. It is not a reliable sign of a mass lesion in the posterior fossa. 2 = posterior choroidal arteries. 3 = thalamoperforating arteries. 0 = both vertebral arteries.

even the posterior cerebral arteries (Fig. 5–96). The cerebellar tonsillar herniations may displace the posterior inferior cerebellar artery below the foramen magnum (Fig. 5–97). (This may be seen, however, without herniation.)

Pontine and "angle" tumors may displace the superior cerebellar artery and the posterior cerebral artery (Fig. 5–98). Angle tumors may also displace or obliterate the petrosal sinus.[208] Smaltino claims to recognize angiographic changes in the course of the auditory artery.[197]

Extra-axial tumors can be distinguished from tumors of the pons and midbrain by vertebral angiography. In pontine lesions, the basilar artery may be in its normal position or displaced against the clivus, whereas in lesions originating in the clivus, such as meningioma, chordoma, or cholesteatoma, the basilar artery will be displaced backward (Fig. 5–99). Backward displacement of the basilar artery may also occur in infantile hydrocephalus.[108]

Thalamic tumors and tumors in the region of the pineal body may displace the posterior choroidal arteries upward, widening their curve. The great vein of Galen may be compressed and depressed by tumors in this area (Fig. 5–88). Severe compression of this vessel may result in poor visualization during angiography.

The basilar artery also may be depressed and become accordion-like. This displacement may represent a large midline mass lying directly above the tip of the basilar artery.[176] The anterior choroidal artery, which usually has a curvilinear course with its convexity medially, will have to take a more oblique course around an uncal herniation and will appear stretched in the lateral projection.

Angioarchitecture of Tumor

The vascular architecture of and the rate of blood flow through a tumor will influence the angiographic appearance and often supply a histological diagnosis. Astrocytomas are usually less vascular than normal brain tissue, whereas glioblastomas, meningiomas, secondary deposits, and hemangioblastomas usually have an enriched blood supply.

GLIOMAS. These form the bulk of primary intracerebral tumors. Those of the glioblastoma multiforme group are highly vascular tumors consisting of tumor vessels

FIGURE 5–97 A vertebral angiogram in a patient with a posterior fossa metastatic deposit. The posterior inferior cerebellar artery (pica) has been displaced below the foramen magnum. This is evidence of tonsillar herniation, but is not a very reliable sign since so many variations of the anatomy occur.

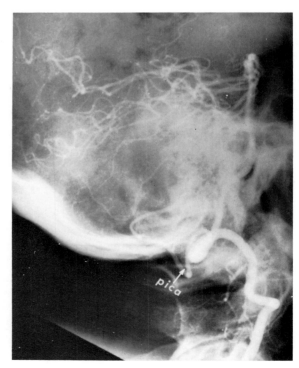

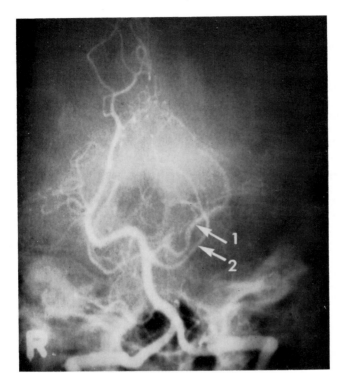

FIGURE 5–98 Vertebral angiogram in left acoustic neuroma. Note displacement of posterior cerebral artery (1) and superior cerebellar artery (2). A film taken three seconds later demonstrated tumor vessels.

FIGURE 5–99 Typical displacement of the basilar artery by an extra-axial lesion. Note the displacement of the basilar artery away from the clivus produced by a clivus chordoma. Other extra-axial masses may produce similar changes. (Courtesy of J. W. D. Bull, National Hospital, Queen Square, London.)

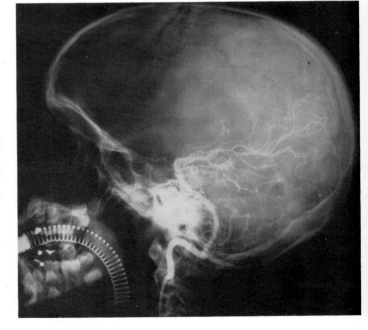

arranged haphazardly. These vessels are of different sizes and shapes, and many arteriovenous shunts are present within the tumor mass (Figs. 5–80 and 5–92). The tumor fills during the arterial phase of the angiogram. Due to the vascularity of the mass and the arteriovenous shunts, the tumor may have emptied completely during the venous phase. It may sometimes be difficult to distinguish between a very vascular glioma and an arteriovenous malformation. The large feeding arteries and draining veins are usually more evident in malformations, which are usually not space-occupying unless they have hemorrhaged and a hematoma has formed.

Malignant gliomas frequently undergo degenerative changes and may contain necrotic areas, cysts, and hemorrhage. This may manifest itself radiologically in a hypervascularized area surrounding an avascular zone. This "ring sign" is seen most frequently in glioblastoma, but may also be present in metastatic deposits; it results from tumor vessels surrounding an area of necrosis (Fig. 5–83). In cysts and abscesses, a false ring sign may be present, but here the hypervascularized halo consists of compressed normal cerebral vessels, and no abnormal tumor vessels can be identified.

Some malignant gliomas have tumor vessels not unlike those just described, but with no visible communications between the arteries and veins. In these cases contrast filling of veins does not occur during the arterial phase. Greitz and Lindgren state that in this group, with the use of rapid serial angiography, the pathological drainage veins will be seen filled before the normal cerebral veins.[67] Some glioblastomas have a vascular supply poorer in vessels than normal adjacent brain, and others may have no difference in their vascular architecture.

The astrocytomas have a poorer blood supply than other gliomas. The angiographic demonstration of tumor vessels is rare, and, in fact, the brain may be less vascularized over this area. Arteriovenous fistulae are absent, and the diagnosis must be made on vessel displacements and areas of avascularity.

MENINGIOMAS. These tumors have angiographic characteristics that are recognizable in over half the cases.[113] Meningiomas are usually attached to the dura and show sites of predilection along the sagittal sinus, sphenoid ridge, and olfactory groove (Figs. 5–81, 5–84, 5–87, and 5–89). Rarely, these tumors are situated within the ventricles, where their characteristic appearances may be present (Fig. 5–100). In a review of 250 confirmed cases of meningio-

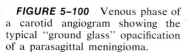

FIGURE 5–100 Venous phase of a carotid angiogram showing the typical "ground glass" opacification of a parasagittal meningioma.

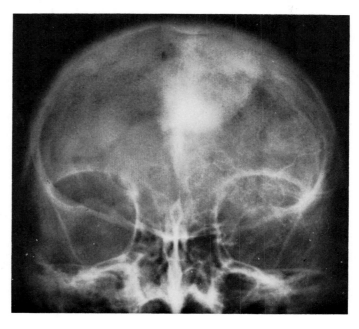

ma by Gassel and Davies, 11 were situated in the lateral ventricles, and carotid angiography (performed in 2 cases) revealed displacement of vessels indicative of a deep mass.[63]

A hypertrophied anterior choroidal artery has been shown to supply the tumor.[7, 47, 82, 220] Rogers reported a case of an intraventricular meningioma diagnosed by vertebral angiography.[163] A right carotid angiogram showed a doubtful displacement of the anterior cerebral artery. In an attempted left carotid arteriogram the needle inadvertently passed into the vertebral artery; the resultant angiogram revealed an intraventricular meningioma supplied by a large elongated posterior choroidal artery. An extensive tumor blush was seen in the venous phase. Intraventricular meningiomas may result in hypertrophy of the anterior choroidal artery (Fig. 5–101). Although other vascular intraventricular tumors may hypertrophy these vessels, the margins of the tumor may not be smooth, and the other

characteristics (persistence of tumor stain, location of tumor at the trigone of ventricle) may not be present. In two cases of intraventricular meningiomas seen by the present author both showed hypertrophy of the anterior choroidal arteries and one showed the characteristic tumor stain. Both were confirmed at postmortem. The tumor vessels of meningiomas usually have regular lumina and are characterized by many capillaries. The vessels may become filled during the arterial phase, and the capillaries usually remain filled until late in the venous phase. The stain is sometimes homogeneous like ground glass. Meningiomas are usually single, although multiple tumors have been reported.

Meningiomas often receive their blood supply from both external and internal carotid arteries (Fig. 5–102). The blood supply from the external carotid artery is usually mediated via the middle meningeal artery, but if the tumor has infiltrated the bone, it may receive supply via the other

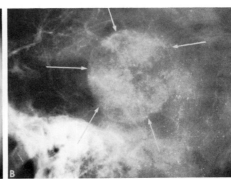

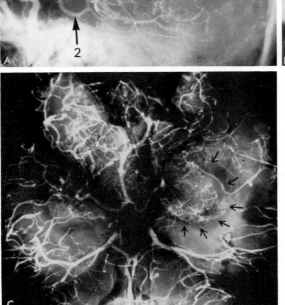

FIGURE 5–101 *A.* Intraventricular meningioma supplied by branches of the internal carotid artery. Note the hypertrophied anterior choroidal artery (1) and hypertrophied posterior cerebral artery (2) supplying the tumor. *B.* Film six seconds later shows homogeneous round smooth-edged area of opacification. Confirmed intraventricular meningioma. *C.* Postmortem angiogram of the intraventricular meningioma. Note the marked vascularity, position, shape, and attachment of the tumor.

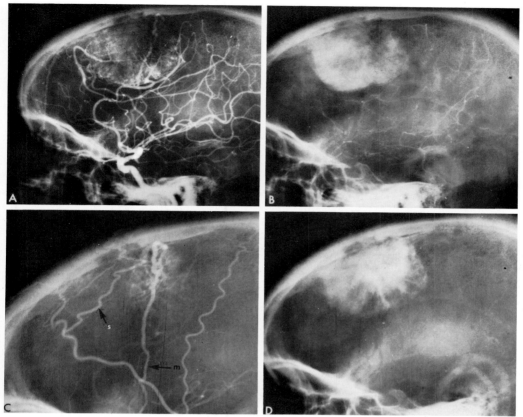

FIGURE 5–102   *A*. Internal carotid angiogram. Note the displacement of branches of the anterior cerebral artery by a large tumor stain. *B*. Later phase of the internal carotid angiogram showing more opacification of the tumor, principally distributed around the outside of the tumor. *C*. External carotid angiogram shows the middle meningeal artery (m) increasing in caliber as it approaches the tumor and involvement also of the superficial temporal artery (s). *D*. A later phase of the external carotid angiogram shows maximum opacification of the tumor in its center. There is less opacification of the periphery of the tumor, which is supplied by the internal carotid artery as is seen in *B*.

branches of the external carotid artery supplying the region (Fig. 5–103). When the tumor receives a supply from these vessels, they hypertrophy, and the segment of the vessel adjacent to the tumor may be larger than the stem vessel.

The tumor stain usually has a regular margin and is well outlined. With differential contrast filling of both the internal and the external carotid arteries, these changes may be more obvious. When the meningioma receives this dual supply the appearance may be quite characteristic, the external meningeal supply will be via the attachment of the tumor and will appear to supply the core of the tumor while the surface of the tumor appears to derive its blood supply from the branches of the

internal carotid artery. The "spoke wheel" angiographic appearance of meningioma referred to by Lindgren results because narrow, regular, tangled vessels are arranged in a radial fashion.[113] This vascular pattern appears to be most common in intraventricular and cerebellopontine angle meningiomas.

Even in the absence of tumor stain there are two situations in which the displacement of vessels is such that the diagnosis of a meningioma is almost certain. Falx meningiomas displace the main stem of the anterior cerebral artery to the contralateral side while the callosomarginal branches may be displaced ipsilaterally (Fig. 5–87). Similarly, tentorial meningiomas may displace the posterior cerebral arteries upward

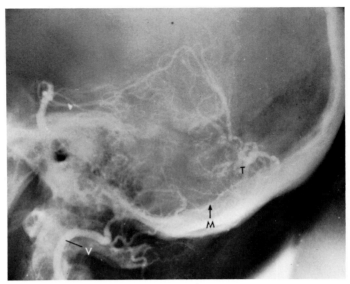

FIGURE 5–103   Posterior meningeal branch (m) of the vertebral artery (v) supplying a tentorial meningioma (t).

and the superior cerebellar arteries downward in the same patient (Fig. 5–104).[185]

METASTASES.   These tumors are usually round and well circumscribed. Hypernephromas are sometimes extremely vascular and may resemble glioblastomas (Fig. 5–82). When multiple separate accumulations of vessels are seen, the diagnosis of secondary deposits is most likely (Fig. 5–105).

HEMANGIOBLASTOMAS.   These are usually situated in the cerebellum and are frequently multiple. Vascular displacement by these tumors is extremely slight, even in the presence of large cysts. In most cases these are, from the pathological standpoint, cystic lesions with a cherry-red mural nodule. The mural nodule consists of a conglomerate of vessels with regular lumina. A vertebral angiogram may demonstrate a hypertrophied vessel leading to the tumor with no obvious draining veins, which distinguishes it from an angioma. The tangle of vessels usually shows up as a dense, small, round, opacified nodule that may be surrounded by an avascular area resembling a cyst (Fig. 5–106). The appearance of these tumors is usually characteristic.[143]

PAPILLOMAS.   These may show fine regular vessels not unlike those of a meningioma. The surface may be circumscribed but umbilicated. The lobulated surface of the papilloma may be seen during pneumoencephalography with air lying within the ventricle. The vessel supplying the tumor may be hypertrophied, as seen in Figure 5–107. Matson and Crofton state that the pneumographic demonstration of an intraventricular mass, in the presence of communicating hydrocephalus, is pathognomonic of this tumor.[125]

ACOUSTIC NEURINOMAS.   Displacement of vessels is more common than the demonstration of tumor vessels (Fig. 5–98). Olsson reviewed his vertebral angiographic findings in 14 acoustic nerve tumors.[142] In all cases the superior cerebellar artery ran an abnormal course. Nine cases showed abnormal tumor vessels related to the mass. Displacement or nonfilling of the petrosal vein is a significant finding in angle tumors.[208]

TUMORS IN THE REGION OF THE PINEAL GLAND.   If these tumors are large enough, they will displace the great vein of Galen downward and the posterior choroidal arteries upward and backward.[116] Tumors in this region include pinealoma or teratoma, thalamic glioma, aneurysm of the great vein of Galen, meningioma of the free margins of the tentorium, and tumors of the quadrigeminal plate and splenium of the corpus callosum.

ORBITAL TUMORS.   Krayenbühl has emphasized the value of carotid angiography in orbital lesions.[99] Displacements of the

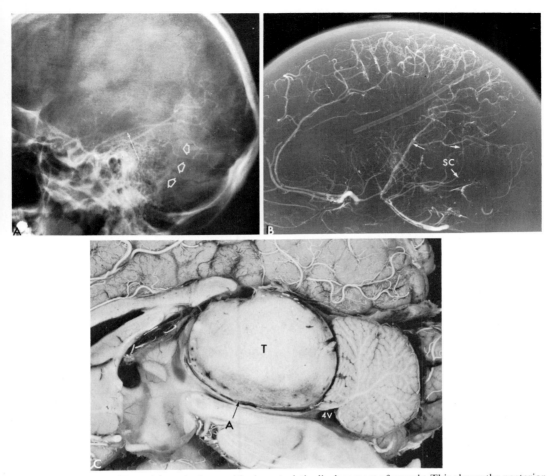

FIGURE 5–104 *A.* Tentorial meningioma with characteristic displacement of vessels. This shows the posterior cerebral artery displaced superiorly (*arrows*), while the superior cerebellar artery is displaced down and back (*arrowheads*). *B.* Postmortem angiogram showing in more detail the characteristic displacement of the posterior cerebral artery and the superior cerebellar artery (sc). *C.* The brain sliced in the sagittal plane through the midline shows the tumor (T), the aqueduct (A), and the fourth ventricle (4V).

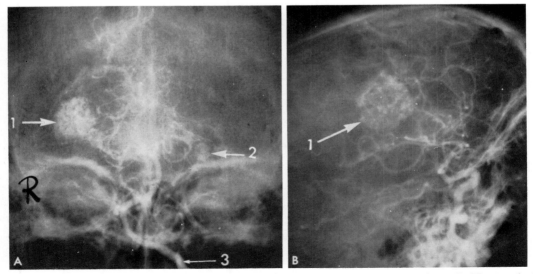

FIGURE 5–105 *A.* Vertebral angiogram showing two discrete areas of tumor vessels (1, 2). The vertebral artery (3) is filled with contrast medium. *B.* Carotid angiogram in the same patient showing a third discrete area of tumor opacification, hypernephroma of kidney with metastatic deposits outlined.

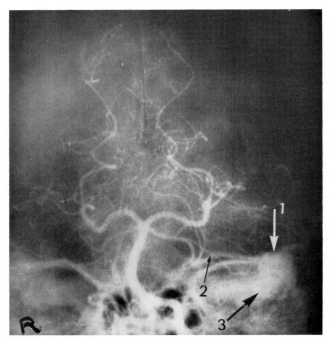

FIGURE 5-106 Vertebral angiogram demonstrating a hemangioblastoma. Note blood supply from branches of superior cerebellar artery (1, 2) and the posterior inferior cerebellar artery. (3) = the opacified tumor. (Reproduced by kind permission of Dr. Bernard Wolf.)

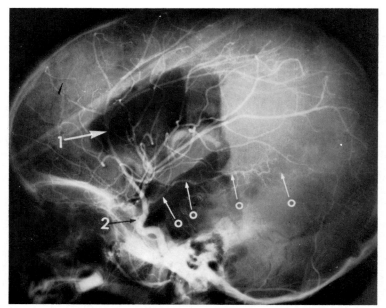

FIGURE 5-107 Carotid angiogram in a child with a papilloma of the choroid plexus of the lateral ventricle. Note the hypertrophy of the anterior choroidal artery (O, O, O, O), which supplies the plexus. The stretched wideswept anterior cerebral artery (1) is an expression of the ventricular dilatation. 2 = internal carotid artery.

ophthalmic artery may be recognized, and vascular intraorbital tumors may fill from the ophthalmic artery. The ophthalmic artery may hypertrophy to supply tumors involving the roof and confines of the orbit.[36] Orbital phlebography and orbitography may be very helpful here, and may enhance the diagnostic potential considerably.

CEREBRAL ABSCESS. This lesion has no characteristic appearances. Vessels may be displaced, revealing an avascular mass.

PARASITES. Hydatid cysts will show displacement and marked stretching of vessels around completely avascular areas.

Raised Intracranial Pressure

In marked elevation of intracranial pressure the circulation of contrast medium through the head is slowed. In a series of 17 cases reported by Pribram, in which narrowing of the carotid artery was seen in the neck and very little contrast medium entered the cerebral circulation, no organic disease was seen in the cervical vessels (Fig. 5–104A and B).[152] All were patients who had experienced an acute rise in intracranial pressure. The similarity of the angiographic appearances to those of carotid occlusion is stressed. The narrowing of the column of contrast medium in the neck is probably accounted for by layering in a slow circulation (Fig. 5–67), and not due to a narrowed lumen of the vessel.[181]

Herniation

Tentorial "Up" Herniation

These may occur with any posterior fossa expanding lesion. The superior cerebellar arteries may be displaced up through the tentorial opening. The posterior cerebral arteries, normally located above the tentorium, may be displaced further upward in severe herniations (Fig. 5–96).

Tonsillar Herniation

These may occur with supratentorial or infratentorial lesions that have resulted in increased intracranial pressure.

The caudal loop of the posterior inferior cerebellar artery passes under the cerebellar tonsil and may be displaced through the foramen magnum with tonsillar hernia-

tions (Fig. 5–97). This is not a very reliable sign, since a loop of the posterior inferior cerebellar artery is not infrequently seen below the foramen magnum unassociated with tonsillar herniations.

Tentorial "Down" Herniations

Tentorial herniations may be either up or down. Herniations of the temporal lobe down through the tentorial opening may occur with cerebral hemisphere swelling or supratentorial space-occupying lesions. In down herniations, the posterior communicating artery and the posterior cerebral artery may be displaced through the tentorial opening. The vessel, in order to negotiate the opening in the tentorium, must also be displaced medially. The artery may be displaced down in a bold curve or may show a stop-wedge deformity (Fig. 5–108). Filling of the posterior cerebral artery occurs in only one third of carotid angiograms, but the basal vein of Rosenthal is usually opacified. Since this vein follows the same course as the posterior cerebral artery, similar displacement of this vessel will occur. Since the veins are more easily compressed than the artery, opacification may be absent or difficult to recognize.

Trauma

The death toll in the United States in 1962 from motor accidents was 40,800. In 1964 in the United States, 10,000,000 disabling injuries occurred, killing almost 1,000,000 people. During 1967, an estimated 3,096,000 persons sustained injuries in moving motor vehicle accidents for which they required medical attention. With high-speed travel a routine of daily living, the major source of injuries in adults has moved to the highway and away from military accidents, industrial accidents, and sporting accidents. In 70 per cent of fatal highway accidents, brain damage was the cause of death.

Blunt trauma to the neck may result in thrombosis of the carotid arteries. This is due to subintimal tears of the intima with thrombus formation.[105, 135] Penetrating injuries to the neck are usually the result of stab wounds and missile injuries. False aneurysms of the carotid artery may occur,

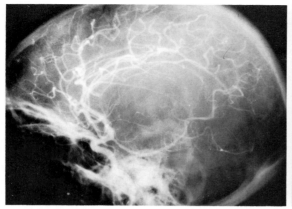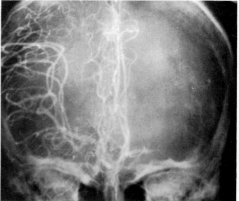

FIGURE 5–108 Temporal lobe tumor. Note the marked elevation of the middle cerebral artery complex, with stretching of these vessels and displacement toward the midline. There is marked transtentorial herniation of the temporal lobe revealed by the very marked displacement downward and to the midline of the posterior cerebral artery.

but these are usually simple to manage.[184] When a major vessel such as the vertebral artery or the carotid artery is torn with the adjacent accompanying veins, an arteriovenous fistula may result. These are major surgical problems and may be very difficult to treat. Unless all the contributing arteries and draining veins are outlined, the operative management becomes complicated, often necessitating repeated operative attacks.[236]

Head injuries, open or closed, may result in raised intracranial pressure and may cause a situation in which blood flow in the cervical internal carotid artery is very slow. This may be due to thrombus formation in the internal carotid artery. Other mechanisms, however, are usually present to account for this pseudothrombosis. The raised intracranial pressure offers resistance to the passage of blood (and blood–contrast medium mixture) through the intracranial circulation. The passage of the column of contrast medium progresses to the base of the skull and then tapers to a very thin stream; little, if any, passes intracranially. The passage through the external carotid artery will, however, appear normal. In the experience of the author, such slow circulation has invariably been a sign of impending death. This phenomenon must be present bilaterally to invoke the agonal flow phenomena. Before making this diagnosis, therefore, it is incumbent to perform bilateral carotid angiography. That organic changes are not present in the neck vessels

in these patients has been proved by us in postmortem studies on patients coming to autopsy. These studies included postmortem angiography using barium gelatin injections and dissection of these vessels (Fig. 5–109).[141] However, when the intracranial vessels are not demonstrated sufficiently well in such patients to exclude an extracerebral hematoma (a remediable condition), a bilateral exploration is indicated. Traumatic aneurysms of the superficial temporal artery were more common in the days of "blood letting" and fencing.[46, 78] Selective angiography of the external carotid artery will demonstrate the lesion (Fig. 5–110). This should not be confused with an aneurysm of the middle meningeal artery.[68] Nontraumatic aneurysms of the middle meningeal artery usually arise at points where the vessel branches.

The value of angiography in the management of head trauma is well established. Post-traumatic lesions that may be demonstrated by this technique are:

1. Subdural hematomas.

2. Epidural hematomas (middle meningeal) with significant accumulation of hematoma, with fistula formation between artery and accompanying dural venous or diploic channels, or with formation of false aneurysm.

3. Intracerebral mass lesions, including cerebral contusion and edema and intracerebral hematoma.

4. Caroticocavernous fistula.

5. Aneurysm of carotid artery in its extracranial course and carotid-jugular fistula.

Additional information may be obtained about:

1. Alterations in blood flow due to thrombosis of carotid or vertebral artery, pseudothrombosis (poor arterial filling due to raised intracranial or low systemic pressure or both), temporary occlusion of vessels (complete and incomplete, by spasm, herniation, and hematoma), and superior sagittal sinus thrombosis.

2. Presence of lesion unrelated to trauma.

Most authorities have accepted the value of angiography and have relegated the multiple blind burr hole exploration to the past. Even the most astute clinicians and skillful surgeons agree that, on occasion, even well-placed burr holes may miss a collection of blood that will be recognized on angiograms. Angiography may also reveal unsuspected lesions.

In cases of post-traumatic intracranial mass lesions, angiograms may occasionally be unrevealing to those unfamiliar with the radiographic principles involved. An understanding of these principles and recognition of some of the misconceptions of angiographic interpretation enhance the diagnostic value of the examination.

Trauma to the vessels outside the head has already been dealt with and we now direct our attention to lesions within the head.

Subdural Hematoma

The acute subdural hematoma is usually caused by tearing of the cortical veins as they enter the superior sagittal sinus. A

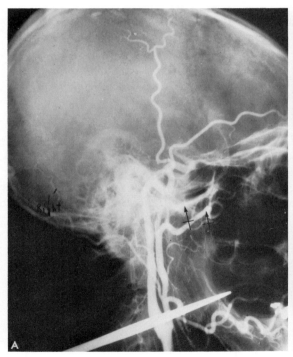
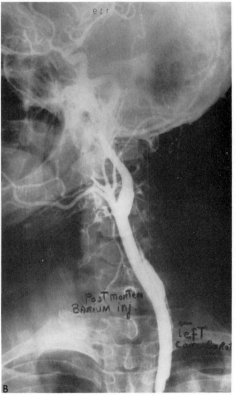

FIGURE 5–109 *A.* Common carotid angiogram in patient who has sustained severe head trauma. Agonal flow due to intracranial hypertension shows filling of external carotid artery and its peripheral branches (*arrows*), whereas the internal carotid artery is not opacified beyond the point of its passage beyond the anterior clinoid process. This phenomenon was present bilaterally. *B.* Postmortem angiogram reveals no organic obstruction in the vessels of the neck or head.

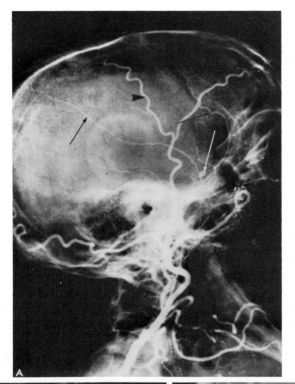

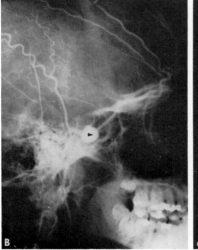

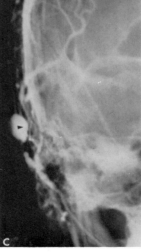

FIGURE 5–110 A. Right common carotid angiogram, lateral view. This patient has an occlusion of the internal carotid artery at its origin. The white arrow points to an aneurysm of the middle meningeal artery (*black arrows*), thought to be of congenital origin. The black arrowhead points to a branch of the superficial temporal artery. B. Right external carotid angiogram, lateral view. The small black arrowhead overlies a pseudoaneurysm of the superficial temporal artery. Note that this pseudoaneurysm is superimposed on the middle meningeal artery, which is intact. C. Right external carotid angiogram, anteroposterior view. The pseudoaneurysm is indicated by the small black arrowhead. This projection clearly shows the pseudoaneurysm arising from the superficial temporal artery and not from the middle meningeal artery.

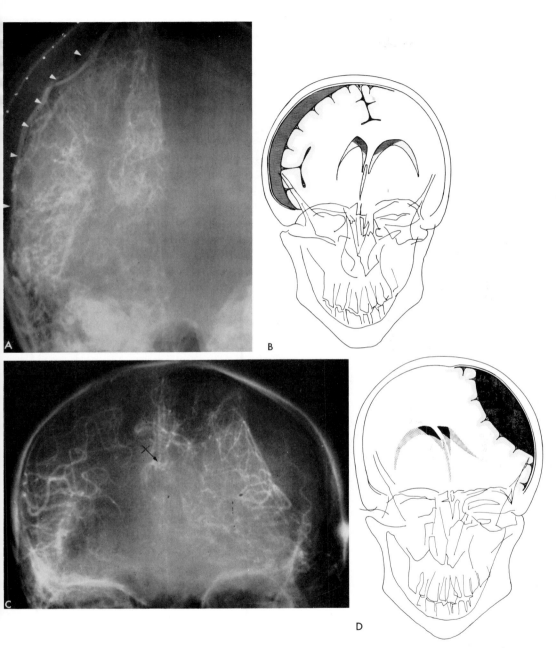

FIGURE 5–111. *A.* Acute subdural hematoma. Note that in the intermediate phase of the carotid angiogram a cortical vein outlines the surface of the brain and that vessels are prevented from reaching the inner table of the skull by the collection of blood. The "bare" area is crescentic in shape. *B.* Schematic representation of an acute subdural hematoma. *C.* Chronic subdural hematoma. The "bare" area is lentiform. Note crowding of branches of the middle cerebral artery and the shift across the midline of the anterior cerebral artery with "falcine" hernia-tion (*arrow*). *D.* Schematic representation of a chronic subdural hematoma. Note the lentiform bare area.

fracture of the skull is usually not present. The fluid collection of blood spreads diffusely over the surface of the brain, displacing it in a more or less uniform fashion away from the inner table of the skull. In a short time, about a week, a membrane begins to form. Theories of the pathogenesis of the chronic subdural hematoma have been proposed, but these are not universally accepted. Putnam and Cushing believed that recurrent fresh hemorrhages into the hematoma account for its progressive enlargement.[153] Gardner suggested that osmotic attraction of cerebrospinal fluid through the semipermeable membrane is responsible for its growth.[61] Chronic subdural hematomas may present without a history of trauma, and the expanding mass may produce signs and symptoms indistinguishable from those produced by any expanding tumor in the head. The pathological distinction between an acute and chronic subdural hematoma is the presence of a membrane. As the diffuse subdural accumulation of blood becomes limited by this membrane and begins to expand in

size, its shape changes from a thin blood clot with a concave medial surface to a lentiform shape (Fig. 5–111). The basis for Norman's angiographic differentiation between acute and chronic subdural hematoma depends on the shape of the bare area recognized angiographically.[138] A criticism of Norman's system of differentiation is offered later. Care must be exercised in the interpretation of these findings. The bare area may be missed completely if the central beam of the x-ray does not strike part of the fluid collection tangentially. Parietal lesions may be best examined with the head in a true anteroposterior position and the central x-ray beam displaced to the appropriate side. Lesions in the frontal region are best seen with the head turned toward the side of the lesion, and posterior lesions with the head turned away from the side suspected (Figs. 5–1 to 5–8 and 5–112).

The intermediate phase of the angiographic series shows opacification of the smaller vessels of the brain and is perhaps the most useful in recognizing these bare

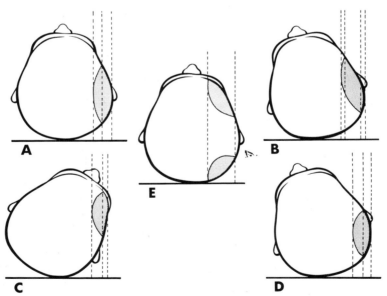

FIGURE 5–112   The shaded area represents the subdural collection of fluid or blood clot. In the anteroposterior projection *A*, a temporoparietal lesion will be recognized since the anterior and posterior margins of the depressed brain are projected within the margin of the vault of the skull. *B*. Note that the bare area in the same position will appear shallower since the head is inappropriately rotated and the beam is no longer projected tangentially to the bare area. *E*. One hematoma situated anteriorly and one situated posteriorly. Note that both of these may be missed in the anteroposterior projection. *C*. The optimal position of the head for an anteriorly located lesion. *D*. The optimal position of the head for a posteriorly located lesion.

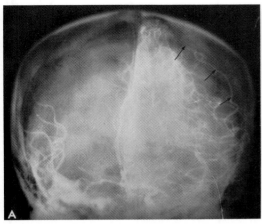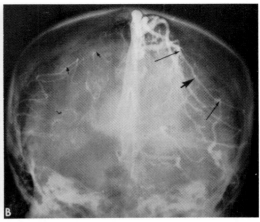

FIGURE 5–113 *A.* The arterial phase of a subdural hematoma. Since the most peripheral branches of the middle cerebral artery, representing the anterior margin of the trough, have an outward convex shape, the erroneous diagnosis of an acute subdural hematoma may be made. *B.* The venous phase shows cortical veins outlining the margin of a chronic subdural hematoma with a characteristic shape (*large arrows*). Note the disproportionate shift of the anterior cerebral artery and the presence of a chronic subdural hematoma on the opposite side (*small arrows*).

areas. Caution in the interpretation of the films is mandatory since three shadows may be projected onto the x-ray film: the anterior margin of the trough, the bottom of the trough, and the distal margin. Occasionally a chronic subdural hematoma may be mistaken for an acute one if a tangential view is not obtained. The venous phase, however, may be more revealing and show the characteristic biconvex shape (Fig. 5–113).[43, 234] Frontal hematomas in the anteroposterior projection may only demonstrate a lateral displacement of the anterior cerebral artery without evidence of the classic bare area. However, on the lateral film one sees displacement posteriorly of the segment of the anterior cerebral artery distal to the anterior communicating artery, and one may occasionally be led to suspect a subdural hematoma because of the demonstration of a bare area between well-developed frontopolar branches and the inner table of the skull.

Since oblique films were discussed in the evaluation of the presence and shape of a subdural hematoma, it must be said that the "acute" shape of Norman's scheme may represent a chronic subdural hematoma. The author has no quarrel with the specificity of the "chronic" shape for chronic subdural hematoma, except that this may also represent an epidural hematoma (Fig. 5–114). The following observations support our contention: (1) not infrequently the

"acute" shape is present in a patient with a history of trauma over four weeks previously, and with well-formed membranes as seen at operation; (2) postmortem observations have revealed the presence of membranes unassociated with a significant collection of fluid; and (3) Gannon has angiographically documented the resolution of a chronic subdural hematoma with a change in the shape from "chronic" to "acute."[60]

Hematomas at sites other than over the frontal, temporal, or parietal regions may be recognized angiographically. An interhemispheric hematoma may separate the two anterior cerebral arteries or the pericallosal and callosomarginal branches of the same anterior cerebral artery, displacing the pericallosal artery to the contralateral side and the callosomarginal artery to the ipsilateral side. This will produce the angiographic appearance of a bare area lying adjacent to the falx (Figs. 5–85 and 5–115). Jacobsen first described this angiographic sign.[90] Campbell and Campbell have angiograms taken after evacuation of an interhemispheric hematoma, which show return of the anterior cerebral artery to its normal position and disappearance of the bare area.[21]

Infratemporal subdural hematomas elevate the branches of the middle cerebral artery and the basal vein of Rosenthal but are difficult to distinguish from intratemporal hematomas. When vessels appear

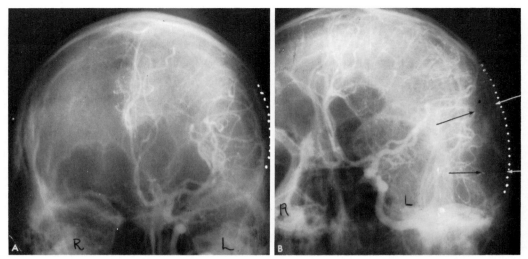

FIGURE 5–114 *A.* Left carotid angiography. Anteroposterior Towne view. There is a slight shift of the midline. No avascular space is demonstrated laterally. *B.* Left carotid angiography with the patient's head turned toward the opposite side. The posteriorly situated epidural hematoma is now demonstrated as an avascular space (*between white and black arrows*).

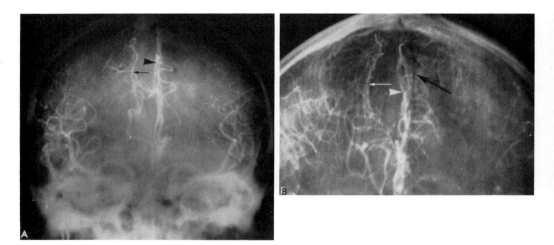

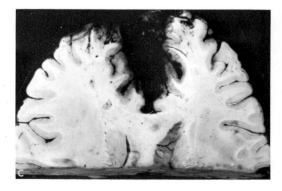

FIGURE 5–115 *A.* Right carotid angiography with compression of the left carotid artery, anteroposterior Towne view. Note the separation of the pericallosal artery (*black arrowhead*) and the callosal-marginal artery (*small black arrow*) by an interhemispheric subdural hematoma. *B.* Right carotid angiography with compression of the left carotid artery. The black arrow points to a linear fracture. This is another patient with an interhemispheric subdural hematoma separating the pericallosal artery on the right (*white arrowhead*) from the callosal-marginal artery (*small white arrow*). *C.* Note the large interhemispheric subdural hematoma. (Specimen by kind permission of Dr. LeMay.)

stretched rather than displaced, an intra-cerebral situation is favored. There may be a minimal shift of the anterior cerebral artery in these lesions.

Vertebral angiography has been less helpful in the recognition of the rare posterior fossa subdural and epidural hematoma. In a recent publication, however, the suspected presence of a posterior fossa epidural hemorrhage was confirmed by vertebral angiography.[148] The posterior meningeal artery was displaced away from the table of the skull and was torn in several places, leaking contrast medium. The branches of the posterior inferior cerebellar artery were displaced away from the inner table of the skull. An epidural hematoma in the posterior fossa was successfully removed.

One usually examines the other side angiographically in head trauma, particularly when there is a disproportionate shift of the anterior cerebral artery across the midline relative to the depth of the bare area representing the extracerebral hematoma. Contralateral compression is useful to compare the two sides simultaneously, but should not be used as an excuse to neglect examining the opposite side in two projections.

Factors to be considered with a disproportionate shift of the anterior cerebral artery include: (1) a subdural or epidural collection fluid on the opposite side (Fig. 5–116); (2) contusion, with swelling of the opposite cerebral hemisphere; (3) a low-placed middle fossa hematoma; (4) atrophy of the underlying brain allowing for accumulation of fluid without shift of the midline; and (5) resolution of the subdural collection.

Epidural Hematoma

These usually result from a tear of the meningeal arteries or veins, but may also originate from the dural sinuses and diploic channels. Although the initial tear may result in slow venous bleeding (the so-called chronic epidural hematoma), small arteries may be torn as the dura is stripped from the skull, and the bleeding becomes both venous and arterial.

Although early investigators doubted the

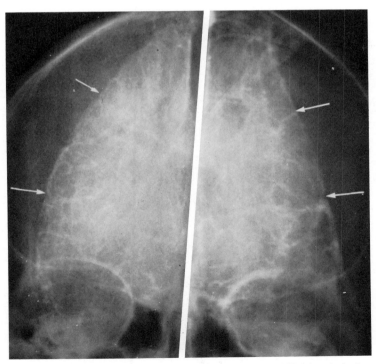

FIGURE 5–116 Bilateral chronic subdural hematomas. Note that the midline is relatively undisplaced, being balanced between the collections of fluid on either side.

feasibility of distinguishing angiographically between an epidural hematoma and a subdural hematoma, recognizable angiographic criteria exist that make such a distinction possible. They are:

1. Displacement inward of a meningeal artery.

2. Displacement of the sagittal sinus, torcular, or transverse sinus.

3. Lentiform bare area with a history compatible with acute hematoma.

4. Irregular margin of the surface of the epidural hematoma.

5. Disproportionate shift of the anterior cerebral artery.

6. Leaking of contrast material from the torn vessel.

7. Fracture line crossing a vascular groove that accommodates a meningeal vessel.

Displacement of the meningeal arteries from the inner table of the skull is pathognomonic of an epidural hematoma, and the diagnosis depends upon the certainty with which the meningeal branches can be identified. A selective internal and external carotid angiogram is desirable and will facilitate this recognition, while a common carotid injection, although of less value, may also allow this distinction to be made (Fig. 5–117). Occlusion of the middle cerebral artery may produce an avascular area, and if common carotid angiography has been performed, the normal meningeal arteries superimposed over the bare area may produce a picture that could be mistaken for an epidural hematoma (Fig. 5–118).

Epidural hematomas are rare in infants and children because of the marked adherence of the dura to the inner table of the skull.[22] In the posterior fossa the dura may normally strip very easily from the inner table of the skull. The dura is less adherent in adults, but limits the spread of an accumulation of blood so that the collection assumes a lentiform shape. The angiographically bare area resembles the "chronic" subdural shape, and in the presence of a recent history is suggestive of an epidural hematoma, especially if a skull fracture transversing a meningeal channel is demonstrated (Fig. 5–114).

Irregularity of the medial surface of the lentiform bare area has been reported with epidural hematomas. This is presumably due to strands of dural tissue that limit its complete separation from the surface of the vault.

Since epidural hematomas have a limited surface area, being confined by the adherence of the dura to the skull, a small-volume

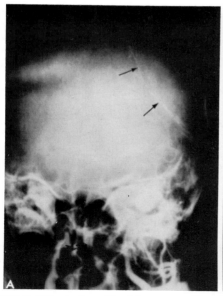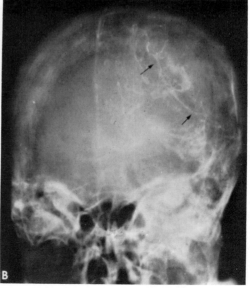

FIGURE 5–117 *A.* An epidural hematoma. Note filling of branches of the external carotid artery with inward displacement of the middle meningeal artery (*arrows*). *B.* This shows disproportionate shift of the anterior cerebral artery with pronounced inward displacement of the middle meningeal artery (*arrows*).

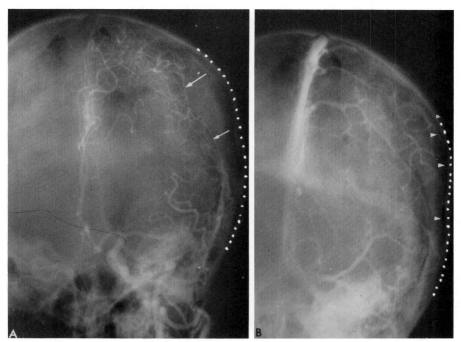

FIGURE 5–118   *A*. Left carotid angiogram, anteroposterior Towne view. There is an avascular space between the vascularized brain (*upper white arrow*) and the inner table of the skull (*white dots*). The middle meningeal artery (*lower white arrow*) is fortuitously superimposed on the inner border of this avascular space. Thus superficially there appears to be an epidural hematoma present, but in fact, the diagnosis here is occlusion of a branch of the middle cerebral artery. No extracerebral hematoma is present. *B*. Venous phase of angiographic series. The proximity of cortical veins (*white arrowheads*) to the inner table of the skull (*white dots*) rules out diagnosis of an extracerebral hematoma.

hematoma that is lentiform in shape may be much thicker than an acute subdural hematoma of a much larger volume. Subdural hematomas tend to spread and occupy a larger surface area. There is, therefore, less shift of the midline structures in epidural hematomas than in subdural hematomas of comparable thickness. This accounts for the disproportionate shift of the middle structures in epidural hematomas (Fig. 5–114).

Separation of the superior sagittal sinus from the inner table of the skull is another pathognomonic angiographic sign of epidural hematoma and was first demonstrated by Wickbom (Fig. 5–119).[223] Bonnal described displacement of the torcular Herophili by a posterior fossa epidural hematoma, and Petit-Dutaillis et al. published a radiogram illustrating displacement of the torcular Herophili and sagittal sinus by a posterior fossa epidural hematoma (Fig. 5–120).[14, 149] Other reports of separation of the sagittal sinus from the skull

have appeared by Pecker et al., Tiwisina and Stecker, McKissock and co-workers, and Alexander.[2, 126, 146, 215] Caution must be exercised in the interpretation of this sign, since slight rotation of the skull in the lateral projection may cause misinterpretation of displacement of the sagittal sinus, or a superior sagittal sinus that is situated a little to the side may be mistakenly interpreted as a displaced sinus. Separation of the superior sagittal sinus from the skull in the anteroposterior projection is unequivocal (Fig. 5–120*B*).

Lohr recommended common carotid angiography to outline the middle meningeal artery.[118] Although he did not demonstrate leaking of contrast material from a torn meningeal vessel, he did demonstrate leaking from a branch of the middle cerebral artery. Since the majority of rapidly evolving epidural collections are recognized clinically and subjected to operation without angiography, and those of a more benign nature have angiograms made quite

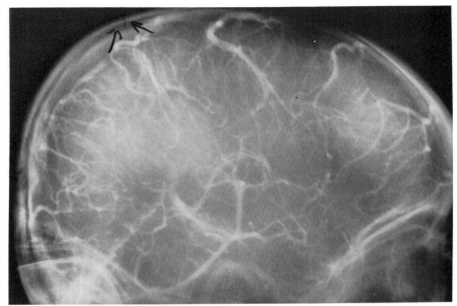

FIGURE 5–119 The two black arrows indicate a fracture extending across the midline to either side. Note that the superior sagittal sinus is displaced away from the inner table of the skull by an acute epidural hemorrhage.

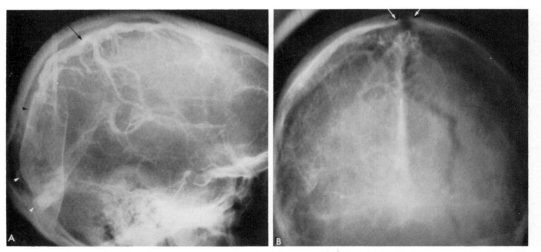

FIGURE 5–120 An epidural hematoma extending into the posterior fossa. Note the fracture extending into the sagittal suture (*white arrows*). Also note the separation of the superior sagittal sinus from the inner table of the skull. The transverse sinuses and the torcular Herophili have also been displaced from the inner margin of the skull (*black and white arrowheads*). Note separation of the superior sagittal sinus in the anteroposterior projection. This is an unequivocal sign of an epidural hematoma.

a few hours after the initial trauma, angiographic recognition of the bleeding site is unusual. Huber states that leaking contrast medium is not usually recognized when angiography is performed more than six hours after the initial trauma.[83] This, however, was not true in the author's experience.

The extradural bleeding may originate from torn meningeal arteries, veins, dural sinuses, or diploic channels. The bleeding site usually identified at operation is the middle meningeal artery or one of its branches.

The rapidity with which the leaking contrast material appears and disappears during angiography usually precludes its entering only the epidural space, since a tremendous hematoma beyond all reasonable proportions would build up. Other workers, the author among them, have indicated that the leaking contrast material and blood is not a simple affair. As reports of this entity have accumulated in the literature, an analysis of the cases has led to the formulation and promulgation of rather rigid clinical diagnostic criteria.

Today it is generally accepted that the clinical spectrum seen with epidural hematomas is wide. Thus, although classic descriptions of the symptomatology include the "lucid interval," such a history is obtained less than 50 per cent of the time — and although the classic description includes progression to a fatal outcome within hours, exceptions are fairly common.[88,127,167]

The explanation for this variability is complex. Certain anatomical factors may be responsible in part. One such is the strength of attachment of the dura to the skull. The dura is more adherent in children, especially along suture lines, and in females and in elderly people. Bradley, commenting on this fact in 1952, observed that certain subjects seem to be "immune" to epidural hemorrhage.[16] Another anatomical factor is the strength of the walls of the middle meningeal vessels. Hassler described congenital defects in the wall of the middle meningeal artery.[73] In addition to these anatomical factors, certain pathological features related to the injury influence the clinical picture. Two key ones are the site of the epidural hemorrhage (temporal location has the most rapidly progressive course) and the severity of injury to the underlying brain.

The use of angiography in epidural hemorrhage has revealed certain other factors that influence the clinical course. Observations of contrast material that has extravasated from a torn meningeal artery led to the following classification:

1. The extravasated contrast material may pass into the epidural space to form an epidural hematoma that progressively enlarges (Figs. 5–121 *A* and 5–122).

2. The extravasated medium may pass out of the epidural space through the adjacent fracture line into the subgaleal area (Figs. 5–121 *A* and 5–122).

3. The extravasated contrast material may be walled off by the formation of a pseudoaneurysm (Figs. 5–121 *C* and 5–123).

4. The extravasated contrast material may pass into adjacent venous channels, thereby indicating the presence of an arteriovenous fistula. These venous channels may be within the diploë of the skull (Figs. 5–121 *D* and 5–124) or they may be the veins that accompany the meningeal artery (Figs. 5–121 *B* and 5–125).

Many reports of the extravasation of contrast material from the middle meningeal artery have been published.[83,111,117,215,219] Arteriovenous fistulae involving the middle meningeal vessels as a result of trauma or "spontaneous" fistulae shown angiographically have been reported.[12,53,87,109,121,170,225,238] Also, pseudoaneurysm formation of the middle meningeal artery has been reported.*

Of particular importance is the time interval between the injury and the angiographic studies. It is of special importance also that, in most of these cases, large amounts of contrast material were seen to leave the torn meningeal artery. Cases in which a tremendous outpouring of contrast material was seen many hours after the episode of trauma, without an epidural hematoma of a size commensurate with the production of the equation — flow times hours after injury — must clearly have had a "protective mechanism in operation."

---

*See references 37, 80, 97, 104, 122, 145, 151, 169, 188, and 237.

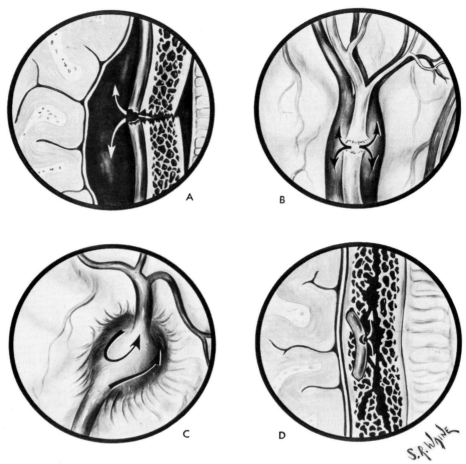

FIGURE 5–121   *A*. In this drawing the middle meningeal artery is not accompanied by a venous channel. A tear in the middle meningeal artery allows the extravasation of blood and contrast material into the epidural space or through the fracture line into the subgaleal space. (See also Fig. 5–122.) *B*. Where the middle meningeal artery is accompanied by a venous channel, blood and contrast material pass out of the torn meningeal artery into the venous channel. This fistula is a type of "protective mechanism." (See also Fig. 5–125.) *C*. A blood clot has sealed off a tear in the middle meningeal artery, forming a "pseudoaneurysm." This is another type of "protective mechanism." (See also Fig. 5–123.) *D*. A tear in the middle meningeal artery as it traverses the diploic space in the temporal area allows passage of blood and contrast material into the venous diploic channels. (See also Fig. 5–124.)

These findings with regard to the presence of extravasation many hours after the episode of trauma are not in accord with those of Huber.[83]

At this point, consideration is given to anatomical factors that the author believes to be responsible for the pattern emerging in any given case in which torn meningeal vessels initiate an episode of hemorrhage. The determining factor is the situation of the meningeal artery at the site of leakage. It may be encased by bone at this point, so that the extravasated material may find its way into diploic channels; the artery may be accompanied by venous channels at the site of the tear, resulting in fistula formation of the arteriovenous variety; finally, there may be no venous channel present adjacent to the torn meningeal artery, in which instance the extravasated material can accumulate only in the epidural space — unless the fracture site itself allows decompression. The anatomical relationships mentioned here are all presented in Figures 5–121 through 5–125.

The basis for an understanding of what is involved in fistula formation lies in the work of Jones.[94, 95] This anatomist was

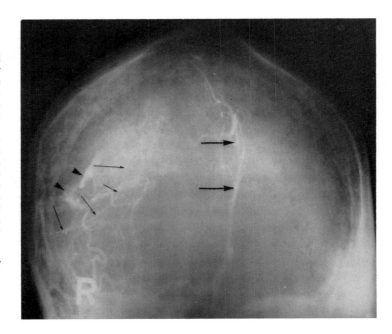

FIGURE 5-122 Right carotid angiogram, anteroposterior Towne view of arterial phase. An epidural hematoma is demonstrated here displacing the middle meningeal artery (*small black arrows*). The black arrowheads indicate collections of contrast material with the epidural space. On the lateral films these collections had a globular appearance. The large black arrows point to the right anterior cerebral artery, which is displaced to the left. The amount of displacement, however, is not commensurate with the thickness of the epidural hematoma (this is one of the radiological signs of the presence of an epidural hematoma).

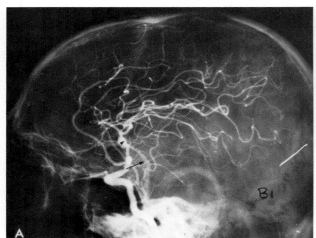

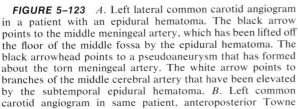

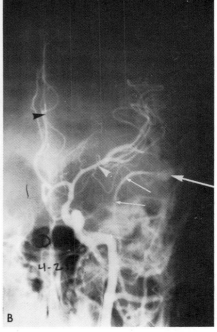

FIGURE 5-123 *A*. Left lateral common carotid angiogram in a patient with an epidural hematoma. The black arrow points to the middle meningeal artery, which has been lifted off the floor of the middle fossa by the epidural hematoma. The black arrowhead points to a pseudoaneurysm that has formed about the torn meningeal artery. The white arrow points to branches of the middle cerebral artery that have been elevated by the subtemporal epidural hematoma. *B*. Left common carotid angiogram in same patient, anteroposterior Towne view. The large white arrow points to the pseudoaneurysm. The small white arrows point to the displaced middle meningeal artery. The white arrowhead points to the displaced middle cerebral trunk. The black arrowhead indicates the left anterior cerebral artery, which is displaced only slightly. Angiography in this patient was performed 168 hours after the episode of trauma.

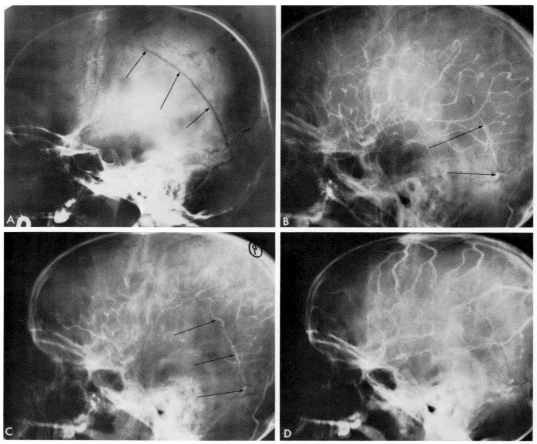

FIGURE 5–124 *A*. Lateral skull film of a 12-year-old boy who was struck by a baseball bat. The black arrows point to a linear fracture. *B*. Left common carotid angiogram in same patient. The black arrows point to extravasated contrast material along the fracture line. The extravasated contrast material has come from a torn meningeal vessel. *C*. Later film of the lateral angiographic series in same patient. The black arrows point to the accumulation of more extravasated contrast material along the fracture line. *D*. Later film of the angiographic series in same patient. Very little extravasated contrast material is still visible. Carotid angiography in this patient was performed 24 hours after the episode of trauma. The anteroposterior angiographic series showed no significant displacement of cerebral vessels and so no operation was performed for removal of extracerebral hematoma. The patient made a complete recovery without any form of surgical intervention. The extravasated contrast material (and blood) is presumed to have run out of the middle meningeal artery, through the fracture, and into the subgaleal space, where a large hematoma was present.

intrigued by the anatomical explanation for the grooves on the inner table of the skull and found that the major channels accounting for these grooves were the accompanying meningeal veins rather than the meningeal artery itself (Fig. 5–126). According to Jones, this fact was discovered at an earlier date, but lost sight of for a time. Figures 5–121 through 5–125 illustrate passage of contrast material from a meningeal artery to an accompanying meningeal vein.

In pseudoaneurysm formation extrav-

asated blood from a torn vessel becomes walled off by a covering made up of fibrinous clot. Thus, the wall of the vessel does not form the wall of the aneurysm.

The lesions that must be considered in the differential diagnosis of a torn meningeal vessel with its resultant fistula formation or pseudoaneurysm formation are: (1) congenital aneurysms of the middle meningeal artery, (2) traumatic pseudoaneurysms of a branch of the external carotid artery in the scalp, and (3) extravasation of

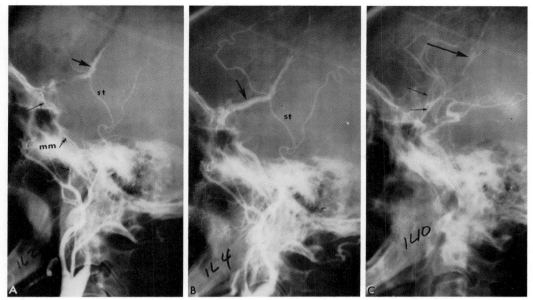

FIGURE 5–125 *A*. Left carotid angiogram, lateral view. The small black arrows point to the middle meningeal artery (mm). The large black arrow points to extravasated contrast material coming from this artery. The superficial artery is labeled st. *B*. Same patient as in A. More contrast material (*large black arrow*) has leaked out of the middle meningeal artery. *C*. Later phase of angiographic series in same patient. The large black arrow points to extravasated contrast material. The small black arrows point to contrast material that has found its way into the meningeal venous channels accompanying the meningeal artery. During this series contrast material in the internal carotid artery has slowly passed into the middle and anterior cerebral arteries. At the time of operation no significant collection of blood was noted in the epidural space.

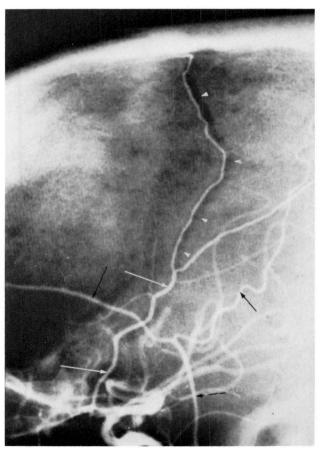

FIGURE 5–126 Left common carotid angiogram. Lateral view. The small white arrows point to the main stem of the middle meningeal artery. The white arrowheads point to the vascular groove in the skull, which is much larger than the lumen of the middle meningeal artery and, in fact, is much larger than the lumen and walls of the artery. This is because the groove accommodates various channels as well as the arterial channel. Note that there are also branches of the middle meningeal artery that do not run in the area of the large venous channels grooving the skull. The small black arrows point to branches of the superficial temporal artery, which here are mainly unrelated to the groove in the skull.

contrast medium from a lacerated cerebral vessel such as the middle cerebral artery.

"Congenital aneurysm" of the middle meningeal artery is a rare phenomenon.[11, 143, 237] Figure 5–110 *A* illustrates such an aneurysm thought to be of congenital origin.

Angiograms demonstrating a pseudoaneurysm of a branch of the external carotid artery in the scalp have been presented by Wortzman.[232] Such pseudoaneurysms usually result from open injury, but may result from closed injury. Clinically, there is generally no difficulty in determining whether such a pseudoaneurysm is present, but angiographically they may overlie a meningeal artery and simulate a pseudoaneurysm of the middle meningeal artery (Fig. 5–110 *B*).

Case reports of extravasation of contrast medium from torn cerebral vessels are extremely rare.[100, 118, 186] Another reported case is illustrated in Figure 5–127.

Intracerebral Mass Lesions

CEREBRAL CONTUSION AND EDEMA. The temporal, frontal, and occipital lobes are the areas most frequently affected in cerebral trauma. The contrecoup phenomenon may result in greater damage on the side opposite the site of direct injury. An associated subdural or epidural hematoma may accompany the brain contusion and will produce the angiographic appearance of a mass lesion with appropriate displacement of vessels. Poor filling of cerebral vessels has been attributed by some to spasm. Swollen brain may account for failure of the midline angiographic structures to return to the midline after evacuation of epidural and subdural hematomas.

A localized segment of vascular narrowing or generalized spasm may result from trauma.[56] Angiograms will show the caliber of the vessels to be considerably narrowed, and the rate of flow of contrast through the cerebral circulation will be delayed. Repeat angiograms at a later date may reveal a return to normal of the caliber of the involved vessels.

INTRACEREBRAL HEMATOMA. These hematomas act as space-taking lesions that are angiographically avascular. Although some regression of vascular displacement may occur when contusion subsides, some displacement persists for a much longer

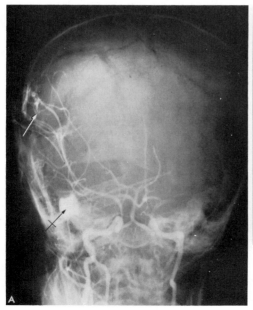

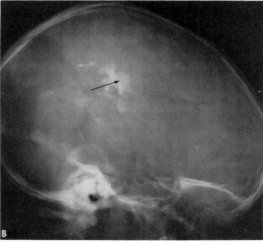

FIGURE 5–127 A young boy suffered severe head trauma with comminuted fractures of the skull. Angiography revealed displacement of intracranial vessels and a tear of a cortical branch of the middle cerebral artery with extravasation of contrast medium (*arrows*) over the cerebral cortex, pooling in cerebral sulci (*B*). ⊢→ = artefact.

period. These lesions may not be recognized without the benefit of angiography.[70]

Traumatic Occlusion of the Middle Cerebral Artery

This has been infrequently reported. Wolpert and Schechter reported four cases of traumatic middle cerebral artery occlusion demonstrated angiographically.[230] Collateral circulation from other vessels was established in three of these cases. The possible pathological factors to explain the occlusions include thrombosis of the middle cerebral artery, embolism of the middle cerebral artery, intracerebral hemorrhage causing direct arterial compression, arterial compression, arterial spasm, and a dissecting aneurysm of the middle cerebral artery.

Caroticocavernous Fistula

These usually result from a fracture involving the base of the skull, which may tear either the wall of the carotid artery as it passes through the cavernous sinus, or more frequently the branches of the internal or external carotid arteries as they enter the cavernous sinus. Penetrating wounds may also be responsible. Carotid and vertebral angiography should be performed to facilitate planning the proposed therapy. Unsuspected collateral channels have been responsible for some of the poor results of operation. In a recent series of cases reported by Rosenbaum and Schechter a fistula involving only branches of the external carotid artery was seen in one case.[164] Selective internal and external carotid angiography showed filling from the

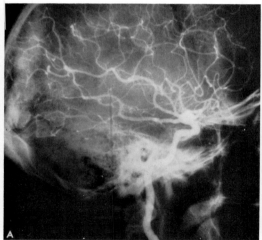
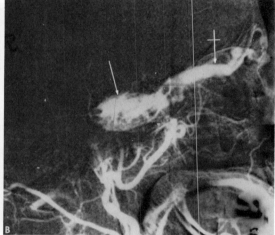
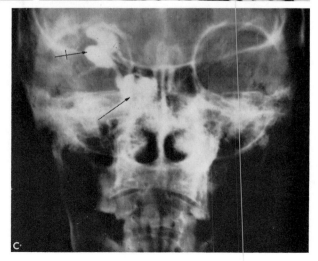

FIGURE 5-128 *A.* Right internal carotid angiogram in a patient with a carotid-cavernous fistula. Note that there is no opacification of the cavernous shunt. *B* and *C.* An external carotid angiogram shows filling of the branches of the external carotid artery and filling of the cavernous sinus (*arrow*) via numerous branches of an external carotid artery. The engorged orbital veins (⊢→) are well opacified.

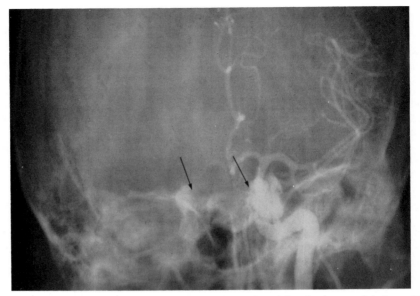

FIGURE 5–129 Left internal carotid angiogram in a patient with a left pulsating exophthalmos. Note filling of the left cavernous sinus with contrast medium and filling also of the right cavernous sinus (*arrows*).

external carotid artery alone with no contribution from the internal carotid artery. The conventional trap procedure, as could be anticipated from the angiogram, did little to the fistulous communications (Fig. 5–128).

The dramatic sudden onset of a pulsating exophthalmos is due to a communication between the branches of the carotid artery and the cavernous sinus. Contrast medium introduced into the carotid artery passes into the cavernous sinus and outlines the engorged ophthalmic veins (Fig. 5–128 B and C). The cavernous sinus on both sides usually fills via the venous communications that are normally present between the cavernous sinuses of both sides (Fig. 5–129).[77, 209]

REFERENCES

1. Alexander, E., Jr., Wigser, S. M., and Davis, C. H.: Bilateral extracranial aneurysms of the internal carotid artery. J. Neurosurg., 25:437–442, 1966.
2. Alexander, G. L.: Extradural hematoma of the vertex. J. Neurol. Psychiat., 24:381–384, 1961.
3. Alpers, B. J., Berry, R. G., and Paddison, R. M.: Anatomical studies of the circle of Willis in normal brain. Arch. Neurol. Psychiat., 81: 409–418, 1959.
4. Anderson, McD., and Schechter, M. M.: A case of spontaneous dissecting aneurysm of the internal carotid artery. J. Neurol. Neurosurg. Psychiat., 22:195–201, 1959.
5. Aronson, N. I.: Traumatic arteriovenous fistula of the vertebral vessels. Neurology, 11:817–823, 1961.
6. Askenasy, H. M., Kosary, I. Z., and Braham, J.: Thrombosis of the longitudinal sinus. Diagnosis by carotid angiography. Neurology, 12: 288–292.
7. Bagchi, A. K.: Lateral ventricle tumors. J. Indian M. Ass., 29:425–432, 1957.
8. Baker, H. L.: Angiographic investigation of cerebrovascular insufficiency. Radiology, 77: 399–405, 1961.
9. Bauer, R., Sheehan, S., and Meyer, J. S.: Arteriographic study of cerebral vascular disease. Arch. Neurol., 4:119–131, 1961.
10. Berk, M. E.: Combined carotid-vertebral angiography. A selective procedure—preliminary report. Brit. J. Radiol., 33:780–783, 1960.
11. Berk, M. E.: Aneurysm of the middle meningeal artery. Brit. J. Radiol., 34:667–668, 1961.
12. Berkay, F.: A rare and interesting case of arteriovenous fistula between the middle meningeal artery and the greater petrosal sinus and surgical treatment. (In Turkish) Tip Fak. Mec., 26:64–71, 1963.
13. Boldrey, E., and Miller, E. P.: Arteriovenous fistula (aneurysm) of the great cerebral vein (of Galen) and the circle of Willis. Report on two patients treated by ligation. Arch. Neurol. Psychiat., 62:778–783. 1949.
14. Bonnal, J.: Hématome extradural de la fosse cérébelleuse. Rev. Neurol., 85:439–443, 1951.
15. Boyd-Wilson, J. S.: The association of cerebral angiomas with intracranial aneurysms. J. Neurol. Neurosurg. Psychiat., 22:218–223, 1958.

16. Bradley, K. C.: Extra-dural hemorrhage. Aust. New Zeal. J. Surg., *21*:241–260, 1959.
17. Bull, J. W. D.: Personal communication, 1960.
18. Bull, J. W. D.: Contributions of radiology to the study of intracranial aneurysms. Brit. Med. J., *2*:1701–1708, 1962.
19. Bull, J. W. D.: Short history of intracranial aneurysms. London Clin. Med. J., *3*:47–61, 1962.
20. Bull, J. W. D., and Schunk, H.: The significance of displacement of the cavernous portion of the internal carotid artery. Brit. J. Radiol., *35*:801–814, 1962.
21. Campbell, J. A., and Campbell, R. L.: Angiographic diagnosis of traumatic head and neck lesions. J.A.M.A., *175*:761–768, 1961.
22. Campbell, J. B., and Cohen, J.: Epidural hemorrhage and the skull of children. Surg. Gynec. Obstet., *92*:257–280, 1951.
23. Castellanos, A., and Pereiras, R.: Retrograde or counter current aortography. Amer. J. Roentgen., *63*:559–565, 1950.
24. Conley, J. J., Chusid, J. G., and Schechter, M. M.: Angiography in head and neck surgery. Arch. Surg., *89*:609–619, 1964.
25. Contorni, L: Il Circulo collaterale vertebro-vertebrale nella obliterazione dell'arteria subclavia alle sua origine. Minerva Chir., *15*:268–271, 1960.
26. Crawford, T.: Some observations on the pathogenesis and natural history of intracranial aneurysms. J. Neurol. Neurosurg. Psychiat., *22*:259–266, 1959.
27. Cronqvist, S.: Vertebral catheterization via the femoral artery. Acta Radiol., *55*:113–118, 1961.
28. Cronqvist, S.: *In* Third International Symposium on Cerebral Circulation. Thule. Salzburg, 1966.
29. Cushing, H., and Bailey, P.: Tumors Arising from Blood Vessels of the Brain. Angiomatous Malformations and Haemangioblastomas. Springfield, Ill., Charles C Thomas, 1928.
30. Dandy, E. W.: Ventriculography following the injection of air into the cerebral ventricles. Ann. Surg., *68*:5–11, 1918.
31. Dandy, E. W.: Roentgenography of the brain after the injection of air into the spinal canal. Ann. Surg., *70*:397–403, 1919.
32. Daseler, E. H., and Anson, B. J.: Surgical anatomy of the subclavian artery and its branches. Surg. Gynec. Obstet., *108*:149–174, 1959.
33. DeBakey, M. E., Crawford, E. S., and Fields, W. S.: Surgical treatment of patients with cerebral arterial insufficiency associated with extracranial arterial occlusive lesions. Neurology, *11*:145–149, 1961.
34. DeGaris, C. F., Black, I. H., and Riemenschneider, E. A.: Patterns of the aortic arch in American white and Negro stocks with comparative notes on certain other mammals. J. Anat., *67*:599–619, 1933.
35. DeKleyn, A.: Some remarks on vestibular nystagmus. Confin. Neurol., *2*:257, 1939.
36. Di Chiro, G.: Ophthalmic arteriography. Radiology, *77*:948–957, 1961.
37. Dilenge, D., and Wuthrich, R.: Traumatic aneurysm of the middle meningeal artery. (In French). Neurochirurgia, *4*:202–206, 1962.
38. Dotter, C. T.: Left ventricular and systemic arterial catheterization. A simple percutaneous method using a spring guide. Amer. J. Roentgen., *83*:969–984, 1960.
39. Dotter, C. T., and Gensini, C. G.: Percutaneous retrograde catheterization of the left ventricle and systemic arteries of man. Radiology, *75*:171–184, 1960.
40. du Boulay, G.: Some observations on the natural history of intracranial aneurysms. Brit. J. Radiol., *38*:721–757, 1965.
41. Eastcott, H. H. G., Pickering, G. W., and Rob, C. G.: Reconstruction of internal carotid artery in a patient with intermittent attacks of hemiplegia. Lancet, *2*:994–996, 1954.
42. Ecker, A.: The Normal Cerebral Angiogram. Springfield, Ill., Charles C Thomas, 1951.
43. Ecker, A., and Riemenschneider, P. A.: Angiographic Localization of Intracranial Masses. Springfield, Ill., Charles C Thomas, 1955.
44. Engeset, A.: Cerebral angiography with Per-Abrodil. Acta Radiol., Suppl. 56, 1944.
45. Engstrom, H., and Hamberger, C. A.: Bilateral tumor of the carotid body. Acta Otolaryng., *48*:390–396, 1957.
46. Erb, K. H., and Hahn, E.: Aneurysmen des Arteria temporalis als Folge von Mensurverletzungen. Zbl. Chir., *58*:2610–2613, 1931.
47. Falk, B.: Radiologic diagnosis of intra-ventricular meningiomas. Acta Radiol., *46*:171–177, 1956.
48. Fawcett, E., and Blackford, J. V.: The circle of Willis: an examination of 700 specimens. J. Anat. Physiol., *40*:63–70, 1906.
49. Feindel, W., and Perot, P.: Red cerebral veins. A report on arteriovenous shunts in tumors and cerebral scars. J. Neurosurg., *22*:315–325, 1965.
50. Fetterman, G. H., and Moran, T. J.: Anomalies of the circle of Willis in relation to cerebral softening. Arch. Path., *32*:251–257, 1941.
51. Fields, W. S., Crawford, E. S., and DeBakey, M. E.: Surgical considerations in cerebral arterial insufficiency. Neurology, *8*:801–808, 1958.
52. Fields, W. S., Edwards, W. H., and Crawford, E. S.: Bilateral carotid artery thrombosis. Arch. Neurol., *4*:369–383, 1961.
53. Fincher, E. G.: Arteriovenous fistula between the middle meningeal artery and the greater petrosal sinus. Case report. Ann. Surg., *133*:886–888, 1951.
54. Fisher, A. G. T.: A case of complete absence of both internal carotid arteries. J. Anat. Physiol., *48*:37–46, 1913.
55. Fisher, M.: Occlusion of carotid arteries. Arch. Neurol. Psychiat., *72*:187–204, 1954.
56. Freidenfelt, H., and Sundstrom R.: Local and general spasm in the internal carotid system following trauma. Acta Radiol. (Diagn.), *1*:278–283, 1963.
57. Gabriele, O. F., and Bell, D.: Ophthalmic origin of the middle meningeal artery. Radiology, *89*:841–844, 1967.
58. Galloway, J. R., Greitz, T., and Sjogren, S. E.:

Vertebral angiography in the diagnosis of ventricular dilatation. Acta Radiol. (Diagn.), 2: 321–333, 1964.

59. Gannon, W. E.: Valves of the common carotid artery during angiography. Amer. J. Roentgen., 86:1050–1057, 1961.

60. Gannon, W. E.: Interhemispheric subdural hematoma. J. Neurosurg., 18:829–830, 1961.

61. Gardner, W. J.: Traumatic subdural hematoma with particular reference to the latent interval. Arch. Neurol. Psychiat., 27:847–858, 1932.

62. Gass, H. H.: Kinks and coils of the cervical carotid artery. Surg. Forum, 9:721–724, 1959.

63. Gassel, M. M., and Davies, H.: Meningiomas in the lateral ventricles. Brain, 84:605–626, 1961.

64. Glynn, L. E.: Medial defects in circle of Willis and their relation to aneurysm formation. J. Path. Bact., 51:213–222, 1940.

65. Gooddy, W., and Schechter, M. M.: Spontaneous arteriovenous fistula of the vertebral artery. Brit. J. Radiol., 33:709–711, 1960.

66. Greenspan, R. H., Simon, A. L., Rickells, H. J., Rojas, R. H., and Watson, J. C.: In vivo magnification angiography. Invest. Radiol., 2:419–431, 1967.

67. Greitz, T., and Lindgren, E.: Angiographic determination of brain tumor pathology. In Abrams, H. L., ed.: Angiography I. Boston, Little Brown and Co., 1961.

68. Gutstein, R. A., and Schecter, M. M.: Aneurysms and arteriovenous fistulas of the superficial temporal artery. In preparation.

69. Hanafee, W. N.: Personal communication, 1963.

70. Hancock, D. O.: Angiography in acute head injuries. Lancet, 2:745–747, 1961.

71. Harrison, J. H., and Davalos, P. A.: Cerebral ischemia. Surgical procedure in cases due to tortuosity and buckling of the cervical vessels. Arch. Surg., 84:85–94, 1962.

72. Hasegawa, T., Ravens, J. R., and Toole, J. F.: Precapillary arteriovenous anastamosed "thoroughfare channels" in the brain. Arch. Neurol., 16:217–224, 1967.

73. Hassler, O.: Medial defects in the meningeal arteries. J. Neurosurg., 19:337–340, 1962.

74. Hassler, O., and Saltzman, G. F.: Histologic changes in infundibular widening of the posterior communicating artery. Acta Path. Microbiol. Scand., 46:305–312, 1959.

75. Hassler, O., and Saltzman, G. F.: Angiographic and histologic changes in infundibular widening of the posterior communicating artery. Acta Radiol. (Diagn.), 1:321–327, 1963.

76. Hauge, T.: Catheter vertebral angiography. Acta Radiol., suppl. 109, 1954.

77. Hayes, G. J.: External carotid-cavernous sinus fistulas. J. Neurosurg., 20:692–700, 1963.

78. Heister, L.: General System of Surgery. London, 1750.

79. Hirano, A., and Terry, R. D.: Aneurysm of the vein of Galen. J. Neuropath. Exp. Neurol., 17:424–429, 1958.

80. Hirsch, J. F., David, M., and Sachs, M.: Les anévrysmes artériels traumatiques intracrâniens. Neurochirurgie, 8:189–201, 1962.

81. Huang, Y. P., and Wolf, B. S.: The veins of the posterior fossa—superior or galenic draining group. Amer. J. Roentgen., 95:808–821, 1965.

82. Huang, Y. S., and Araki, C.: Angiographic confirmation of lateral ventricle meningiomas. A report of 5 cases. J. Neurosurg., 11:337–352, 1954.

83. Huber, P.: Die Verletzungen der Meningealfasse bein Epiduralhamatöm im Angiogramm. Fortschr. Röntgenstr., 96:207–220, 1962.

84. Hurwitt, E. S., Carton, C. A., Fell, S. C., Kessler, L. A., Seidenberg, B., and Shapiro, J. H.: Critical evaluation and surgical corrections of obstructions in the branches of the aortic arch. Ann. Surg., 152:472–484, 1960.

85. Hutchinson, E. C., and Yates, P. O.: The cervical portion of the vertebral artery. A clinicopathological study. Brain, 79:319–331, 1956.

86. Hutchinson, E. C., and Yates, P. O.: Caroticovertebral stenosis. Lancet, 1:2–8, 1957.

87. Jackson, D. C., and du Boulay, G. H.: Traumatic arterio-venous aneurysm of the middle meningeal artery. Brit. J. Radiol., 37:788–789, 1964.

88. Jackson, I. J., and Speakman, T. J.: Chronic extradural hematoma. J. Neurosurg., 7:444–447, 1950.

89. Jackson, J. R., Tindall, G. T., and Nashold, B. S.: Rupture of an intracranial aneurysm during carotid arteriography. A case report. J. Neurosurg., 17:333–336, 1960.

90. Jacobsen, H. H.: An interhemispherically situated hematoma. Case report. Acta Radiol., 43:235–236, 1955.

91. Jaeger, R., and Whiteley, W. H.: Cerebral angiography by an intravascular intubation technique. Amer. J. Roentgen., 73:735–747, 1955.

92. Jamieson, K. G.: Unusual case of extra-dural haematoma. Aust. New Zeal. J. Surg., 21:304–307, 1952.

93. Johansson, C.: The central veins and deep dural sinuses of the brain. Acta Radiol., suppl. 107, 1954.

94. Jones, F. W.: Grooves upon ossa parietalia commonly said to be caused by arteria meningea media. J. Anat. Physiol., 46:228–238, 1912.

95. Jones, F. W.: Vascular lesion in some cases of middle meningeal haemorrhage. Lancet, 2:7–12, 1912.

96. Karras, B. G., Cannon, A. H., and Ashby, R. N.: Percutaneous left brachial aortography. Personal communication, 1960.

97. Kia-Noury, M.: Traumatisches intrakranielles Aneurysma der Arteria meningica media nach Schadelbasis-fraktur. Zbl. Neurochir., 21:351–357, 1961.

98. Krayenbühl, H.: Cerebral venous thrombosis: diagnostic value of cerebral angiography. Schweiz. Arch. Neurol. Psychiat., 74:261–287, 1954.

99. Krayenbühl, H.: The diagnostic value of orbital angiography. Brit. J. Ophthal., 42:180–190, 1958.

100. Krayenbühl, H., and Richter, H. R.: Die Zerebrale Angiographie. Stuttgart, Georg Thieme, 1952.

101. Krayenbühl, H., and Yasargil, M. G.: Die Vaskularen Erkrankungen in Gebiet der Arteria

Vertebralis und Arteria Basialis. Stuttgart, Georg Thieme, 1957.

102. Krayenbühl, H., and Yasargil, M. G.: Das Hirnaneurysma. Basel, J. R. Geigy, 1958.

103. Kuhn, R. A.: The normal brachial cerebral angiogram. Amer. J. Roentgen., 84:78–87, 1960.

104. Kuhn, R. A., and Kugler, H.: False aneurysms of the middle meningeal artery. J. Neurosurg., 21:92–96, 1964.

105. Lai, M. D., Hoffman, H. B., and Adamkiewicz, J. J.: Dissecting aneurysm of the cervical portion of the internal carotid artery secondary to non-penetrating neck injury. Acta Radiol. (Diagn.), 5:290–295, 1966.

106. Laine, E., Delandtsheer, J. M., Galibert, P., and Delandtsheer-Arnot, G.: Phlebography in tumours of the hemispheres and central grey matter. Acta Radiol., 46:203–214, 1956.

107. Lassen, N. A.: The luxury perfusion syndrome and its possible relation to acute metabolic acidosis localized within the brain. Lancet, 2:1113–1115, 1966.

108. La Torre, E., Occhipinti, E., and Pollicita, A.: Backward displacement of the upper part of the basilar artery in infantile hydrocephalus. Acta Radiol. (Diagn.), 8:385–399, 1969.

109. Leslie, E. V., Smith, B. H., and Zoll, J. G.: Value of angiography in head trauma. Radiology, 78:930–939, 1962.

110. Lindgren, E.: Percutaneous angiography of the vertebral artery. Acta Radiol., 33:389–405, 1950.

111. Lindgren, E.: Röntgenologie. Band II. In Olivecrona, H., and Tonnis, W., eds.: Handbuch der Neurochirurgie. Berlin, Springer-Verlag, 1954.

112. Lindgren, E.: Another method of vertebral angiography. Acta Radiol., 46:257–262, 1956.

113. Lindgren, E.: Radiologic examination of the brain and spinal cord. Acta Radiol., suppl. 151, 1957.

114. Litvak, J., Yahr, M. D., and Ransohoff, J.: Aneurysms of the great vein of Galen and midline cerebral arteriovenous anomalies. J. Neurosurg., 17:945–954, 1960.

115. Liverud, K.: Technique in percutaneous carotid and vertebral angiography with polyethylene catheters. J. Oslo City Hosp., 8:220–242, 1958.

116. Lofgren, O. F.: Vertebral angiography in the diagnosis of tumors in the pineal region. Acta Radiol., 50:108–124, 1958.

117. Lofstrom, J. E., Webster, J. E., and Gurdjian, E. S.: Angiography in the evaluation of intracranial trauma. Radiology, 65:847–855, 1955.

118. Lohr, W.: Hirngefassverletzungen in arteriographischer Darstellung. Zbl. Chir., 63:2466–2482, 1936.

119. Lombardi, G.: Radiology in Neuro-Ophthalmology. Baltimore, Md., Williams & Wilkins Co., 1967.

120. Luckett, W. H.: Air in the ventricles of the brain following a fracture of the skull. J. Nerv. Ment. Dis., 40:326–328, 1913.

121. Markham, J. W.: Arteriovenous fistula of the middle meningeal artery and the greater petrosal sinus. J. Neurosurg., 18:847–848, 1961.

122. Markwalder, H., and Huber, P.: Aneurysmen der Meningealarterien. Schweiz. Med. Wschr., 91:1344–1347, 1961.

123. Maslowski, H. A.: Vertebral angiography. Percutaneous lateral atlanto-occipital method. Brit. J. Surg., 43:1–8, 1955.

124. Maslowski, H. A.: International Meeting Society of British Neurological Surgeons and La Societé de Neurochirurgiens de Langue Française, 1960.

125. Matson, D. D., and Crofton, F. D. L.: Papilloma of the choroid plexus in childhood. J. Neurosurg., 17:1002–1027, 1960.

126. McKissock, W., Taylor, J. C., Bloom, W. H., and Till, K.: Extradural hematoma. Observations on 125 cases. Lancet, 2:167–172, 1960.

127. McLaurin, R. L., and Ford, L. E.: Extradural hematoma. Statistical study of 47 cases. J. Neurosurg., 21:364–371, 1964.

128. Mones, R.: Vertebral angiography. An analysis of 106 cases. Radiology, 76:230–236, 1961.

129. Moniz, E.: L'encephalographie artérielle, son importance dans la localization des tumeurs cérébrales. Rev. Neurol., 342:72–90, 1927.

130. Moniz, E., and Alves, A.: L'importance diagnostique de l'arteriographie de la fosse posterieure. Rev. Neurol., 40:91–96, 1933.

131. Morris, L.: Arteriographic demonstration of the vertebral artery with special reference to percutaneous subclavian puncture. Brit. J. Radiol., 32:673–679, 1960.

132. Mount, L. A., and Taveras, J. M.: Arteriographic demonstration of the collateral circulation of the cerebral hemispheres. Arch. Neurol. Psychiat., 78:235–253, 1957.

133. Murphy, F., and Shillito, J., Jr.: Avoidance of false angiographic localization of the site of internal carotid occlusion. J. Neurosurg., 16:24–31, 1959.

134. New, P. F. J.: True aneurysm of the middle meningeal artery. Clin. Radiol., 16:236–240, 1965.

135. New, P. F. J., and Momose, K. J.: Traumatic dissection of the internal carotid artery on the atlantoaxial level secondary to non-penetrating injury. Radiology, 93:41–46, 1969.

136. Newton, T. H., and Couch, R. S. C.: Possible errors in the arteriographic diagnosis of internal carotid artery occlusion. Radiology, 75:766–773, 1960.

137. Norlen, G., and Paly, N.: Aneurysms of the vertebral artery. J. Neurosurg., 17:830–835, 1960.

138. Norman, O.; Angiographic differentiation between acute and chronic subdural and extradural hematomas. Acta Radiol., 46:371–378, 1956.

139. O'Brien, M. S., and Schechter, M. M.: Arteriovenous malformations involving the galenic system. In preparation.

140. Odman, P.: Percutaneous selective angiography of the main branches of the aorta. Preliminary report. Acta Radiol., 45:1–14, 1956.

141. Okay, N. H.: Angiographic studies of the factors causing cervical and intracranial flow. Brit. J. Radiol., 42:676–681, 1969.

142. Olsson, O.: Vertebral angiography in the diagnosis of acoustic nerve tumors. Acta Radiol., *39*:265–272, 1953.

143. Olsson, O.: Vertebral angiography in cerebellar hemangioma. Acta Radiol., *40*:9–16, 1953.

144. Padget, D. H.: The circle of Willis: its embryology and anatomy. *In* Dandy, W. E., ed.: Intracranial Arterial Aneurysm. Ithaca, N.Y., Comstock Publishing Co., 1944.

145. Paillas, J. E., Bonnal, J., and Lavielle, J.: Angiographic images of false aneurysmal sac caused by rupture of median meningeal artery in the course of traumatic extradural hematomata. Report of three cases. J. Neurosurg., *21*:667–671, 1964.

146. Pecker, J., Javalet, A., and Stabert, C.: L'angiographie dans les traumatismes crâniens. J. Radiol. Electr., *40*:623–628, 1959.

147. Perret, G., and Nishioka, H.: Cerebral angiography. An analysis of the diagnostic value and complications of carotid and vertebral angiography in 5,484 patients. J. Neurosurg., *25*:98–114, 1966.

148. Perrot, P., Ethier, R., and Wong, A.: An arterial posterior fossa extradural hematoma demonstrated by vertebral angiography. Case report. J. Neurosurg., *26*:255–260, 1967.

149. Petit-Dutaillis, D., Guiot, G., Pertuiset, B., and LeBesnerais, Y.: Les hématomes extraduraux de la fosse cérébelleuse. Presse Méd., *64*:521–524, 1956.

150. Poppen, J. L., and Avman, N.: Aneurysms of the great vein of Galen. J. Neurosurg., *17*:238–244, 1960.

151. Pouyanne, H., Leman, P., Got, M., and Gouaze, A.: Traumatic arterial aneurysm of the left middle meningeal artery: Rupture one month after the accident; Temporal intracerebral hematoma; intervention. (In French). Neurochirurgie, *5*:311–315, 1959.

152. Pribram, H. F. W.: Angiographic appearances in acute intracranial hypertension. Neurology, *11*:10–21, 1961.

153. Putnam, T., and Cushing, H.: Chronic subdural hematoma. Arch. Surg., *11*:329–393, 1925.

154. Pygott, F., and Hutton, C. F.: Vertebral angiography by percutaneous brachial artery catheterization. Brit. J. Radiol., *32*:114–119, 1959.

155. Quattlebaum, J. K., Upson, E. T., and Neville, R. L.: Stroke associated with elongation and kinking of the internal carotid artery: report of three cases treated by segmental resection of the common carotid artery. Ann. Surg., *150*:824–832, 1959.

156. Radner, S.: Intracranial angiography via the femoral artery. Preliminary report of a new technique. Acta Radiol., *28*:838–842, 1947.

157. Radner, S.: Vertebral angiography by catheterization. A new method employed in 221 cases. Acta Radiol., suppl. 87, 1951.

158. Reivich, M., Holling, H. E., Roberts, B., and Toole, J. F.: Reversal of blood flow through the vertebral artery and its effects on cerebral circulation. New Eng. J. Med., *265*:878–885, 1961.

159. Ring, B. A.: Variations in the striate and other

160. Riser, M., Geraud, J., Ducoudray, J., and Ribaut, L.: Dolichocarotide interne avec syndrome vertigineux. Rev. Neurol., *85*:145–147, 1951.

161. Rivaglia, cited by Perrig, H.: Zur Anatomie, Klinik and Therapie der Verletzungen und Aneurysmen der Arteria vertebralis. Beitr. Klin. Chir., *154*:272–307, 1931.

162. Rob, C. G., and Wheeler, E. B.: Thrombosis of internal carotid artery treated by arterial surgery. Brit. Med. J., *2*:264–266, 1957.

163. Rogers, V.: Vertebral angiography in the diagnosis of meningioma within the lateral ventricle. Brit. J. Radiol., *33*:326–328, 1960.

164. Rosenbaum, A. E., and Schechter, M. M.: Carotid-cavernous fistulae. Acta Radiol. (Diagn.) in press.

165. Rossi, P.: Personal communication, 1967.

166. Rossi, P.: Transaxillary selective catheterization of the carotid and vertebral arteries. Acta Radiol. (Diagn.), *5*:458–464, 1966.

167. Rowbotham, G. F., and Whalley, N.: Prolonged compression of the brain resulting from an extradural hemorrhage. J. Neurol. Neurosurg. Psychiat., *15*:64–65, 1952.

168. Roy, P.: Percutaneous catheterization of the axillary artery. Tenth International Congress of Radiology, 1962.

169. Ruggiero, G., and Jay, M.: Une technique pour l'arteriographie de l'artere carotide externe. Acta Radiol., *50*:453–459, 1958.

170. Ruggiero, G., Calabro, A., Metzger, J., and Simon, J.: Arteriography of the external carotid artery. Acta Radiol. (Diagn.), *1*:395–403, 1963.

171. Rydell, J. R., and Jennings, W. K.: The surgical treatment of carotid aneurysm in the neck. West. J. Surg., Obstet. Gynec., *64*:385–390, 1956.

172. Saltzman, G. F.: Circulation through the posterior communicating artery in different compression tests. Acta Radiol., *51*:10–16, 1959.

173. Saltzman, G. F.: Infundibular widening of the posterior communicating artery studied by carotid angiography. Acta Radiol., *51*:415–421, 1959.

174. Saltzman, G. F.: Angiographic demonstration of the posterior communicating and posterior cerebral arteries. I: Normal angiography. Acta Radiol., *52*:1–20, 1959.

175. Scatliff, J. H., Hyde, I., and Gantot, H. J.: Vertebral artery reflux: a laboratory investigation of the non-obstructive causes of retrograde flow of contrast material in the contralateral vertebral artery. Radiology, *88*:63–74, 1967.

176. Scatliff, J. H., Kier, E. L., Zingesser, L. H., and Schechter, M. M.: Terminal basilar artery deformity secondary to suprasellar masses and third ventricular dilatation. Amer. J. Roentgen., *101*:61–67, 1967.

177. Schechter, M. M.: Total vertebrobasilar arteriography using a single vertebral puncture technique. J. Neurosurg., *18*:74–78, 1961.

cerebral veins affecting measurement of the "venous angle." Acta Radiol., *52*:433–447, 1959.

178. Schechter, M. M.: Percutaneous carotid catheterization. Acta Radiol. (Diagn.), *1*:417–426, 1963.

179. Schechter, M. M., and Chusid, J. G.: Chemodectomas of the carotid bifurcation. Acta Radiol. (Diagn.), *5*:488–508, 1966.

180. Schechter, M. M., and De Gutierrez-Mahoney, C. G.: Vertebral angiography. Exhibited at International Congress of Neurosurgery, 1961.

181. Schechter, M. M., and Elkin, M.: The layering effect in cerebral angiography. Acta Radiol., *1*:427–435, 1963.

182. Schechter, M. M., and Zingesser, L. H.: The radiology of basilar thrombosis. Radiology, *85*:23–32, 1965.

183. Schechter, M. M., and Zingesser, L. H.: The anterior spinal artery. Acta Radiol. (Diagn.), *3*:489–495, 1965.

184. Schechter, M. M., and Zingesser, L. H.: The spinal arteries. Acta Radiol. (Diagn.), *5*:1124–1131, 1966.

185. Schechter, M. M., Zingesser, L. H., and Rosenbaum, A. E.: Tentorial meningiomas. Amer. J. Roentgen., *104*:123–131, 1968.

186. Schmidt, H., and Rossi, U.: Intracerebrale extravasation nach Hirnkortusion im Karotisangiogramm. Fortschr. Röntgenstr., *94*:505–508, 1961.

187. Schneider, H. J., and Felson, B.: Buckling of the innominate artery simulating aneurysm and tumor. Amer. J. Roentgen., *85*:1106–1110, 1961.

188. Schulze, A.: Seltene verlaufsformen epiduraler Hematome. Zbl. Neurochir., *17*:40–47, 1957.

189. Sears, A. D., Miller, J. E., and Kilgore, B. B.: Diagnosis of cerebral atrophy from the anteroposterior carotid phlebogram. Amer. J. Roentgen., *85*:1128–1133, 1961.

190. Seldinger, S. I.: Catheter replacement of the needle in the percutaneous arteriography. A new technique. Acta Radiol., *39*:368–376, 1953.

191. Sergent, P., Rougerie, J., Pertuiset, B., and Petit-Dutailis, D.: L'angiographie vertebrale percutanée cervicale anterieure d'après 130 cas. Technique et bases de l'interpretation des cliches. Presse Méd., *60*:1415–1418, 1952.

192. Sheehan, S., Bauer, R. B., and Meyer, J. S.: Vertebral artery compression in cervical spondylosis, arteriographic demonstration during life of vertebral artery insufficiency due to rotation and extension of the neck. Neurology, *10*:968–986, 1960.

193. Shimidzu, K.: Beitrage zur Arteriographie des Gehirns einfache percutane Methode. Arch. Klin. Chir., *188*:295–316, 1937.

194. Silvan (1913): Quoted by Krayenbühl and Yasargil, see ref. 101.

195. Silverstein, A., Lehrer, G. M., and Mones, R.: Relation of certain diagnostic features of carotid occlusion to collateral circulation. Neurology, *10*:409–417, 1960.

196. Sjögren, S. E.: Anterior choroidal artery. Acta Radiol., *46*:143–157, 1956.

197. Smaltino, F.: Personal comments.

198. Spatz, E. L., and Bull, J. W. D.: Vertebral arteriography in the study of subarachnoid hemorrhage. J. Neurosurg., *14*:543–547, 1957.

199. Stehbens, W. E.: Intracranial arterial aneurysms. Aust. Ann. Med., *3*:214–218, 1954.

200. Stopford, J. S. B.: The arteries of the pons and medulla oblongata. J. Anat., *50*:131–164, 1916.

201. Sugar, O., Holden, L. B., and Powell, C. B.: Vertebral angiography. Amer. J. Roentgen., *61*:166–182, 1949.

202. Sutton, D.: Anomalous carotid basilar anastomosis. Brit. J. Radiol., *23*:617–619, 1950.

203. Sutton, D.: Discussion on the clinical and radiological aspects of diseases of the major arteries. Proc. Roy. Soc. Med., *49*:559–571, 1956.

204. Sutton, D.: Vertebral arteriography by percutaneous brachial artery catheterization. Note to the Editor. Brit. J. Radiol., *32*:283, 1959.

205. Sutton, D.: Arteriography, London, E. & S. Livingstone, Ltd., 1962.

206. Swann, G. F.: Vertebral arteriography using the Sheldon needle and modifications of it. Brit. J. Radiol., *31*:23–27, 1958.

207. Takahashi, K.: Die percutane Arteriographie der Arteria vertebralis und ihrer Versorgungsgebiete. Arch. Psychiat., *111*:373–379, 1940.

208. Takahashi, M., Wilson, G., and Hanafee, W.: Significance of petrosal vein in diagnosis of cerebellopontine angle tumors. Radiology, *89*:834–840, 1967.

209. Taptas, J. N.: Les anévrismes arterio-veineux carotido-caverneux. Neurochirurgie, *8*:385–394, 1963.

210. Tatelman, M.: Pathways of cerebral collateral circulation. Radiology, *75*:349–362, 1960.

211. Taveras, J. M., and Poser, C. M.: Roentgenologic aspects of cerebral angiography in children. Amer. J. Roentgen., *82*:371–391, 1959.

212. Taveras, J. M., and Wood, E. H.: Diagnostic Neuroradiology. Baltimore, Md., Williams & Wilkins Co., 1964.

213. Taveras, J. M., Mount, L. A., and Friedenberg, R. M.: Arteriographic demonstration of external-internal carotid anastomosis through the ophthalmic arteries. Radiology, *63*:525–530, 1954.

214. Tindall, G. T., and Culp, H. B., Jr.: Vertebral arteriography by retrograde injection of the right common carotid artery. Radiology, *76*:742–747, 1961.

215. Tiwisina, T., and Stecker, A. D.: The fresh cranio-cerebral injuries in vascular picture. (In German). Chirurg, *30*:344–349, 1959.

216. Tori, G., and Garusi, G. F.: Left carotid-jugular arteriovenous fistula. Radiol. Clin., *30*:76–85, 1961.

217. Ullrich, D. P., and Sugar, O.: Familial cerebral aneurysms including one extracranial internal carotid aneurysm. Neurology, *10*:288–294, 1960.

218. vander Eecken, H. M., and Adams, R. D.: The anatomy and functional significance of the meningeal arterial anastomosis of the human brain. J. Neuropath. Exp. Neurol., *12*:132–157, 1953.

219. Vaughan, B. F.: Middle meningeal haemorrhage demonstrated angiographically. Brit. J. Radiol., 32:493–494, 1959.

220. Wall, A. E.: Meningiomas within the lateral ventricle. J. Neurol. Neurosurg. Psychiat., 17:91–103, 1954.

221. Weiner, I. H., Azzato, N. M., and Mendelsohn, R. A.: Cerebral angiography. J. Neurosurg., 15:618–626, 1958.

222. Wickbom, I.: Angiography of the carotid artery. Acta Radiol., suppl. 72, 1948.

223. Wickbom, I.: Angiography by post-traumatic intracranial hemorrhages. Acta Radiol., 32:249–258, 1949.

224. Wickbom, I., and Bartley, O.: Arterial spasm in peripheral arteriography using the catheter method. Acta Radiol., 47:433–448, 1957.

225. Wilson, C. B., and Cronic, F.: Traumatic arteriovenous fistulas involving the middle meningeal vessels. J.A.M.A., 188:953–957, 1964.

226. Wolf, B. S., Huang, Y. P., and Newman, C. M.: Superficial sylvian venous drainage system. Amer. J. Roentgen., 89:398–410, 1963.

227. Wollschlaeger, P. B., and Wollschlaeger, G.: Personal communication, 1968.

228. Wollschlaeger, P. B., and Wollschlaeger, G.: The interhemispheric subdural or falx hematoma. Amer. J. Roentgen., 92:1252–1254, 1964.

229. Wolman, L.: Cerebral dissecting aneurysms. Brain, 82:276–291, 1959.

230. Wolpert, S. M., and Schechter, M. M.: Traumatic middle cerebral artery occlusion. Radiology, 87:671–677, 1966.

231. Wood, E. H.: Angiographic identification of the ruptured lesion in patients with multiple cerebral aneurysms. J. Neurosurg., 21:182–198, 1964.

232. Wortzman, G.: Traumatic pseudo-aneurysm of the superficial temporal artery. A case report. Radiology, 80:444–446, 1963.

233. Yates, P. O.: Pathological changes following proximal vertebral arterial stenosis. Proc. Roy. Soc. Med., 50:663–665, 1957.

234. Zaclis, J., and Tenuto, R. A.: Diagnóstico angiográfico dos hematomas subdurais. Valor de fase venuso em incidência sagital. Arq. Neuropsiquiat., 13:273–295, 1955.

235. Zielke, K., and Weidner, H.: Eine einfache und ungefährliche Punktionsmethode zue Kontrastmittelfüllung der Arteria vertebralis. Acta Neurochir., 9:87–101, 1960.

236. Zilkha, A.: Les fistules arterioveineuses traumatiques du carr. Presented at the Eighth Neuroradiological Symposium. Paris, 1967.

237. Zingesser, L. H., Schechter, M. M., and Rayport, M.: Truths and untruths concerning the angiographic findings in extracerebral haematomas, Brit. J. Radiol., 38:835–847, 1965.

238. Zingesser, L. H., Bernstein, J., Schechter, M. M., and Wollschlaeger, G.: The neuroradiologic significance of anomalies of the aortic arch. Presented at the meeting of the Association of University Radiologists, New Haven, Conn., 1963.

6

ENCEPHALOGRAPHY

PNEUMOENCEPHALOGRAPHY

Radiographic demonstration of the ventricular system was first obtained in 1912.[6] The patient was a man who had sustained trauma in a streetcar accident. As a consequence of a fracture in the posterior wall of the frontal sinus, air had entered the ventricular system. Radiograms demonstrated the air-filled ventricles. It was not until 1918–1919, however, that Walter Dandy deliberately introduced air into the ventricles and into the subarachnoid space of the spinal canal for the purpose of demonstrating the intracranial cerebrospinal fluid-containing spaces.[2, 3]

Pneumoencephalography and ventriculography are thus the oldest neuroradiological diagnostic modalities save for the application of the method of Röntgen to the examination of the bones and soft tissues of the head itself. These procedures remained the mainstay of neuroradiological diagnosis, even after the introduction of angiography, until relatively safe contrast media were discovered. Today, cerebral angiography has largely supplanted pneumography in the investigation of intracranial neurological disease. There are, however, lesions of various sorts that are best diagnosed by means of air studies. Advances in our knowledge of the arteriographic and venographic anatomy relating to the ventricular and cisternal anatomy have enabled the expert who is well versed in the interpretation of angiographic studies to make well-informed statements about the exact situation and state of most parts of the ventricular system and cisterns, but the complete demonstration of all parts of the ventricular system and cisterns is possible only with the replacement of spinal fluid with contrast material, which may be either opaque or nonopaque. Thus, certain tumors that are large enough only to protrude into the subarachnoid cisterns, intraventricular lesions, juxtaventricular lesions, certain congenital anomalies, and conditions associated with atrophy of the brain are best studied in this manner (Figs. 6–1 and 6–2).

On the other hand, the angiographic techniques allow the investigation of space-occupying lesions to proceed without alteration of the pressures that have resulted from the intracranial mass lesion. The replacement of cerebrospinal fluid with air or even the addition of air to the cerebrospinal fluid spaces without removal of spinal fluid is the first in a series of events that may lead to shifts in the position of the brain and the mass lesion that will further jeopardize the patient's condition. At times, such shifts in the ventricular system may also give a false impression as to the location of a mass lesion.[12] This is true particularly when cerebral atrophy is present. Situations in which these considerations are vital and ways to minimize these effects are discussed in greater detail later in this chapter.

Preparation of the Patient

A wide variety of medications has been used to prepare the patient for pneumoencephalography. These are given to allay apprehension and to minimize the effects of the study on the vegetative nervous system. Intake of food and fluid should be restricted

L. H. ZINGESSER
M. M. SCHECHTER

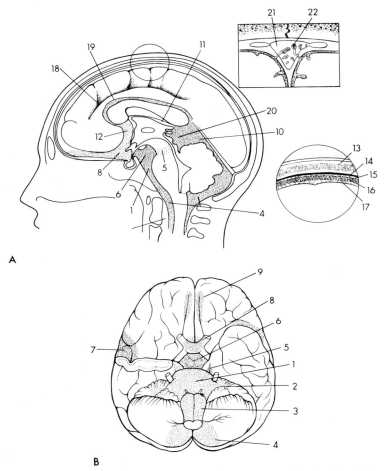

FIGURE 6–1 *A*. Sagittal view of subarachnoid cisterns. *B*. Basal view of subarachnoid cisterns. 1. Pontine cistern. 2. Pontocerebellar cistern. 3. Medullary cistern. 4. Cisterna magna (vallecular portion communicates with outlet foramina of fourth ventricle). 5. Ambient cistern. 6. Interpeduncular cistern. 7. Cistern of the sylvian fissure. 8. Chiasmatic cistern. 9. Cistern of the olfactory tract. 10. Superior cerebellar cistern. 11. Velum interpositum (when filled with air is called the cavum veli interpositi). 12. Cistern of the lamina terminalis. 13. Calvarium. 14. Dura mater. 15. Subdural space. 16. Arachnoid. 17. Subarachnoid space. 18. Cistern of the cingulate sulcus. 19. Cistern of the corpus callosum. 20. Cistern of the quadrigeminal plate or cistern of the great vein of Galen. 21. Superior sagittal sinus. 22. Arachnoid villus.

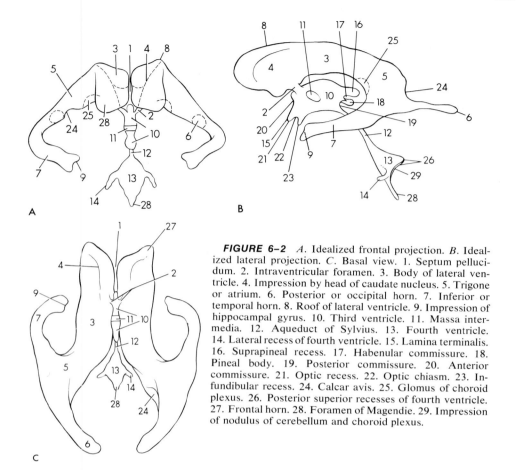

FIGURE 6-2 *A.* Idealized frontal projection. *B.* Idealized lateral projection. *C.* Basal view. 1. Septum pellucidum. 2. Intraventricular foramen. 3. Body of lateral ventricle. 4. Impression by head of caudate nucleus. 5. Trigone or atrium. 6. Posterior or occipital horn. 7. Inferior or temporal horn. 8. Roof of lateral ventricle. 9. Impression of hippocampal gyrus. 10. Third ventricle. 11. Massa intermedia. 12. Aqueduct of Sylvius. 13. Fourth ventricle. 14. Lateral recess of fourth ventricle. 15. Lamina terminalis. 16. Suprapineal recess. 17. Habenular commissure. 18. Pineal body. 19. Posterior commissure. 20. Anterior commissure. 21. Optic recess. 22. Optic chiasm. 23. Infundibular recess. 24. Calcar avis. 25. Glomus of choroid plexus. 26. Posterior superior recesses of fourth ventricle. 27. Frontal horn. 28. Foramen of Magendie. 29. Impression of nodulus of cerebellum and choroid plexus.

for several hours before the study is begun. A combination of barbiturates and atropine has, in the authors' experience, been the simplest and most effective way of preparing patients for the study. Problems may arise in elderly individuals in whom the effect of barbiturates may be excitatory rather than sedative and in young persons in whom more medication may have to be used than seems appropriate for the weight of the patient. A dosage schedule of medication for pediatric patients is included here (Table 6-1).[4, 9] It must be emphasized that there is a variability in response from patient to patient. In general, the younger the patient, the higher the per kilogram dose requirements.

General anesthesia is seldom used by the authors, for the morbidity of the procedure is probably increased in this way, but this may not be so in certain uncontrollable pa-tients and where the general anesthetic is administered by experienced personnel.

Technique of Pneumoencephalography

The examination can be carried out via the lumbar or the cisternal route. There is usually no advantage to the cisternal route except when the lumbar route is blocked. The spinal puncture should be performed several days after any previous spinal puncture. Otherwise the spinal fluid that issues from the needle may be coming from a pool in the subdural space rather than from the subarachnoid space.

Selection of the proper needle is of great importance. The smaller the needle, the smaller the hole remaining when the needle is removed, and the less leakage of spinal

TABLE 6-1 *PEDIATRIC*
NEURORADIOLOGIC PREMEDICATION

Age (yr.)	Secobarbital (mg/kg)	Chlorpromazine (mg/kg)	Atropine (mg/kg)
PNEUMOENCEPHALOGRAMS AND VENTRICULOGRAMS			
Newborn − 2 yr.	10–8	1.0	0.01
2–4	7–6	1.0	0.01
5–8	6–5	1.0	0.01
9–15	4–3	0.75–0.5	0.01 (up to 0.4 mg per patient)
ANGIOGRAMS AND MYELOGRAMS			
Newborn − 2 yr.	8–7	1.0	0.01
2–4	6–5	1.0	0.01
5–8	5–4	1.0	0.01
9–15	4–3	0.75–0.5	0.01 (up to 0.4 mg per patient)

fluid. This is an important consideration in patients with increased intracranial pressure. A 20-gauge needle in adults and a 22-gauge needle in children are recommended. The bevel of the needle should be short. This is very important, for the risk of injection of air into the subdural space is minimized with the short-beveled needle.

If it is necessary to collect spinal fluid for laboratory assay, this fluid should be collected immediately. A cellular response occurs very rapidly after the introduction of air, and the protein value may be altered also. Generally it is best to remove as little fluid as possible, especially in the early stages of the examination, and it is best to remove no fluid if intracranial pressure is raised.

The needle is introduced in the conventional way in the lumbar area and the usual sensations are felt as the needle penetrates the theca. When the stylet is removed, the spinal fluid should flow freely. If it does not, gentle manipulation of the needle may be required, for a fold of arachnoid or a nerve root may be blocking the needle even though it is centrally placed within the spinal canal. When a long-beveled needle is used, free flow of spinal fluid does not guarantee that the air introduced is going to pass into the subarachnoid space. Some workers believe that the needle should be introduced so that the bevel is longitudinally oriented. It is claimed that in this way the fibers of the dura are separated and not interrupted.

The patient should be comfortably seated. A "military" position of the head and neck is usually effective in directing the first air into the vallecular portion of the cisterna magna and thence into the foramen of Magendie. If the patient's neck and head are overflexed, the bulk of the air will pass over the surface of the cerebellum, which is desirable only if the pathological condition to be studied is located in that area. With overextension of the head and neck the bulk of the air will pass into the pontine cistern, and then go through the interpeduncular cistern to pass through a membrane usually located in that area to enter the cisterns at the base of the brain. From that location the air will pass around the lateral and anterior portions of the brain as it ascends to the high convexity.

The first films are critical in that they will indicate whether the needle is correctly placed, whether tonsillar herniation exists, and whether the posterior fossa is free of disease. Also, on later films cisternal air may obscure the aqueduct. The radiographic equipment that is employed should therefore provide for the necessity of obtaining horizontal and half-axial films of good quality with the patient erect. Apparatus that includes an upright Bucky grid for the half-axial films is a necessity. The lateral films obtained with a high-quality stationary grid, however, will be satisfactory. Some workers find the use of polaroid films or image-intensification equipment to be advantageous in following the early passage of the air.

On these early films, careful attention is paid to the craniocervical junction. The cervical cord itself is evaluated, and one looks for evidence of tonsillar herniation. At times, the lobe of the ear overlies this area and simulates tonsillar herniation; it is advantageous to tape the ears forward in order to obviate this difficulty.

According to the path followed by the air on these early films, an adjustment in the position of the head and neck may have to be made to direct the air to the foramen of Magendie. If a large cisterna magna is present, considerable air may have to be introduced before the air-fluid level drops below the foramen of Magendie and air enters the fourth ventricle.

There are occasions when, in spite of

proper positioning of the patient and correct placement of the needle (so that there is no evidence of subdural injection of air), the air does not enter the fourth ventricle. As long as there is no evidence of tonsillar herniation the study should be continued, introducing a total of at least about 30 cc of air. Oftentimes, the changes in the subarachnoid cisterns will afford valuable information. A tumor may be demonstrated in the cistern, and the size of the ventricles can be estimated if the air passes into the cistern of the corpus callosum. Disease in the fourth ventricle may account for the absence of filling of the ventricular system in some cases, but there are a significant number of cases in which nonfilling of the system occurs when the lesion is not in the posterior fossa. When the reason for nonfilling of the ventricles is thought to be increased intracranial pressure, an infusion of a hypertonic solution such as urea or mannitol may be helpful in getting the ventricles to fill.[11] Brow-up and brow-down films should be obtained even though the ventricles do not fill when the patient is erect because some air may enter the ventricles when the patient is repositioned for these views.

The patient with nonfilling of the ventricular system should be regarded with a high index of suspicion. A significant percentage of these patients will be shown, on other studies, to have an intracranial mass lesion. Dilatation of certain subarachnoid cisterns, particularly the wings of the ambient cisterns and the pericallosal cistern is especially significant (in conjunction with nonfilling of the ventricular system) as an indication of pressure hydrocephalus (Fig. 6–3).

The air should be fractionally introduced in increments of about 10 cc. The first film should be taken after the introduction of the first 10 cc. It should be a lateral film that is coned to show the posterior fossa and craniocervical junction.

The second film should be a tomogram or autotomogram of the posterior fossa. Equipment for doing midline tomography with the patient in the erect position is not generally available. Since autotomography is a most valuable and yet simple technique for the clear demonstration of the fourth ventricle and aqueduct free of confusing bone shadows caused by the overlying mastoid air cells, its technique is described. The patient rests his forehead against a sponge taped to the headstand, and the head is rocked from side to side either by the patient himself or with the assistance of the examiner. An exposure

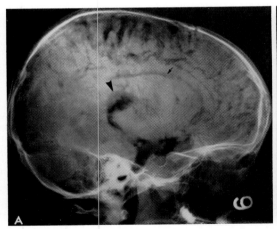 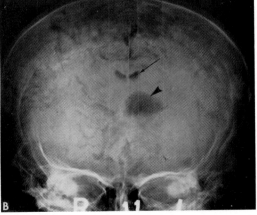

FIGURE 6–3   Lateral, *A*, and anteroposterior Towne, *B*, projections of patient with nonfilling of the ventricular system following the introduction of air via the lumbar route. The large arrowhead points to air in a portion of the wing of the ambient cistern. This cistern is dilated. The small arrow points to a dilated cistern of the corpus callosum. Note also the sulci of the convexity. The changes indicated here are *not* the result of atrophy, but usually indicate the presence of a tumor in the midline of the posterior fossa. Further studies – angiography or ventriculography – are needed to demonstrate the lesion in this case, but cisternal air may at times outline a portion of the tumor.

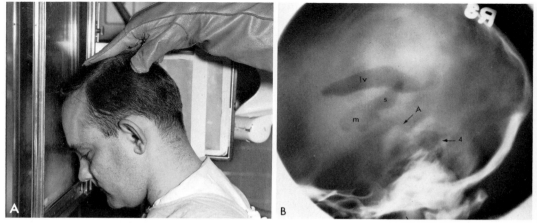

FIGURE 6-4 A. Patient positioned for autotomography. The patient's head will be rocked back and forth while his forehead is pressed against the head unit. B. Autotomogram taken after the introduction of 10 cc of air. Structures outlined are the fourth ventricle (4), aqueduct (A), third ventricle (containing m, the massa intermedia, and s, the suprapineal recess), and a lateral ventricle (lv).

time of two or three seconds is used. The film so obtained will show in sharp focus those midline structures along the axis of rotation passing through the odontoid. Structures that are lateral to the axis of rotation will be blurred. It is desirable to obtain delineation of these structures before the cisterns have been flooded with air, for the air in the cisterns adjacent to the aqueduct will otherwise obscure the aqueduct (Fig. 6-4).

The fourth ventricle contains a number of recesses, the two lateral recesses, and the posterior superior recess. These compartments may be appreciated only in a general way on the initial films of the air study, which include a lateral film showing the passage of the first air into the fourth ventricle, an autotomogram, and a reverse Towne (half-axial) view (Fig. 6-5). Appreciation of these various compartments is enhanced when tomography in the coronal

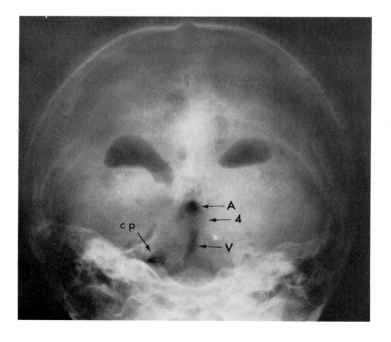

FIGURE 6-5 Reverse Towne projection. The vallecula (V), the fourth ventricle (4), and the point of entry of the aqueduct (A) into the fourth ventricle are demonstrated. In addition there is air in the right cerebellopontine angle (cp).

plane is employed, but since it is laborious and time-consuming, this procedure is not warranted unless disease is suspected in this area of the fourth ventricle. Information obtained from the routine films is sufficient in most cases. The rostral portion of the fourth ventricle (anterior medullary velum) generally is flat or convex inferiorly. The posterior portion of the fourth ventricle (posterior medullary velum) has a distinct convexity inward. The "indentation" should be recognized as normal, being due to the nodulus of the cerebellum and to the choroid plexus in the area. There are various measurements that relate the position of the fourth ventricle to bony landmarks. One of the most useful of these is based on Twining's line: A line is drawn connecting the tuberculum sella and the torcular Herophili. The line is bisected. The midpoint should fall within and lie close to the floor of the fourth ventricle.[13]

The aqueduct should describe a gentle curve paralleling the curve of the inner table of the skull. Occasionally one sees a slight normal "kink" in the region of the quadrigeminal plate. A useful method of locating the position of the normal aqueduct is the Lysholm or Sahlstedt system. A line is drawn from the dorsum sellae to a point on the inner table of the skull. (The point may be selected anywhere along the inner table; the line that is thereby determined will pass through the aqueduct.) This line is then divided into thirds. The aqueduct should lie at the junction of the proximal and middle thirds.[7] In the posteroanterior half-axial projection, the fourth ventricle (including the lateral recesses), the aqueduct, and the posterior part of the third ventricle can be identified in the midline as the air passes through them.

In addition to the positions of the parts of the ventricular system just mentioned, the following cisterns should be demonstrated on these early films with the patient erect: the cisterna magna and the medullary, pontine, interpeduncular, ambient, crural, and chiasmatic cisterns. Extension of the head at the time the air is introduced may be necessary to direct the air into them. Reversing this maneuver (flexing the head) may be helpful when it is desired to direct air into cisterns above the cerebellum.

After all these structures have been demonstrated, an additional lateral film is obtained to demonstrate the roof of the lateral ventricles, and to ascertain whether

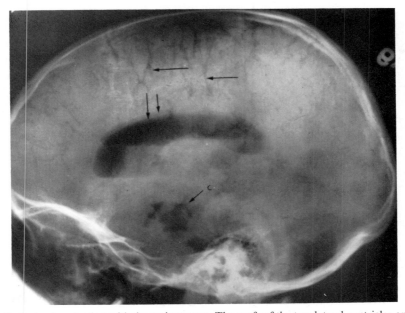

FIGURE 6–6 Lateral projection with the patient erect. The roofs of the two lateral ventricles are well demonstrated (*two vertical arrows*). The two horizontal arrows indicate a few of the sulci that are outlined by air. The arrow labeled c indicates the region of the interpeduncular cistern, which merges with the chiasmatic cistern anteriorly and the pontine cistern inferiorly.

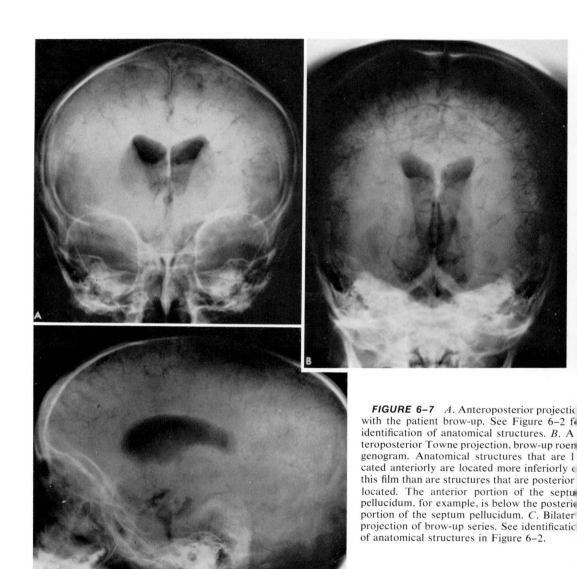

FIGURE 6–7 *A.* Anteroposterior projectic with the patient brow-up. See Figure 6–2 fe identification of anatomical structures. *B.* A teroposterior Towne projection, brow-up roen genogram. Anatomical structures that are l cated anteriorly are located more inferiorly this film than are structures that are posterior located. The anterior portion of the septu pellucidum, for example, is below the posteric portion of the septum pellucidum. *C.* Bilater projection of brow-up series. See identificatic of anatomical structures in Figure 6–2.

there is enough ventricular air to carry out the remainder of the study. To expand on these two points, midline lesions such as parasagittal or falx meningiomas in the posterior frontal area may be demonstrated better on this than on subsequent lateral films mainly because the portion of the lateral ventricle affected most by such lesions is best displayed on this erect lateral film (Fig. 6–6). The second reason for taking this film is to ascertain whether enough air is present for the remainder of the examination. As a rough guide, enough air should be present within the lateral ventricles so that when the patient is turned brow-up the air-fluid level extends several centimeters posterior to the foramen of Monro. More air will be required in some patients than in others. Although the normal adult ventricular system contains only about 21 cc, most studies will require that twice this amount be introduced in order to obtain sufficient ventricular filling, and sometimes substantially more is required. This is so mainly because of the not inconsiderable fraction of air that passes into the cisterns rather than into the ventricular system.

It is important that the examination of the posterior fossa should be accomplished as rapidly as possible to minimize the amount of time the patient spends in the sitting position. This is especially true when the systemic blood pressure is low and when the intracranial pressure is elevated.

The next part of the examination is carried out with the patient in the brow-up position. Several films are obtained at this point including two frontal views, an anteroposterior view, a Towne projection, and a lateral view (Fig. 6–7). On these films the anterior horns and a portion of the bodies of the lateral ventricles are demonstrated. Structures adjacent to these portions of the ventricular system, i.e., the genu and rostrum of the corpus callosum, the heads of the caudate nuclei, anterior portions of the thalamus making up the floor of the lateral ventricles, and the lateral wall of the body of the lateral ventricles should be identified. The septum pellucidum can be identified here and should be inspected because its displacement may indicate the presence of a mass lesion and also because it may be the primary site of a pathological process.

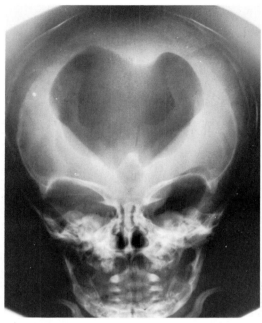

FIGURE 6–8 Brow-up anteroposterior film of patient with the Arnold-Chiari malformation. Absence of the septum pellucidum is demonstrated. The lateral ventricles are dilated and have a more pointed configuration anteriorly and inferiorly than is normal. Both these features are frequently seen in the Arnold-Chiari malformation.

The type of displacement of the septum pellucidum may do more than indicate the presence of a mass lesion—it may indicate in a fairly precise way whether the lesion is high or low and whether it is anterior or posterior. Anterior or posterior placement of the lesion is, however, usually best indicated on the Towne projection, as this film displays the anterior portion of the septum pellucidum inferiorly and the more posterior portion of the septum pellucidum superiorly. An assessment of whether a lesion is high or low in location is best carried out by utilizing the configuration of the lateral angle of the lateral ventricle as well as the septum pellucidum and the anterior portion of the third ventricle.

Primary pathological conditions involving the septum pellucidum include a wide range of diseases. The septum may be congenitally absent (Fig. 6–8). It may be extremely thin as, for example, in patients with marked hydrocephalus, or it may be perforated as, for example, in boxers or because of the thinning resulting from extreme hydrocephalus. The septum may appear abnormally thick, and if this is so, a differentiation must be made between a cavum septi pellucidi, a primary tumor of the septum pellucidum, and a hemispheric lesion extending into the septum pellucidum, perhaps by way of the corpus callosum.

A cavum of the septum pellucidum may or may not fill with air at the time of the initial study. If it does not, it is not uncommonly filled on films taken a number of hours or a day later. Such a lesion, when fluid filled, does not usually bulge asymmetrically into the medial portions of the anterior horns. A primary tumor of the septum will usually, but not always, demonstrate some asymmetry. Features that would lead one to suspect that a thickening of the septum pellucidum is caused by a tumor extending into the septum pellucidum from the corpus callosum are abnormalities such as indentations along the roof of the lateral ventricle and perhaps the demonstration of an abnormally thick corpus callosum as indicated by the air in the cistern of the corpus callosum and its distance from the air within the ventricles. Irregularity of the roof of the lateral ventricles may be a normal finding. In the interpretation of their meaning, degree and configuration of the irregular areas must be taken into account.

After the three brow-up films have been obtained, additional maneuvers should be carried out to demonstrate anterior portions of the ventricular system that may not have been clearly visualized. The first of these is designed to demonstrate the anterior portion of the third ventricle to advantage. With the patient brow-up (sometimes with his head hanging back in order to direct air from the lateral ventricles into the anterior portion of the third ventricle), the patient's head is rocked from side to side while a two- or three-second exposure is carried out in the lateral projection. This film usually demonstrates well the two recesses of the anterior third ventricle—the optic and the infundibular recesses (Fig. 6–9). There are times, however, when these recesses are obscured by air in the cisterns adjacent. If the maneuver just described is repeated 24 hours following the

introduction of the air, most or all of the cisternal air will have been absorbed so that the anterior third ventricle will no longer be obscured. Identification of these recesses within the third ventricle, the lamina terminalis, and the anterior commissure, and more posteriorly, the massa intermedia can then be made. The massa intermedia is quite variable in size. Confusion with a colloid cyst of the third ventricle (occurring just behind the foramen of Monro) is sometimes possible. A large massa intermedia and diverticulum of the anterior portion of the third ventricle as well as an absence of the septum pellucidum may be seen in patients with the Arnold-Chiari malformation. An accessory bundle of fibers (Meynert's commissure) may be seen in the anterior third ventricle in the Arnold-Chiari malformation (cf. Fig. 6–13).[5]

The other portion of the ventricular anatomy to be demonstrated with the patient in the brow-up position is the tip of the temporal horn. Both temporal tips may be demonstrated if the patient's head is extended as far posteriorly as possible (off the edge of the table) and a film is taken with the beam directed through the orbits. Frequently, the lateral and supracornual clefts of the temporal horns can be identified if there is enough air in the temporal horns (Fig. 6–10). If this maneuver is unsuccessful because not enough air leaves the body of the lateral ventricle, then the horns can be filled one at a time. This is accomplished by turning the head to one side, then dropping the head below the edge of the table, and then turning the head brow-up into a neutral position. The perorbital view is again obtained in order to demonstrate each temporal horn.

After the anterior portions of the ventricular system have been demonstrated, the patient is turned into the brow-down position and three more films are obtained. These should include a posteroanterior view, a reverse Towne view (half-axial), and a lateral view (Fig. 6–11). Here the posterior portion of the bodies of the lateral ventricles, the occipital horns (when they are present), and the posterior portions of the temporal horns will be displayed. The term specifying the juncture of these por-

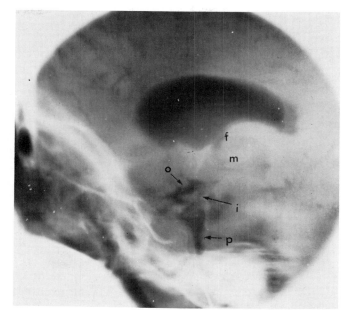

FIGURE 6-9 Brow-up autotomogram. The optic (o) and infundibular (i) recesses of the anterior portion of the third ventricle are visualized through the air in the chiasmatic cistern. The foramen of Monro is labeled f, the pontine cistern, p, and the massa intermedia, m.

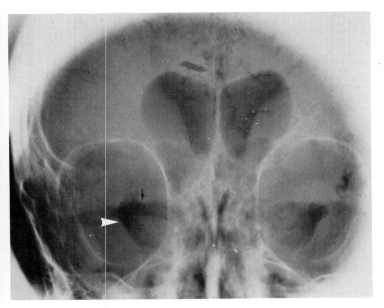

FIGURE 6-10 Anteroposterior projection of the temporal horns through the orbits. The large arrowhead indicates the lateral cleft and the small arrow indicates the supracornual cleft.

tions of the ventricles is the "trigone"; sometimes the term "atrium" is used to denote this area. Two features of the normal anatomy seen best on these views include the glomus of the choroid plexus of the lateral ventricle and the calcar avis.

The examination is usually complete at this point, but at times other views may be required. If the middle segment of the temporal horn has not been demonstrated, it may be necessary to turn the patient into the decubitus position in order to obtain views of the temporal horn with a horizontal and a vertical x-ray beam. It may even be necessary to obtain films with the patient suspended upside down in order to trap considerable air in the temporal horns.

Films obtained 24 hours after injection of the air may be of aid in specific circumstances. As has been mentioned, cisternal air has largely disappeared by this time, and a better view of portions of the ventricular anatomy may be possible. Another reason for obtaining late films is that a porencephalic cyst may be demonstrated even when it did not fill previously. Also, a cyst of the septum pellucidum may require some time to fill with air. The ventricles usually appear larger at this time (Fig. 6–12).

Space allotted precludes all but an abbreviated presentation of lesions that may be demonstrated pneumoencephalographically. The illustrations selected show mainly those lesions that require an air study for optimal demonstration; most of them are closely related to the ventricular system (Figs. 6–13, 6–14, 6–15, 6–16, and 6–17).

Air in the cisterns or the absence of air in the cisterns may be of primary importance in neuroradiological diagnosis, as is indicated by the next set of illustrations. Atrophy of gray matter is indicated by dilation of sulci and by separation of cerebellar folia. Tumors may be large enough to be recognized in the cisterns, and yet they may have not reached a size sufficient to displace a portion of the ventricular system. Finally, the passage of air through the tentorial notch and up over the cerebral convexities is to be expected if the examination is properly conducted, and absence of these events may indicate a block in the subarachnoid pathways.

At times, it may be thought desirable to employ a gas other than air for the demonstration of the ventricular anatomy. A variety of gases has been employed, including carbon dioxide and nitrous oxide. Claims have been made for lesser morbidity with these gases than with air. Their absorption is more rapid, and in any event the gas that is found in the lateral ventricles after a period of time is a result of the partial pressures of these gases in the blood. In the authors' institution, carbon dioxide is used only to study a child with a ventricular-vascular shunt, and it must be stated that even in this circumstance, there is no report of an air embolus resulting from a pneumoencephalographic examination performed with air.

A discussion of the morbidity and mortality that may result from pneumoencephalography should include the following considerations: tonsillar herniation, air embolism, extracerebral hematoma formation, and meningitis, as well as the common events such as headache, nausea, and vomiting.

Tonsillar herniation is most apt to occur as a result of increased intracranial pressure. Further, it is more apt to occur in patients who have increased intracranial pressure as a result of a supratentorial mass lesion than in those who have increased intracranial pressure as a result of a mass lesion in the posterior fossa. It may be desirable to perform an air study by a spinal puncture in a patient who has increased intracranial pressure because the information obtained from cisternal air contrast is required or because it is considered unwise to go through the steps of ventriculographic procedure. In this situation, certain precautions should be observed. These include having the equipment and the personnel available for tapping the ventricles if evidence of tonsillar herniation develops. As always, the air should be introduced fractionally and in small increments. An inspection of early lateral films should be made for evidence of tonsillar herniation. No more air should be introduced than is necessary to demonstrate the lesion (and sometimes to exclude other lesions). After the diagnosis has been made, in patients with a high degree of intracranial pressure, it is advisable to follow the diagnostic procedure with the appropriate

Text continued on page 222.

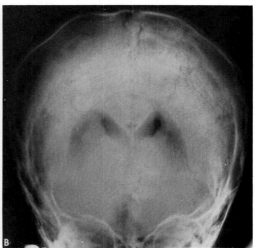

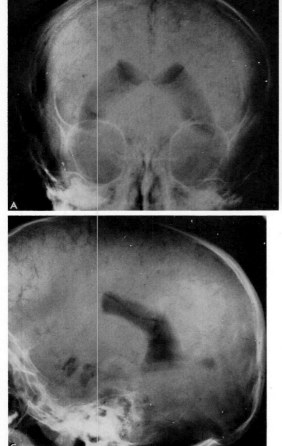

FIGURE 6-11 *A*. Posteroanterior projection, brow-down series. See identification of anatomical structures in Figure 6–2. *B*. Reverse Towne projection of brow-down series. *C*. Bilateral projection of brow-down series.

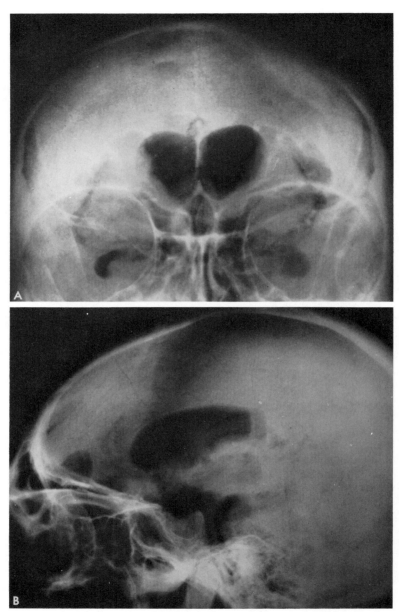

FIGURE 6–12   *A* and *B*. Anteroposterior and lateral films of patient with large porencephalic cyst in the left temporal lobe.

Illustration continued on opposite page.

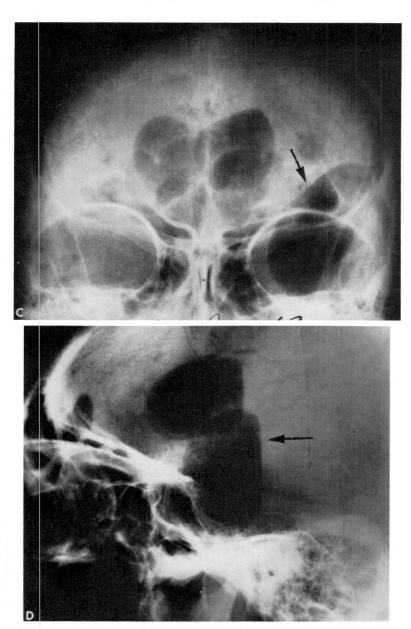

FIGURE 6-12 *(Continued)*   *C* and *D*. Same patient 24 hours later. The porencephalic cyst has filled with air.

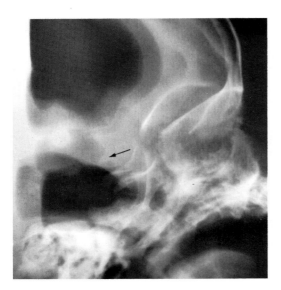

FIGURE 6-13   Same patient as in Figure 6–8. The arrow points to an accessory bundle of fibers (Meynert's commissure). This also is a common finding in the Arnold-Chiari malformation.

FIGURE 6-14   Autotomogram with the patient's head hanging back ("hanging-head autotomogram"). Air has spilled from the lateral ventricles into the anterior third ventricle. The recesses are splayed by a tumor (T) that was not demonstrated angiographically. The tumor, which was removed, proved to be a craniopharyngioma.

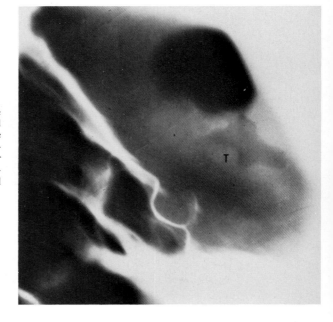

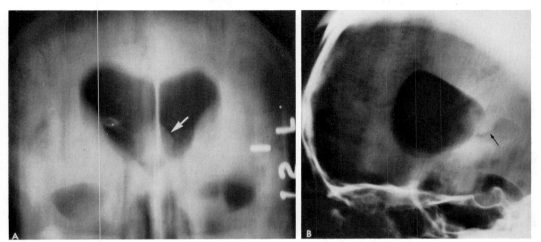

FIGURE 6–15 *A*. Brow-up anteroposterior tomogram demonstrating a colloid cyst of the third ventricle (*arrow*). These lesions may sometimes be diagnosed angiographically because of changes in the venographic phase that indicate a third ventricular mass lesion. They are best delineated with air, however. Note also the shunt tube in the right lateral ventricle. *B*. Same patient as in Figure 6–15 *A*, hanging-head lateral view. Air outlines the anterior aspect of the colloid cyst (*arrow*), which is located just behind the foramen of Monro.

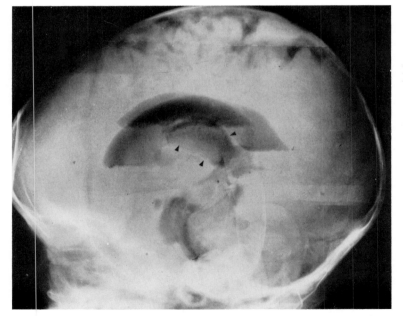

FIGURE 6–16 Lateral projection, patient erect. The arrowheads indicate a cavum veli interpositi above the third ventricle. This space communicates with the cisterns of the quadrigeminal plate posteriorly. This differentiates it from a cavum vergae, which fills after the ventricles fill and is always associated with a cavum septi pellucidi.

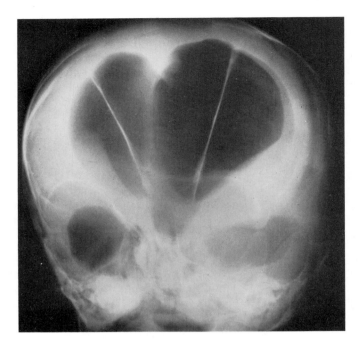

FIGURE 6-17 Ventricular bands in hydrocephaly resulting from ependymitis.

operative therapy, or to institute ventricular drainage if the operation is to be delayed. The bad reputation that pneumoencephalography acquired in the investigation of patients with increased intracranial pressure is due, in part, to the fact that large increments of air were introduced with no radiological control and that patients were put to bed for a considerable time after the completion of the procedure before operation was undertaken. The condition of a patient who has a ventriculographic study because of increased intracranial pressure may also deteriorate if the study is not followed with appropriate operative therapy.

Air embolization is an extremely serious complication of improperly conducted encephalographic examination. It occurs only when large amounts of air are introduced into the subdural space and will not occur if one adheres to correct technique. One should not be trapped into introducing large quantities of air into the subdural space in persistent attempts to "adjust" the needle so that the air may be introduced into the subarachnoid space. Frequently, the subarachnoid space is collapsed as more and more subdural air is introduced so that it becomes virtually impossible to

achieve what is desired. It is best to terminate the study and to delay any further attempts to study the patient via this route for a period of several days.

Another serious complication that may occur is the production of an extracerebral (particularly a subdural) hematoma. This also is more apt to occur in a situation in which considerable subdural air has been introduced. It is even more likely if there is pre-existing cerebral atrophy. Bridging veins are more susceptible to injury if these factors are present. Another factor that may be important in this context is anticoagulation. Anticoagulation is a relative contraindication to pneumoencephalography.

A mild or moderate meningitis of the aseptic variety frequently follows pneumoencephalography, and this is indicated by a low-grade fever and by a cellular response in the spinal fluid. A more severe chemical meningitis may result if there are contaminating chemicals on the needle or tubing used in the performance of the procedure. Bacterial meningitis is infrequent. In an attempt to avoid this complication, some authorities have advocated using air that is filtered. There is no adequate proof that filtering the air will reduce the already low incidence of bacterial meningitis as a complication of pneumoencephalography.

The minor complications such as headache and vomiting are common and will subside after a relatively short period of time. These complications are often quite distressing to the patient and may preclude his cooperation in other neuroradiological studies. It is for this reason that pneumoencephalography is sometimes called a "sign-out procedure." It is interesting that headache seems to result mainly from air in the cisterns rather than in the ventricles. In fact, patients do not usually complain of headache until a quantity of air reaches the cisterns. It is also of interest, although not easy to explain, that patients with atrophy may experience no headache whatsoever. Some workers believe that introducing the air without removing spinal fluid reduces the incidence and severity of headache. However, experience does not confirm this belief.

VENTRICULOGRAPHY

Dandy, in 1918, succeeded in demonstrating the ventricular system in hydrocephalic infants by inserting a needle through an area of sutural diastasis, and then through the brain into the ventricular system.[2] In adults, the puncture is carried out through twist drill holes or through burr holes in the calvarium. The hole may be placed posteriorly so that the atrium of the ventricle is entered, but there is danger that the needle may enter the vascular glomus lying on the floor of the atrium and cause a hematoma.

Often, the hole is made anteriorly through the coronal suture and 2.5 cm from the midline on the side of the nondominant hemisphere. Ventriculography may be performed through twist drill holes, and the contrast material introduced via a Scott cannula. A drill bit of adequate size to introduce the Scott cannula should be selected, and the hole should be drilled at the same angle at which the cannula is to be introduced. The cannula is directed toward the nasion and is slowly introduced until a "give" is felt; then the obturator is removed. Free flow of ventricular fluid indicates correct placement. Several sutures are placed around the hub of the cannula to affix the device to the scalp. Next, air is introduced; this can be done with the patient either brow-up or brow-down. It is best to do the exchange in the brow-up position if it is desired to study all parts of the ventricular system rather than just the posterior portions of the lateral ventricles, third ventricle, aqueduct, and fourth ventricle. If the air is to be introduced with the patient supine, the head should be turned so that the ventricle containing the tip of the cannula is dependent. In that position, more air can be introduced. Fractional instillation of air and removal of fluid can then be carried out. Enough air is instilled to carry out the study, and at the end-point, the pressure is allowed to equilibrate with the atmosphere.

The first films are obtained with the patient's head hanging somewhat so that the air is able to find its way through the foramen of Monro into the third ventricle. Brow-up, anteroposterior, and lateral films are obtained, and if better definition of the anterior portion of the third ventricle is desired than is obtained on the lateral film, then autotomography (mentioned earlier in the section on pneumoencephalography) or tomography is carried out.

If there is a block in the foramen of Monro, but no associated perforation of the septum pellucidum, then a puncture of the opposite lateral ventricle may have to be performed in order to establish the diagnosis firmly.

If the lesion is caudad to the anterior portion of the third ventricle, the brow-down films will be of importance. The patient is rapidly turned from the supine into the prone position so that the air in the anterior third ventricle passes into the posterior third ventricle and not (as will often happen if he is turned slowly) back through the foramen of Monro into the uppermost lateral ventricle. Four films are obtained as soon as possible after the patient is brow-down. It is advantageous to have the tube and film positioned for the first of these—the lateral film—before the patient is turned. If the aqueduct is large the air will pass rapidly through this structure, making its demonstration difficult; if the aqueduct is partially or completely blocked, however, then the timing is not so critical. After the lateral film is obtained, autotomography or tomography is carried out in order to better display the midline portions of the ventricular system. When properly performed this has the further virtue of demonstrating a shift of normally midline structures, for these structures will then be out of focus on the autotomogram or midline tomogram. Finally, a reverse Towne view and a posteroanterior view are obtained. At times the reverse somersault maneuver may be required to demonstrate the aqueduct and fourth ventricle.

If there is no obstruction to the ventricular system and the air passes out of the fourth ventricle into the cisterna magna, then by bending the patient's head and neck far forward, one can bring it into the spinal canal and then up again so that the cisterns may be studied. As indicated in the section on pneumoencephalography, the study of the cisterns may yield information that is of importance in establishing the diagnosis.

In the discussion on pneumoencephalography, mention was made of the place of ventriculography, and some of the fallacies about "risks" of pneumoencephalography, especially in the presence of increased intracranial pressure, were discussed. In situations in which there is nonfilling of the ventricular system with air introduced from below by spinal puncture, ventriculography is indicated if the nonfilling is not due to such "technical reasons" as subdural placement of the air, and if the cisternal air present does not allow exact localization of the lesion. Also, if tonsillar herniation is present on preliminary pneumoencephalographic films, it may be wise to tap the ventricular system to relieve the pressure and either to continue the examination from below or to carry out the remainder of the examination from above.

There will be occasional instances when the ventriculographic examination will be greatly facilitated if an opaque contrast agent is used instead of air. The opaque material may be nonsoluble (and heavier than spinal fluid) as for example iophendylate (Pantopaque), or it may be soluble meglumine iothalamate (Conray).[1] A modification of the technique using a nonsoluble contrast agent such as Pantopaque is to use an emulsion of Pantopaque in ventricular fluid, which is then introduced into the ventricular system to coat the walls of the ventricles.[10]

If one is fortunate in placing the ventricular cannula, the tip will lie adjacent to the foramen of Monro. Introduction of Pantopaque into the third ventricle is then easily accomplished. If the tip of the cannula is not in such a position, the patient must be positioned so that the Pantopaque passing through the cannula will gravitate into the anterior horn of the lateral ventricle.

Only a few milliliters of Pantopaque are required for the complete demonstration of the aqueduct and fourth ventricle. With the Pantopaque in the anterior horn of a lateral ventricle the patient's head and neck, which are flexed, are gradually straightened and the head is tilted slightly to the side so that the lateral ventricle containing the Pantopaque is uppermost. As the head is gradually extended, about the time a neutral position is reached, the Pantopaque will pass through the medially placed foramen of Monro into the third ventricle. Then the patient is placed in the supine position, and lateral, anteroposterior, and Towne (half-axial) films are obtained. If these maneuvers are correctly performed, the Pantopaque will be in position to demonstrate the posterior part of the third ventricle and distal structures. Serial films may be required over a period of hours if maximal information is desired about the aqueduct in special circumstances.

If for some reason the Pantopaque has not entered the foramen of Monro with this maneuver, it will come to lie in the trigone or occipital horn, and can then be moved back into the frontal horn either by turning the patient upside down or by hanging his head back and turning it to the side so that the Pantopaque-containing ventricle is dependent. The Pantopaque will move into the body of the lateral ventricle; rapidly turning the patient into the prone position will cause the Pantopaque to flow into the anterior horn once more. Gradually, with the patient sitting, the flexed head and neck are again extended.

If a water-soluble contrast agent such as Conray is introduced rather than Pantopaque, serial films must be obtained fairly rapidly in order to demonstrate the passage of this material through the ventricular sys-

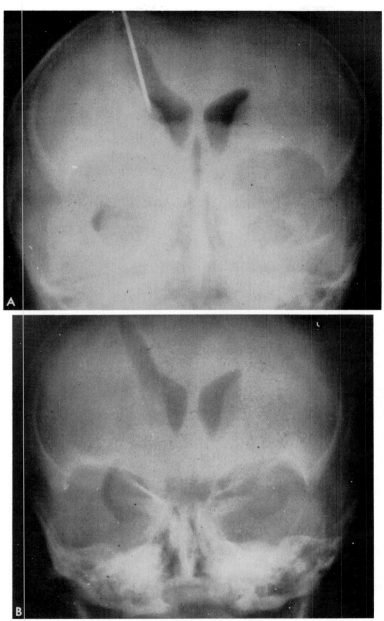

FIGURE 6-18 This set of anteroposterior roentgenograms taken during, *A*, and after, *B*, the introduction of air into the ventricular system illustrates the formation of an area of porencephaly along the needle tract.

tem. A biplane angiographic unit may easily be programmed for this kind of study. Water-soluble agents presently used seem to evoke little inflammatory response within the ventricular system, but passage of these substances into the cisterns may provoke a chemical meningitis.

Complications of ventriculography include epidural hematoma, cerebral hemorrhage, and formation of porencephalic diverticula along the needle tract (most apt to occur in hydrocephalics) (Fig. 6–18).

EXAMINATION OF THE CEREBELLOPONTINE ANGLE WITH PANTOPAQUE

This procedure has its greatest usefulness in studying patients who are suspected of having a small lesion that is extra-axial in location and that is involving the eighth cranial nerve alone, or perhaps the eighth cranial nerve and other near-by nerves. Such a lesion may be confined entirely to the internal auditory meatus. The procedure should be undertaken after tomographic examination of the internal auditory meatuses in order to confirm or to supplement the results of this examination.

If the lesion is large and is suspected to lie primarily in the brain stem or cerebellum, then it is probably preferable to perform pneumoencephalography rather than an examination with Pantopaque, for more of the posterior fossa anatomy will be displayed with air than will be displayed with Pantopaque, especially if the examination with the opaque substance is conducted only with the patient in the prone position.

Examination of the cerebellopontine angle with Pantopaque carries with it a lesser morbidity than examination with air. There will probably be no discomfort or little discomfort, and for this reason the examination seems more appropriate in the patient who has only an impairment of hearing that might or might not be due to a small mass lesion. The examination procedure begins with the introduction of a few milliliters of Pantopaque into the lumbar subarachnoid space through a lumbar puncture.[14] The oily opaque material is then brought up into the cervical canal by tilting

the patient head down while the head and neck are extended (patient's chin on sponge). In this way the opaque medium is brought over the hump in the thoracic area into the trough in the cervical area produced by the extension of the head and neck. No opaque medium will pass into the head as long as the tilt of the inclined table is not too steep. When sufficient opaque medium has been pooled in the cervical area, the examination may proceed. The inclined fluoroscopic table should at this time be in the neutral position. The sponge supporting the patient's chin is then removed, and the chin is tucked down toward the patient's chest. The Pantopaque will then begin to flow up onto the clivus. When the Pantopaque there begins to outline the area of juncture of the vertebral arteries, the patient's head is turned so that the side with the suspected lesion is lowermost. Pantopaque will run into the cerebellopontine angle. A slight tilt of the table may be required to bring the necessary amount of opaque medium into this location, but the tilt should be minimized so that the contrast agent does not escape the posterior fossa to pass into the middle fossa. The end-point of the examination is reached when opaque medium has either penetrated deeply into the internal auditory meatus, or when it is clearly blocked by a lesion in this area. A bony ridge, the crista falciformis, is demonstrated at the depth of the meatus. Patients often experience a twinge of pain in the ear when the Pantopaque penetrates deeply into the meatus. Spot films are obtained with the patient's head in this oblique position, and also with the patient's head turned back to neutral. If the chin remains tucked down, the meatus will be displayed through the orbit, and there will be no problem in interpreting the examination.

If the opposite meatus must be examined as well, then this side of the patient's head is placed against the table, and the opaque medium is pooled in this angle and meatus. Spot films are again obtained with the patient positioned obliquely, and then again with his head in neutral position.

For orientation it may be helpful to place a wax pellet containing an opaque substance, such as a piece of solder, within the patient's external auditory meatus at the beginning of the examination. This helps to

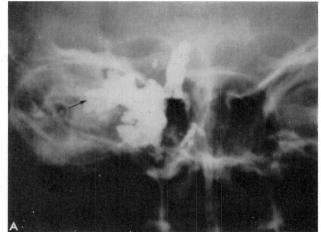

FIGURE 6–19 *A*. Perorbital view with the patient in right decubitus position. Pantopaque in the right internal auditory meatus is in contact with the crista falciformis (*arrow*), separating the vestibular and cochlear divisions of the eighth cranial nerve. *B*. Base view of patient in right lateral decubitus position. The crista falciformis (*arrow*) is again demonstrated. This study was performed to exclude a small eighth nerve tumor on the right as a cause for hearing loss.

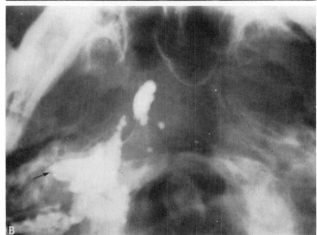

identify the internal auditory meatus when the patient is in the oblique position.

Finally, the opaque medium should be recovered by tilting the head of the table upward. Small droplets may lodge against vascular structures or nerves; these can be dislodged by having the patient rock or shake his head from side to side.

The examination can be conducted without fluoroscopy if the patient is placed in the decubitus instead of the prone position. Tilting the patient so that the head is dependent, and then neutralizing this angle directs the opaque medium into the appropriate meatus. In this technique, tomography may be used as a further refinement (Fig. 6–19).

When the examination of the cerebellopontine angle with Pantopaque is attempted in patients with large tumors, one commonly finds that the opposite meatus cannot be demonstrated. The brain stem is shifted in such a way as to block the access of the contrast medium to the contralateral cerebellopontine angle. This is one type of false positive result. Another source of false positive results is the variation in the depth of penetration of the subarachnoid space into the internal auditory meatus. Because of these problems, there may be a small percentage of false positives, even when the examination is conducted by an experienced person.

On the other hand, the low rate of morbidity associated with the procedure and the clarity of demonstration of the anatomy of the area recommend this technique, particularly in the diagnosis of small lesions.

RHOMBOENCEPHALOGRAPHY

This is a technique of examination of the posterior fossa with an oily opaque medium that was described by Mones and Werman (1958).[8] In this procedure about 9 ml of Pantopaque is introduced into the lumbar subarachnoid space. The needle is then removed and the patient is placed in the supine position. He is tilted head downward about 80 degrees while his head is flexed. After about a minute in this position, he is brought back to about 70 degrees. Lateral and anteroposterior films are then obtained. The posterior foramen magnum, tonsils, fourth ventricle, and aqueduct may be clearly demonstrated in this fashion.

There are few instances in which the information obtainable with this procedure cannot be obtained in some other way, but it has the advantage at times of providing definition and clarity in difficult cases without resorting to Pantopaque ventriculography. The procedure has not gained widespread popularity, probably because of the fear of being unable to recover all of the Pantopaque from the head. Patients are likely to experience moderate to severe headache if the Pantopaque cannot be recovered.

REFERENCES

1. Campbell, R. L., et al.: Ventriculography and myelography with absorbable radioopaque medium. Radiology, 82:286, 1964.
2. Dandy, W.: Ventriculography following the injection of air into the cerebral ventricles. Ann. Surg., 68:5, 1918.
3. Dandy, W.: Roentgenography of the brain after the injection of air into the spinal canal. Ann. Surg., 70:397, 1919.
4. Erenberg, G.: Personal communication.
5. Goodling, C., et al.: New ventriculographic aspects of the Arnold-Chiari malformation. Radiology, 89:626, 1967.
6. Luckett, W. H.: Air in the ventricles of the brain following a fracture of the skull. Surg. Gynec. Obstet., 213, 1913.
7. Lysholm, E., et al.: Das ventriculogramm. Acta Radiol. Suppl. 26, 1935.
8. Mones, R., and Werman, R.: Pantopaque fourth ventriculography via lumbar route (REG). J. Mount Sinai Hosp., N.Y., 25:201, 1958.
9. Nellhaus, G., and Chutorian, A.: Narcosis for neuroradiologic procedures in children. Arch. Neurol., 10:485, 1964.
10. Portera, A., et al.: Emulsified Pantopaque ventriculography. J. Neurosurg., 21:422, 1964.
11. Ruggiero, G.: Encephalography today. Acta Radiol., 5:715, 1966.
12. Schechter, M. M., et al.: Dynamic displacements of intracranial structures simulating mass lesions. Amer. J. Roentgen., 98:535, 1966.
13. Twining, E. W.: Radiology of the third and fourth ventricles. Parts I and II. Brit. J. Radiol., 12: 385 and 569, 1939.
14. Valvassori, G.: Abnormal internal auditory canal: the diagnosis of acoustic neuroma. Radiology, 92:449, 1969.

7

SURGICAL CONSIDERATIONS OF VENTRICULOGRAPHY

HISTORICAL BACKGROUND

It is interesting that contrast ventriculography did not come into use earlier than it did. At the turn of the century, sites of election for benign ventricular puncture through silent areas of the brain had been determined. The external landmarks of Kocher and Keen provided, respectively, access to the frontal horn and the ventricular trigones. Cushing and others considered ventricular puncture useful for the sampling of cerebral spinal fluid under certain circumstances and for temporary relief of increased intracranial pressure.[4, 21]

In 1913, W. H. Luckett inadvertently demonstrated an air-filled ventricular system in a patient who had sustained a compound frontal fracture.[23] However, the diagnostic implication of air contrast within the ventricular system remained unrecognized until 1918 when Walter Dandy reported his technique of "ventriculography."[5]

Dandy had long recognized the need for greater accuracy in tumor localization and had performed experimental ventriculography in dogs with the renal contrast materials of the day. These substances proved uniformly fatal. However, Halstead's reminder of "the remarkable power of intestinal gases to perforate bone on x-ray" prompted Dandy's choice of air as a suitable contrast medium.

The same clinical experience that led to the early reports of major morbidity and an up to 8 per cent mortality rate surrounding ventriculography, also later provided guidelines for the prevention of these complications.[2, 15, 25] Thus, Dandy's original technique of air ventriculography has survived essentially without modification until today.[27, 30, 31]

Despite Dandy's disappointments with iodide contrast materials, the search continued for a positive contrast substance that would prove superior to air for demonstrating the midline ventricular system. Iodized oil (Lipiodol) and thorium dioxide (Thorotrast) were among the substances that were tried and abandoned. The need for precise landmarks for stereotaxic operations has been a renewed stimulus in the evolution of midline contrast ventriculography. Iophendylate (Pantopaque) and meglumine iothalamate (Conray 60) have proved acceptable agents but have some limitations. The physical properties of these materials have required advances in their technical placement, including direct transfrontal cannulation of the foramen of Monro.[32]

INDICATIONS AND CONTRAINDICATIONS FOR VENTRICULOGRAPHY

Except in infants and young children, arteriography and isotope brain scanning have replaced ventriculography as the procedure of choice in localizing supratentorial mass lesions. Ventriculography, however, is often used for further elucidation when these more benign procedures yield equivocal results, and it remains the procedure of choice for the demonstration of the third ventricle, aqueduct, and fourth

J. T. ROBERTSON
I. C. DENTON, JR.

229

ventricle. Ventriculography is used routinely in stereotaxic operations and frequently is used in patients having emergency operations for cerebral trauma.

Providing the patient is a candidate for an operation, there are essentially no contraindications to ventriculography. The single most important guideline is that ventriculography should never be undertaken without preparation for subsequent operative intervention.

TECHNIQUES FOR VENTRICULOGRAPHY

Although the same basic principles of ventriculography apply to both children and adults, the technical approach to the ventricular system varies before and after closure of the cranial sutures.

In infants, ventriculography is usually performed by introducing an 18-gauge spinal needle through the scalp, which has been scrubbed and prepared for an operative procedure and injected with local anesthetic. The coronal suture is open and can be penetrated with ease. The needle is held in the sagittal plane on a line with the pupil while being advanced on a coronal plane in a line toward the inner canthus of the eye. It is advanced slowly and the stylet withdrawn at intervals. The appearance of cerebrospinal fluid should identify the ventricle at a depth not greater than 4 cm. Since repeated needle passes may increase the risk of hemorrhage and cortical damage,

only in unusual circumstances should more than three attempts at ventricular puncture be made on either side without shifting to the opposite one. Occasionally the air will not communicate with the opposite ventricle, and bilateral puncture may be necessary for a satisfactory exchange of air and ventricular fluid. In all cases, ventricular fluid pressure should be either estimated or measured and a small aliquot of fluid withdrawn for analysis.

If air ventriculography is performed in infants for purposes other than evaluation of hydrocephalus, complete fluid-air exchange will insure the best results. In order to maintain relatively normal pressure relationships, equivalent amounts of fluid and air should be exchanged in repeated aliquots of a few cubic centimeters. Adequate exchange is facilitated by positioning the head to create drainage of the fluid by gravity. In studying the patient with hydrocephalus, the smallest amount of air that will provide an adequate diagnosis should be used. The same principles of fluid-air exchange should be observed, but total exchange of air and fluid in the patient with hydrocephalus seldom is needed and can cause harm. In all cases, the exchanged room air should be filtered through several layers of sterile surgical sponge fitted around the stopcock.

In adults and in older children whose sutures are approaching closure, access to the ventricular system is provided by trephination (Fig. 7–1). Three standard points for the placement of trephines are recog-

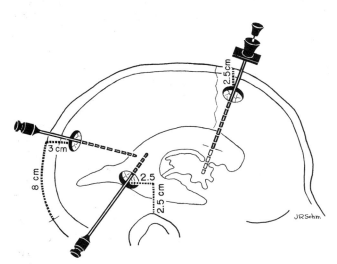

Figure 7–1 The three standard trephination sites used to gain access to the lateral ventricles. The anterior site or Kocher's point is 3 cm posterior to the normal hair line and 2.5 cm lateral to the midline. The Keen's point trephine opening permits tapping of the trigone of the lateral ventricle. It is 2.5 cm behind and 2.5 cm above the external auditory meatus. The posterior aspect of the lateral ventricle is approached through a posterior parietal trephine opening which is 8 cm above the inion and 2.5 to 3 cm lateral to the midline.

nized. Posterior parietal trephine openings, perhaps the most commonly used, are placed 8 cm above the inion at a point 2.5 to 3 cm lateral to the midline. The needle is directed along a line toward the inner aspect of the eye within the transverse plane of the supraorbital ridge. A Keen's point trephine opening 2.5 cm behind and 2.5 cm above the external auditory meatus provides access to the trigone of the lateral ventricle when the needle is directed at right angles to the cortex. The frontal horn of the ventricle may be approached by trephination at Kocher's point 3 cm posterior to the normal hair line and 2.5 cm lateral to the midline. This position allows penetration of the anterior horn at its widest point.

Depending upon the trephination site that is selected, ventriculography may be performed in the sitting, semi-sitting, prone, or supine positions. If the patient is cooperative, an attempt should be made to use local anesthesia. Following placement of the trephine openings, usually bilaterally, the dura is incised in cruciate fashion and the brain is punctured through a gyrus. Meticulous hemostasis should be obtained. The galea and skin may be closed prior to or after the ventricular puncture. Usually the initial attempt to place the needle in the ventricle is made on the side of the brain opposite to the one that is suspected of harboring the disease. The normal side of the brain is more likely to have the ventricle in a normal position and configuration. A blunt ventricular needle is considered safer than a sharp one and it affords a keen sensation of pressure as tissues of varying density are traversed. It transmits a distinct sensation of increased and then suddenly eased resistance as the ventricular wall is encountered.

When the needle is satisfactorily placed in the ventricle, a small amount of air should be instilled immediately in order to prevent possible ventricular collapse. The general principles already enumerated concerning repeated needle punctures, the estimation of cerebrospinal fluid, collection of fluid for analysis, and fluid exchange apply in the adult also.

In both children and adults, positive contrast ventriculography is used to best advantage in demonstrating alterations of midline ventricular configuration. The value of contrast ventriculography in stereotaxic operations is unquestioned. Several points concerning positive contrast ventriculography are noteworthy.

For positive contrast ventriculography, the technique of ventricular puncture should be modified so that a rubber catheter on a stylet may be directed into the third ventricle or placed near the foramen of Monro. Thus, through frontal burr holes, the catheter is directed in the coronal plane toward the inner canthus of the eye and on a sagittal plane toward the opposite external auditory meatus. When the ventricle is encountered a small bubble of air is introduced. The flexible catheter without its stylet, when introduced another 1 to 2 cm, will follow the floor of the frontal horn into the foramen of Monro. Prior to introducing the contrast material, a lateral skull film should be taken to confirm the presence of the air bubble in the frontal horn.

Pantopaque and Conray 60 are the most frequently used contrast materials at the present time. As a general rule, the amount of contrast material used should be restricted to the amount necessary to achieve a satisfactory study. Three to four milliliters of undiluted Pantopaque will suffice. For an adequate Pantopaque study, head manipulation may be required to direct the transit of this nondispersible substance into the third ventricle, through the aqueduct, and into the fourth ventricle. Air-Pantopaque studies may be useful in evaluation of patients with hydrocephalus.[26] Conray 60 may be injected after diluting 4 to 6 ml of this substance with an equal amount of spinal fluid. This highly dispersible material readily circulates throughout the ventricular system. It is widely accepted among neurosurgeons that no more than 10 to 12 ml of Conray 60 should be used at any one time. Greater quantities have, however, been used in the study of patients with hydrocephalus.[3]

COMPLICATIONS OF VENTRICULOGRAPHY

It is convenient to divide the complications of ventriculography into those of major and those of minor consequence.

Subjective disturbances and seizure activity constitute the bulk of the minor complications. Pain, nausea, vomiting, and prostration are far less common with ventriculography than with pneumoencephalography. Nevertheless, minor degrees of discomfort do occur and may be associated with some alteration in vital signs such as mild temperature elevation and signs of meningeal irritation. These complaints are minimized if the contrast material does not get over the surface of the brain. Although transient electrocardiographic abnormalities may accompany fluid-air exchange, subjective complaints of palpitations or chest discomfort and objective electrocardiographic changes occurring some hours subsequent to ventriculography usually are related to cardiac disease rather than to the procedure.[8] Seizures occasionally occur with air ventriculography and are easily controlled in most cases. They occur far more frequently after the use of Conray 60 than after the use of air as the contrast medium.[29] These seizures are of two types. The most common is the generalized seizure occurring if the substance comes in contact with the cortex of the brain; these usually are easily controlled and self-limited. The second type of seizure is thought to be due to the irritation of the spinal cord or brain stem, resulting from excessive contrast material around these structures. These seizures, fortunately rare, require careful management. Respiratory support following pharmacological paralysis may be required to prevent the patient from becoming exhausted. This "spinal seizure" is likewise self-limited, usually disappearing within 24 hours.

The major complications of ventriculography fall into four general groups: infection, complications resulting from alterations in fluid dynamics, visual complications, and hemorrhage. As with any intracranial procedure, contamination of the operative field may lead to meningitis or brain abscess. The problem of infection very likely exceeds its reported incidence.[18] Nevertheless, with careful sterile techniques, significant complications from infections as a result of ventriculography are most unusual. If air is used, filtration of the air through multiple layers of an operative sponge before its introduction into the ventricular system effectively reduces the bacterial count of the ambient room air.[19] The use of oxygen for ventriculography would probably further reduce this likelihood of contamination. Theoretically, certain rare complications of ventriculography, such as cerebritis or ventriculitis, might occur in patients with septicemia or meningitis.[28] Such complications, however, appear to be quite rare. Ventricular tapping in the presence of an infected myelomeningocele may alter cerebral fluid dynamics, promoting an ascending infection.

The complications resulting from alterations of fluid dynamics are directly related to increased intracranial pressure and ventricular size.[20, 24] In children with increased pressure, the development of a traumatic porencephalic diverticulum following ventricular puncture may occur with an incidence of approximately 9 per cent.[22] Multiple needle punctures at the same site also predispose to this complication. The porencephalic diverticulum assumes the form of a truncated cone with its base confluent with the ventricles and the apex beneath the gray matter. These diverticula may not be entirely innocuous; some authors have considered them responsible for seizure disorders and occult hemiparesis.[9]

Despite careful attention to air-fluid exchange, alterations of fluid dynamics may allow compartmental shifts. For example, an upward herniation of the posterior fossa contents may occur in the presence of a posterior fossa mass. Likewise the supratentorial compartments are subject to such shifts.[11] Clinical deterioration may herald these disturbing events; they demand immediate craniotomy.

Visual complications are usually due to repeated attempts at ventricular puncture through the occipital cortex when posterior trephine openings are used. Typically, such complications may occur in cases with pseudotumor cerebri, in which small ventricles make it difficult to perform successful ventricular puncture without multiple needle passes. Although small permanent visual field defects may persist, most visual difficulties clear within a few days. In some cases with increased intracranial pressure, however, ventriculography may be followed by sudden blindness. One cause of blindness under such circumstances is compression of the posterior artery by cerebral herniation. Another cause of this sudden visual loss is presumed to be sudden pressure alterations resulting in blood flow shifts that promote optic nerve ischemia.

Intracerebral, intraventricular, subdural, and epidural hemorrhages have all been observed after ventriculography. Intracerebral hemorrhage is unusual when a blunt ventricular needle is used. Occult hemorrhage may not be manifested by bright bleeding through the needle at the time of ventricular puncture. However, at the time of x-ray studies of the ventricle, hemorrhage may be perceived as a mass in the region of cortical puncture. Intraventricular hemorrhage resulting from needle puncture may be due to injury of the glomus of the choroid plexus.[12] The radiographic demonstration of an intraventricular mass in the region of the choroid plexus signifies this complication. Most of these hemorrhages resolve spontaneously and do not require operative intervention. At a later date, benign calcification of the needle tract may attest to a previous hemorrhagic lesion incurred at the time of ventriculography.[13]

Although subdural hemorrhage may complicate pneumoencephalography, the development of a subdural hematoma following ventriculography is rare. Epidural hemorrhage, although unusual, may follow ventriculography.[10, 16, 17] Epidural hemorrhage in young people 16 years old or less has been reported at sites distant from the site of trephination, usually frontotemporal. At this age, the dura is usually quite elastic and less firmly applied to the inner table of the calvarium than it is in adults. It is presumed that epidural bleeding distant from the site of trephination results from traction on the dura by bridging cortical vessels following partial ventricular collapse. Subsequent hemorrhage occurs from the stripped calvarium. Experimental evidence from dog studies suggests that only 90 gm of nonpulsatile force is required to strip the dura from the calvarium, and once a collection is formed, the force required to expand the mass is further reduced.[14] The seriousness of this complication in young people undergoing ventriculography cannot be overemphasized, for only two survivors have been reported.[1]

Since the dura of adults is more adherent than that of children, they rarely, if ever, manifest this complication.

In adults, epidural hemorrhage is more likely to occur at the trephination site where dural dissection may result from procedural factors. Benign epidural hemorrhage occurring at the site of trephination is frequently attested by button-like calcifications noted on x-rays taken at a later date.[33] Fortunately significant epidural hemorrhage at the site of trephination is a rare entity.

In both groups, the complication of epidural hemorrhage bears a direct relationship to ventricular size. In the patient with markedly enlarged ventricles, massive accumulations may occur before their presence is suggested by clinical deterioration. Unexplained anemia in a patient with hydrocephalus may offer a diagnostic clue to occult hemorrhage prior to clinical deterioration.[34] Epidural hemorrhage can best be avoided by proper fluid-air exchange. Its presence may be detected radiographically at a late date, if the air has not been fully absorbed.

The overall number of deaths due to ventriculography is difficult to assess. The greatest factor compromising the accuracy of mortality rate figures after ventriculography is that the seriously ill patient frequently requires a subsequent craniotomy. For the same reason the incidence of seizures following ventriculography is difficult to define. The single most important principle concerning ventriculography is that immediate operative intervention must follow the demonstration of a mass lesion. Adherence to this and other principles has reduced the earlier mortality rate of 8 per cent to near zero per cent.

REFERENCES

1. Arias, B. A., and Voris, H. C.: Extradural hemorrhage after ventriculography. Amer. J. Surg., *116*:109–112, 1968.
2. Cairns, H.: Observations on the localization of intracranial tumors: The disclosure of localizing signs following ventriculography. Arch. Surg., *18*:1936–1944, 1929.
3. Cornejo, S. G.: Positive contrast ventriculography using water soluble media (Conray). Presented at the meeting of the American Academy of Neurological Surgery. Mexico City, November 18–21, 1970.

4. Cushing, H.: *Keen Surgery*. W. W. Keen, ed. Philadelphia and London, W. B. Saunders Co., 1908, Vol. III, p. 172.

5. Dandy, W. E.: Ventriculography following the injection of air into the cerebral ventricles. Ann. Surg., 68:5–11, 1918.

6. Davidoff, L. M., and Dyke, C. G.: The Normal Pneumoencephalogram. Philadelphia, Lea & Febiger, 1937.

7. Davidoff, L. M., and Epstein, B. S.: The Abnormal Pneumoencephalogram. 2nd Ed. Philadelphia, Lea & Febiger, 1955.

8. Davie, J. C.: EKG alterations observed during fraction pneumoencephalography. J. Neurosurg., 20:321–328, 1963.

9. Dekabon, A. S.: Is needle puncture of the brain entirely harmless? Neurology (Minneap.), 8:556–557, 1958.

10. Del Viron, R. E., and Armenesse, B.: Ematoma epidurale acutospontaneo depo decompress ventriculari in corso di idrocephalo. Minerva Neurochir., 5:43–48, 1961.

11. Dyke, C. G.: Acquired subtentorial pressure diverticulum of a cerebral lateral ventricle. Radiology, 39:167–174, 1942.

12. Dyke, C. G., Elsberg, C. A., and Davidoff, L. M.: Enlargement in the defect in the air shadow following ventriculography. Amer. J. Roentgen., 33:736–743, 1935.

13. Falk, B.: Calcification in the track of the needle following ventricular puncture. Acta Radiol., 35:304–308, 1951.

14. Ford, L. E., and McLaurin, R. L.: Mechanism of extradural hematoma. J. Neurosurg., 20:760–769, 1963.

15. Grant, F. C.: Ventriculography: A review based on the analysis of 392 cases. Arch. Neurol. Psychiat., 14:513–522, 1925.

16. Haft, H., Liss, H., and Mount, L. A.: Massive epidural hemorrhage as a complication of ventricular drainage. J. Neurosurg., 17:49–54, 1960.

17. Higazi, I.: Epidural hematoma as a complication of ventricular drainage. Report of a case and review of literature. J. Neurosurg., 20:527–528, 1963.

18. Hook, E. B.: Central nervous system infection in hydrocephalic children following ventriculography. Clin. Pediat., 481–483, 1965.

19. Hook, E. B., and Vesley, D.: The efficacy of sterile gauze as a filter of air ventriculography in pneumoencephalography. Neurology (Minneap.), 15:1078–1080, 1965.

20. Jefferson, G.: The balance of life and death in cerebral lesions. Surg. Gynec. Obstet., 93:444–458, 1951.

21. Keen, W. W.: Exploratory trephining and puncture of the brain. Med. News, 53:603–609, 1888.

22. Lorber, J., and Emery, J. L.: Intracerebral cyst complicating ventricular needling in hydrocephalic infants: A clinical pathologic study. Develop. Med. Child Neurol., 6:125–139, 1964.

23. Luckett, W. J.: Air in the ventricles of the brain following a fracture of the skull. Surg. Gynec. Obstet., 17:237–240, 1913.

24. Marini, G., and Taveras, J. M.: Influence of ventricular size on mortality and morbidity following ventriculography. Acta Radiol., 1:602–608, 1963.

25. Masson, C. B.: The disturbances in vision and in visual fields after ventriculography. Bull. Neurol. Inst. N.Y., 3:190–209, 1934.

26. Papatheodorou, C. A., and Teng, P.: Air-Pantopaque ventriculography in congenital hydrocephalus and myelomeningocele. Acta Radiol. [Diag.] (Stockholm), 91:647–655, 1964.

27. Pendergrass, E. P.: Indications and contra-indications of encephalography and ventriculography. J.A.M.A., 94:408–411, 1931.

28. Petersdorf, R. G., Swarner, P. R., and Garcia, M.: Studies on the pathogenesis of meningitis. II. J. Clin. Invest., 41:320–327, 1962.

29. Picaza, J. A., Hunter, S. E., and Cannon, B. W.: Axial ventriculography. J. Neurosurg., 33:297–303, 1970.

30. Riggs, H. W.: The dangers and mortality of ventriculography. Bull. Neurol. Inst. N.Y., 3:210–231, 1934.

31. Walker, E. A.: A History of Neurological Surgery. New York, Hafner Pub. Co., 1967, pp. 27–29.

32. Vinas, F. J.: Iodoventriculography by direct catheterization of third ventricle in posterior fossa lesions of childhood. J. Neurosurg., 21:492–496, 1964.

33. Whisler, W. W., and Voris, H. C.: Ossified epidural hematoma following posterior fossa exploration. J. Neurosurg., 23:214–216, 1965.

34. Youmans, J. R., and Schneider, R. C.: Post-traumatic intracranial hematomas in patients with arrested hydrocephalus. J. Neurosurg., 17:590–597, 1960.

8

RADIOLOGY OF THE SPINE

A great deal of knowledge concerning the radiology of the spine and its contents has accumulated over the years. For a more comprehensive review than is given in this chapter, the reader is referred to the standard texts on the subject.[8, 10, 15, 17, 26, 28]

The technique for the examination of the spine should include views taken to outline the odontoid peg, the bodies of the vertebrae, the pedicles and laminae, the spinous processes, the articular facets, the spinal canal dimensions, the intervertebral spaces, the intervertebral foramina, and the lateral masses. These requirements should be met by the open-mouth view for the odontoid peg, oblique views for the intervertebral foramina, by drawing the shoulders downward to visualize the lower cervical spine (see Fig. 8–40), and by angulation of the tube for a view of the lateral masses. For accurate assessment of the extent of the disc space, the x-ray beam must be directed individually through each intervertebral space. An extended Water's skull projection often will allow an unobstructed view of the odontoid process through the foramen magnum. Extension and flexion films may be indicated on occasion. This is particularly true in the cervical and lumbar region. Also laminagraphy and cinematography will enhance the anatomical details and are helpful in diagnosis in some patients.

A valuable indication of the dimensions of the spinal canal may be obtained using the following measurements. In the anteroposterior projection the interpedicular distances may be measured and compared with the charts compiled by Elsberg and Dyke.[7] Reference may also be made to Hinck et al. for spinal canal measurements in children.[12] In the lateral projection the anterior-posterior dimensions of the canal may also be measured.[13] While measuring the interpedicular distances it should be noted that the shape of the pedicles normally changes from an indistinct round shadow in the cervical region to a kidney-shaped structure in the thoracic region and to a round structure in the lumbar region. The inner margin is always convex inward.

The intervertebral foramen at C2–C3 is usually larger than the other cervical foramina. This is important when evaluating the possible presence of a dumbbell tumor.

Smith has summarized the various figures presented in the literature concerning the dimensions of the cord and spine at various levels.[29] As a general rule the interpedicular distance increases and becomes progressively wider from C2 to C6. From C6 to T4 there is progressive diminution, and from T4 downward it progressively increases. In the anteroposterior diameter the canal progressively narrows. Wolf et al. state that a sagittal diameter of 10 mm or less of the cervical spinal canal is likely to be associated with cord compression.[33] However, it is not always possible to be certain of the exact location of posterior projecting spines in relation to the midline (Figs. 8–1, 8–2, and 8–3).

CONGENITAL ANOMALIES

In an evaluation of the cervical spine the following anomalies may be encountered. In basilar invagination there is indentation of the upper cervical vertebra into the base of the skull. Various lines and measurements are available in the literature to de-

M. M. SCHECHTER

E. L. KIER

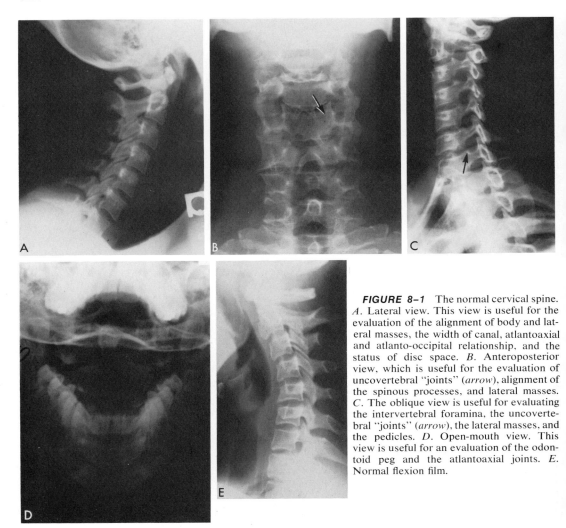

FIGURE 8–1 The normal cervical spine. *A.* Lateral view. This view is useful for the evaluation of the alignment of body and lateral masses, the width of canal, atlantoaxial and atlanto-occipital relationship, and the status of disc space. *B.* Anteroposterior view, which is useful for the evaluation of uncovertebral "joints" (*arrow*), alignment of the spinous processes, and lateral masses. *C.* The oblique view is useful for evaluating the intervertebral foramina, the uncovertebral "joints" (*arrow*), the lateral masses, and the pedicles. *D.* Open-mouth view. This view is useful for an evaluation of the odontoid peg and the atlantoaxial joints. *E.* Normal flexion film.

termine its presence. McGregor's line extends from the posterior margin of the hard palate to the inferior margin of the occipital squamae. The tip of the odontoid should not extend more than 5 mm above this line. Other measurements for evaluating basilar invagination have been described by Bull, by Chamberlain, and others.[20] The condition may be associated with the various disease entities causing bone softening. Paget's disease is the most common cause and others include the various bony dysplasias (Fig. 8–4).

In occipitalization of the atlas the capacity of the foramen magnum is diminished (Fig. 8–4). The posterior arch of C1 is not visible but is assimilated into the occiput. Partial absence of the arch of C1 should be considered in the evaluation of fractures in this region (Fig. 8–5).

Many anomalies of the odontoid may be encountered. The odontoid ossifies from five primary and two secondary centers. The ossification is not complete until the second year of life and occasionally remains incomplete. Ossification may be a prolonged process, and because of the many centers involved, anomalies do occur. These should not be interpreted as fractures or fracture-dislocations (Fig. 8–6). The dens may be congenitally absent or bifid, and the apex may be unossified or unfused to the rest of the odontoid. The odontoid may remain unfused to the body of C2.

Failures of normal segmentation will result in many anomalies including the Klippel-Feil syndrome, Sprengel's deformity, hemivertebrae, and blocked vertebrae, all of which have classic appearances (Fig. 8–7). The blocked vertebrae should be distinguished from destruction of the disc space by infection and trauma. In acquired blocked vertebrae, other evidence of trauma or infection is present. In addition, the total height of the two fused vertebrae is less than that of the congenital blocked vertebrae because of destruction of the disc space (Fig. 8–8).

Spina bifida may occur as an isolated defect in bony fusion, but it may also be associated with a congenital anomaly that may include a meningomyelocele (Fig. 8–9), a lipoma, a dermoid, or any other defect associated with spinal dysplasia. Segmentation anomalies of the lumbar sacral region may present as a sacralized L5 or a lumbarized S1. The only way to determine the exact anatomy is to count down from C1. The presence of a large sacral canal may suggest an occult sacral meningocele.

TRAUMA

Fractures of the spinal column are usually associated with certain types of injuries. The cervical spine is most commonly involved in trauma. Certain types of trauma affect parts of the arch, making them vulnerable to further injury. The trauma may involve the odontoid peg (Figs. 8–10 and *Text continued on page 244.*

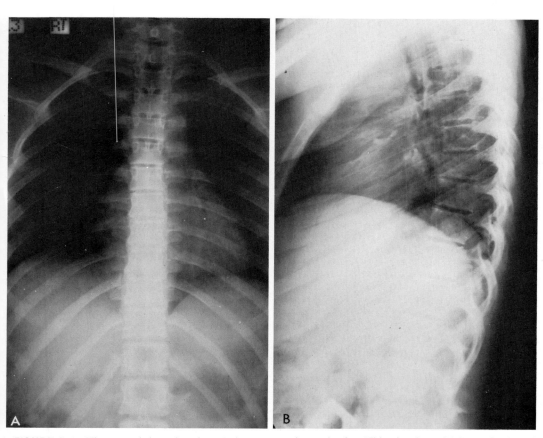

FIGURE 8–2 The normal thoracic spine. *A.* Anteroposterior projection. This view is useful for evaluation of the pedicles, interpedicular distances, alignment of spinous processes, paraspinal masses. *B.* Lateral projection. This view is useful for an evaluation of disc spaces and pedicles.

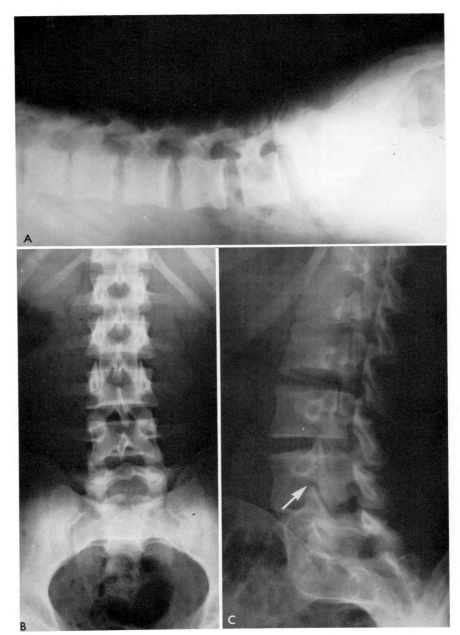

FIGURE 8–3 The normal lumbar spine. *A*. Lateral projection for evaluation of disc spaces, bodies, alignment. *B*. Anteroposterior projection for evaluating disc space, shape and integrity of pedicles and spinous processes, integrity of sacrum, and sacroiliac joints. *C*. Oblique view for pedicles, articular facets, pars interarticularis (*arrow*).

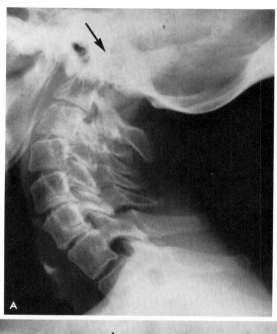

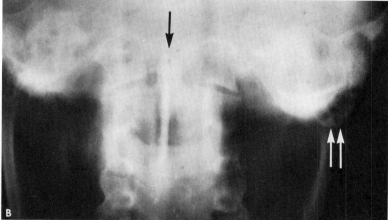

FIGURE 8-4   Basilar invagination (Paget's disease). *A*. Note that the odontoid peg (*arrow*) extends above the foramen magnum. There is occipitalization of the posterior arch of C1. *B*. Anteroposterior projection showing the odontoid peg (*black arrow*) high above the mastoid processes (*white arrows*).

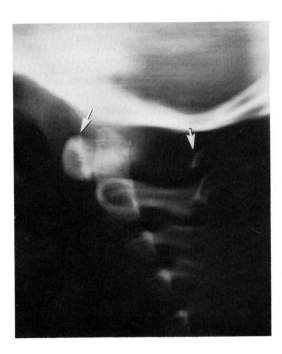

FIGURE 8-5 Anomaly of first cervical vertebra. Part of the posterior arch of C1 is absent (*right arrow*). Note the normal relationship of the odontoid to the anterior arch of C1 (*left arrow*).

FIGURE 8-6 Infant cervical spine. Note the normally large distance between the incompletely ossified odontoid peg and the anterior arch of the atlas. The odontoid is not fused to the body of C2.

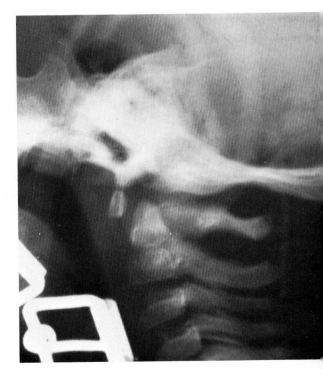

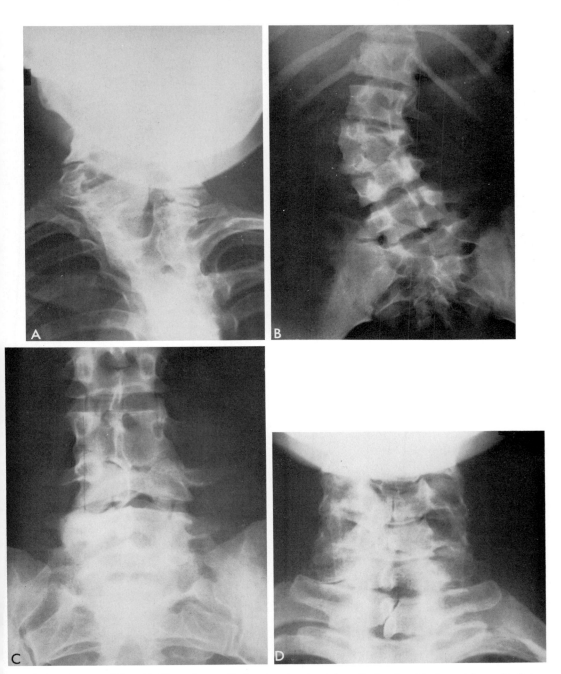

FIGURE 8–7 *A*. Klippel-Feil syndrome. *B*. Lumbar hemivertebra. *C*. Lumbar block vertebrae. *D*. Spina bifida occulta.

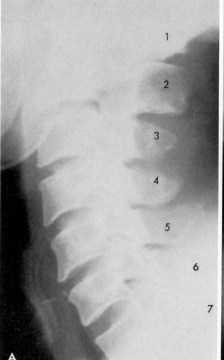
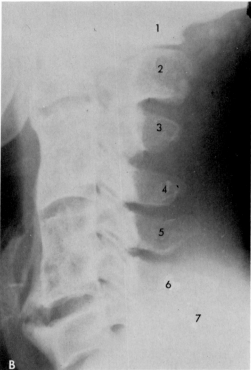

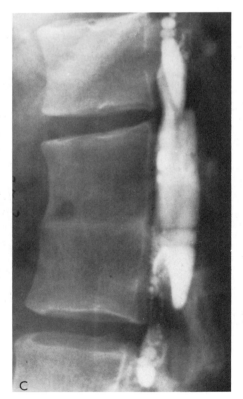

FIGURE 8–8 Acquired block vertebrae. *A* and *B*. Preoperative and postoperative views of cervical spine showing two pairs of block vertebrae from surgical fusion. *C*. Block vertebrae secondary to infection.

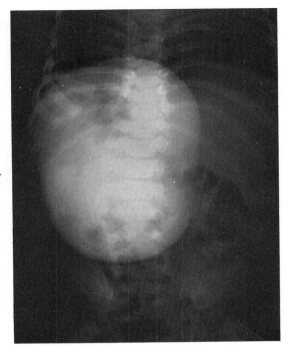

FIGURE 8-9 Meningomyelocele. The large soft tissue density is obvious. Note multiple anomalies of the thoracolumbar spine.

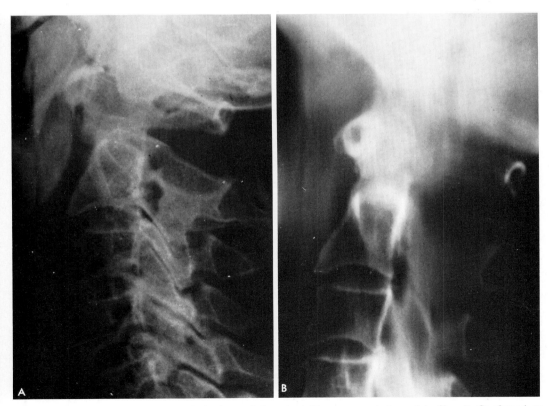

FIGURE 8-10 *A*. Fracture through the base of the odontoid peg suspected on plain film. *B*. Confirmed on laminagraphy.

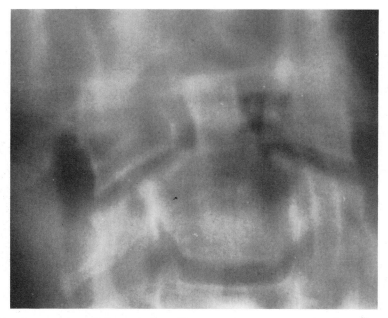

FIGURE 8–11 Fracture through base of odontoid peg seen on anteroposterior view. Note the atlantoaxial dislocation.

8–11), the body of the vertebrae, the intervertebral disc, the neural arch, or the transverse and spinous processes.

Fractures of the lower cervical and upper thoracic vertebral bodies can be missed. Unless an effort is made to pull the shoulders down these vertebral bodies will not be visualized in a large number of patients (Fig. 8–13). In the obese patient with a short neck, pulling the shoulders down is inadequate and spinal alignments are difficult to evaluate in the swimmer's projection. A special double exposure technique is necessary to visualize the cervical thoracic junction.[9] It is imperative to make an all-out effort to visualize the lower cervical region, especially in the unresponsive patient. Occasionally an intoxicated patient admitted for trauma will be rendered quadriparetic as a result of manipulation that was considered safe because of a "negative" cervical spine examination that did not include the cervical-thoracic junction (Fig. 8–14). Blurring of the cervical prevertebral fat stripe may help in the detection of a fracture.[32] Oblique anteroposterior projections may demonstrate unsuspected fractures of the lateral masses.[30] Occasionally cervical spine trauma results from

trauma to the skull. Thus, every patient with head trauma should have a careful examination of the cervical spine.

The following fractures occur in the cervical spine: (1) Jefferson's fracture of the atlas; (2) fractures of the axis at the base of the odontoid; fractures through laminae and pedicles; and (3) fractures through C3–C7, which may include a fracture-dislocation without vertebral body compression as well as fracture with body compression.

Fractures of the spinous processes and transverse processes may result from sudden traction of ligaments and muscles. These may be recognized in the routine projections, or special projections may be necessary.

The majority of thoracic-lumbar fractures involve T12, L1, and L2. These are increasing in frequency in automobile accidents involving cars in which abdominal seat belts are used (Figs. 8–15 and 8–16). Thoracic-lumbar fractures may result in wedging of the vertebral bodies, disruption of the posterior elements, and fractures of the transverse processes. Compression fractures may result in the extrusion of disc material through the disrupted posterior ligaments and anulus. Dislocation occurs when the

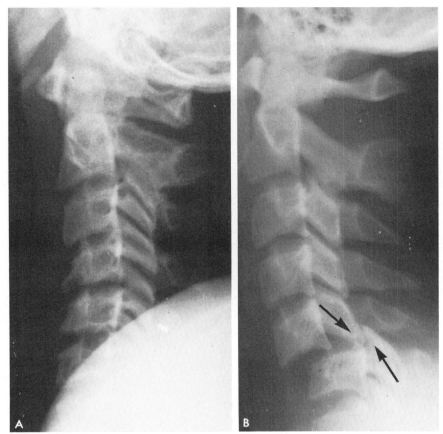

FIGURE 8-12 *A*. Compression fracture of C4 and C5. *B*. Fracture-dislocation of C5 and C6 with locking of articular facets (*arrows*).

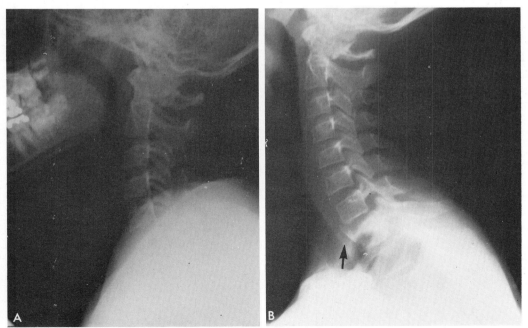

FIGURE 8-13 *A*. Compression fracture of T1 was missed on initial examination because shoulders were not pulled down. *B*. The fracture is obvious in the examination with the shoulders pulled down.

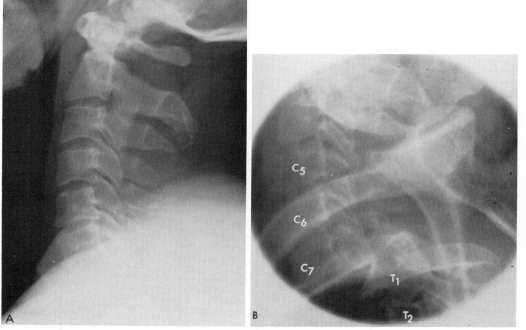

FIGURE 8–14 *A*. Severe fracture-dislocation of C7, T1 was missed. Since the fracture was not suspected after the initial roentgenogram, manipulations of the neck resulted in pressure on the cord and paraplegia. *B*. Double exposure technique shows the severe fracture-dislocation.

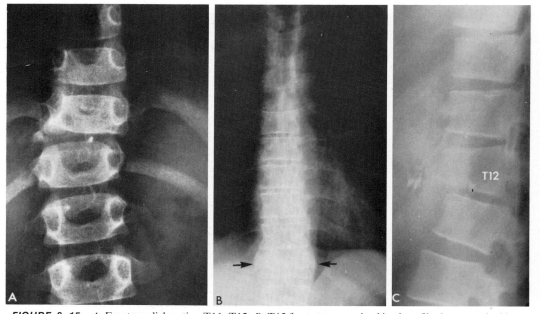

FIGURE 8–15 *A*. Fracture-dislocation T11, T12. *B*. T12 fracture recognized in chest film by paraspinal hematoma (*arrows*). *C*. Seat belt fracture of T12. Compression injury. Radiogram was taken with patient lying on her back and with a horizontal beam. The important trauma to the posterior elements was not detected. This illustrates the need to raise the patient off the table top to include these structures in the roentgenogram.

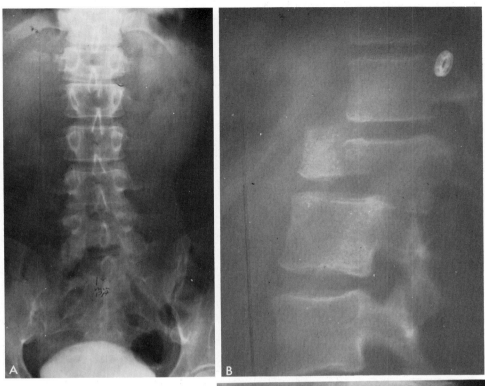

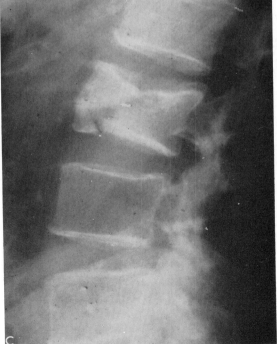

FIGURE 8–16 *A.* Patient was involved in an accident, but was neurologically intact. This film was part of an intravenous pyelogram series. Note loss of disc space and malalignment of the spinal processes. There are fractures through both transverse processes. *B.* Lateral roentgenogram of same patient taken because of findings in *A.* Note the severe fracture-dislocation. *C.* Compression fracture of L3.

inferior articular facet of an upper cervical segment slides forward on the upper articulating facet of an adjacent lower cervical segment. These may be locked in this abnormal position (see Fig. 8–12). Rotatory dislocation of C1 on C2 is still a controversial entity.[34]

Spondylolisthesis is presently considered to be a result of trauma (Fig. 8–17). The vertebral body moves forward leaving the posterior elements behind. In the minor degrees no defect is present in the pars interarticularis and degeneration of the disc may be sufficient to allow the minor movements. When the dislocation is great, however, a defect may be recognized in the pars interarticularis. Oblique views should be taken routinely when this situation is

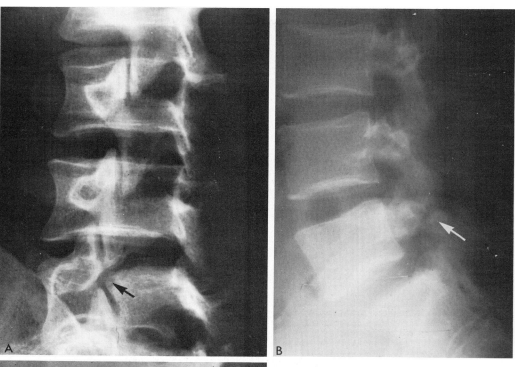

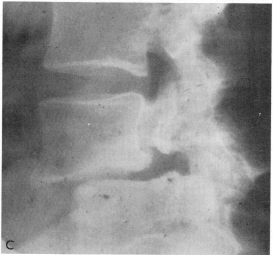

FIGURE 8–17 Spondylolisthesis. *A.* Oblique view of lumbar spine demonstrating a defect in the pars interarticularis. Note the translucent line running across the "neck of the scotty dog." *B.* Defect of pars interarticularis seen in lateral projection. *C.* Long-standing spondylolisthesis showing narrowing of disc space with movement of the vertebral body forward.

suspected and the defect sought (Fig. 8–17*A*).

In lateral roentgenograms of the cervical spine with the neck flexed there is frequently a slight displacement anteriorly with respect to the subjacent vertebrae. In infants and children this may be exaggerated. This should not be mistaken for a dislocation; flexion and extension of the neck will show that the movements are normal.[21]

Various types of traumatic subarachnoid disruption may occur (see Fig. 8–39). Avulsion of the brachial nerve roots may occur as a result of severe trauma to the shoulder. The arachnoid and dura forming the nerve root sleeve are torn, leaving a pocket in which the contrast medium may collect. Various traumatic communications between the subarachnoid space and the thoracic and abdominal cavities may occur. Subarachnoid mediastinal fistulae are extremely rare.[35] Traumatic extradural cysts of the spine may result from tears of the dura during lumbar disc surgery.[27]

INFECTIONS

There is a tendency not to consider seriously the possibility of infectious diseases of the spine. This attitude has been propagated by the antibiotic era. Awareness of the possibility of an infectious process may alert the physician to it in time to avoid the serious complications of spinal cord damage associated with it.

Usually pyogenic infection of the vertebrae is staphylococcal and of hematogenous spread. The radiological changes due to infection may manifest themselves weeks after the onset of symptoms. The infection usually begins in the vertebral body near the disc, which shows early involvement. The characteristic changes are loss of definition of the margins of the vertebral bodies with slight narrowing of the disc spaces (Fig. 8–18). Prolonged infection is marked by bony proliferation, which may end in fusion of the bodies. A paravertebral mass occasionally is seen and may be one of the early changes and the only clue to the bony disease. In the later stages the breakdown of the infected material may calcify, leaving a signature of the disease process. In tu-

berculous infection the process is much more prolonged with caseation going on to granulomatous changes. There may be rupture of pus through the ligaments with tracking and the formation of a cold abscess. The abscess and tracks may later calcify. Severe spinal deformity may occur and may include scoliosis and a pronounced kyphoscoliosis. Other infectious processes such as syphilis, brucellosis, actinomycosis, toxoplasmosis, and typhoid may involve the spine without any specific characteristic changes. Charcot's spine, a neuropathic joint disease, is usually due to syphilis, diabetes, tumors, paraplegia, syringomyelia, or transverse myelitis. The neuropathic joint changes consist of a marked articular cartilaginous destruction and a haphazard proliferation of subchondral bone with osteophytes and complete disorganization of the joint.

OSTEOARTHRITIS

Osteoarthritis results from the aging process of the disc, which is the precipitating factor in the production of this condition. Dehydration, disintegration, and fragmentation of the disc occurs, causing bulging of the disc, increasing traction at the attachment of the longitudinal ligaments, and secondary formation of spurs. As the disc continues to degenerate and narrow, abnormal movements and contact of exposed adjacent bony structures result in secondary spur formation. These ridges and spurs may encroach upon the spinal canal and on the intervertebral foramina, causing cord compression or root compression respectively (Fig. 8–19). The vertebral artery may be compromised by encroachment upon its lumen, particularly when the head and neck are rotated. The most common sites of cervical disc degeneration are at C5–C6 and C6–C7. These bony ridges may be recognized in the plain radiograms. Oblique projections must be taken to outline the intervertebral foramina.

Ankylosing spondylitis is also known as Marie-Strümpell disease. The pathological process of this disease involves the sacroiliac and other spinous joints with eventual ligamentous ossifications (Fig. 8–20).

The most important aspect of rheuma-

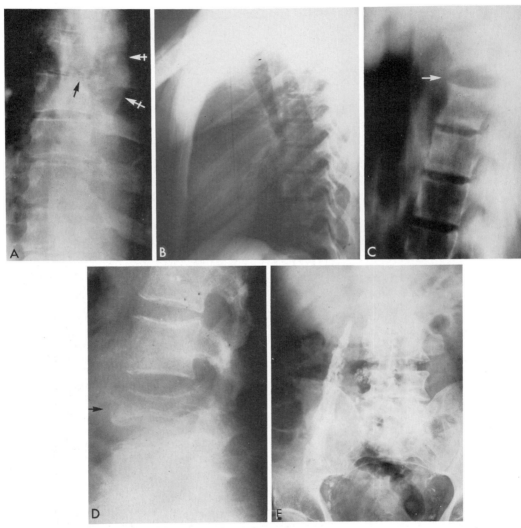

FIGURE 8–18 Infection. *A.* Pyogenic infection with loss of the disc space (*single arrow*) and a paraspinal mass (*arrows with crossed shaft*). *B.* Tuberculous destruction of a vertebral body was missed in the routine lateral chest film but recognized in the laminagram, *C,* in which the body is seen to have virtually disappeared, leaving what looks like a wide disc space (*arrow*). *D.* Pyogenic osteomyelitis simulating metastatic disease. Note collapse of the body (*arrow*) with intact disc spaces. *E.* Calcified psoas abscess, a late manifestation of tuberculosis osteomyelitis.

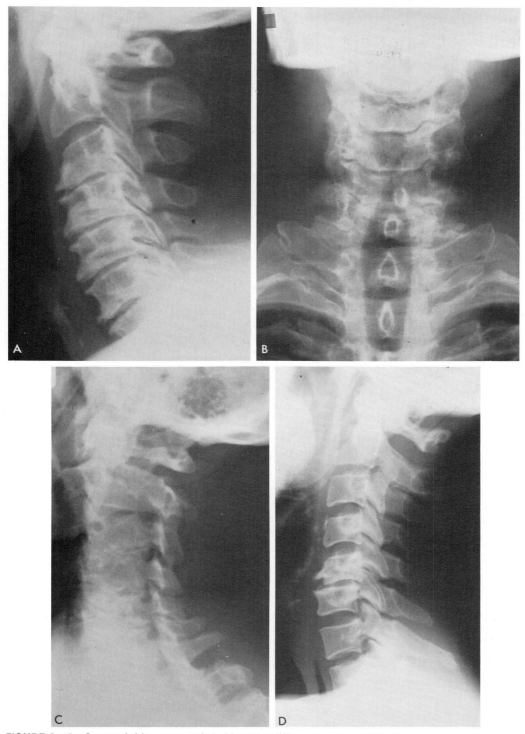

FIGURE 8–19 Osteoarthritis. *A, B,* and *C.* Note the diffuse narrowing of the disc spaces, spur formation, eburnation of bone, and encroachment on intervertebral foramina. *D.* Isolated involvement of C5 and C6.

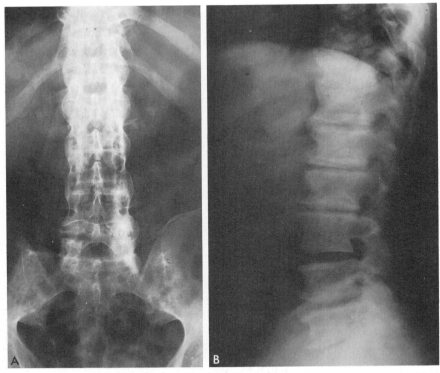

FIGURE 8–20 *A*. Ankylosing spondylitis—note changes in sacroiliac joints and the typical bamboo spine with ossification of the longitudinal ligaments. *B*. Advanced Paget's disease.

toid arthritis of the spine is its effect on the synovial joint between the dens and the anterior arch of the atlas. The resulting ligamentous involvement, which at times is accompanied by odontoid peg destruction, may cause atlantoaxial dislocation. This should not be mistaken for trauma to this region (Fig. 8–21).

PAGET'S DISEASE

Paget's disease is often unsuspected and occurs mainly in the spinous body. It is a disease of unknown etiology. Pathological changes in the spine include bone softening, resorption, and disorganized bony reformation. The result is a widened, dense vertebral body, which may fracture and may cause cord compression (see Fig. 8–20 *B*). Malignant degeneration may occur but is rare.

TUMORS

Although spinal cord tumors are only one sixth as common as brain tumors, over 50 per cent of them are benign and great effort should be made to recognize them. The usual classification of spinal tumors is: extradural, intradural-extramedullary, and intradural-intramedullary. The myelographic criteria for deciding in which group a specific tumor belongs are discussed later. The grouping is not of academic interest alone since the determination of the compartment involved usually gives a clue to the type of tumor. Over 90 per cent of extradural tumors are malignant, 75 per cent of extradural lesions are metastatic, and over 50 per cent of intradural lesions are benign.

Neurofibromas and meningiomas constitute more than 90 per cent of intradural lesions. Eighty per cent of spinal meningiomas occur in women of an average age of 50 years and favor the thoracic area. Calcification that can be detected in plain films is infrequent in meningiomas. They are rarely extradural.[3]

Schwannomas are slightly more common than meningiomas. There is no sexual or site predilection. Occasionally they are multiple. Seventy per cent of schwannomas are intradural, 15 per cent are dumbbell (intradural and extradural), and 15 per cent are extradural. Bone changes are more frequent than in meningiomas and usually occur with the dumbbell tumors. The bony changes include erosion of the pedicles, widening of the interpedicular distance, and scalloping of the posterior surface of the vertebral body.

Over 95 per cent of intramedullary lesions are gliomas. These may cause a widening of the spinal canal involving more than one segment. Intramedullary metastatic lesions are rare, but 160 cases have been reported in the literature. Half of these were from primary lung carcinoma.

Metastatic disease is the most common cause of tumor of the spine. As metastatic hematogenous spread affects the spongiosa first and since the radiological density of the body resides in the cortical bone, a large part of the body may be involved without showing any radiological change.

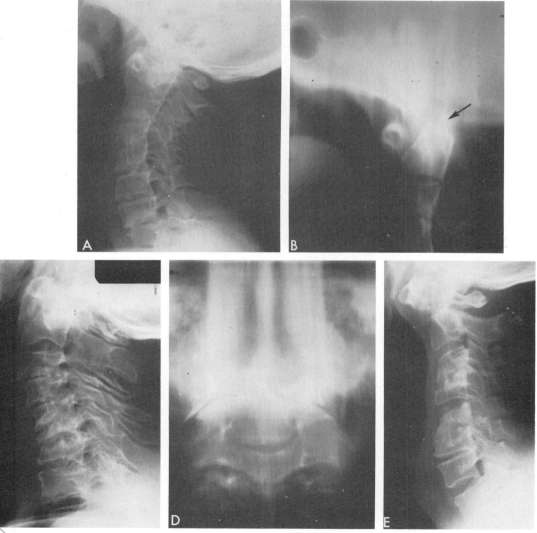

FIGURE 8-21 Rheumatoid arthritis. *A.* Rheumatoid arthritis with destruction of odontoid process. *B.* Tomography shows the area of destruction to better advantage (*arrow*). *C.* Another case of rheumatoid arthritis showing less destruction of the odontoid peg but more changes in movement in the cervical spine. *D.* Tomography in the anteroposterior projection showing the odontoid changes. *E.* C3–C4 and C5–C6 fusion secondary to rheumatoid arthritis.

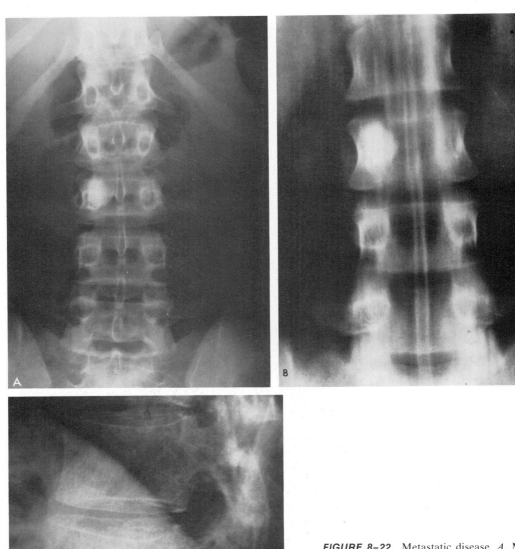

FIGURE 8–22 Metastatic disease. *A*. Metastatic disease involving pedicle only. *B*. Tomogram showing the osteoblastic metastatic deposit to better advantage. *C*. Osteoblastic metastatic disease from prostate.

Only when the cortex is involved will radiological changes be appreciated.

The most common tumors to metastasize to the spine are those of the breast, prostate, thyroid, kidney, and lung. The bone reaction depends on the nature of the primary neoplasm. Breast and prostate tumors are usually osteoblastic (Fig. 8–22). While those of the thyroid and kidney are usually osteolytic, any combination may be present (Fig. 8–23). Pedicular involvement is important to recognize since it may be associ-

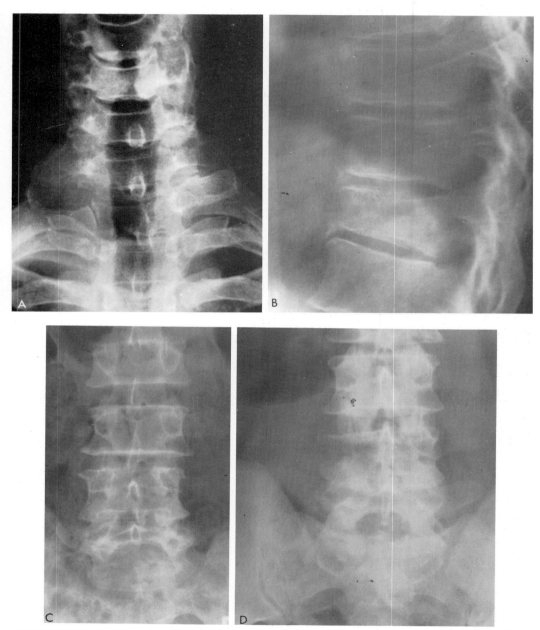

FIGURE 8–23 *A.* Osteolytic metastatic disease destroying the lateral transverse process of T1. *B.* Partial collapse of a vertebral body involved in metastatic disease. *C.* Unsuspected sacral and iliac destruction in patient with clinical diagnosis of herniated disc. *D.* Lytic vertebral body destruction secondary to adjacent soft tissue sarcoma.

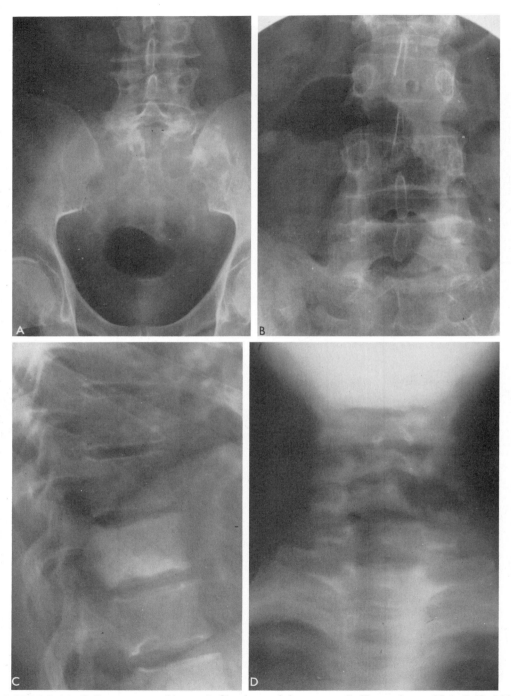

FIGURE 8–24   Solitary tumors of bone. *A*. Chordoma of the sacrum. *B*. Hemangioma of L4. *C*. Hodgkin's disease involving only T11. *D*. Reticulum cell sarcoma involving C6.

ated with cord compression and is usually due to metastatic disease. Multiple myeloma may resemble metastatic disease closely and usually it is not possible to distinguish between them.

Certain solitary tumors have characteristic changes, such as sarcomas, aneurysmal bone cyst, hemangiomas, and osteoid osteomas (Fig. 8–24). The diffuse disseminated diseases at times may have characteristic changes but often cannot be distinguished from one another or from metastatic diseases (Fig. 8–25).

A condition simulating an intraspinal neoplasm is the dural ectasia that may occur as an isolated manifestation of neurofibromatosis (Fig. 8–26). This ectasia with associated bone changes may involve one or several vertebral segments. The backs of the vertebral bodies assume a scalloped appearance, and there may also be thinning of the pedicles. Other manifestations of neurofibromatosis are severe kyphoscoliosis, spondylolisthesis, and intrathoracic meningoceles.

MYELOGRAPHY

Myelography may be undertaken using positive or negative contrast medium. Pantopaque (iodophenylundecylic acid) is usually the contrast medium of choice although gas myelography is increasing in popularity. Pantopaque is not the ideal contrast medium, but it is the least irritating and safest of the positive contrast agents that are available at the present time. Systemic reactions and local reactions have been reported. Because of the irritating effects of the Pantopaque it is important to remove it at the end of the procedure.

Since Pantopaque is hyperbaric it must be manipulated into position. No other positive contrast medium in use today may be passed from the sacral sac to the basilar subarachnoid system. Emulsified Pantopaque has not gained popularity because of the incidence of increased meningeal reactions.[19] One of the disadvantages of regular Pantopaque, which contains 30 per cent iodine by weight, is the potential to mask

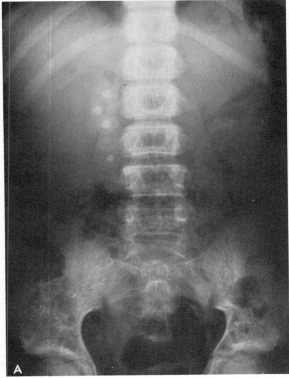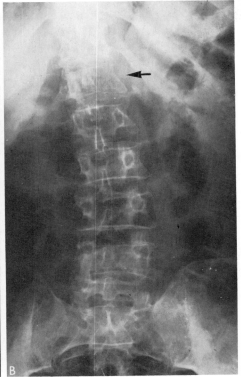

FIGURE 8–25 *A*. Sickle cell disease. *B*. Multiple myeloma. Note absence of T12 pedicle.

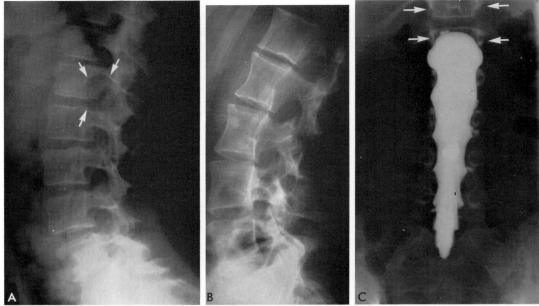

FIGURE 8-26 Neurofibromatosis. *A*. Enlarged intervertebral foramen (*arrows*) as a result of a dumbbell neurofibroma. *B*. Neurofibromatosis showing dysplasia of bone. The spinal canal is widened; there is pedicular erosion and scalloping of the posterior margins of the vertebral bodies simulating a spinal tumor. An ependymoma may resemble this. *C*. Dural ectasia showing thinning of pedicles (*arrows*) and outpouchings of contrast medium.

intraspinal masses because of its density. This prompted several investigators to use less dense Pantopaque.[11, 16] The disadvantages of the less dense Pantopaque are its poor radiographic density and its reduced rate of flow, which make the examination tedious. A water-soluble contrast medium has been used extensively in Europe. Its major disadvantage is its irritant effect, necessitating spinal anesthesia. Another disadvantage is that it can only be used in the lumbar region.

Recently water-soluble meglumine iothalamate (Conray) has been used as a myelographic agent. However, numerous serious side reactions have been reported.[22]

Gas myelography is used extensively in Scandanavia. The technique is much more exacting than Pantopaque myelography and requires more sophisticated equipment and meticulous care in performance and interpretation.[15, 31] The gas produces little irritation, is completely absorbed in a short time, and may be used for any region of the spine. The examination can be repeated as often as desired and there is no residual contrast agent present to obscure the pic-

ture. The discomfort some patients have may be a disadvantage of this technique. In experienced hands this medium has shown its greatest versatility in demonstrating lesions that may not be recognized with other contrast media. Gas myelography is of special value in the detection of cystic spinal cord lesions that communicate with the subarachnoid space and for detecting cord atrophy (see Fig. 8–42).[4]

Technique

Undoubtedly the most important aspect of myelography is the introduction of the entire amount of desired contrast into the subarachnoid space. This requires a meticulous technique. The patient may be placed in the lateral decubitus position with the knees drawn toward the forehead. In this position the spinal spaces are opened to allow easiest introduction of the needle. The myelographer may prefer to place the patient prone on the table with a pillow under the abdomen or to have him sitting with the back flexed. The smallest possible gauge needle should be used, but the viscosity of the medium precludes using anything smaller than 20-gauge. An 18- or 19-gauge needle facilitates the removal of the Pantopaque. Meticulous attention to technique obviates the need for the various specialized myelographic needles. A short-

bevel needle is preferred because the contrast medium can be introduced into a single compartment. Furthermore, it facilitates the Pantopaque removal. The disadvantages of a short-bevel needle are that it is harder to introduce and may tear the arachnoid.

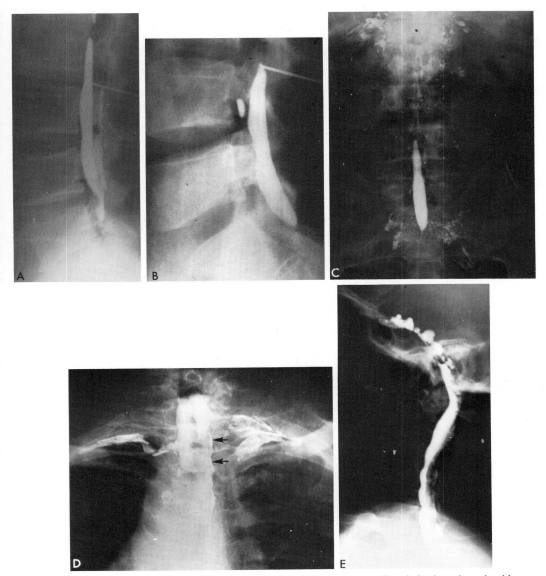

FIGURE 8–27 *A.* The patient is lying prone. The bulk of the contrast medium is in the subarachnoid space. A second collection is in the subdural space. *B.* The patient is lying prone, but the contrast medium is not against the back of the spinal bodies. This is the typical appearance of subdural contrast. A repeat myelogram with contrast medium in the subarachnoid space revealed the presence of a diseased lumbar disc missed on the first study. *C.* Epidural contrast medium showing the classic appearance of tracking along nerve roots. This may occur during the study or after the removal of the needle. *D.* Pantopaque in the three compartments—subarachnoid, subdural, and epidural. The arrows point to the subdural collection—the thin dense line. *E.* Cervical myelogram. Improper position of head has resulted in spillage of contrast into the middle fossa.

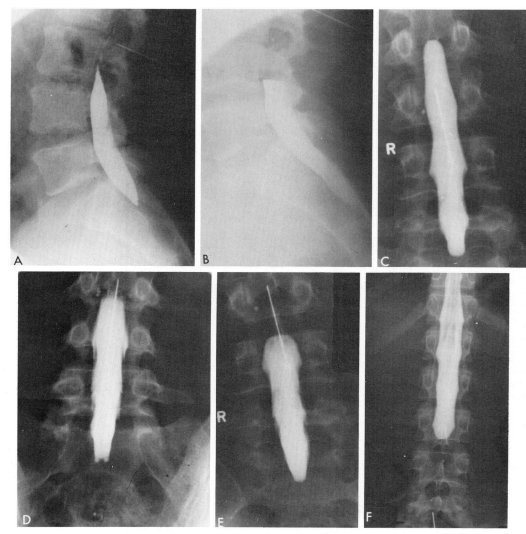

FIGURE 8-28   Lumbar myelogram. *A.* Lateral view. *B.* Lateral view with patient standing in hyperextension. This is done to accentuate bulge of anulus. *C.* Posteroanterior view. *D.* Posteroanterior view with tube angled toward feet. This is done for better visualization of sac. *E.* Posteroanterior view with patient erect. *F.* View of conus.   *Illustration continued on opposite page.*

The site of puncture is usually at L2–L3 since this is below the level of the cord and above the majority of herniated discs. Occasionally the puncture site has to be lower when an upper lumbar lesion is suspected. In cases of total block or when the upper extent of a lesion is to be outlined, a cisternal puncture or a lateral cervical puncture may be used.[23] Fluoroscopic control of the entire procedure is absolutely essential. This monitors the position of the needle for the correct midline introduction and the desired level of puncture.

A small amount of Pantopaque should be introduced and its movement observed under screen control. If the Pantopaque remains around the needle tip when the patient is tilted it is imperative to stop. The position of the test injection may then be ascertained by fluoroscopic visualization or by a cross-table roentgenogram. When the examiner is satisfied that the contrast

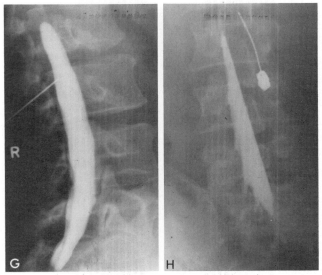

FIGURE 8-28 *(Continued)* *G.* Oblique view. *H.* Lateral decubitus view.

is in the proper compartment and moving satisfactorily, the remainder of it can be introduced. It should be remembered that the flow may be slow in a spondylotic canal. By taking other views and ascertaining that the contrast is in the appropriate compartment, needless cancellation of the examination may be avoided.

It should be noted that a normal rate of flow of the Pantopaque can occur in the subdural space. A film to ascertain the position of the test dose of Pantopaque will insure the correct placement of the contrast medium. When Pantopaque is outside the subarachnoid space the needle should be withdrawn and a new puncture two spaces removed should be undertaken (Fig. 8–27). A myelogram should not be performed, if delay is at all possible, within seven days of a previous lumbar puncture because of collapse of the subarachnoid space.

The amount of Pantopaque used depends upon the personal preference of the examiner, the area of examination, and the width of the spinal canal. Usually 6 to 9 ml is used for the lumbar region, 12 to 15 ml for the cervical region, and 15 to 20 ml for the thoracic region.

The routine examination of the lumbar region includes anteroposterior, oblique, and lateral projection films. Occasionally films are taken with the patient standing with extension and flexion of the spine. The count of vertebral level should be included in each study (Fig. 8–28). In the thoracic region, fluoroscopy is more essential because the contrast medium usually passes fairly rapidly over the thoracic kyphosis. The best way to examine the thoracic cord is to place the patient in the supine position after removing the needle. Again anteroposterior and lateral projections should be taken. Lateral decubitus films may be useful to show filling of the nerve root pouches (Fig. 8–29).

In the cervical area, anteoposterior, lateral, and oblique views should be taken. Films may also be taken in extension and flexion of the neck. To fill the cervical subarachnoid canal the head must be well extended during the passage of the contrast medium from the lumbar region. The table is tilted head down and the neck extended maximally. After the contrast has pooled in the cervical region, the table may be placed horizontally and the neck placed in a neutral position between flexion and extension (see Fig. 8–27). Cervical myelography is incomplete if C7 is not outlined in the lateral projection. To do this the shoulders may be pulled down or the swimmer's projection may be used. The double

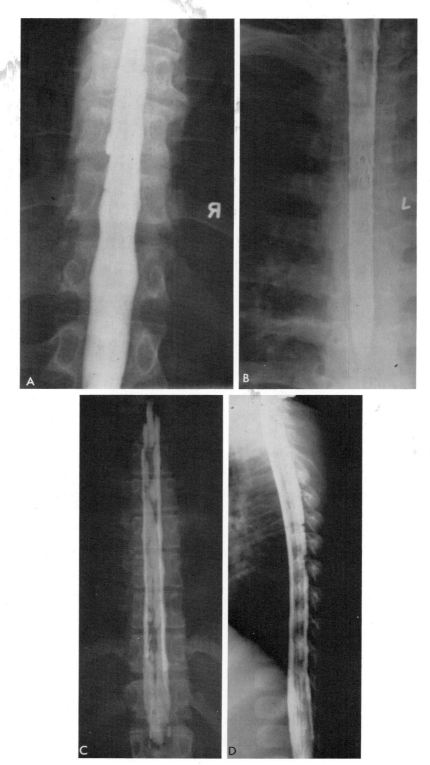

FIGURE 8–29 Thoracic myelogram. *A*. Prone position showing lower thoracic region. *B*. Prone position showing upper thoracic region. *C*, with needle removed and patient supine, making an anteroposterior projection. This is the best view for visualizing the thoracic cord and to demonstrate abnormal vascularity. *D*. In decubitus film with vertical beam and with enough Pantopaque, the entire cord may be outlined. Overpenetration film may be taken to reveal anatomy obscured by dense Pantopaque.

262

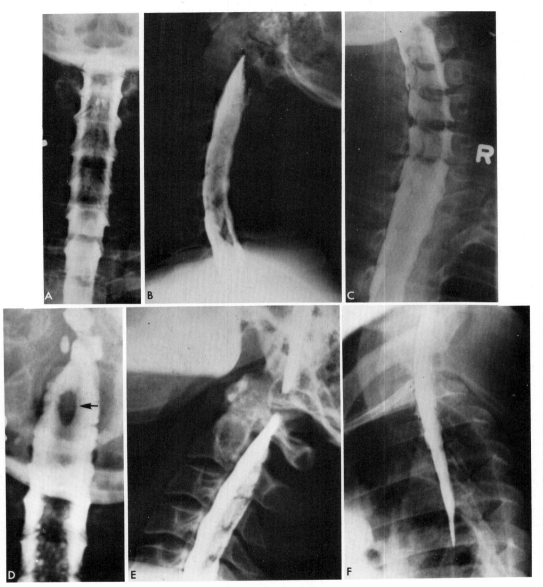

FIGURE 8–30 Cervical myelogram. *A*. Normal posteroanterior projection of cervical myelogram. *B*. Lateral cervical myelogram. *C*. Oblique projection. *D*. Upper cervical area. Note defect of odontoid peg (*arrow*). *E*. Lateral view showing the normal "skip area" around the odontoid peg and ligaments with some contrast medium on the clivus. *F*. Swimmer's position. A useful view for the cervicothoracic junction when obesity or the shoulder shadows might obscure the anatomy of this region.

exposure technique may be helpful in the lateral projection (Fig. 8–30).

When a vascular lesion of the cord is suspected the patient must be examined in the supine position, since these lesions are predominantly on the back of the cord.[6] For lesions around the foramen magnum the patient must be examined in both the prone and the supine positions.

Whenever possible an attempt should be made to remove the contrast medium. This is best achieved under fluoroscopic control, particularly when only a milliliter or two remains and may be pooled under the tip of the needle. The siphonage technique facilitates removal.[8] When a complete block is present, it is the usual practice not to attempt to remove the contrast medium. In the thoracic region a reference point on the skin is helpful to the surgeon to show the level of the block.

Cisternography

The value of positive contrast cisternography resides in its applicability to the investigation of angle tumors. Tiny acoustic neuromas may defy recognition in air studies even with careful laminagraphy.

Two milliliters of Pantopaque is introduced into the subarachnoid space and is manipulated into the internal auditory meatus, preferably under screen control (Fig. 8–31).[2] Both canals should be ex-

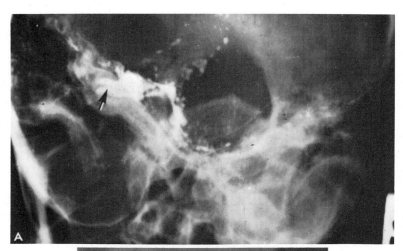

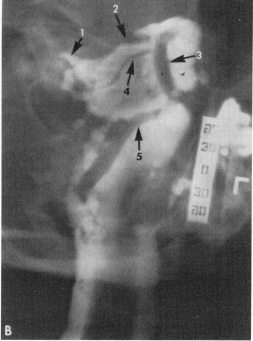

FIGURE 8–31 Normal cisternal myelography. *A.* Study with 2 ml of Pantopaque demonstrating contrast in internal auditory meatus. Note defect formed by crista (*arrow*). *B.* Large volume cisternogram. Note the structures visualized: 1, internal auditory canal; 2, fifth cranial nerve; 3, basilar artery; 4, anterior inferior cerebellar artery; 5, vertebral artery.

amined. Occasionally the canal will not fill because of normally large nerves or because the subarachnoid space does not extend into the canal. To visualize the entire cerebellopontine angle a larger amount of Pantopaque is necessary. Angle lesions, however, will be recognized with air studies (Fig. 8–31).[1, 25]

Air Myelography

Air myelography entails replacing the spinal subarachnoid fluid with air. The technique as first described by Lindgren involves puncturing the cisterna magna with the patient in the lateral decubitus position with the table tilted head down 30 to 40 degrees.[18] The cerebrospinal fluid is replaced by air and the space is distended by the introduction of air to a pressure of 200 mm of water. Tomographic cuts are then undertaken to include the whole length of the cord. Other modifications for the cervical region include using a lumbar puncture rather than a cervical puncture and trapping air in the cervical subarachnoid space.[14]

Myelographic Appearance of Specific Lesions

The width of the shadow of the cord is an important indicator of spinal cord disease.[5] Because of magnification factors the proportionate size relative to the width of the subarachnoid space is much better for the evaluation of cord abnormalities than the absolute measurements. Space-taking lesions may be epidural, subdural, subarachnoid, or intramedullary. Each has a characteristic appearance in the myelogram (Figs. 8–32 to 8–49). Occasionally the lesion may be in more than one compartment (Fig. 8–33).

Text continued on page 283.

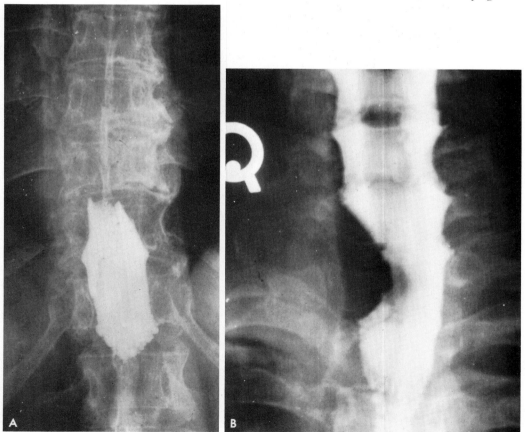

FIGURE 8–32 Tumors. *A.* Epidural metastases showing the column of contrast displaced medially with tapering of the column of contrast showing the "bundle of faggots" appearance and displacement of the cord. *B.* Metastatic deposit. An epidural lesion showing medial displacement of the Pantopaque column.

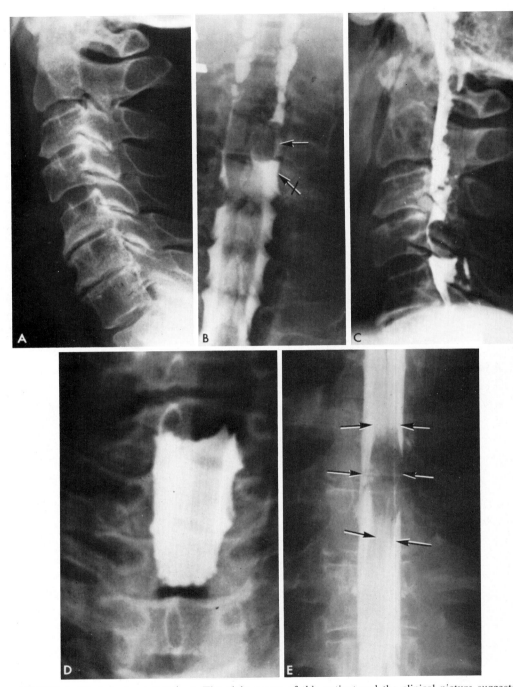

FIGURE 8–33　Intradural tumor. *A.* The plain x-rays of this patient and the clinical picture suggested the diagnosis of osteoarthritis. *B.* The myelogram reveals the classic appearance of an intradural extramedullary lesion with displacement of the cord and widening of the subarachnoid space (*arrow with crossed shaft*) at the level of the lesion (*arrow*), which is capped by contrast medium. There was a partial block permitting contrast medium to pass beyond this point, and an effort was made to cap the upper extent of the tumor. *C.* Lateral projection demonstrating the capped lesion. *D.* Unusual case of an intradural metastatic deposit with capping, displaced cord, and widened subarachnoid space. Metastatic disease may simulate a benign lesion myelographically when it is located in the intradural compartment. *E.* Thoracic disc in which widening of the cord shadow in the antero-posterior projection simulates an intramedullary lesion.

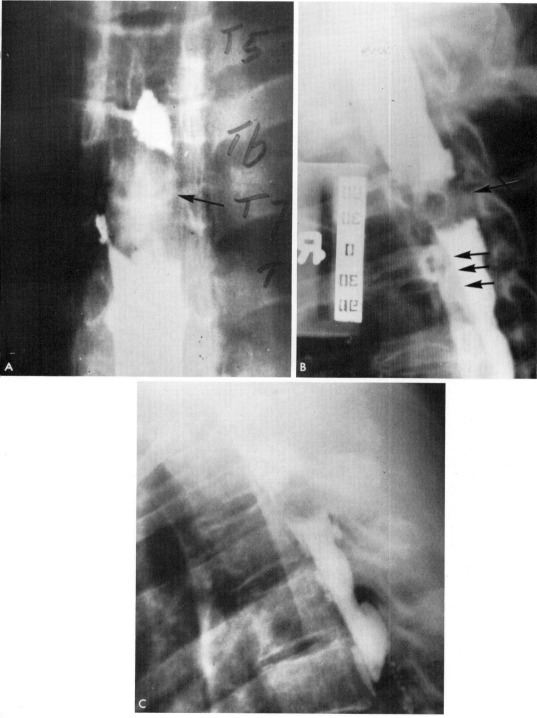

FIGURE 8–34 *A.* Spinal thoracic meningioma in a woman. Film shows calcification of tumor (*arrow*) and capping with Pantopaque. *B* and *C.* Thoracic meningioma in a woman showing characteristic displacement of the cord (*arrows*) with widening of the subarachnoid space and capping of the lesion (*arrow with crossed shaft*).

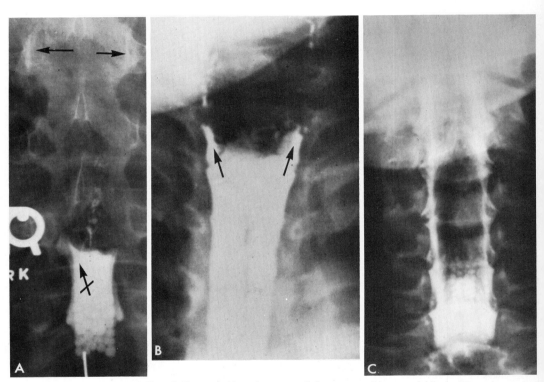

FIGURE 8–35 Intramedullary lesions. *A*. Ependymoma of the conus with a total block. There is marked thinning of the pedicles (*arrows*) above the level of the Pantopaque block, evidence of the extent of the tumor. Margins of the contrast medium are displaced outward (*arrow with crossed shaft*). *B*. Glioma of cervical cord with almost total block but showing the extreme narrowing of the Pantopaque column with its margins displaced laterally (*arrows*). *C*. Spinal cord hematoma from a diving accident. Note wide shadow of cord.

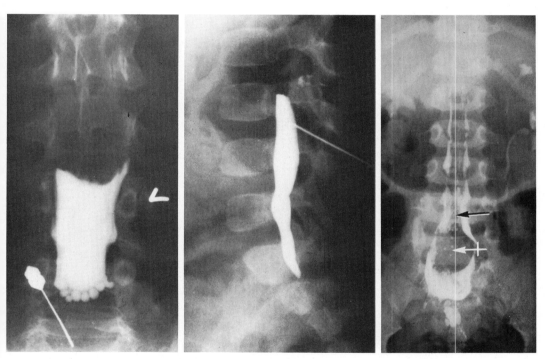

FIGURE 8–36 *A*. Epidermoid. Multiple lumbar punctures were performed in the past. The Pantopaque reveals a large round tumor lying within the dura. *B*. Spinal lipoma with tethering of cord. Patient was erect and the lesion was not demonstrated. *C*. Same case as *B* with patient supine following removal of needle. The lipoma (*arrow with crossed shaft*) was now visualized. Note the low tethered cord.

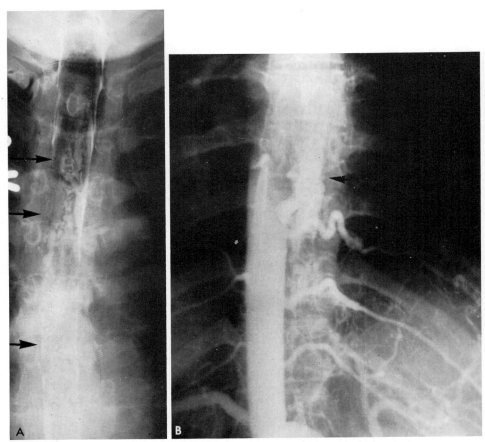

FIGURE 8–37 Spinal angioma. *A.* Supine myelogram demonstrating a widened cord and serpiginous shadows representing tortuous large spinal vessels (*arrows*). *B.* An aortogram showing the large spinal angioma (*arrow*).

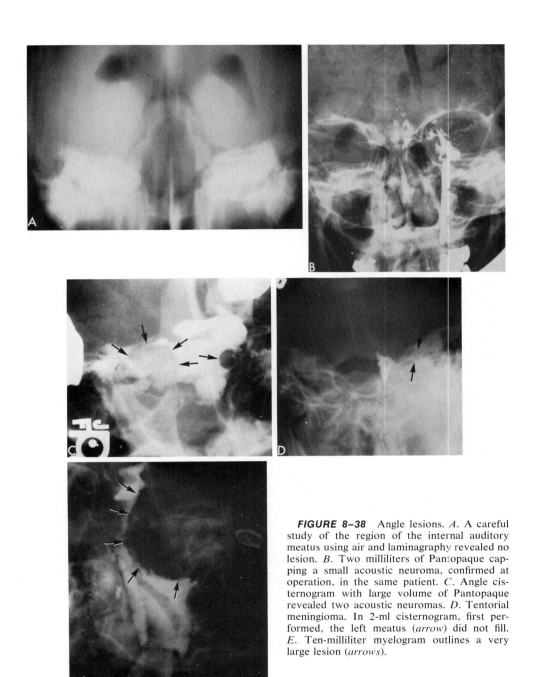

FIGURE 8–38 Angle lesions. *A.* A careful study of the region of the internal auditory meatus using air and laminagraphy revealed no lesion. *B.* Two milliliters of Pantopaque capping a small acoustic neuroma, confirmed at operation, in the same patient. *C.* Angle cisternogram with large volume of Pantopaque revealed two acoustic neuromas. *D.* Tentorial meningioma. In 2-ml cisternogram, first performed, the left meatus (*arrow*) did not fill. *E.* Ten-milliliter myelogram outlines a very large lesion (*arrows*).

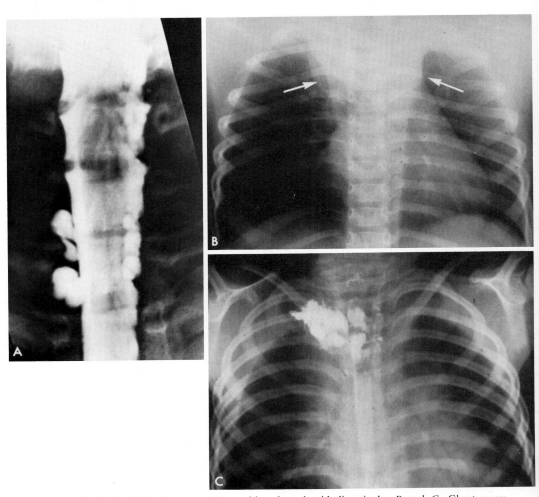

FIGURE 8–39 *A*. Brachial plexus avulsion with subarachnoid diverticula. *B* and *C*. Chest x-ray showing an abnormal density (*arrows*) in the upper mediastinum in a child who suffered severe trauma. The myelogram shows Pantopaque outside the subarachnoid space and loculated within the mediastinum.

Illustration continued on opposite page.

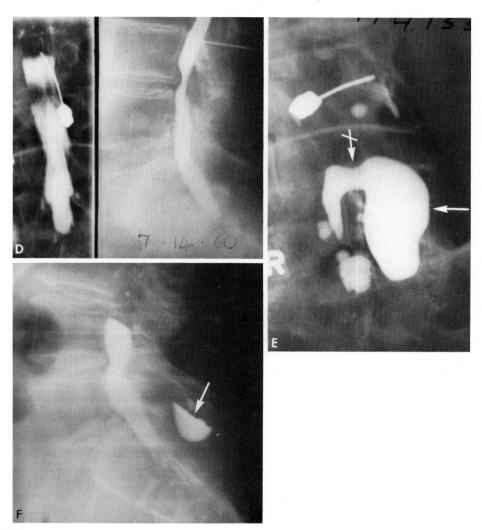

FIGURE 8-39 *(Continued)* *D.* Myelogram showing disc protrusion. A laminectomy showed a large protruded disc, which was removed. *E* and *F.* Myelogram made three years later showing large extradural cyst *(arrow)* communicating with the lumbar subarachnoid space *(crossed-shaft arrow)*. Confirmed at operation.

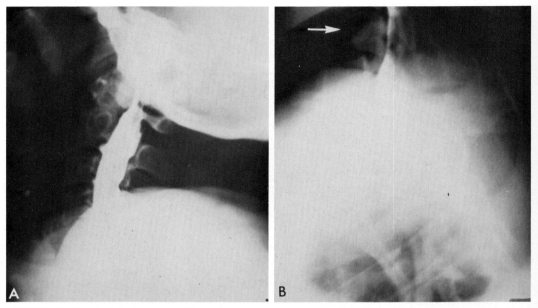

FIGURE 8–40   *A*. Spinal trauma with cord compression was missed on first myelogram because no attempt was made to visualize the lower cervical region. *B*. A repeat myelogram with the double exposure technique revealed a compression fracture of a lower cervical body compressing the cord.

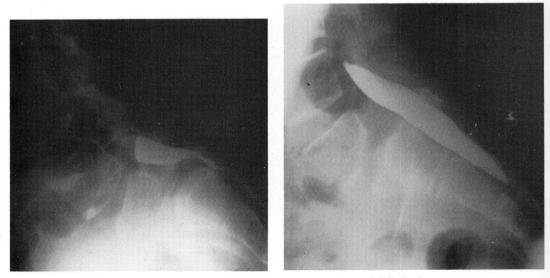

FIGURE 8–41   Myelographic appearance of spondylolisthesis.

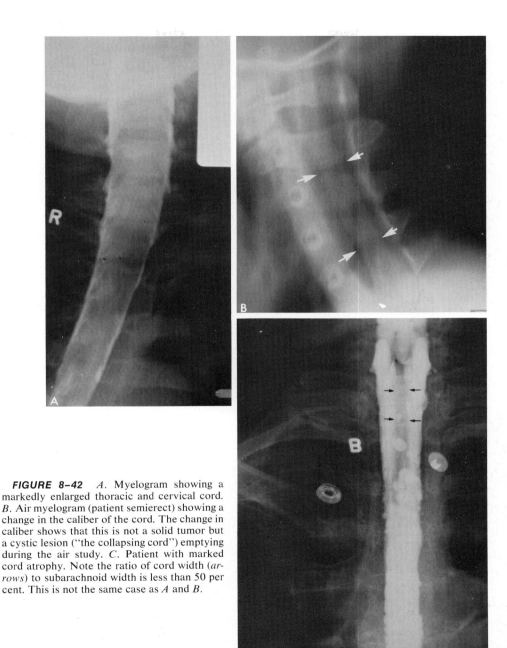

FIGURE 8–42 *A.* Myelogram showing a markedly enlarged thoracic and cervical cord. *B.* Air myelogram (patient semierect) showing a change in the caliber of the cord. The change in caliber shows that this is not a solid tumor but a cystic lesion ("the collapsing cord") emptying during the air study. *C.* Patient with marked cord atrophy. Note the ratio of cord width (*arrows*) to subarachnoid width is less than 50 per cent. This is not the same case as *A* and *B*.

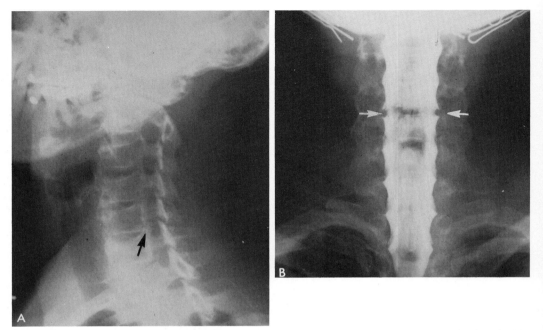

FIGURE 8–43 *A.* Forty-year-old woman referred with a diagnosis of amyotrophic lateral sclerosis. Note uncovertebral osteophytes in this oblique projection at the C5–C6 level. *B.* Myelogram. Note the presence of a bar defect and nerve root amputations at the same level. Patient markedly improved following operation.

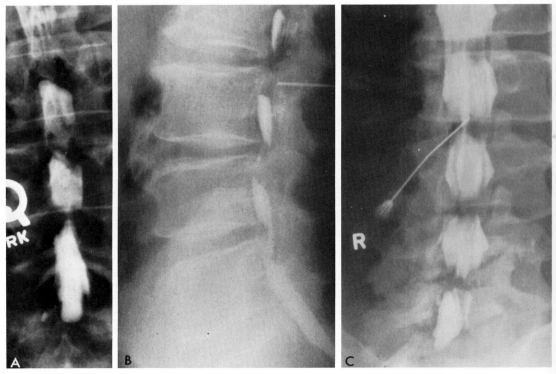

FIGURE 8–44 Lumbar spondylosis. Washboard appearance in the lumbar region is due to lumbar spondylosis. Although this is considered a classic picture, multiple discs may resemble this closely. The flow may be slow during myelography since the Pantopaque has to negotiate each hump opposite the disc spaces.

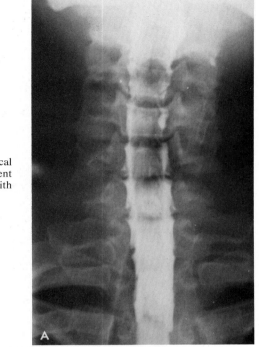

FIGURE 8–45 Cervical spondylosis. *A*. Cervical spondylosis with multiple bar defects and encroachment on nerve root sleeves. *B* and *C*. Severe spondylosis with cord compression.

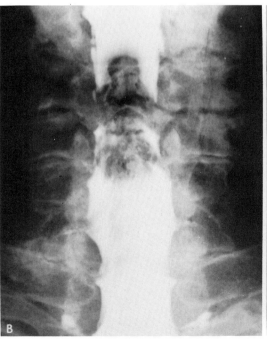

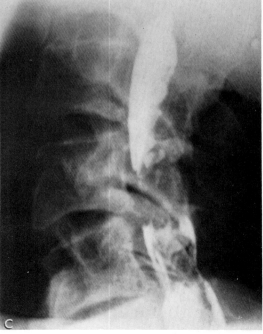

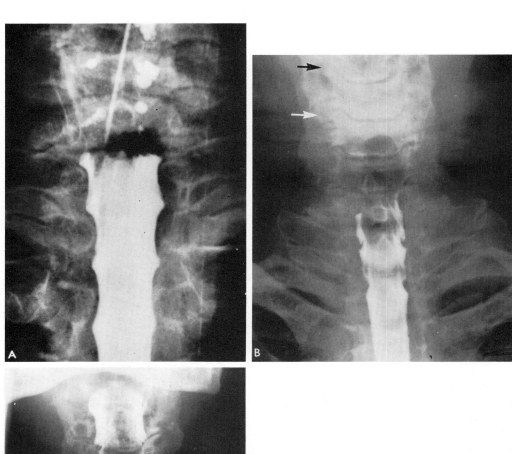

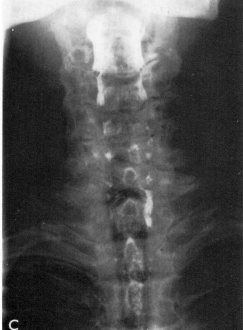

FIGURE 8-46 *A.* Myelogram from below showing complete block at C7–T1 due to severe spondylosis with disc herniation. An exploratory operation at this level produced no improvement. A re-exploration revealed a disc herniation two spaces higher. *B* and *C.* A patient with extensive cervical spondylosis showed a block at C6–C7 when Pantopaque was introduced from the lumbar region, *B.* Only after introduction of Pantopaque from above was another block outlined at C3–C4. Note the uncovertebral "joints" (*arrows*), associated with the degeneration of the disc and collapse of the disc space.

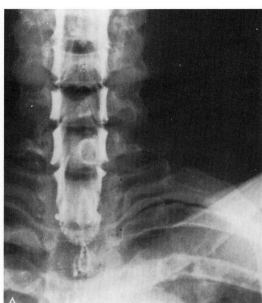

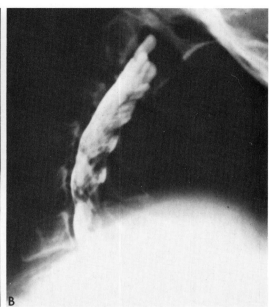

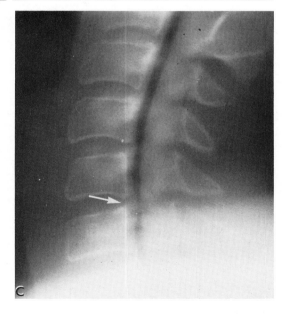

FIGURE 8–47 The value of air myelography. Patient was referred for myelography because of an anterior spinal artery syndrome. *A* and *B*. Pantopaque myelography demonstrates changes at C5–C6 that were not considered significant enough to explain her clinical picture. *C*. Air myelogram via a C1–C2 lateral cervical puncture clearly demonstrates a ridge impinging on the anterior margin of the cord (*arrow*).

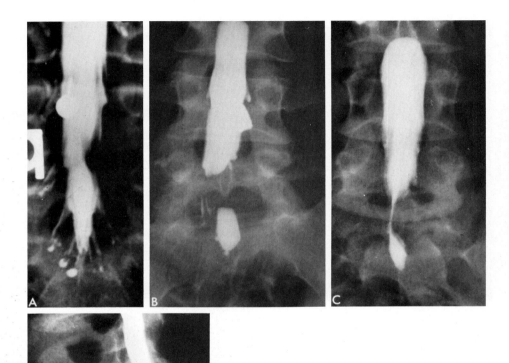

FIGURE 8–48 *A.* Lumbar myelogram showing amputation of a nerve root sleeve and a lateral defect in the column of contrast. A few sacral diverticula are seen. *B.* Lumbar myelogram showing L5–S1 disc with almost total block. *C* and *D.* Disc extrusion at L5–S1 with posterior migration and presenting with a posterior defect (*arrow*).

Illustration continued on opposite page.

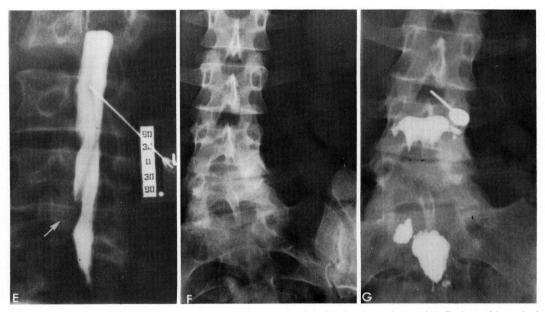

FIGURE 8–48 *(Continued)*   *E.* Oblique view demonstrating L4–L5 disc *(arrow)*. *F* and *G*. Patient with marked L4–L5 disc space narrowing and vertebral body sclerosis. Myelography demonstrates almost complete block secondary to large herniated disc.

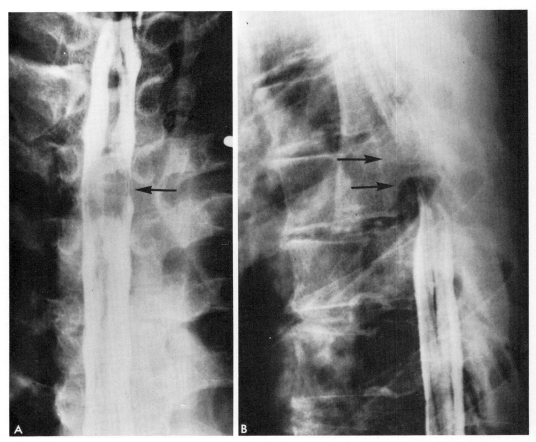

FIGURE 8–49 *A*. Thoracic disc widening the cord (*arrow*) simulating an intramedullary lesion in the anterior projection. *B*. The lateral projection shows posterior displacement of the cord and Pantopaque opposite a disc space.

Spondylosis usually occurs in the cervical and lumbar regions.[29] The familiar myelographic appearance is the "stepladder" appearance caused by multiple bulgings of the disc space (Fig. 8–41 and 8–44). The lateral projection will show this to best advantage. Occasionally spondylosis may occur at one level with a single defect.

Recognition of herniated disc material depends upon certain changes in the Pantopaque column. These appearances vary with the level of the pathological changes. Thus in the low lumbar region, there may be amputation of nerve roots. At higher levels, there may be amputation of a nerve root with encroachment on the major column of contrast suggesting root involvement and cord involvement (Fig. 8–48). In the cervical region, compression of the column of contrast in the anteroposterior diameter may widen the cord shadow and suggest an intramedullary lesion. The lateral projection will reveal the extradural nature of the compressive lesion. It should be mentioned that a large disc fragment may be extruded without deforming the myelographic picture and also that deformities may be present in the Pantopaque column in the absence of symptoms.

REFERENCES

1. Baker, H. L.: Myelographic examination of the posterior fossa with positive contrast medium. Radiology, *81*:791–801, 1963.
2. Britton, B. H., Hitselberger, W. E., and Hurley, B. J.: Iophendylate examination of posterior fossa in diagnosis of cerebellopontine angle tumors. Arch. Otolaryng., *88*:608–617, 1968.
3. Bull, J. W. D.: Spinal meningiomas and neurofibromas. Acta Radiol., *40*:283, 1953.
4. Conway, L. W.: Hydrodynamic studies in syringomyelia. J. Neurosurg., *27*:501–514, 1967.
5. Di Chiro, G., and Fisher, R. L.: Contrast radiography of the spinal cord. Arch. Neurol., *11*:125–143, 1964.
6. Djindjian, R.: Angiography of the Spinal Cord. Baltimore, Md., University Park Press, 1970.
7. Elsberg, C. A., and Dyke, C. G.: The diagnosis and localization of tumors of the spinal cord by means of measurements made on the x-ray films of the vertebra and the correlation of clinical and x-ray findings. Bull. Neurol. Inst., New York. *3*:359, 1934.
8. Epstein, B. S.: The Spine, 3rd Ed. Philadelphia, Lea and Febiger, 1969.
9. Febbroriello, M.: Double exposure of the lateral cervical spine. Presented at the Connecticut Society of X-ray Technologists, 1963.
10. Hadley, L. A.: Anatomico-Roentgenographic Studies of the Spine. Springfield, Ill., Charles C Thomas, 1964.
11. Heinz, E. R., Brinker, R. A., and Taveras, J. M.: Advantages of a less dense Pantopaque contrast material for myelography. Acta Radiol. (Diagn.), *5*:1024–1031, 1966.
12. Hinck, V. C., Clark, W. M., Hopkins, C. E.: Normal interpediculate distances (minimum and maximum) in children and adults. Amer. J. Roentgen., *97*:141–153, 1966.
13. Hinck, V. C., Hopkins, C. E., Savara, B. S.: Sagittal diameter of the cervical spinal canal in children. Radiology, *79*:97–108, 1962.
14. Jirout, J.: Pneumographic investigation of the cervical spine. Acta Radiol., *50*:221–225, 1958.
15. Jirout, J.: Pneumomyelography. Springfield, Ill., Charles C Thomas, 1969.
16. Kieffer, S. A., Peterson, H. O., Gold, L. H. A., and Binet, E. F.: Evaluation of dilute Pantopaque for large-volume myelography. Radiology, *96*:69–74, July 1970.
17. Koehler, A.: Borderlines of the Normal and Early Pathologic in Skeletal Roentgenology, 10th Ed. New York, Grune & Stratton, 1956.
18. Lindgren, E.: Radiologic examination of brain and spinal cord. Acta Radiol., Stockholm, suppl. 151, 1957.
19. Maupin, R. A., Baker, H. L., and Kerr, F. W. L.: Emulsified Pantopaque: Its possible application for myelography. Radiology, *86*:509–514, 1966.
20. McRae, D. L.: The significance of abnormalities of the cervical spine; Caldwell lecture, 1959. Amer. J. Roentgen., *84*:3–25, 1960.
21. Penning, L.: Functional Pathology of the Cervical Spine. Baltimore, Md., Williams & Wilkins Co., 1968.
22. Praestholm, J., and Lester, J.: Water-soluble contrast lumbar myelography with meglumine iothalamate (Conray). Brit. J. Radiol., *43*:303–308, 1970.
23. Rosomoff, H. L., Carroll, F., Brown, J., and Sheptak, P.: Percutaneous radiofrequency cervical cordotomy: Technique. J. Neurosurg., *23*:639–644, 1965.
24. Ruge, D.: Spinal Cord Injuries. Springfield, Ill., Charles C Thomas, 1969.
25. Scanlan, R. L.: Positive contrast medium (iophendylate) in diagnosis of acoustic neuroma. Arch. Otolaryng., *80*:698–706, 1964.
26. Schmorl, G., and Junghanns, H.: The Human Spine in Health and Disease. New York & London, Grune & Stratton, 1959.
27. Shahinfar, A. H., and Schechter, M. M.: Traumatic extradural cysts of the spine. Amer. J. Roentgen., *98*:713–719, 1966.
28. Shapiro, R.: Myelography. 2nd Ed. Chicago, Year Book Medical Publishers, 1968.
29. Smith, B. H.: Cervical Spondylosis and Its Neurological Complications. Springfield, Ill., Charles C Thomas, 1968.
30. Vines, F. S.: The significance of "occult" fractures of the cervical spine. Amer. J. Roentgen., *107*:493–504, 1969.

31. Westberg, G.: Gas myelography and percutaneous puncture in the diagnosis of spinal cord cysts. Acta Radiol. (Diagn.) (Stockholm), suppl. *252*:1–67, 1966.

32. Whalen, J. P., and Woodruff, C. L.: The cervical prevertebral fat stripe. Amer. J. Roentgen., *109*:445–451, July 1970.

33. Wolf, B. S., Khilnani, M., and Malis, L.: The sagittal diameter of the bony cervical spinal canal and its significance in cervical spondylosis. J. Mount Sinai Hosp., N.Y., *23*:283–292, 1956.

34. Wortzman, G., and Dewar, F. P.: Rotary fixation of the atlantoaxial joint: Rotational atlantoaxial subluxation. Radiology, *90*:479–487, 1968.

35. Zilkha, A., Reiss, J., Shulman, K., and Schechter, M. M.: Traumatic subarachnoid mediastinal fistula. J. Neurosurg., *32*:473, 1970.

9

RADIONUCLIDE IMAGING STUDIES

With the advent of radiopharmaceuticals and radiation-detecting instrumentation another modality has been added for the diagnosis of disease. Intracranial tumor detection was among the first outstanding products of this development. Brain scanning has become a prominent and reliable contributor to the present-day practice of neurosurgery.

The increasing sophistication of nuclear medicine has carried with it a growing terminology applied to the instrumentation, tracers, and procedures used. This has created an expanding vocabulary. In the interest of brevity and common understanding, the term "brain scan" is used throughout this chapter. This applies to the images obtained with a rectilinear moving detector, as well as to the cerebral images produced by stationary imaging devices.

HISTORICAL BACKGROUND

Several early radioactive tracer studies were developed around stable element dye compounds used for various clinical laboratory tests. An example is diiodofluorescein labeled with iodine-131, reported by Moore in 1948 as a radionuclide tracer for brain tumor localization.[72] This development followed the observation that sodium fluorescein when administered intravenously exhibited a consistent affinity for brain tumors.[71] Erickson et al. and Selverstone et al. in the same year reported studies of brain tumor tissue concentration of phosphorus-32.[39, 94] Chou et al., in 1951, reported iodine-131-labeled human serum albumin as a suitable agent for tumor localization.[23]

Historically there have been parallel areas of investigation contributing to the present state of brain imaging with radionuclides. These areas are instrumentation and radiopharmaceutical development. The technique for detection and localization involved point counting with a Geiger-Müller tube positioned at symmetrically located points over the calvarium. Later scintillation detectors with their greater sensitivity for gamma emissions were introduced. When these scintillation detectors were coupled to rectilinear scanning mechanisms, by Cassen et al., the brain scan as a cartographic display came into being.[20] Much of the success of this mechanized scanning technique is owed to the use of the heavy shielding, collimators, and spectrometers reported by Allen and Risser, Francis et al., and Shy et al.[2, 43, 95] Concurrently positron emitters, such as arsenic-74 and copper-64, with coincidence counting techniques were used to advantage.[16, 118]

Subsequent instrumental developments in 1955, 1956, and 1959 were photorecording modifications for scan data presentation on film.[12, 52, 56] Three other notable imaging devices for radioactivity distribution recording were developed in this period. These were the scintillation camera invented by Anger in 1957, the autofluoroscope invented by Bender and Blau in 1960, and the Ter-Pogossian camera developed in 1963.[5, 6, 13, 105]

A continuing search for radionuclide

J. K. GOODRICH

R. H. WILKINSON, Jr.

tracers with greater tumor affinity led to the development of mercury-203-labeled chlormerodrin by Blau and Bender in 1963.[14] The low-energy, shorter half-life radiopharmaceutical, mercury-197-labeled chlormerodrin, introduced clinically by Sodee in 1963, served as a widely used brain scanning agent until the development of technetium-99m sodium pertechnetate by Harper et al. in 1964.[48, 96] More recently, indium-113m (a daughter product of tin-113) when chelated to form indium-113 diethylenetriamine pentaacetic acid (DTPA) was reported by Stern et al. as a suitable brain scanning agent.[98] Technetium-99m pertechnetate remains the most widely used radionuclide tracer for brain scanning.

INDICATIONS FOR BRAIN SCAN

The brain scan as a diagnostic screening procedure should be considered when a careful neurological history and physical examination lead the clinician to suspect intracranial disease. As a screening effort, the scan has proved useful in patients with primary or metastatic neoplasms, cerebral vascular accidents, inflammatory lesions, and head trauma.

As a more definitive study, the brain scan often serves to detail the size and location of various intracranial lesions. This is a particularly useful aid in selecting the optimal neuroradiographic procedures to follow. In some instances, e.g., multiple

TABLE 9–1   INDICATIONS FOR BRAIN SCANNING

Brain tumor
Primary neoplasm
Metastatic foci
Cerebrovascular disease
Arteriovenous malformations
Intracranial hemorrhage
Cerebral ischemia
Cerebral infarction
Hematoma: subdural, epidural, or intracerebral
Venous sinus thrombosis
Cerebral contusion
Inflammatory cerebral disease
Meningitis
Cerebritis
Abscess
Other benign (intracranial) disorders
Hydrocephalus
Porencephaly
Cysts

metastatic lesions, the scan has obviated the need for further diagnostic studies. Furthermore, the scan may assist in determining the feasibility of surgical intervention. The brain scan provides the radiation therapist with a means for selecting the size and position of his external beam treatment portals. As a follow-up examination, the brain scan serves as an innocuous study suited to outpatient care. Here it is especially useful in determining recurrence of brain tumors, resolution of intracranial abscesses, and appearance of new foci of metastatic disease.

Table 9–1 lists some of the specific entities most commonly encountered.

RADIOPHARMACEUTICAL TRACERS

The first radionuclide tracer, ^{131}I diiodofluorescein, was introduced for brain tumor localization in 1948.[72] Since this initial work, a multitude of various radiopharmaceuticals have been applied to brain scanning. The agents that have been effective enough to warrant wide use are iodine-131-labeled human serum albumin, chlormerodrin labeled with mercury-203 or mercury-197, and technetium-99m pertechnetate.

Iodine-131 human serum albumin has been shown in many reports to have a significantly prolonged biological retention within tumors as compared to normal cerebral tissue. In order to obtain a favorable tumor to non-tumor activity ratio, a delay of at least 24 hours was required prior to scanning.[95] This proved to be a clinical disadvantage that was compounded by the long study periods necessitated by the small allowable tracer dose.

Mercury-203 chlormerodrin, while displaying a favorable tissue concentration ratio in the tumor and non-tumor, carried a renal cortical irradiation dose that was reported as high as 75 rads per millicurie. Its counterpart, mercury-197 chlormerodrin, delivered a considerably lower renal irradiation dose of approximately 5 rads per millicurie. This tracer had a weaker gamma emission, which somewhat reduced the definition of lesions by its scatter within the calvarium. Mercury-203 chlormerodrin has been restricted by the Atomic Energy

Commission to the investigation of suspected deep-seated intracranial lesions.

Technetium-99m pertechnetate is the most practical single cerebral imaging tracer in use today. Those features that have led to its popularity are: (1) Its simple elution from the sterile molybdenum-99/technetium-99m generator; (2) its short half-life, which permits administration of a larger dose and hence a greater photon density in imaging; (3) the brief pre-imaging delay following tracer administration; (4) its relatively low patient exposure dosage; and (5) its ready incorporation into various compounds whose characteristics permit the imaging of other organs.

Investigators using technetium-99m-labeled human serum albumin have combined the favorable biological properties of iodine-131 human serum albumin with the markedly superior photon density of the short half-life tracer, technetium-99m pertechnetate. The necessity for on-the-scene chemical preparation of technetium-99m human serum albumin has, however, interfered with its widespread use.

Several investigators, including Di Chiro et al., have reported that some brain lesions that were not demonstrated by technetium-99m pertechnetate were identified when other tracers were employed.[33]

Attempts at more definitive brain lesion diagnosis have employed multiple tracers administered in tandem. From a practical standpoint, use of multiple tracers can add only a small improvement in the overall accuracy of disease detection when compared with technetium-99m pertechnetate used alone. Repeat brain scans using an alternate tracer may provide desirable information in circumstances in which neuroradiographic procedures are limited or delayed. Currently, interest has been directed toward an imaging delay of one to four hours following the injection of technetium-99m pertechnetate. Gates, et al. report an increase in positive results as well as better definition of initially equivocal lesions.[43a]

Recently, the short-lived tracer, indium-113m, when chelated with diethylenetriamine pentaacetic acid (DTPA) has been shown to be effective as a brain scan agent.[98] Its significant attribute by comparison with technetium-99m pertechnetate is its failure to concentrate in choroid plexus and salivary glands. Although millicurie doses equal to those of technetium-99m provide high photon yields for scanning, the nearly threefold greater gamma energy necessitates scan detector collimation that reduces detector efficiency for collimator assemblies of equal resolution. As in the case of technetium-99m human serum albumin, the indium-113m DTPA must be formulated in the licensee's laboratory. The present Atomic Energy Commission regulations limit the use of this radionuclide tracer to broadly licensed institutions.

Some preliminary work has been reported by a small number of investigators, using intra-arterially injected iodine-131-labeled macroaggregated human serum albumin for the detection of intracerebral lesions.[54, 55, 74, 90] These investigators cite the tracer's advantages as being better posterior fossa disease detection and more rapid imaging capability. The reported and potential complications as well as the necessity for arterial puncture appear to outweigh these advantages.[55]

Table 9–2 reviews the salient features of the more frequently employed radionuclide tracers for brain scanning.

The question of how the commonly employed radiopharmaceuticals accumulate in or about neoplastic lesions has not been fully resolved. The generally accepted explanation for the appearance of radioactive tracers within the majority of cerebral lesions has been ascribed to a breakdown in the "blood-brain barrier." A precise and basic understanding of the "blood-brain barrier" remains to be elucidated. Bakay has reviewed the complex and oftentimes conflicting opinions and data relevant to this subject.[7, 8] He classified the evidence into the following categories: (1) blood content of tumor tissue, (2) permeability of central nervous system membrane by passive diffusion or active carrier transport or both, (3) pinocytosis, (4) neoplastic blood vessel structure, (5) extracellular space, (6) peritumoral or tumoral edema or both, and (7) cellular metabolism. It would appear that more than one of these factors are involved in the accumulation and retention of tracer. Furthermore, the factors involved may vary with the tracer employed.

TABLE 9–2 *RADIOPHARMACEUTICALS FOR BRAIN SCANNING AND CISTERNOGRAPHY*

Radiopharma-ceuticals	Physical Half-Life	Principal Gamma Energy (kev)	Route of Adminis-tration	Dosage	Premedication	Interval Until Examination Time	Length of Examination	Total Body Dose (Rads)	Target Organ and Dose (Rads)
BRAIN SCANNING									
131I human serum albumin	8.05 d	364	IV	375 μc	Lugol's solution	24 hr	3–4 hr	0.7	blood 2.5
203Hg Chlor-merodrin	45.7 d	280	IV	10 μc/kg 750 μc/ max.	Mercuhydrin 1 ml IM	1–3 hr	3–4 hr	0.46	kidney* 75
197Hg Chlor-merodrin	67 hr	72 (mean)	IV	14μc/kg max. 1 mc	Mercuhydrin 1 ml IM	1–3 hr	3–4 hr	0.1	kidney* 5
99mTc per-technetate	6.13 hr	140	IV	7.5 mc to 15 mc	Lugol's solu-tion or per-chlorate or nothing	15 min–4 hr	1½ hr	0.12	large bowel 2
113mIn DTPA	1.7 hr	393	IV	10 to 15 mc	None	None	1½ hr	0.09	bladder 6
99mTc human serum albumin	6.13 hr	140	IV	10 mc	None	30 min–24 hr	1½ hr	0.17	blood 0.47
CISTERNOGRAPHY									
131I human serum al-bumin (high specific activity)	8.05 d	364	Cisterna magna or Lumbar in-trathecal	100 μc (no more than 2 mg of albumin)	Lugol's solu-tion	Serial views after 1–2 hr	Once daily for 3–4 d	0.1	CNS 1.0
99mTc human serum albu-min	6.13 hr	140		2 mc (no more than 2 mg of albumin)	None	Serial views after 1–2 hr	6 hr to 1 d	—	CNS 0.26

*Without stable mercury premedication.

At present, there is no tracer that will localize within a tumor to a greater degree than it will in certain organs elsewhere in the body. Thus the relative paucity of activity in normal brain tissue makes the "increased" level of tracer activity within the neoplasm a "positive" area. Tator has pointed out that the phrase "absence of blood-brain barrier" should replace the phrase "breakdown in the blood-brain barrier" in the case of meningiomas and acoustic neuromas because these are areas in tissue that do not have a blood-brain barrier.[8] For a more detailed discussion and references on this subject, the reader is referred to Bakay.[7, 8]

INSTRUMENTATION

The instrumentation for radionuclide portrayal of intracranial disease may be classified as moving detector and stationary detector imaging devices. Moving detectors include 3-inch or 5-inch diameter scintillation crystal probes mechanically and electronically linked to recording devices. These produce images of the tracer distribution in the field under study. The recording may be placed on photographic (x-ray) film, paper, or oscilloscope or computer-type tape. Any combination of these records may be produced. Pictorial records may range from black and white, shades of gray to black, or even multiple color renditions arranged according to activity levels perceived by the detector. Dual moving detector "scanners" have become commercially available and permit simultaneous recording of opposing scan views.

The stationary scintillation detector assembly, while having a limited field of view, portrays activity distribution patterns from any particular area of the body. The image is displayed on oscilloscope or television monitors, which may be photographed for permanent record. Computer or video tape recording may also be used. The capability of this scintillation camera to record from all its fields of view at once provides imaging of rapidly changing sequential events. This has an application to rapid serial image recording of the passage of a radioactive tracer bolus into the cerebral circulation, which results in a gross low-resolution "angiogram."

With the advent of sophisticated data retrieval instruments, kinetic recordings may be quantitated for region-to-region comparison.

SCANNING TECHNIQUE

The variety of commercial instruments for brain scanning prevents a detailed discussion of scanning technique. However, certain basic tenets should be observed. These are as follows: (1) careful daily calibration of the instrument, (2) proper detector collimator selection according to tracer and desired image detail, (3) premedication as indicated for sedation or when certain tracers are employed (see Table 9–2), (4) attention to proper patient positioning and comfortable immobilization, and (5) the use of a standardized photorecording technique that depicts as much information as is available from the count rates that are present.

NORMAL BRAIN SCAN

The normal appearance of the technetium-99m pertechnetate brain scan is portrayed in Figure 9–1. Rectilinear scans as well as images recorded by stationary detectors may be considered to present the cranial vault delineated in the sagittal and coronal planes. Detailed descriptions of normal anatomy may be found in several articles and texts.[79, 108, 110]

Brain scanning using the tracer technetium-99m pertechnetate produces an image of tracer concentration within the choroid plexus in a significant number of cases. This choroidal concentration can be blocked effectively by oral premedication with 200 to 500 mg of sodium or potassium perchlorate.[53, 114, 116] Choroid plexus blockade with Lugol's solution may be used, but is reported to be less effective.[116]

Figure 9–1 illustrates a scan obtained after the patient received sodium perchlorate premedication. Frequent normal scan variations are: unilateral dominance of the transverse sinus on posterior and lateral views; peripheral frontal tracer concentrations adjacent to the superior sagittal sinus, which are attributable to prominent irregular venous drainage pathways; and

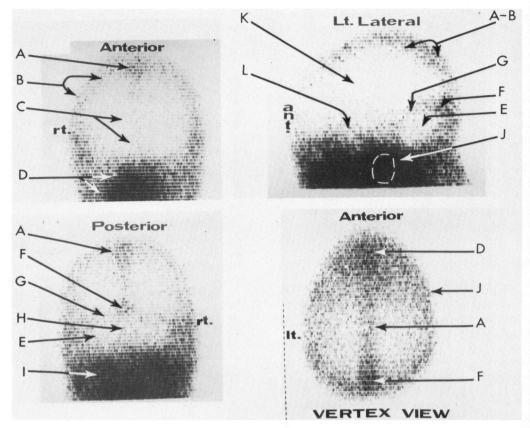

FIGURE 9–1   Normal ^{99m}Tc pertechnetate brain scan anatomy. Superior sagittal sinus (A), scalp, diploë, and meningeal vascularity (B), midline vasculature (C), oronasopharynx (D), posterior fossa (E), torcular Herophili (F), transverse sinus (G), straight sinus (H), nuchal vascularity (I), parotid gland (J), hemisphere (K) and sella turcica (L).

vascular activity at the periphery of the cranium, which overlies the sellar region on the lateral view.

Technetium-99m pertechnetate ion contained in saliva, gastric contents, and tears may, on occasion, produce a false focus of activity by surface contamination.

APPEARANCE OF DISEASE

The brain diseased by tumor or vascular insult may be expected to evidence the abnormality by retention of radioactive tracer. This results in a relatively higher concentration of radioactivity in diseased tissue than in surrounding normal brain. The scan recording technique is designed to display this activity differential. There are, however, uncommon lesions that may be detected by the converse. Cysts, for example, having little or no vascularity to allow tracer entry may present as areas of reduced tracer concentration by comparison with activity in a contralateral hemispheric region.[69]

Typically, Grade III and Grade IV astrocytomas and meningiomas are seen as dense tracer concentrations. The detectable concentration of tracer activity appears to vary with the tumor type or the duration of the cerebrovascular accident. Metastatic lesions are distinctive when multiple, but the tracer levels in the individual lesions may range from barely perceptible to dense concentrations. Cerebrovascular lesions are occasionally definable by the anatomical distribution of the greater tracer concentration in the region of the vessel system involved. This appearance may be mimicked by a neoplasm. Thus, a specific lesion diagnosis cannot be made on the basis of the scan appearance alone.

Neoplastic Lesions

Although the positive brain scan does not dictate the specific nature of intracranial disease, there are often salient features that may serve as clinical clues. They are as follows: (1) tracer concentration in the lesion in relation to adjacent normal activity levels, (2) configuration of the abnormal focus, (3) definition of lesion margins, (4) location within the cranial vault, and (5) multiplicity of foci.

From a practical standpoint, the positive brain scan may be considered to confirm the clinical suspicion of disease and direct the selection of subsequent neuroradiographic studies. Thus, attention may be focused on specific areas for selective angiographic or pneumoencephalographic investigation.

Table 9–3 presents a collation of 12 clinical series reporting brain scan results in confirmed intracranial neoplastic disease.

The detection of intracranial disease by brain scanning is greater than 90 per cent successful for meningiomas (Fig. 9–2), astrocytomas, Grades III and IV (Fig. 9–3), and oligodendrogliomas. The brain scan feature common in the majority of these lesions is the tumor tracer concentration, which equals or is greater than the activity in the scalp, superior sagittal sinus, or retro-orbital pool areas. Occasionally in large lesions, central necrosis may produce a "doughnut" configuration of lower central activity surrounded by peripheral higher activity levels in the lesion (Fig. 9–3). This central defect of tracer concentration may also be found on occasion in intracerebral abscess.

More than 80 per cent of metastatic lesions and medulloblastomas have been reported detectable by scanning. The tracer concentrations in metastases are highly variable. The presence of multiple foci of abnormal tracer activity is strongly suggestive of metastatic disease when a primary tumor has been discovered (Fig. 9–4). The multiplicity of arteriovenous malformations and other vascular lesions may mimic metastatic disease. Medulloblastomas bear no singular scan characteristic beyond age incidence and location. This lesion is about twice as difficult to detect by scanning as the cerebellar astrocytoma.[104]

Astrocytomas, Grades I and II, and ependymomas have been demonstrated in approximately 70 per cent of the proved cases as shown in Table 9–3.

TABLE 9–3 *COMPILATION OF REPORTED BRAIN SCAN RESULTS IN NEOPLASTIC LESIONS*

NEOPLASM	AUTHORS (See References)	NUMBER OF CASES REPORTED	INCIDENCE OF ALL TUMORS (Per Cent)	NUMBER OF POSITIVE CASES*	PER CENT OF POSITIVE CASES
All gliomas	1, 17, 19, 36, 46, 59, 75, 78, 86, 91, 109, 116	616	42.7	513	83.3
Astrocytomas (grades I and II)	17, 19, 36, 46, 59, 78, 86, 91, 109, 116	235	16.4	169	71.9
Astrocytomas (grades III and IV)	17, 19, 36, 46, 59, 75, 78, 86, 91, 109, 116	288	20.0	264	91.7
Ependymomas	1, 17, 36, 46, 78, 86, 116	12	0.8	8	75
Oligodendrogliomas	1, 36, 46, 91, 109, 116	11	0.7	10	92.8
Medulloblastomas	1, 17, 46, 59, 91, 116	11	0.7	9	81.8
Other gliomas	17, 36, 46, 75, 86, 91, 109	14	01.0	11	78.6
Meningiomas	1, 17, 19, 36, 46, 59, 75, 78, 86, 91, 109, 116	232	16.1	218	94.0
Craniopharyngiomas	1, 19, 46, 78, 86	11	0.7	6	55
Pituitary adenomas	1, 19, 46, 78, 86, 109, 116	57	4.0	28	49.1
Acoustic neuromas	1, 17, 46, 59, 78, 86, 109, 116	21	1.4	12	57.1
Metastases	1, 17, 19, 36, 46, 59, 75, 78, 86, 91, 109	365	25.3	303	83.0
Miscellaneous	1, 17, 19, 46, 75, 78, 86, 91, 109, 116	142	9.8	89	62.7
Total		1444		1169	81

*All equivocal cases were recorded as negative.

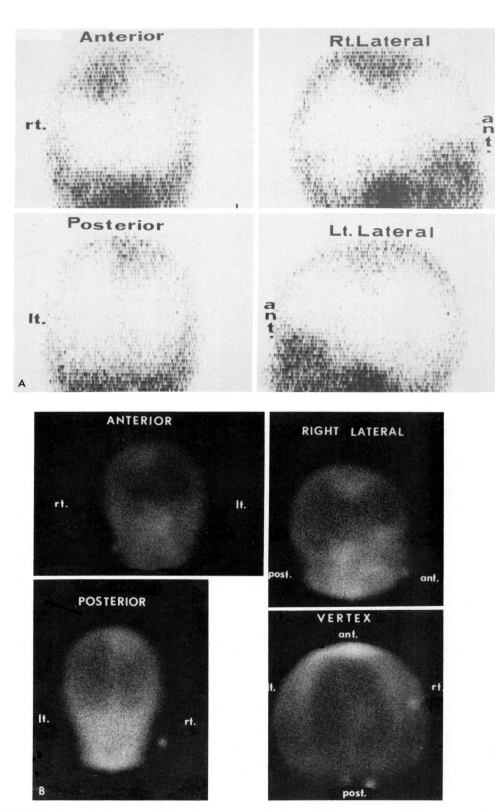

FIGURE 9–2 *A*. Right parasagittal meningioma recorded by rectilinear scanner. *B*. The same meningioma recorded by scintillation camera. Note vertex view at lower right.

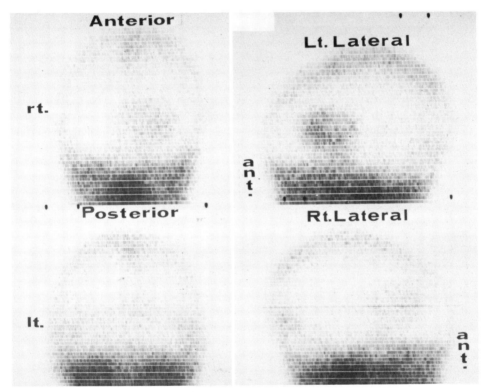

FIGURE 9-3   Astrocytoma, Grade IV (glioblastoma multiforme). Note central clear zone in the lesion (the "doughnut sign").

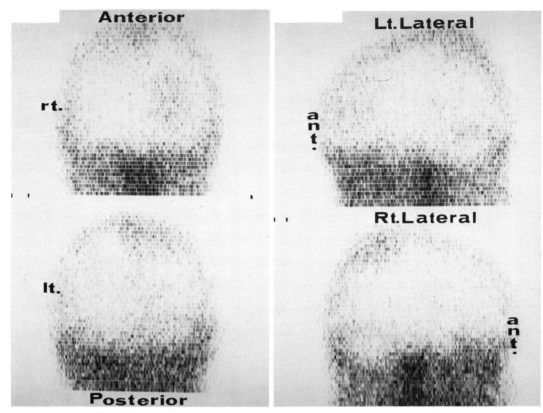

FIGURE 9-4 Metastatic lesions in left frontal and right posterior parietal area.

There has been a wide variation in reported identification of acoustic neurinomas by scanning (Fig. 9–5). Failure to detect these tumors when they are small may be attributed to their proximity to the parotid gland and other physiological pools of activity at the base of the calvarium. DeLand and Wagner reported the successful identification of 12 of 14 proved cases studied.[26] This accuracy is not reflected by the 21 neurinomas reported in Table 9–3.

Pituitary adenomas (Fig. 9–6) and craniopharyngiomas, and occasionally meningiomas, are the midline sellar and suprasellar tumors detected by scanning. Here too the proximity of these lesions to physiological pools of tracer activity may render them more difficult to discern by scanning.

The miscellaneous group in Table 9–3 encompasses the incidence of the less frequently encountered neoplasms. Examples of these include hemangioblastoma, pinealoma, and sarcoma.

Post-treatment Brain Scanning

Patients who have received surgical or radiation therapy may be followed by brain scanning at appropriate intervals.[42, 111] These intervals may be governed by the post-treatment clinical course. In each case an early post-treatment baseline scan is desirable. This is particularly true following craniotomy, when postoperative tissue changes will result in a positive tracer uptake. The abnormal appearance due to surgery may persist for months or years. Thus the baseline study will serve for comparison with subsequent scans searching for recurrence of disease.

Nonneoplastic Disease

The features of scan findings in nonneoplastic disease are essentially the same as those described for neoplasms. Reports of scanning results from seven authors have been summarized in Table 9–4.

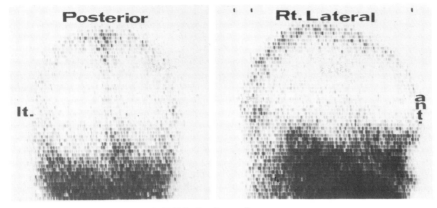

FIGURE 9-5 Acoustic neuroma.

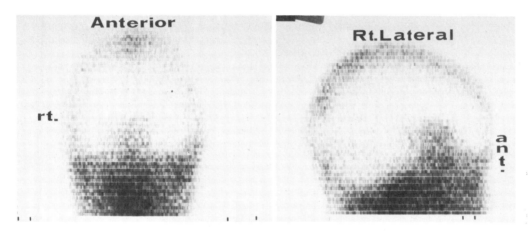

FIGURE 9-6 Chromophobe adenoma.

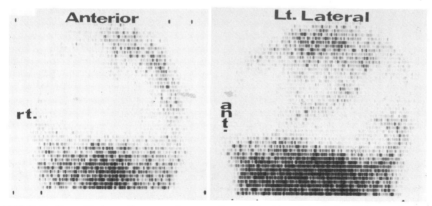

FIGURE 9-7 Scan 16 days after a cerebrovascular accident involving left middle cerebral artery.

TABLE 9–4 *COMPILATION OF REPORTED BRAIN SCAN RESULTS IN NONNEOPLASTIC LESIONS*

LESION	AUTHORS (See References)	NUMBER OF CASES REPORTED	NUMBER OF POSITIVE CASES*	PER CENT OF POSITIVE CASES
Cerebral infarction	24, 57, 77, 113, 115	236	95	40
A-V malformation	24, 36, 57, 73, 77, 115	56	40	71
Intracerebral hematoma	24, 36, 73, 77, 115	34	24	71
Cerebral abscess	36, 57, 77, 113, 115	15	14	93
Epidural and subdural hematoma and abscesses†	24, 36, 73, 77, 113, 115	52	41	79

*All equivocal cases were recorded as negative.
†This grouping is made necessary by the manner in which these cases were reported.

Cerebrovascular Accidents

Cerebrovascular accidents have been reported to demonstrate a definite correlation between positive scan results and the amount of time that has passed since the onset of clinical symptoms. Table 9–5 summarizes this correlation. The scan image of cerebrovascular accidents may reveal a lesion clearly within the distribution of a specific intracerebral artery (Fig. 9–7). This is not always the case, however, and multiple areas of hemorrhagic infarction may be found. If scans of suspected cerebrovascular accidents are negative in the first 10 days, they should be repeated in the third or fourth week after the onset of symptoms to improve the probability of lesion detection. Tow et al. have reported their series of serially scanned cerebrovascular accident patients.[107] In their series the cerebral hemorrhage patients had an earlier onset of positive scan findings as well as a higher overall percentage of positive studies compared to patients who had cerebral thrombosis. Serial scans may differentiate cerebrovascular accidents from tumor because the scan image of a cerebrovascular accident will return to normal by three months in contrast to that of a tumor, which will remain abnormal. This presumes of course, that additional cerebrovascular insult has not occurred in the interval.

Intracranial Hematomas

Experience has shown the brain scan to be a significant detector for subdural hematomas. Epidural hematomas may also be detected. The unilateral hematoma presents as a tracer collection that widens the convexity of the brain scan image (Fig. 9–8). Bilateral subdural hematomas are a more difficult problem because identification often depends on comparison of opposing convexities of the cranial image. The anterior and posterior scan views are the projections most likely to demonstrate the existence of a subdural hematoma. The lateral views may show a diffuse increase of tracer activity over the brain or give no evidence of any abnormality. The crescent

TABLE 9–5 *PERCENTAGE OF POSITIVE BRAIN SCANS AT WEEKLY INTERVALS AFTER CEREBROVASCULAR ACCIDENTS*

	1ST WEEK	2ND WEEK	3RD WEEK	4TH WEEK	COMBINED 5TH–12TH WEEKS	AFTER 12 WEEKS
Authors (see references)	45, 47, 70, 107	45, 47, 70, 107	45, 47	45, 47, 70, 107	45, 77	45, 73, 77
Total number of cases	87	78	26	27	47	30
Number of positive cases*	24	35	13	16	20	0
Percentage of positive cases	27.6	45	50	59	42.5	0

*All equivocal cases were recorded as negative.

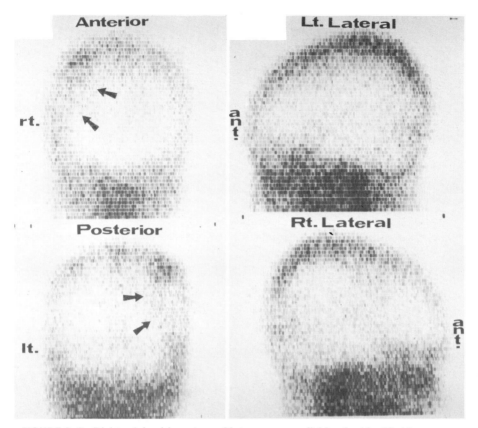

FIGURE 9-8   Right subdural hematoma. Note convex medial border identified by arrows.

appearance of peripheral cranial activity was originally believed pathognomonic of subdural hematoma. This is not true. Heiser et al. reported such a pattern in cerebrovascular accident, craniotomy defect, granulomatous pachymeningitis, meningioma, metastatic breast lesion, extracranial trauma, and other lesions.[50]

Some workers have concluded that the tracers, iodine-131 human serum albumin and mercury-203 chlormerodrin, demonstrate greater concentrations within the subdural membrane than in the subdural fluid contents.[37, 44, 66, 67] One may assume from this that better scan detection of subdural hematomas may be made after the formation of an enclosing membrane. Other investigators using mercury-197 chlormerodrin tracer have shown the subdural fluid to contain the greater tracer activity.[112, 119]

Intracerebral hematomas may also be identified by scanning. These lesions are indistinguishable from neoplasms and most cerebrovascular accidents.

Brain Abscesses

Intracerebral abscesses may be detected by brain scanning; a limited number were reported in the brain scan series recorded in Table 9-4.

In the light of a clinically suspected cerebral inflammatory process and the presence of a focal area of abnormal tracer activity, the clinician may be tempted to assign these findings solely to abscess. It should be remembered, however, that both cerebritis and meningitis may present a similar picture. Thus, neuroradiographic studies are of significant value in the determination of the presence of a mass lesion effect accompanying abscess formation. The scan appearance of meningitis and cerebritis is most often that of a diffuse irregular tracer retention. A subdural empyema cannot be distinguished from the subdural hematoma by scan alone. Further, the clinician should be alert to the appearance of peripheral tracer activity that accompanies a diagnostic fontanelle tap in children.

Arteriovenous Malformation

A majority of authors have reported greater success in detection of arteriovenous malformations by scanning immediately after tracer injection. Budabine, Schlesinger et al., and Planiol and Ackerman reported excellent results using iodine-131 human serum albumin for this purpose.[18, 83, 93] Budabine reported that delayed scans using mercury-197 chlormerodrin were much less successful.[18] Thus, one explanation of early positive scan results is the recording of the tracer in abnormal blood pools of the vascular malformation. Evidence that more than blood pool activity alone enters into this scan search has been given by Afifi et al., who reported a small series of abnormal scans performed four hours after injection of mercury-203 chlormerodrin.[1] A static brain scan image of an arteriovenous malformation is shown in Figure 9–9.

Maynard reported 22 positive studies in 26 patients who had proved arteriovenous malformations. He emphasized that no lesions over 2 cm in diameter were missed when the tracer, technetium-99m pertechnetate, was used.[63] Rosenthall and Maynard et al. have performed rapid-sequence serial brain scintiphoto studies using the scintillation camera as a scintiangiographic device (Fig. 9–10).[64, 88] With this system they have localized arteriovenous malformations with the characteristic appearance of an early "blush" of radioactivity within the vascular malformation followed by a fading of the tracer "blush" in the late phase of the sequence.

Trauma

Trauma producing scalp contusion or laceration, skull fracture, or cerebral contusion will generally yield a positive scan image. The scan may not allow clear differentiation of these entities, however. Coincident skull fracture and cerebral contusion cannot be separately identified unless there is contrecoup contusion. Cerebral contusions generally present as relatively localized areas of tracer activity. The positive scan in cerebral contusion occurs early after trauma and may be expected to resolve in 6 to 10 weeks according to Gilson and Gargano.[44] Intracerebral hematomas and contusions are indistinguishable by scanning. Appropriate interpretation of the brain scan in cases of trauma may be made only after review of the skull x-rays and examination of the patient's scalp for signs of topical damage.

Skull Lesions

Positive brain scans have been reported to occur in lesions of the skull. The skull lesions that may produce positive scans include primary bone neoplasms, metastases, Paget's disease, hyperostosis frontalis interna, cholesteatoma, dermoid cysts, fibrous dysplasia, hemangiomas, fractures, inflammatory lesions, and craniotomy defects.[65]

Charkes and Sklaroff reported a case in which a meningioma with considerable bone invasion produced a positive mercury-203 chlormerodrin scan, but a nega-

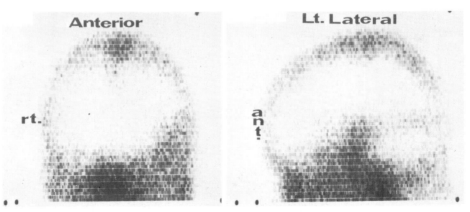

FIGURE 9–9 Arteriovenous malformation.

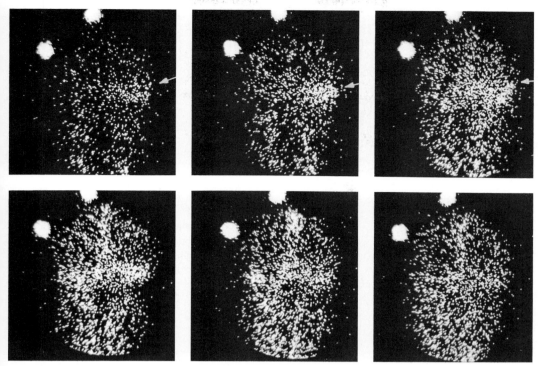

FIGURE 9-10   Rapid-sequence serial scintiphotos recording an arteriovenous malformation at the arrow.

tive strontium-85 bone scan.[21] This might suggest that a primary brain tumor could be distinguished from a lesion arising in bone. However Tow and Wagner reported the relative tracer activity of bone lesions and brain tumors using strontium-85 or strontium-87m and technetium-99m in laboratory animals and humans.[106] They determined that it may be possible to distinguish peripheral intracerebral lesions from skull lesions by this technique. It is evident that skull films are useful and necessary adjuncts in the proper interpretation of brain scans.

BRAIN SCANNING AFTER CAROTID ARTERIOGRAPHY

Several authors have indicated that cerebral arteriography may produce a falsely positive brain scan.[11, 58, 97] Subsequently, Heinz et al. reported 10 cases of brain scans performed before and after arteriography with no apparent falsely positive scan results.[49] They concluded that careful arteriographic technique would prevent a false positive study. Anderson and Seimsen reviewed a series of 116 scans and found nothing to indicate angiographically induced positive scans.[3] Planiol did not observe any adverse effects on the scan following cerebral arteriography in 800 cases.[82]

BRAIN SCANNING IN CHILDREN

With the advent of shorter-lived, lower-energy gamma-emitting radiopharmaceuticals, the reluctance to use brain scanning in children has been much reduced. The brain scan has become a significant screening procedure in recent years.

Tefft reported the results of 1500 brain scans in children.[104] Premedication consisted of 100 mg of potassium perchlorate for children under 12 years and 250 to 500 mg for older children. The dose of technetium-99m pertechnetate varied from 2 to 10 mc.

In Tefft's series, supratentorial lesions gave positive scan results in 85 to 90 per cent of patients with Grade III and IV gliomas and 15 to 20 per cent of patients with Grade I and II gliomas. Sixty-five per cent of the optic gliomas were demonstrated. Infratentorial neoplasms were positive in approximately 45 per cent of the patients with medulloblastoma, in comparison with 90 per cent of the cerebellar astrocytomas. Only 10 per cent of the craniopharyngiomas and lesions in the pons were identified. Tefft reported that 30 per cent of children with acute leukemia with cerebral signs and symptoms had positive scans.

In the series reported by Lorentz et al., two false negative scans were encountered in five infratentorial neoplasms.[57] Maynard reported 80 per cent of brain tumors in 25 children were detectable by scanning.[62]

The authors feel that the judicious use of brain scanning in children with suspected cerebral disease is clearly worthwhile. The "routine" request for the pediatric brain scan should not be encouraged because of the danger of radiation exposure to the juvenile. So long as the risks of such radiation exposure have not been adequately delineated, the benefits must be weighed against the limitations to guide the clinician's judgment.

SERIAL RAPID-SEQUENCE STUDIES

With the advent of stationary imaging devices such as the Anger scintillation camera, the Autofluoroscope, and the Ter-Pogossian camera, the ability to take rapid-sequence serial images has become a reality.[6, 13, 105] Several groups have reported recording the vascular flow pattern in cerebral studies. The diagnostic value of this procedure in the occlusion of the carotid or major cerebral arteries has been amply shown by many investigators.[41, 84, 87, 89] A vascular occlusion results in decreased tracer perfusion in the region of the affected vessel or vessels. The striking feature has been that in vascular occlusion, the rapid-sequence studies were frequently positive when the routine scans were negative (Fig. 9–11). The serial study is of clinical importance in the early postocclusive period when the static cerebral scan is ordinarily negative. Maynard et al. have noted

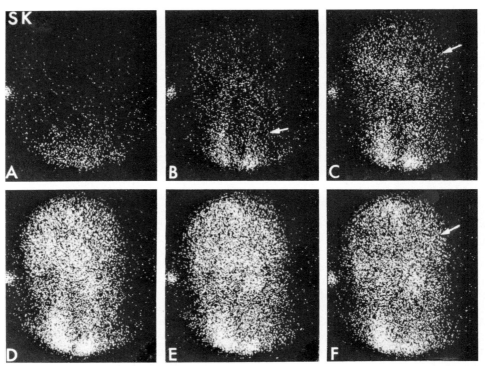

FIGURE 9–11 Rapid-sequence serial scintiphotos following a left cerebrovascular accident. Arrow in frame *B* indicates left carotid and vertebral artery activity. Arrow in frame *C* indicates decreased activity in the ischemic left hemisphere. Arrow in frame *F* demonstrates delayed perfusion into the ischemic area.

decreased activity in instances in which there was tumor displacement of normal vessels.[64] This might simulate a lesion secondary to cerebrovascular occlusion. As noted earlier, the arteriovenous malformations show increased activity early in the arterial phase, but lose activity in the late venous phase.[64, 88] Meningiomas and astrocytomas of Grade III and Grade IV may produce a prompt "blush" of tracer activity that persists throughout the study. Current investigative work in the quantification of cerebral blood flow studies offers further expansion of the intracerebral use of radionuclide tracers.

RADIONUCLIDE CEREBROSPINAL FLUID STUDIES

Early studies applying radionuclides to describe the physiology of the cerebrospinal fluid were reported by several groups. Sweet et al. counted serial samples of cerebrospinal fluid, blood, and urine following the intrathecal injection of the tracer.[99] Chou and French employed external counting in the determination of the rate of diffusion, absorption, and clearance of intrathecally injected iodine-131 human serum albumin.[22] Crow et al. reported localizing cerebrospinal fluid fistulae by counting the radioactivity on cotton wool pledgets placed in the nasopharynx after injection of sodium-24 into the cisterna magna.[25] A further review of the early development of the intrathecal use of radionuclides may be found in articles by Di Chiro et al.[32, 34]

Di Chiro and Tator et al. have detailed the course of normal flow of cerebrospinal fluid labeled with iodine-131 human serum albumin.[32, 101] When the labeled tracer was injected into the lumbar subarachnoid space it was carried to the basal cisternae within two hours. At six hours the tracer was seen in the sylvian cisternae and along the interhemispheric fissure. Within 24 hours the tracer accumulated along the superior sagittal sinus, and at 48 hours most of the radioactivity had disappeared. In normal cases, no significant radioactivity was recorded in the ventricular system.

When iodine-131 human serum albumin was injected into the cisterna magna, the majority of the tracer passed around the medulla to the cisterna medullaris and up into the cisterna pontis. Some of the tracer descended into the spinal subarachnoid space. Usually all basal cisternae could be identified by scanning the tracer within one hour after injection. Within four hours the sylvian cisternae, the cisterna lamina terminalis, and the callosal cisternae could be recorded by scanning. At 24 hours the tracer had collected over the cerebral hemispheres in the parasagittal areas and in the interhemispheric fissure.

Several authors have reported the use of iodine-131 human serum albumin as a variation of the myelogram.[9, 10] This myeloscintigram, however, lacks the image detail of the radiographic air or opaque contrast material myelogram.

The most popular radioactive tracer agent for cisternography or ventriculography is human serum albumin labeled with iodine-131 or technetium-99m. This tracer must have a high specific activity in the order of 50 to 100 μc of iodine-131 per milligram of albumin and 1 mc of technetium-99m per milligram of albumin; high specific activity material was cited by Di Chiro in order to reduce the incidence of protein irritation of the meninges. The two cases of aseptic meningitis reported in the literature occurred after intrathecal injection of 27 mg of albumin in one case and 100 to 130 mg of albumin in the other case.[27, 76] We have experienced several occurrences of minor transient meningeal irritation when using 1 to 3 mg of albumin labeled with technetium-99m. We have not encountered this with the use of iodine-131 human serum albumin in quantities not exceeding 2 mg of albumin. Di Chiro has recommended doses of albumin on the order of 4 mg or less for intrathecal injection.[29] Oldham and Staab have reported two cases of aseptic meningitis following the intrathecal injection of less than 2 mg of ^{131}I human serum albumin.[76a] The more common clinical applications of radionuclide cerebrospinal fluid studies include the cerebrospinal fluid leak localization, evaluation of communicating and noncommunicating hydrocephalus, and evaluation of shunt patency.

Cerebrospinal Fluid Leak Study

The cerebrospinal fluid leak study was developed as a parallel technique to dye studies using indigo carmine. Localization of cerebrospinal fluid leaks relied on the staining of cotton pledgets carefully placed at the orifices of the paranasal sinuses and near the cribriform plate. In the authors' experience a positive radionuclide cerebrospinal fluid leak study has required cotton pledgets from a particular area to have four to five times the count rate of the other pledgets. It should be noted that some radioactivity will appear on all pledgets because of the free unbound tracer ions and the release of tracer ions from the albumin label and their subsequent appearance in the nasal secretions.

In addition to counting the cotton pledgets, serial image recording of the cerebrospinal fluid leak may be of value. Rectilinear scans or scintiphotos, in the authors' experience, have recorded gross leaks (Fig. 9–12). Small and intermittent leaks were more difficult or impossible to localize by the imaging technique. Di Chiro et al. and Ashburn et al. have published interesting illustrations of cerebrospinal fluid leaks using the Anger camera.[4, 35]

Cerebrospinal Fluid Circulation Study

The radionuclide cisternogram applied to the normotensive hydrocephalic patient may be performed by lumbar intrathecal injection or by the direct instillation of the tracer into the cisterna magna. The scan image may record activity in the dilated ventricles within the first 24 hours. Subsequent 48-hour and 72-hour scans in normotensive communicating hydrocephalus will generally not show any evidence of activity distributed over the superior cortical surface and in the area of the superior sagittal sinus.[102] Some authorities report ventricular tracer activity in other forms of communicating hydrocephalus.[80] They feel that the distinguishing factor between normotensive communicating hydrocephalus and the other forms of communicating hydrocephalus with ventricular activity is the presence of cortical surface activity and parasagittal sinus activity in the latter group. While pneumoencephalography may show patency of the subarachnoid space, it does not depend on the active circulation of the spinal fluid. The radionuclide tracer, however, must be distributed by active cerebral spinal fluid flow.[102] Hence, the radionuclide cisternogram may be a more sensitive test for distinguishing normotensive communicating hydrocephalus from other forms of hydrocephalus. Unlike the pneumoencephalogram, the radionuclide cisternogram requires no special positioning of the patient to insure circulation of the tracer used for imaging. An example of normotensive hydrocephalus is illustrated in Figure 9–13.

Radionuclide ventriculography obtained by instilling the tracer directly into the ventricle has assisted in the evaluation of shunt patency and in the identification of a spontaneous cerebrospinal fluid shunt.[31] Evaluation of the hydrocephalic child by intrathecal tracer injection and scanning has been reported as a useful procedure.[60]

CONCLUSION

Brain scanning has considerable value in the detection of the majority of malignant cerebral neoplasms. It also evidences a significant diagnostic relevance in the detection of several nonneoplastic diseases. An appreciation of its limitations must accompany its acceptance as a diagnostic procedure. This understanding will enhance its diagnostic usefulness.

The accuracy of scanning in the detection of cerebral neoplasms may be compared with other diagnostic procedures in Table 9–6, which is a compilation of several comparative reports. This defines its value as a screening procedure as well as a major diagnostic tool. The authors have reviewed and reported their findings in over 1000 brain scans, which included 112 cerebral neoplasms. These results parallel the cumulative results reported in this chapter.[46a]

While the attributes of brain scanning are evident, this or any single neuroradiographic procedure should not be used as a sole determinant of the presence of intracranial disease. The studies should be considered mutually complementary. The combination of physical examination, skull films, electroencephalography, and brain scanning should produce as nearly perfect a screening study series as is available at this time.

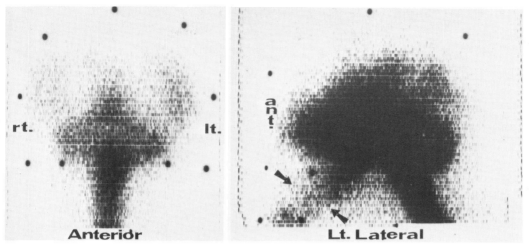

FIGURE 9–12 Anterior and left lateral scans following intrathecal injection of 1 mc ^{99m}Tc human serum albumin. Arrows identify the cerebrospinal fluid leak arising from the middle fossa.

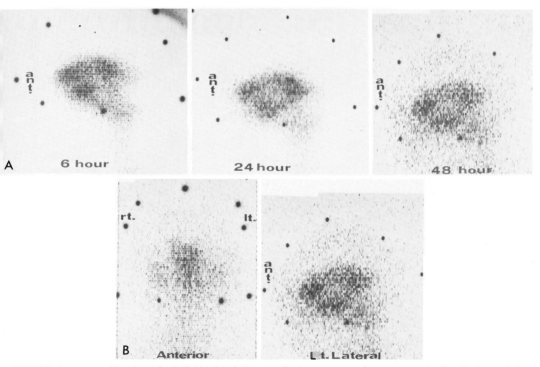

FIGURE 9–13 *A*. Cerebrospinal fluid circulation study in normotensive communicating hydrocephalus. *B*. Anterior and left lateral scans at 48 hours record the tracer activity in lateral ventricles and basal cisterns. Note absence of significant activity over the cerebral convexity and parasagittal regions in particular.

TABLE 9-6 *RESULTS OF DIAGNOSTIC TESTS FOR BRAIN TUMORS*

	AUTHORS (See References)	TOTAL	POSITIVE*	PER CENT CORRECT
Scans	1, 36, 46, 75, 78, 109, 115	519	432	83
Neurologic examination	46	118	110	93
Skull films	1, 46, 78, 109, 115	381	144	38
Carotid and brachial arteriogram	1, 36, 46, 78, 109, 115	325	277	85
Pneumoencephalogram	1, 46, 78, 115	38	32	84
Ventriculogram	1, 36, 46, 78	34	33	97
Combined pneumo- and ventriculogram	1, 36, 46, 78, 109, 115	121	106	88
EEG	1, 46, 75, 78, 109, 115	289	222	77

*All equivocal cases were recorded as negative.

Investigation in the areas of instrument design and tracer development in the coming years will produce combinations of capabilities that will provide means for finer image production and ultra-high-speed kinetic data acquisition. Thus, more sophisticated diagnoses by innocuous radionuclide tracer methods may be expected.

REFERENCES

1. Afifi, A. R., Morrison, R. R., Sahs, A. L., and Evans, T. C.: A comparison of chlormerodrin Hg-203 scintiencephalo-scanning with neuro-radiology and electroencephalography for localization of intracranial lesions. Neurology, *15*:56–63, 1965.
2. Allen, H. C., Jr., and Risser, J. R.: Simplified apparatus for brain tumor surgery. Nucleonics, *13*:28–31, 1955.
3. Anderson, W. B., and Siemsen, J. K.: Brain scanning after cerebral angiography. Radiology, *89*:492–494, 1967.
4. Ashburn, W. L., Harbert, J. C., Briner, W. H., and Di Chiro, G.: Cerebrospinal fluid rhinorrhea studied with the gamma scintillation camera. J. Nucl. Med., *9*:523–529, 1968.
5. Anger, H. O.: The scintillation camera: A new instrument for mapping the distribution of radioactive isotopes. U.C.R.L. Report 3845, 1957.
6. Anger, H. O.: The scintillation camera with multichannel collimators. J. Nucl. Med., *5*:515–531, 1964.
7. Bakay, L.: Basic aspects of brain tumor localization by radioactive substances. J. Neurosurg., *27*:239–245, 1967.
8. Bakay, L., and Klein, D. M., eds.: Brain Tumor Scanning with Radioisotopes. Springfield, Ill., Charles C Thomas, 1969.
9. Bauer, F. K., and Yuhl, E. T.: Myelography by means of I-131: The myeloscintigram. Neurology (Minneap.), *3*:341–346, 1953.
10. Bell, R. L.: Automatic contour myelography in infants. J. Nucl. Med., *3*:288–292, 1962.
11. Bender, M. A.: Discussion of papers: Medical Radioisotope Scanning. Int. Atomic Energy Comm., Vienna, 1959, p. 208.
12. Bender, M. A., and Blau, M.: A versatile high-contrast photoscanner for the localization of human tumors with radioisotopes. Int. J. Appl. Radiat., *4*:154, 1959.
13. Bender, M. A., and Blau, M.: Autofluoroscope: The use of a nonscanning device for tumor localization with radioisotopes. J. Nucl. Med., *1*:105, 1960.
14. Blau, M., and Bender, M. A.: Clinical evaluation of Hg-203 neohydrin and I-131 albumin in brain tumor localization. J. Nucl. Med., *1*:106–107, 1960.
15. Brown, A. J., Zingesser, L., and Scheinberg, L. C.: Radioactive mercury labeled chlormerodrin scans in cerebrovascular accidents. Neurology, *17*:405–412, 1967.
16. Brownell, G. L., and Sweet, W. H.: Localization of brain tumors with positron emitters. Nucleonics, *11*:40–45, 1953.
17. Bucy, P. C., and Ciric, I. S.: Brain scans in diagnosis of brain tumors scanning with chlormerodrin Hg-203 and chlormerodrin Hg-197. J.A.M.A., *191*:93–99, 1965.
18. Budabine, M.: Diagnostic value of RIHSA and chlormerodrin Hg-197 brain scanning in intracranial arteriovenous malformations. J. Nucl. Med., *8*:879–890, 1967.
19. Bull, J. W. D., and Marryat, J.: Isotope encephalography: Experience with 100 cases. Brit. Med. J., *1*:474–480, 1965.
20. Cassen, B., Curtis, L., Reed, C., and Libby, R.: Instrumentation for I-131 use in medical studies. Nucleonics, *9*:46–50, 1951.
21. Charkes, N. D., and Sklaroff, D. N.: Early diagnosis of metastatic bone cancer by photoscanning with strontium-85. J. Nucl. Med., *5*:168–179, 1964.
22. Chou, S. N., and French, L. A.: Systemic absorption and urinary excretion of RISA from subarachnoid space. Neurology (Minneap.), *5*:555–557, 1955.
23. Chou, S. N., Aust, J. B., Moore, G. E., and Peyton, W. T.: Radioactive iodinated human serum albumin as tracer agent for diagnosing and localizing intracranial lesions. Proc. Soc. Exp. Biol. Med., *77*:193–195, 1951.
24. Ciric, I. S., Quinn, J. L., and Bucy, P. C.: Mercury 197 and technetium-99m brain scans in the diagnosis of non-neoplastic intracranial lesions. J. Neurosurg., *27*:119–125, 1957.

25. Crow, H. J., Keogh, C., and Northfield, D. W. C.: Localization of cerebrospinal fluid fistulae. Lancet, *2*:325–327, 1956.

26. DeLand, R. H., and Wagner, H. N., Jr.: Brain scanning as a diagnostic aid in the detection of eighth nerve tumors. Radiology, *92*:571–575, 1969.

27. Detmer, D. E., and Blacker, H. M.: A case of aseptic meningitis secondary to intrathecal injection of I-131 human serum albumin. Neurology, *15*:642–643, 1965.

28. Di Chiro, G.: RISA encephalography and conventional neuroradiologic methods. A comparative study. Acta Radiol. (Stockholm), suppl. 201, 1961.

29. Di Chiro, G.: Specific activity of radioiodinated human serum albumin for intrathecal injection. A correction. Neurology, *15*:950, 1965.

30. Di Chiro, G.: Observations on the circulation of the cerebrospinal fluid. Acta Radiol. Diagn., *5*:988–1002, 1966.

31. Di Chiro, G., and Grove, A. S., Jr.: Evaluation of surgical and spontaneous cerebrospinal fluid shunts by isotope scanning. J. Neurosurg., *24*:743–748, 1966.

32. Di Chiro, G., Ashburn, W. L., and Briner, W. H.: Technetium Tc-99m serum albumin for cisternography: The use of high specific activity technetium Tc-99m serum albumin as a tracer for subarachnoid and ventricular scintiphotography. Arch. Neurol., *19*:218–227, 1968.

33. Di Chiro, G., Ashburn, W. L., and Grove, A. S., Jr.: Which radioisotope for brain scanning? Neurology, *18*:225–236, 1968.

34. Di Chiro, G., Reames, P. M., and Matthews, W. B., Jr.: RISA ventriculography and RISA cisternography. Neurology, *14*:185–191, 1964.

35. Di Chiro, G., Ommaya, A. K., Ashburn, W. L., and Briner, W. H.: Isotope cisternography in the diagnosis and followup of cerebrospinal fluid rhinorrhea. J. Neurosurg., *28*:522–529, 1968.

36. Dugger, G. S., and Pepper, F. D.: The reliability of radioisotopic encephalography. A correlation with other neuroradiological and anatomical studies. Neurology, *13*:1042–1053, 1963.

37. Dunbar, H. S., and Ray, B. S.: Localization of brain tumors and other intracranial lesions with radioactive iodinated human serum albumin. Surg. Gynec. Obstet., *98*:433–436, 1969.

38. Engbring, N. H.: Brain scan artifact from saliva contamination. J.A.M.A., *199*:861, 1967.

39. Erickson, T. C., Larson, F. C., and Gordon, E. S.: Uptake of radioactive phosphorus by glioblastoma multiforme and therapeutic application. Trans. Amer. Neurol. Ass., *73*:112, 1948.

40. Feindel, W., Yamamato, Y. L., McRae, D. L., and Zanelli, J.: Contour brain scanning with iodine and mercury compounds for detection of intracranial tumors. Amer. J. Roentgen., *92*:177–186, 1964.

41. Fish, M. B., Pollycove, M., O'Reilly, S., Khentigan, A., and Koch, R. L.: Vascular characterization of brain lesions by rapid sequential cranial scintiphotography. J. Nucl. Med., *9*:249–259, 1968.

42. Flipse, R. C., Vuksanovic, M., and Fonts, E. A.: Sequential brain scanning in radiation therapy of malignant tumors of the brain. Amer. J. Roentgen., *102*:88–92, 1968.

43. Francis, J. E., Bell, P. R., and Harris, C. C.: Medical scintillation spectrometry. Nucleonics, *13*:82–88, 1955.

43a. Gates, G. F., Dore, E. R., and Taplin, G. V.: Interval brain scanning with sodium pertechnetate Tc-99m for tumor detectability. J.A.M.A., *215*:85–88, 1971.

44. Gilson, A. J., and Gargano, F. D.: Correlation of brain scans and angiography in intracerebral trauma. Amer. J. Roentgen., *94*:819–827, 1965.

45. Glasgow, J. L., Currier, R. D., Goodrich, J. K., and Tutor, F. T.: Brain scans of cerebral infarcts with radioactive mercury. Radiology, *88*:1086–1091, 1967.

46. Goodrich, J. K., and Tutor, F. T.: The isotope encephalogram in brain tumor diagnosis. J. Nucl. Med., *6*:541–548, 1965.

46a. Goodrich, J. K., and Wilkinson, R. H., Jr.: The effectiveness of brain scanning for detecting intracranial disease. *In* Central Nervous System Investigation with Radionuclides. Proceedings of the Second Annual Nuclear Medicine Seminar, Miami Beach, Fla., March 19–23, 1970. Springfield, Ill., Charles C Thomas, 1970, pp. 365–374.

47. Gutterman, P., and Shenkin, H. A.: Cerebral scans in completed strokes. Value in prognosis of clinical course. J.A.M.A., *207*:145–147, 1969.

48. Harper, P. V., Beck, R., Charleston, D., and Lathrop, K. A.: Optimization of a scanning method using Tc-99m. Nucleonics, *22*:50, 1964.

49. Heinz, E. R., Brylski, J. R., Izenstark, J. L., and Weens, H. S.: Post-angiography isotope brain scanning: Positive or negative? Amer. J. Roentgen., *98*:336–344, 1963.

50. Heiser, W. J., Quinn, J. L., and Mollihan, W. V.: The crescent pattern of increased radioactivity in brain scanning. Radiology, *87*:483–488, 1966.

51. Holmes, R. A., Herron, C. S., and Wagner, H. N., Jr.: A modified vertex view in brain scanning. Radiology, *88*:498–503, 1967.

52. Horwitz, N. H., and Lofstrom, J. E.: Photographic recording method for scintillation scanning. Nucleonics, *13*:56, 1955.

53. Jaskar, D. W., Griep, R. T., and Nelp, W. B.: The uptake and concentration of the pertechnetate by the choroid plexus. J. Nucl. Med., *8*:387, 1967.

54. Kennady, J. C., and Taplin, G. V.: Albumin macroaggregated for brain scanning experimental bases and safety in primates. J. Nucl. Med., *6*:566–581, 1965.

55. King, E. G., Wood, D. E., and Morley, T. P.: The use of macroaggregates of radioiodinated human serum albumin in brain scanning. Canad. Med. Ass. J., *95*:381–389, 1966.

56. Kuhl, D. E., Chamberlain, R. H., Hale, J., and Gorson, R. O.: A high contrast photographic recorder for scintillation counter scanning. Radiology, *66*:730–739, 1956.

57. Lorentz, W. B., Simon, J. L., and Benua, R. S.:

Brain scanning in children. J.A.M.A., *201*:5–7, 83–85, 1967.

58. McAfee, J. G.: *In* Quinn, J. L., III, ed.: Scintillation Scanning in Clinical Medicine. Philadelphia, W. B. Saunders Co., 1964.

59. McClintock, J. T., and Dalrymple, G. V.: The value of brain scans in the management of suspected intracranial lesions. J. Nucl. Med., *5*:189–192, 1964.

60. McCullough, D. C., and Luessenhop, A. J.: Evaluation of photoscanning of the diffusion of intrathecal RISA in infantile and childhood hydrocephalus. J. Neurosurg., *30*:673–678, 1969.

61. Mack, J. F., Webber, M. M., and Bennett, L. R.: Brain scanning: Normal anatomy with technetium-99m pertechnetate. J. Nucl. Med., *7*:633–640, 1966.

62. Maynard, C. D.: Brain scanning in the pediatric age group. J. Nucl. Med., *8*:390, 1967.

63. Maynard, C. D.: Clinical Nuclear Medicine. Philadelphia, Lea & Febiger, 1969, p. 172.

64. Maynard, C. D., Witcofski, R. L., Janeway, R., and Cowan, R. J.: Radioisotope arteriography as an adjunct to the brain scan. Radiology, *92*:908–912, 1969.

65. Maynard, C. D., Hanner, T. G., and Witcofski, R. L.: Positive brain scans due to lesions of the skull. Arch. Neurol., *18*:93–97, 1968.

66. Mealey, J., Jr.: Radioisotopic localization in subdural hematomas. An experimental study with arsenic-74 and radioiodinated human serum albumin in dogs. J. Neurosurg., *20*:770–776, 1963.

67. Mealey, J., Jr., Dehner, J. R., and Reese, I. C.: Clinical comparison of two agents used in brain scanning radioiodinated serum albumin vs. chlormerodrin Hg-203. J.A.M.A., *189*:260–264, 1964.

68. Miller, M. S., and Simmons, G. H.: Optimization of timing and positioning of the technetium brain scan. J. Nucl. Med., *9*:429–435, 1968.

69. Mishkin, F., and Truksa, J.: The diagnosis of intracranial cysts by means of the brain scan. Radiology, *90*:740–746, 1968.

70. Molinari, G. F., Pircher, F., and Heyman, A.: Serial brain scanning with technetium-99m in patients with cerebral infarction. Neurology, *17*:627–636, 1967.

71. Moore, G. E.: Fluorescein scan agent in the differentiation of normal and malignant tissues. Science, *106*:130–133, 1947.

72. Moore, G. E.: Use of radioactive diiodofluorescein in the diagnosis and localization of brain tumors. Science, *107*:569–571, 1948.

73. Morrison, R. T., Afifi, A. K., Van Allen, M. W., and Evans, R. C.: Scintiencephalography for the detection and localization of non-neoplastic intracranial lesions. J. Nucl. Med., *6*:7–15, 1965.

74. Murphy, E., Cervantes, Q. B., and Maass, R.: Radioalbumin macroaggregate brain scanning: A histopathologic investigation. Amer. J. Roentgen., *102*:88–92, 1968.

75. Murphy, J. T., Gloor, P., Yamamoto, Y. L., and Feindel, W.: A comparison of electroencephalography and brain scan in supratentorial tumors. New Eng. J. Med., *276*:309–313, 1967.

76. Nichols, C. F.: A second case of aseptic meningitis following isotope cisternography using I-131 human serum albumin. Neurology (Minneap.), *17*:199–200, 1967.

76a. Oldham, R. R., and Staab, E. V.: Aseptic meningitis following the intrathecal injection of radioiodinated serum albumin. Radiology, *97*:317–321, 1970.

77. Overton, M. C., III, Haynie, T. P., and Snodgrass, S. R.: Brain scans in nonneoplastic intracranial lesions. Scanning with chlormerodrin Hg-203 and chlormerodrin Hg-197. J.A.M.A., *191*:431–436, 1965.

78. Overton, M. C., III, Snodgrass, S. R., and Haynie, T. P.: Brain scans in neoplastic intracranial lesions. Scanning with chlormerodrin Hg-203 and chlormerodrin Hg-197. J.A.M.A., *192*:747–751, 1965.

79. Overton, M. C., III, Haynie, T. P., Otte, W. K., and Coe, J. E.: The vertex view in brain scanning. J. Nucl. Med., *6*:705–710, 1965.

80. Patten, D. H., and Benson, D. F.: Diagnosis of normal pressure hydrocephalus by RISA cisternography. J. Nucl. Med., *9*:457–461, 1968.

81. Perryman, C. R., Noble, P. R., and Bragdon, F. H.: Myeloscintigraphy: A useful procedure for localization of spinal block lesions. Amer. J. Roentgen., *80*:104–111, 1958.

82. Planiol, T.: Discussion of papers: Medical Radioiostope Scanning. Int. Atomic Energy Comm., 1959, p. 208.

83. Planiol, T., and Akerman, M.: Gamma encephalography in supratentorial arteriovenous malformation: Study of 54 cases. Presse méd., *73*:2205–2210, 1965.

84. Powell, M. R., and Anger, H. O.: Blood flow visualization with the scintillation camera. J. Nucl. Med., *7*:729–732, 1966.

85. Quinn, J. L., III.: Scintillation Scanning in Clinical Medicine. Philadelphia, W. B. Saunders Co., 1964.

86. Quinn, J. L., III, Ciric, I., and Hauser, W.: Analysis of 96 abnormal brain scans using technetium-99m (pertechnetate form). J.A.M.A., *194*:158–160, 1969.

87. Rosenthall, L.: Application of the gamma ray scintillation camera to dynamic studies in man. Radiology, *86*:634–639, 1966.

88. Rosenthall, L.: Radionuclide diagnosis of arteriovenous malformation with rapid sequence brain scans. Radiology, *91*:1185–1188, 1968.

89. Rosenthall, L.: Detection of altered cerebral arterial blood flow using technetium-99m pertechnetate and gamma ray scintillation camera. Radiology, *88*:713–718, 1967.

90. Rosenthall, L., Aguayo, A., and Stratford, J.: A clinical assessment of carotid and vertebral artery injection of macroaggregates of radioiodinated albumin (MARIA) for brain scanning. Radiology, *86*:499–505, 1966.

91. Rhoton, A. L.: Chlormerodrin Hg-197 brain scanning: Selecting the optimal interval between isotope administration and scanning. J. Nucl. Med., *9*:16–18, 1968.

92. Rhoton, A. L., Jr., Carlsson, A. M., and Ter-Pogossian, M. M.: Brain scanning with chlormerodrin Hg-197 and chlormerodrin Hg-203. Arch. Neurol., 10:369–375, 1964.

93. Schlesinger, E. B., DeBaves, S., and Taveras, J.: Localization of brain tumors using radio-iodinated human serum albumin. Amer. J. Roentgen., 87:449–462, 1967.

94. Selverstone, B., and Solomon, A. K.: Radioactive isotopes in study of intracranial tumors; preliminary report of methods and results. Trans. Amer. Neurol. Ass., 73:115–119, 1948.

95. Shy, G. M., Bradley, R. B., and Matthews, W. B., Jr.: External Collimation Detection of Intracranial Neoplasia with Unstable Nuclides. Edinburgh, E. and S. Livingstone Ltd., 1958.

96. Sodee, D. B.: The result of 350 brain scans with radioactive mercurial diuretics. J. Nucl. Med., 4:185, 1963.

97. Spencer, R.: Scintiscanning in space occupying lesions of the skull. Brit. J. Radiol., 38:1–15, 1965.

98. Stern, H. S., Goodwin, D. A., Scheffel, U., and Wagner, H. N., Jr.: In-113m for blood-pool and brain scanning. Nucleonics, 25:62–65, 1967.

99. Sweet, W. H., Brownell, G. L., School, J. A., Bowstis, D. R., Benda, P., and Stickley, E. E.: The formation flow and absorption of cerebrospinal fluid: Newer concepts based on studies with isotopes. Res. Publ. Ass. Nerv. Ment. Dis., 34:101–159, 1954.

100. Tator, C. H., Morley, T. P., and Olszewski, J. A.: A study of the factors responsible for the accumulation of radioactive iodinated human serum albumin (RIHSA) by intracranial tumors and other lesions. J. Neurosurg., 22:60–76, 1965.

101. Tator, C. H., Fleming, J. F. R., Sheppard, R. H., and Turner, V. M.: Studies of cerebrospinal fluid dynamics with intrathecally administered radioidionated human serum albumin (IHSA-131). Canad. Med. Ass. J., 97:493–503, 1967.

102. Tator, C. H., Fleming, J. F. R., Sheppard, R. H., and Turner, V. M.: A radioisotope test for communicating hydrocephalus. J. Neurosurg., 28:327–340, 1968.

103. Tauxe, W. N., and Thorsen, H. C.: Cerebrovascular permeability studies in cerebral neoplasms and vascular lesions: Optimal dose-to-scan interval for pertechnetate brain scanning. J. Nucl. Med., 10:34–39, 1969.

104. Tefft, M.: Radioisotopes in malignancies in children. J.A.M.A., 207:1853–1857, 1969.

105. Ter-Pogossian, M., Kastner, J., and Vest, T. B.: Autofluorography of the thyroid gland by means of image amplification. Radiology, 81:984–988, 1963.

106. Tow, D. E., and Wagner, H. N., Jr.: Scanning for tumors of brain and bone. J.A.M.A., 199:610–614, 1967.

107. Tow, D. E., Wagner, H. N., Jr., DeLand, F. H., and North, W. A.: Brain scanning in cerebral vascular disease. J.A.M.A., 207:105–108, 1969.

108. Wagner, H. N., Jr.: Principles of Nuclear Medicine. Philadelphia, W. B. Saunders Co., 1968.

109. Wang, Y., Shea, F. J., and Rosen, J. A.: Comparison of the accuracy of brain scanning and other procedures used for brain tumor detection. Neurology, 15:1117–1119, 1965.

110. Webber, M. M.: Normal brain scanning. Amer. J. Roentgen., 94:815–818, 1965.

111. Wilkins, R. H., Pircher, F. J., and Odom, G. L.: The value of post-operative brain scan in patients with supratentorial intracranial tumors. J. Neurosurg., 27:111–118, 1967.

112. Williams, C. M., and Garcia-Bengochea, F.: Concentration of radioactive chlormerodrin in the fluid of chronic subdural hematoma. Radiology, 84:745–747, 1965.

113. Williams, J. L., and Beiler, D. D.: Brain scanning in non-tumorous conditions. Neurology, 16:1159–1166, 1966.

114. Witcofski, R. L., Maynard, C. D., and Janeway, R.: Concentration of technetium-99m by the choroid plexus: Experimental demonstration in vivo. Arch. Neurol. (Chicago), 18:301–303, 1968.

115. Witcofski, R. L., Maynard, C. D., and Roper, T. J.: A comparative analysis of the accuracy of the technetium-99m pertechnetate brain scan: Follow-up of 1000 patients. J. Nucl. Med., 8:187–196, 1967.

116. Witcofski, R. L., Janeway, R., Maynard, C. D., Bearden, E., and Schultz, J. L.: Visualization of the choroid plexus on the technetium-99m brain scan. Arch. Neurol. (Chicago), 16:286–289, 1967.

117. Witcofski, R. L., Roper, T. J., and Maynard, C. D.: False positive brain scans for extracranial contamination with 99m technetium. J. Nucl. Med., 6:524–527, 1965.

118. Wrenn, F. R., Jr., Good, M. L., and Handler, P.: The use of positron-emitting radioisotopes for the localization of brain tumors. Science, 113:525, 1951.

119. Zingesser, L. H., Mandell, S., and Schecter, M. M.: The gamma encephalogram in extracerebral hematomas. Acta Radiol., 5:972–980, 1966.

10

LUMBAR PUNCTURE AND ANALYSIS OF CEREBROSPINAL FLUID

HISTORICAL BACKGROUND

Although Quincke is generally considered to have been the pioneer in puncturing the lumbar subarachnoid space in man, Corning, in 1885, actually made the first spinal puncture for the injection of cocaine for anesthesia.[2, 11] Quincke's initial taps were made in 1891 for the purpose of reducing intracranial pressure. His work was paralleled by that of Morton and of Wynter, who independently developed the use of the technique in the same year.[9, 17] It remained for Fürbringer, in 1895, to describe various gross, microscopic, and chemical changes in cerebrospinal fluid in certain pathological conditions.[6] This early work was supplemented by the descriptions of cytological changes in neurological diseases by Widal, Sicard, and Ravaut six years later.[16] Froin, in 1903, first observed spontaneous clotting and xanthochromia in inflammations of the meninges, while the serological spinal fluid test for syphilis was developed by Wassermann in 1906.[5, 15] The first monograph describing the constituents of cerebrospinal fluid in both normal and pathological states was published in 1912 by Mestrezat.[8] Queckenstedt's description of manometric changes occurring in the presence of spinal subarachnoid block was made in 1916.[10] The monograph of Merritt and Fremont-Smith remains a classic reference source for those interested in clinical changes in the cerebrospinal fluid.[7]

Excellent summaries relating to the clinical pathology of the fluid have been made by Adams, Fishman, Schaltenbrand and Wolff, and Schmidt, while the physiology of the fluid is the subject of the magnificent monograph of Davson.[1, 3, 4, 12, 13] The cytology of the cerebrospinal fluid is reviewed by Spriggs and Boddington in their beautifully illustrated work.[14]

VALUE OF LUMBAR PUNCTURE

There is a trend in neurological surgery, and medicine in general, to employ special diagnostic procedures excessively. None is absolutely benign, free of discomfort, or inexpensive, and many add significantly to the duration of hospitalization. Moreover, some kinds of information are nonspecific, are difficult to assess, and can obfuscate rather than cast light upon a correct diagnosis. A traditional approach to the diagnosis of diseases of the nervous system is to include an examination of the cerebrospinal fluid, often as a first measure. While in some situations lumbar puncture is a necessary initial step, in others the indications should be weighed in the light of the development of other planned investigations; in yet others, it is unnecessary or contraindicated.

T. K. CRAIGMILE

K. WELCH

Similarly, the use of lumbar puncture as a therapeutic measure in neurological surgery formerly enjoyed favor that it no longer merits.

INDICATIONS FOR LUMBAR PUNCTURE

Diagnostic Indications

Primary indications for examination of the cerebrospinal fluid occur in suspected cases of diffuse or disseminated infections of the nervous system or meninges, subarachnoid hemorrhage, neoplasms, and demyelinating disease. In bacterial meningitis the finding of turbid fluid, an elevated leukocyte count and protein value, a diminished glucose level, and increased cerebrospinal fluid pressure will tentatively establish a diagnosis that can be confirmed by isolation and identification of the bacterial organism. Sensitivity studies will dictate specific therapy, and the fluid may be examined for bacteriostatic or bactericidal activity as a monitor of the effectiveness of therapy.

Spontaneous subarachnoid hemorrhage, although it can ordinarily be diagnosed from the history and clinical findings, can be verified only by the recovery of uniformly bloody cerebrospinal fluid. Rarely the appearance of blood in the lumbar fluid may be delayed for some hours, so a second diagnostic puncture may be needed to establish its presence.

Multiple sclerosis and other demyelinating diseases, along with luetic infections, may produce an elevation in the gamma globulin protein fraction of the cerebrospinal fluid as well as an alteration in the colloidal gold curve. The leukocyte count, as well, is commonly elevated in such diseases. These special studies are discussed later.

In the presence of an intraspinal tumor the protein content of the cerebrospinal fluid is usually increased, particularly when the tumor has completely or partially occluded the spinal canal. If the obstruction is a total one, the protein content of the fluid may approach plasma levels. Intracranial tumors situated near the ventricular system or the subarachnoid cisterns ordinarily cause elevation in the cerebrospinal fluid protein, while intracerebral lesions may not change its value.

Infectious polyneuritis, the Landry-Guillain-Barré syndrome, produces a marked increase in the cerebrospinal fluid protein level without a corresponding leukocytic response. Diabetic peripheral neuropathy is frequently accompanied by an elevated cerebrospinal fluid protein and glucose content.[28, 33] Hypoparathyroidism may, through obscure means, elevate the protein level in the cerebrospinal fluid.[26] Such protein elevation, along with that accompanying myxedema and other metabolic and infectious processes, may result in papilledema.[22] Although lumbar puncture is often made in patients who have had generalized seizures with no demonstrable organic cause, the findings are usually normal, and the study is probably not warranted as a routine diagnostic measure.

One of the most important indications for lumbar puncture is the need to introduce a contrast medium, air or Pantopaque, for pneumography and myelography. These studies are described in those sections concerning radiographic diagnostic procedures.

Therapeutic Indications

At one time it was common practice to carry out repeated spinal drainage for the control of intracranial hypertension in the period following craniotomy, and there is little question that many patients were made more comfortable by this procedure. Even before the introduction of steroids to control edema of the brain, use of this method of reducing pressure was diminishing, and it is now rarely necessary.

Once the diagnosis of spontaneous subarachnoid hemorrhage has been made, repeated lumbar puncture may be of some value in reducing intracranial pressure and removing blood from the subarachnoid space. The observations of Sprong and Meredith lend little support to the use of this technique insofar as the removal of red blood cells is concerned, and the principal benefit of the puncture is relief of headache.[45, 52]

Antibacterial agents may be injected intrathecally for the treatment of certain forms of meningeal infection. Kempe and his associates have determined which antibiotics may be safely administered by way of the cerebrospinal fluid.[36] These medications, along with permissible concentrations and total dosages, are listed in Table 10–1. Calculation of dosage and concentration of the antibiotic should be duplicated by a second person to avoid error. Similarly, subarachnoid infusion of various chemotherapeutic and radiotherapeutic drugs has been advocated in the therapy of neoplastic processes pervading the cerebrospinal axis.[23, 37, 38, 48, 51] A well-established indication for lumbar puncture is the need for spinal anesthesia in a variety of surgical operations.

The intrathecal administration of a phenol-Pantopaque suspension is helpful in the relief of various forms of intractable pain as well as in the lower extremity spasticity occurring with lesions of the spinal cord.[42, 44, 46, 47] It should be emphasized that a patient who is harboring a malignancy may also have a lumbar disc lesion, and this possibility must be considered and excluded by myelography before a primary pain-relieving measure is carried out.

After a chronic subdural hematoma has been evacuated, particularly in an elderly patient, recovery may be speeded by reducing any tentorial herniation with a lumbar subarachnoid injection of normal saline or other physiological solution.[40] Anyone

who has surgically disimpacted a tentorial herniation, however, may be entitled to some skepticism that the measure is forceful enough to effect a significant reduction. Surgical exposure of cerebral aneurysms and certain tumors is often enhanced by drainage of cerebrospinal fluid at the time of operation. Repeated lumbar puncture is useful in the conservative management of cerebrospinal fluid rhinorrhea. Following surgery for cerebrospinal fluid fistula, its use may be helpful in insuring healing at the operative site by reducing intracranial pressure. The treatment of pseudotumor cerebri by the repeated removal of cerebrospinal fluid, once widely practiced, has been shown to be of limited value.[20]

CONTRAINDICATIONS TO LUMBAR PUNCTURE

Clinical evidence of increased intracranial pressure should give one thoughtful pause in making a decision to do lumbar puncture. When meningitis, encephalitis, or subarachnoid hemorrhage is suspected, the test is an absolute necessity. There are significant hazards in making a puncture when the elevated pressure is due to a space-taking or brain-displacing lesion. The decision must be carefully weighed in each instance, and if it is thought that risks are involved, one must be prepared to decompress the ventricles or institute definitive surgical therapy if necessary. Efforts have been made to show that lumbar puncture is safe in the routine investigation of all cases of suspected intracranial tumor,[39, 41] but this viewpoint is so contrary to our experience that we find it unacceptable. Lumbar puncture is an especially frequent prelude to tentorial herniation and death in acute encephalopathy of childhood, and a decision to proceed should be made with this in mind.

Lumbar puncture is rarely necessary following a craniocerebral injury. The presence of blood in the cerebrospinal fluid or an elevation of cerebrospinal fluid pressure will in no way aid in establishing a diagnosis of intracranial hematoma. The pressure at the lumbar level may not reflect an increase in intracranial pressure if herniated cerebellar tonsils occlude the subarachnoid

TABLE 10–1 *ANTIMICROBIAL THERAPEUTIC AGENTS FOR INTRATHECAL ADMINISTRATION**

DRUG	DOSAGE AND CONCENTRATION
Amphotericin B	0.5–1.0 mg in 10 ml CSF every second day
Bacitracin	Intrathecal or intraventricular, 500–5000 units daily, 1000 units per ml
Gentamicin	Intraventricular, 1 mg daily gives level of 3–5 μg/ml CSF
Penicillin G	5–10 ml daily, 1000 units/ml, intrathecal or intraventricular
Polymyxin B	Patient under 2 years, 2 mg daily or every second day
	Patient over 2 years, 5 mg daily or every second day
	Concentration, 0.5–1.0 mg/ml, intrathecal or intraventricular

*Modified from Kempe, H., and Yeager, A.: *In* Silver, H., Kempe, H., and Bruyn, H., (eds.): Handbook of Pediatrics. 8th Ed. Los Altos, Calif., Lange Medical Pubs., 1969.

space at the foramen magnum, and possibly fatal herniation may follow if cerebrospinal fluid is removed or if it leaks from the puncture site.

Occasionally need for examination of the cerebrospinal fluid following injury may occur later when there is suspicion that a compound injury may have led to a meningitic or other inflammatory process.

Any cutaneous or osseous infection in the lumbar area is an absolute contraindication to the insertion of a needle into the subarachnoid space at this level. This is a rare event, but should it exist and should there be need for analysis of cerebrospinal fluid, the specimen can be obtained by cisternal puncture.

TECHNIQUE OF LUMBAR PUNCTURE

The puncture is ordinarily made in the lateral recumbent position to insure the most accurate pressure determination. The patient's back should be at the edge of the bed or examining table, the vertebral spines parallel to its surface. If there is a dorsolumbar sag it may be corrected by placing a rolled towel or other support beneath the flank. The puncture site should be level with the foramen magnum, and the thighs should be flexed upon the trunk to reduce the lumbar lordosis and widen the interspinous spaces. Excessive flexion of the neck is unnecessary and may result in erroneous pressure measurements, particularly if there is spondylotic or other narrowing of the cervical spinal canal. In the corpulent patient, the sitting position is sometimes helpful since it allows more accurate identification of the spinous processes and interspaces. When there is scoliosis involving the lumbar area the sitting position is also advisable, and the procedure may be further facilitated if radiographs of the spine are examined. Any hair at the puncture site is shaved immediately before the procedure. The application of an organic iodine detergent completes the skin preparation. Aseptic surgical technique is essential.

The often-provided lumbar puncture drape that has an aperture in its midportion is unwieldy since it may easily be displaced and obscure anatomical landmarks or contaminate the sterile field. A folded towel paralleling the midline is an entirely adequate drape.

Any of the lower lumbar interspaces may be employed as a puncture site, but the L5–S1 level affords certain advantages over those more cephalad. Here the interspace is ordinarily wider, as is the arachnoid sac. The spinal canal is more superficially situated, and there are fewer nerve roots to be encountered by the needle tip. The tap should never be done above the L2–L3 interspace since the conus usually extends to the level immediately cephalad. In children and dwarfs the conus is more caudal and the L4 or L5 interspaces should be used. In a few patients the arachnoid sac may narrow significantly in the lower lumbar region or may terminate at an unusually high level to cause an occasional failure to obtain a successful puncture at the L5 space. The presence of a surgical spine fusion requires the use of a higher interspace. When the puncture is made in connection with myelography, the neurological signs may dictate the level of the puncture or the levels to be avoided.

An 18-, 20-, or 22-gauge needle with a well-fitting stylet may be used. If the needle is of the presterilized disposable variety, the possibility of bacterial or chemical contamination of the subarachnoid space is reduced. A new disposable needle should always be used when the intrathecal injection of a therapeutic, anesthetic, or radiographic diagnostic agent is to be made. When there is clinical evidence that intracranial pressure is increased, a 22-gauge needle should be used since it allows fluid to drain more slowly and creates a smaller hole in the arachnoid and dura. Manometric studies may, however, be more accurate when a larger needle is employed. It is generally easier to insert a large, fairly rigid cannula than a slender flexible one.

The intradermal and subcutaneous injection of a few milliliters of a local anesthetic agent reduces the discomfort associated with the introduction of the spinal needle. When the desired interspace is identified, the point at which the needle is to be introduced may be clearly demarcated by indenting the skin with a thumbnail. The needle should be directed exactly in the sagittal plane and slightly cephalad. Occasionally the point will encounter a spinous process or lamina on the first attempt. The needle should then be withdrawn until the tip is in the subcutaneous tissue and be re-inserted with a few degrees of cephalad or caudad adjustment in its direction. Further-more, it is advisable to release manual control of the needle after it has been ad-vanced a few millimeters into the inter-spinous ligament. If it is not then in the sagittal plane, a good puncture is unlikely and it is better to withdraw and reinsert the needle. Rotating the needle so that the bevel parallels the sagittal plane may allow the fibers of the dura to be separated longi-tudinally rather than incised transversely so that the opening will seal more readily.[21]

Often an audible or palpable "pop" will indicate that the dura has been penetrated, and advancing the needle another 2 or 3 mm will place its tip in the subarachnoid space. Further advancement is undesirable since perforation of the dura anteriorly may occur with resultant hemorrhage from an epidural vein that will contaminate the cerebrospinal fluid with blood. Too deep advancement of the needle may also pro-duce inaccurate pressure evaluation owing to the aperture of the needle being partially within and partially outside the arachnoid membrane. Frequently there is no audible or palpable evidence that the cannula has perforated the dura, and in these instances the stylet must be removed several times as the needle is slowly advanced to determine when it is fully within the subarachnoid space.

Once the subarachnoid space has been entered, it is essential that a minimum of cerebrospinal fluid escape before the Ayer manometer is attached to the needle by a three-way stopcock for the initial pressure determination. Firm abdominal compres-sion will ordinarily cause an elevation in the manometric column and thereby indicate that there is a patent communication be-tween the subarachnoid space and the manometer. Failure of the column to rise with abdominal compression is evidence that the needle aperture is not entirely within the subarachnoid space or is being partially occluded by apposition of a nerve root. Careful rotation, advancement, or withdrawal of the needle will ordinarily correct the obstruction. When the initial

pressure recording is made, the patient should be relaxed and the flexion of the thighs reduced. Straining or crying will re-sult in an abnormally high pressure reading.

THE LUMBAR MANOMETRIC TEST

As originally introduced by Quecken-stedt for the detection of spinal block, the examination consisted of observing the re-sponse of cerebrospinal fluid pressure fol-lowing manual jugular compression. At-tempts to standardize the test by timing and charting the rise and fall in pressure were made by Stookey and his colleagues, while Elsberg and Hare recorded the response to the inhalation of amyl nitrite.[25, 53] Measured and timed compression with a sphygmo-manometer was introduced by Grant and Cone.[29]

Normally, with bilateral jugular com-pression, when little or no cerebrospinal fluid has been allowed to escape, there is a prompt rise in intraspinal pressure to a figure 100 to 300 mm higher than the orig-inal pressure, with a prompt return to approximately the original figure when the compression is released. Manual compres-sion must be sufficient to occlude the veins effectively, but not so forceful as to ob-struct carotid blood flow. The use of the sphygmomanometer technique is more accurate and informative since varying reproducible pressures can be exerted and responses measured and recorded. Ini-tially the cuff is inflated to a pressure of 20 mm of mercury for 10 seconds, and the rate and extent of rise of spinal fluid pres-sure is observed. If indicated, observations may be made after inflation of the cuff to 40 to 60 mm levels. In normal circum-stances there is a rapid response to 20 mm compression. When a partially obstructive lesion is present, cerebrospinal fluid pres-sure rises slowly with application of even 40 to 60 mm of jugular compression, and there is no secondary elevation when the block is complete.

The Queckenstedt test should be done only when there is suspicion that a spinal subarachnoid block exists and is due to a tumor or vertebral fracture-dislocation. Too often it is carried out routinely and,

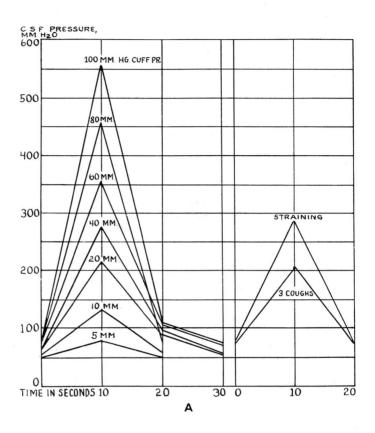

FIGURE 10–1 *A.* Graph obtained in patient with normal response to graduated and timed jugular compression. The initial pressure was 50 mm, and responses vary from 80 mm of water at a cuff pressure of 5 mm of mercury to 550 mm of water at a cuff pressure of 100 mm. *B.* Graph showing responses in a patient with a C5 fracture-dislocation. On the left is depicted the slight response (from 108 to 150 mm of water) from compression of the neck for 10 seconds by cuff pressures from 5 to 80 mm. As shown in the right half of the graph, however, the cerebrospinal fluid pressure rose promptly when the patient coughed or strained. (From Grant, W. T., and Cone, W. V.: Graduated jugular compression in the lumbar manometric test for spinal subarachnoid block. Arch. Neurol. Psychiat., *32*:1194, 1934.)

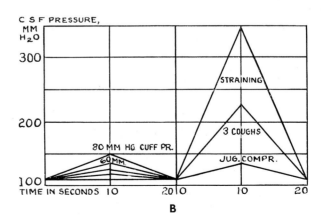

particularly if intracranial pressure is elevated, may be hazardous. When there is manometric evidence of obstruction to the movement of cerebrospinal fluid, it is often desirable to proceed directly with myelography. The indications for the manometric test are generally the same as for myelography, and the latter is a more definitive examination. In the past, the manometric test with unilateral jugular compression was employed in the diagnosis of transverse sinus thrombosis,[54] but its use in this instance has been replaced by improved angiographic techniques.

The Queckenstedt test is unreliable in the presence of a high cervical block because distention of epidural veins beneath the level of the lesion can produce a normal manometric response. Kaplan and Kennedy emphasized the variation in patency of the spinal canal in cervical spondylosis resulting from changes in position of the head.[34]

Because the casual measurement of cerebrospinal fluid pressure has given findings within the range of normal in patients suffering from communicating hydrocephalus, and because of the difficulty in separating these patients from those who have presenile dementia, Katzman and Hussey have devised a test of the absorptive capacity of the cerebrospinal fluid system.[18, 31, 35]

In this method, normal saline is infused at a constant rate two to three times the usual rate of formation of cerebrospinal fluid while the cerebrospinal fluid pressure is monitored. If the cerebrospinal fluid dynamics are normal the infused fluid will be readily absorbed, and there will be only a slight increase in cerebrospinal fluid pressure. In the presence of communicating hydrocephalus the capacity to absorb the infused fluid is impaired and the cerebrospinal fluid pressure rises more promptly and to a greater degree. The technique appears to be useful in the evaluation of communicating hydrocephalus in children and "occult" hydrocephalus in adults. It is of no value in the assessment of internal obstructive hydrocephalus.

COLLECTION OF FLUID

A specimen of cerebrospinal fluid is collected for study after initial pressure recordings are made. The amount of fluid removed is dependent upon the number and nature of diagnostic studies contemplated, but 5 to 10 ml is usually sufficient. Only a small sample of fluid may be needed to establish the diagnosis of subarachnoid hemorrhage or meningitis. The fluid is usually collected in two or three tubes. The specimen that is obtained first is occasionally bloody owing to injury to a vein by the needle. The fluid from such a "traumatic tap" usually becomes clear after a few milliliters has escaped while that in the presence of subarachnoid hemorrhage does not. The cell count should be made promptly since morphological change may occur if there is undue delay.

Before the needle is withdrawn a final pressure is recorded. The patient usually is directed to remain in bed with no elevation of the head for 12 to 24 hours following the examination, but he may be permitted to get up to use the bathroom.

COMPLICATIONS OF LUMBAR PUNCTURE

Herniation of the brain stem and uncus through the incisure of the tentorium or of the cerebellar tonsils into the foramen magnum are the most dire complications of the removal of the spinal fluid. Such herniation, which may result in fatal brain stem compression, is a rare complication and occurs most often when lumbar puncture is unwisely done in the presence of significantly increased intracranial pressure. This untoward event is much more likely to occur when the elevation of pressure is due to a mass lesion instead of to spontaneous subarachnoid hemorrhage or acute bacterial meningitis.

Postpuncture headache is the most common complication, occurring in approximately one fifth of all patients studied.[30] It usually appears during the first day and lasts for as long as a week. Rarely, it is of longer duration and may persist for several weeks. The cause is generally believed to be persistence of the opening in the meninges made by the needle with continuing leakage of fluid. Headache is ordinarily suboccipital, is always worse when the patient is in an erect position, and is usually promptly relieved when he becomes recumbent. It is less likely to follow puncture when a small needle is employed.[26, 55] When the patient lies in the prone position for several hours after the examination, the incidence of headache is reported to diminish.[21]

Meningitis or subdural or epidural abscess may occur when the puncture site is infected or the skin has been improperly prepared. Respiratory droplet contamination has been identified as another source of infection.[50] Chronic constrictive arachnoiditis following diagnostic lumbar puncture is virtually unknown, but it may, rarely, follow intrathecal injection of a therapeutic, diagnostic, or anesthetic substance. Ordinarily such an agent should not be introduced into the subarachnoid space if the cerebrospinal fluid contains blood, since arachnoidal reactions are more likely to occur under such circumstances.[32]

Removal of cerebrospinal fluid below a tumor or other process producing spinal cord compression may result in a prompt worsening of the signs of cord dysfunction and necessitate immediate operation. Intraspinal epidermoid tumors may appear years after the introduction of a fragment of skin by a spinal needle.[43] Such an event occurs more frequently when the needle has an ill-fitting stylet. Injury to the anulus fibrosus by a lumbar puncture needle has been implicated as an etiological factor in lumbar disc herniations.[19, 27] Transitory low back pain may result from the puncture, and irritation of a nerve rootlet by the advancing needle occasionally produces short-lived radiating pain or dysesthesia in the lower extremities.

Chronic subdural hematomas may follow traction injury to a superior cerebral vein. This complication is more common in the elderly and is ascribed to continuing leakage of cerebrospinal fluid with sagging of the brain and consequent avulsion of the vessel. Extraocular palsies may rarely follow removal of cerebrospinal fluid, the sixth nerve being involved more frequently than the others.[24, 49]

PROPERTIES AND COMPOSITION OF CEREBROSPINAL FLUID*

Pressure

The initial cerebrospinal fluid pressure, with the patient in the lateral position, is generally considered to range between 70 and 180 mm of water when a technically satisfactory puncture has been made. Tourtellotte and his associates, however, found these values to be somewhat higher in a series of normal subjects.[106] When the puncture is made with the patient sitting, the height of the fluid in the manometer reaches slightly above the level of the foramen magnum. The measured pressure, therefore, will vary with the height of the individual.

Excursions of the fluid with arterial pulse and respiratory movements indicate that the manometric system is open. The cerebrospinal fluid pulse is transmitted from the vessels of the choroid plexus, brain, and spinal cord, and removal of fluid will reduce the amplitude of pulsation.[62, 63, 68] Pressure changes with breathing reflect changes in venous pressure. The pressure may be elevated in hemorrhagic or inflammatory conditions of the meninges, expanding lesions of the brain (tumor, hemorrhage, abscess, infarction with swelling), conditions causing hydrocephalus, and those resulting in elevation of venous pressure. Pressure may also be increased during and after the administration of hypotonic solutions, the tetracyclines and excessive amounts of vitamin A, during general

TABLE 10–2 *COMPOSITION AND PROPERTIES OF NORMAL CEREBROSPINAL FLUID*

Pressure	70–180 mm water (lateral position)
Quantity (average adult)	140 ml
Specific gravity	1.007
Viscosity	1.05
Cells	0–5 lymphocytes or mononuclear cells
Protein	15–45 mg/100 ml
Glucose	60–75 mg/100 ml
Calcium	4.5–5.5 mg/100 ml
Chloride	120–130 mEq/L
Cholesterol	0.06–0.22 mg/100 ml
Creatinine	0.4–1.5 mg/100 ml
Magnesium	3.3 mg/100 ml
Potassium	3 mEq/L
Nonprotein nitrogen	12–30 mg/100 ml
Urea nitrogen	6–15 mg/100 ml

---

*The following pertains to the fluid in adults. The cerebrospinal fluid in infancy is dealt with separately.

anesthesia, and in the presence of fever. It may be reduced following an earlier lumbar puncture, beneath a foramen magnum or spinal block, during and after the intravenous infusion of hypertonic solutions, in the presence of hypothermia, and rarely spontaneously and unaccountably.

Appearance

The fluid is normally clear and colorless. Occasionally it may contain blood, owing to injury of a vessel by the needle. When this occurs the fluid will usually, but not invariably, become clear after a few milliliters have escaped. Fluid containing blood should be centrifuged immediately and the supernatant layer examined for yellow discoloration. It is only by examining for xanthochromia, which is due to the presence of hemoglobin from lysed cells or bilirubin, that fluid from a traumatic puncture can be distinguished from that obtained after subarachnoid hemorrhage. Varying degrees of turbidity may result from exudative reactions, and fluid with a high protein content may clot.

Quantity of Cerebrospinal Fluid

The average amount is usually estimated to be 140 ml. Half of this may be contained in the ventricles and intracranial subarachnoid spaces and the remainder in the spinal meninges. The amount is increased in hydrocephalus and the various atrophic processes.

The Ayala index, calculated by multiplying the final cerebrospinal fluid pressure by the amount removed and dividing by the initial pressure, gives an estimation of the volume of the cerebrospinal fluid reservoir.[57] The normal value is 5.5 to 6.5. A quotient above 7.0 indicates the reservoir is large, suggesting the presence of communicating hydrocephalus or an atrophic cerebral process. A value less than 5.0 suggests the reservoir is small, as occurs with an intracranial space-taking lesion or a spinal subarachnoid block. The test is no longer considered reliable and is rarely used.

Physical Properties

The specific gravity of cerebrospinal fluid is 1.007.[93, 101] Its viscosity relative to water is 1.05.[101]

Cells

Normal fluid may contain two or three, and rarely as many as five, lymphocytes. Polymorphonuclear leukocytes and other cells are not normally present. The cell contents of cerebrospinal fluid in various pathological states are summarized in Table 10–3. The cell count is made in a hemocytometer chamber immediately after the fluid has been removed. The fluid is ordinarily examined without dilution and the nine large squares counted (0.9 cu mm). Fluid containing extraordinarily large numbers of cells may be diluted, however. A differential count may be made from a stained film or may be made in the hemocytometer chamber, the cells having been stained with polychrome methylene blue.

Cytomorphological Studies

Although counting and identification of cells in the cerebrospinal fluid may be one of the least reliable laboratory studies carried out, in occasional instances identification of malignant tumor cells will obviate further useless diagnostic investigation or surgical treatment.

Tumors that may be diagnosed from cytomorphological examination of the cerebrospinal fluid with a high degree of accuracy are disseminated carcinomas, meningeal melanoblastosis, and medulloblastomas.[85] Diagnosis of certain other neoplasms can be made with less reliability. These include choroid plexus papillomas, glioblastomas, ependymomas, and lymphomas.[85] Intra-axial gliomas, meningiomas, and neurinomas do not shed cells into the cerebrospinal fluid and cannot be identified through such cytological examination.[85, 104]

Marks and Marrack have established the following criteria for identification of malignant cells in cerebrospinal fluid: (1)

The cells should not be those found in normal cerebrospinal fluid or in infection; (2) they are usually more than 20 μ in diameter; (3) they form syncytia; (4) they usually contain more than two nuclei and nucleoli; (5) the nucleus to cytoplasm ratio is high; and (6) active mitoses are common.[90] No single criterion is pathognomonic, and it must be remembered that fluid with a normal cell count may contain abnormal cells.

When only a qualitative assay of abnormal cerebrospinal fluid cells is needed the controlled diffusion technique of Kolar is satisfactory.[85] When accurate differential cell counts are desired the more precise method described by Tourtellotte should be employed.[105] Prompt examination of the fluid is necessary to prevent lysis of the cells. If the cerebrospinal fluid protein is significantly elevated, an anticoagulant should be added to prevent attraction of the cells to the fibrin clot that may result.

Herndon has recently described a method of preparation of cerebrospinal fluid sediment for examination with the electron microscope.[78] His investigation shows that both normal and pathological cells undergo remarkably little distortion with ultra-centrifugation. Although it has not been thoroughly developed, the technique obviously has great potential value.

Solutes

In contrast to plasma, the fluid is poor in protein. Compared to a dialysate of plasma, it is rich in sodium, chloride, and magnesium, but is deficient in potassium, calcium, phosphate, urea, glucose, and amino acids.

Glucose

In human cerebrospinal fluid the concentration of glucose is approximately four fifths that of plasma. When the concentration in plasma is changed, some time is required before the response in the fluid approaches completion. The relative deficiency in the fluid is maintained over a range of plasma concentrations. Experimental studies of the movement of sugars from plasma into the brain have shown selectivity and, for several, saturation and mutual competition.[66, 69, 72, 73, 84, 87, 95] It is believed, therefore, that the transport is carrier mediated. For mixed cerebrospinal fluid similar features have been shown and may, to a large extent, reflect the movement into the brain.[64, 70] Additionally, there is an independent control by the choroid plexus as new fluid is secreted.[100]

From the clinical viewpoint the most interesting feature is the reduced concentration of glucose encountered in bacterial meningitis, diffuse leptomeningeal spread of malignant tumors, and in some instances of subarachnoid hemorrhage.[60, 74, 89, 96, 99, 108] It was assumed for years that in bacterial meningitis the sugar was consumed by bacteria. Then Goldring and Harford showed quantitatively that such consumption could not account for the finding.[74] They measured the rate of decline of glucose due to utilization by leukocytes in fluid removed in experimentally produced aseptic meningitis and found that, in order to produce comparable rates, pneumococci in numbers unheard of in meningeal infection were required. It has been established that there is synergy between bacteria and leukocytes in that phagocytizing white cells utilize glucose at an increased rate.[96] After the establishment of an aseptic meningitis in which glucose levels are maintained, a fall in concentration could be produced by the introduction of organisms or bacterial endotoxin.[96] Recently Prockop and Fishman have studied the question of glucose transport in experimental meningitis.[98] They found impairment in the carrier mediated system, but an increased permeability to entry by diffusion; the net effect of the change could not, however, account for the lowering of glucose concentration. It has recently been suggested that an increased rate of glycolysis by the brain might account for the observed phenomena.[92]

Protein

With certain exceptions, cerebrospinal fluid proteins are qualitatively similar to plasma proteins. Total protein levels vary

TABLE 10-3   *CEREBROSPINAL FLUID SYNDROMES*

CONDITION	PRESSURE	APPEARANCE	CELLS	PROTEIN	GLUCOSE	SPECIAL FEATURES
Normal CSF	70–180 with patient in lateral position	Clear and colorless	0–5 lymphocytes or mononuclear cells	15–45 mg/100 ml	50–80 mg/100 ml	When puncture is done in sitting position, pressure rises to slightly above level of foramen magnum
Normal newborn	Normal to slight increase	Often slightly hemorrhagic or xanthochromic	Several thousand RBC's and 100–200 WBC's	45/100 mg/100 ml	Normal to slight increase	Cellular and protein abnormalities are increased in premature infants
Intracranial tumor	Slight to marked elevation	Usually clear and colorless	Normal to slight increase	Normal to moderate increase	Usually normal Decreased in meningeal carcinomatosis	Pathological cells may be present in metastatic and certain primary malignant tumors Protein particularly increased in acoustic neurinomas and in tumors involving meninges
Intracranial abscess	Slight to great elevation	Clear and colorless Opalescent to purulent if abscess ruptures	Normal to extreme leukocytosis	Normal to marked increase	Normal to reduction with meningeal involvement	Findings in encapsulated abscess may be normal As abscess nears meninges or ruptures into subarachnoid space cell count increases, sugar declines, culture may be positive and bacteria may be identified on smear Cells mainly poly's
Cerebral infarction	Normal to marked increase	Usually clear and colorless	Normal to minimal increase	Normal to minimal increase	Normal	Pressure elevation varies with size of infarct In hemorrhagic infarcts near ependymal or meningeal surfaces, fluid may be slightly bloody and leukocyte count increased
Chronic subdural hematoma	Increased to subnormal	May be xanthochromic	Normal to slight increase	Normal to slight increase	Normal	Lumbar puncture of little value in establishing diagnosis; may be hazardous Pressure determinations unreliable; lumbar CSF pressure may be low
Spontaneous subarachnoid hemorrhage	Normal to extreme elevation (above 600 ml water)	Pink to grossly bloody Rarely clear on first puncture	RBC's moderately to greatly elevated (3,000,000) WBC's elevated	Elevated proportionate to RBC content	Normal to marked reduction	Fluid uniformly bloody in all specimens Supernatant fluid xanthochromic WBC's increase with severity of hemorrhage Marked leukocytosis may persist when RBC absorption nears completion
Benign intracranial hypertension	Moderate to marked increase (300–600 ml water)	Clear and colorless	Usually normal Slight leukocytosis may occur	Normal to slight increase	Normal	Dural sinus thrombosis, obesity, hypoparathyroidism, and chronic pulmonary insufficiency may be etiologic factors Tumor must be excluded by angiography and ventriculography
Lead encephalopathy	Slight to marked increase	Clear and colorless	Normal to moderate increase	Normal to moderate elevation	Normal	Cells are lymphocytes Lead may be qualitatively identified in CSF
Intraspinal tumor	Normal or reduced	Clear and colorless to profound xanthochromia	Normal to slight increase. Occasional subarachnoid hemorrhage	Normal to marked increase	Normal	Protein content depends largely upon degree of subarachnoid space block; is elevated to plasma levels in complete obstruction Clotting may occur in marked protein elevation
Meningeal carcinomatosis	Slight to moderate increase	Normal to increased viscosity May be slightly opalescent or xanthochromic	Leukocytosis to 500–1000 Tumor cells may be present	Slight to marked increase	Normal to marked reduction	Diagnosis suspected from leukocytosis, increased protein, and hypoglycorrhachia; confirmed by recovery of malignant cells

TABLE 10–3 *CEREBROSPINAL FLUID SYNDROMES (Continued)*

CONDITION	PRESSURE	APPEARANCE	CELLS	PROTEIN	GLUCOSE	SPECIAL FEATURES
Herniated intervertebral disc and spondylosis	Normal except in subarachnoid space block	Clear and colorless Xanthochromic beneath complete block	Usually normal	Normal to slight increase Rarely above 100 mg/100 ml	Normal	Clinical findings and myelography confirm diagnosis; CSF usually obtained at myelography Greater protein values beneath complete block
Acute bacterial meningitis	Moderate to great increase	Variable Clear, opalescent, milky, to grossly purulent Clot may form	Marked increase to 10,000–50,000 Largely polymorphonuclears	Moderate to marked increase	Moderate to profound reduction	Bacteria may be seen on smear and identified from culture CSF changes may be used as monitor of effectiveness of treatment With therapy there is relative increase of lymphocytes and mononuclear cells
Tuberculous meningitis	Slight to moderate elevation	Clear to opalescent Pellicle may form	Slight to moderate leukocytosis (5000)	Moderate increase Occasionally to 500 mg/100 ml	Moderate reduction 30–40 mg/100 ml	Cells mainly lymphocytes Chlorides may be reduced Organism may be identified on stained smear; diagnosis must ordinarily be confirmed by culture or animal innoculation
Viral meningoencephalitic infections	Normal to moderate elevation	Clear and colorless	Slight to moderate increase Rarely more than 1000	Normal to slight increase (100 mg/100 ml)	Normal	Cellular response predominantly lymphocytic Virus may be identified by culture; clinical course usually completed before nature of virus is established
Aseptic meningeal reactions	Slight to marked elevation	Ordinarily clear and colorless	Slight to great increase Mainly lymphocytes	Slight to moderate increase Rarely more than 150 mg/100 ml	Normal	Occur following intrathecal injection of diagnostic, therapeutic, or anesthetic agents, with cerebral infarction or venous sinus thrombosis, and in presence of perimeningeal infection
Multiple sclerosis	Normal	Clear and colorless	Slight increase in acute exacerbation Rarely more than 50	Normal to slight increase	Normal	Gamma globulin protein fraction often increased in acute exacerbations Colloidal gold curve change parallels increase in gamma globulin Cells are lymphocytes
Infectious polyneuritis (Landry-Guillain-Barré)	Normal to slight increase	Usually clear and colorless	Usually normal	Moderate to marked increase to 1000 mg/100 ml	Normal	All protein fractions elevated; gamma globulin often disproportionately increased
Diabetes mellitus.	Normal	Clear and colorless	Normal	Slight to moderate elevation	Increased Varies with severity of disease and adequacy of control	Diabetic neuropathy may simulate disc lesions, spondylosis with neurological involvement, or polyneuritis; often must be excluded by myelography and metabolic studies
Early syphilitic infections	Normal to minimal elevation	Clear and colorless	Slight to moderate increase (100–1000)	Normal to slight increase	Normal	Cellular response lymphocytic Wassermann and TPI reactions positive Gamma globulin fraction may be elevated
Meningovascular syphilis	Normal to moderate increase	Clear to slightly turbid	Increased to 100–500, occasionally to 1000–2000	Slight to moderate elevation	Normal	Both lymphocytes and polymorphonuclears seen Gamma globulin increased; all phases of gold curve elevated Serologic tests positive
Treated luetic infections	Ordinarily normal	Clear and colorless	Normal to minimal increase (lymphocytes)	Normal to slight elevation	Normal	Positive serological and gold curve changes may persist Gamma globulin fraction may remain somewhat elevated

from 15 to 45 mg per 100 ml.[93] Ventricular or cisternal fluid has a lower protein content, but, except for the higher prealbumin fraction, it is similar to fluid obtained at lumbar puncture.

Total protein levels, as noted previously, are elevated in a variety of pathological conditions. Abnormality of the blood–cerebrospinal fluid barrier and the blood–brain barrier associated with various infections, tumors, trauma, and hemorrhage may result in an increased protein content. Elevated levels are found below a spinal subarachnoid space obstruction, in several forms of polyneuritis, sometimes in diabetes, and in hypoparathyroidism.

The Pandy test is a quick and convenient method of obtaining qualitative information that the protein level is elevated. The test is conducted by adding a drop of cerebrospinal fluid by pipette to a saturated phenol solution in a watch glass. When the protein content is significantly increased, a heavy cloud of precipitated protein appears. A faint cloud occurs with normal protein values.

Electrophoresis of Cerebrospinal Fluid Proteins

Electrophoresis of cerebrospinal fluid indicates that its proteins are similar to those found in serum. Since cerebrospinal fluid is so dilute, however, it must be concentrated in order to be analyzed by such techniques as electrophoresis on paper, cellulose acetate, or acrylamide. This requires a rather large amount of fluid and, therefore, electrophoresis is not a routine laboratory procedure. In general, plasma proteins appear in cerebrospinal fluid in proportion to their concentration in serum, with restriction of those of greater molecular weight.[88] Therefore, cerebrospinal fluid contains virtually no high molecular weight proteins such as low-density lipoproteins, macroglobulins, or high molecular weight haptoglobin.[83] In addition, the prealbumin fraction of serum is present in relatively large concentrations in the cerebrospinal fluid.[83] The existence of proteins peculiar to cerebrospinal fluid has been both affirmed and denied.

Gamma Globulin Determination in Multiple Sclerosis, Neurosyphilis, and Subacute Sclerosing Panencephalitis

In 1942 Kabat and his co-workers published the first of a series of papers indicating that the gamma globulin fraction of the cerebrospinal fluid protein was elevated in many patients with multiple sclerosis or luetic infections of the nervous system.[81, 82, 83] Subsequent investigations have shown that the gamma globulin fraction is increased only occasionally in the other demyelinating diseases.[103] The Landry-Guillain-Barré syndrome may be accompanied by an abnormally high gamma globulin content along with a markedly raised total protein. Other neurological states producing an increase in the gamma globulin fraction are subacute sclerosing panencephalitis and neuromyelitis optica.[58, 67, 76] The latter is frequently an initial manifestation of multiple sclerosis rather than a disease entity.

The quantitative precipitin method devised by Kabat is complicated, time-consuming, and expensive. Hartley, Merrill, and Claman, in 1966, described a cheaper, simpler, and faster electroimmunodiffusion technique for gamma globulin assay.[77] This method has provided a simple and reliable confirmatory test in suspected cases of multiple sclerosis or neurosyphilis. A gamma globulin fraction that is increased above 14 per cent in an adult, in the presence of a normal total protein value, is strong substantiating evidence for a diagnosis of multiple sclerosis or neurosyphilis.[103] On the other hand, recent studies suggest that a gamma globulin value of 10 per cent of the total protein may be abnormal in a young child suspected of having a demyelinating disease.[94]

Other methods of gamma globulin determination have been employed with varying percentages of gamma globulin being considered abnormal.* These figures range from 10 per cent when the filter paper electrophoresis technique is used, to 29 per cent with the colorimetric zinc sulfate method. Certain of these techniques are not specific for gamma globulin and are generally less

---

*See references 61, 65–76, 80, 81, 86, 97, 102, 107, 111, and 112.

accurate than the electroimmunodiffusion or quantitative precipitin methods.

In general, an elevation in the gamma globulin protein fraction parallels an abnormality in the colloidal gold curve.

CEREBROSPINAL FLUID IN EARLY INFANCY

The composition of cerebrospinal fluid that is considered normal in childhood and adult life is not reached until 3 to 6 months of age. In the newborn some degree of xanthochromia is not abnormal.[75, 79, 110] There are ordinarily several thousand red cells and up to several tens of white cells per cubic millimeter.[75, 79] These features seem to be independent of birth weight, but the total protein, which is considerably higher than is normal in adults, is correlated negatively with birth weight.[56, 59, 75, 79] The following values may be considered normal: adults, 15 to 45 mg per 100 ml; fullterm newborns, 45 to 100 mg per 100 ml; premature infants, a mean of 180 with higher values for birth weight less than 1500 gm.[59]

The character of the protein, as shown by electrophoresis, is similar to that in the adult fluid.[56]

Although its significance is not completely understood, the difference between the fluid in infancy and that in the more mature has been attributed to the incomplete development of the blood–brain barrier.[56, 109]

REFERENCES

Historical and General

1. Adams, R. D.: Cerebrospinal fluid. *In* Page, L. B., and Culver, P. J., eds.: A Syllabus of Laboratory Examinations in Clinical Diagnosis. Cambridge, Harvard University Press, 1961.
2. Corning, J. L.: Spinal anesthesia and local medication of the cord. New York Med. J., *42*: 483, 1885.
3. Davson, H.: Physiology of the Cerebrospinal Fluid. Boston, Little, Brown and Co., 1967.
4. Fishman, R. A.: Cerebrospinal fluid. *In* Baker, A. B., ed.: Clinical Neurology. New York, Hoeber Medical Div., Harper & Row, 1962, pp. 350–384.
5. Froin, G.: Inflammations méningées avec reactions chromatique, fibrineuse, et cytologique

du liquide céphalorachidien. Gaz. Hôp., *76*: 1005, 1903.
6. Fürbringer, P.: Zur klinischen Bedeutung der spinalen Punction. Berlin. Klin. Wschr., *32*: 272, 1895.
7. Merritt, H., and Fremont-Smith, F.: The Cerebrospinal Fluid. Philadelphia, W. B. Saunders Co., 1937.
8. Mestrezat, W.: Le liquide céphalorachidien normal et pathologique. Paris, A. Maloine, 1912.
9. Morton, C. A.: The pathology of tuberculous meningitis, with reference to its treatment by tapping the subarachnoid space of the spinal cord. Brit. Med. J., 2:840, 1891.
10. Queckenstedt, H.: Zur Diagnose der Rückenmark-kompression. Deutsch. Z. Nervenheilk, 55:325, 1916.
11. Quincke, H.: Die Lumbalpunction des Hydrocephalus. Berlin. Klin. Wschr., 28:929, 965, 1891.
12. Schaltenbrand, G., and Wolff, H.: Die Produktion und Zirkulation des Liquors und Ihre Störung. *In* Olivecrona, H., and Tönnis, W., eds.: Handbuch der Neurochirurgie. Berlin, Springer-Verlag, 1959, pp. 91–207.
13. Schmidt, R. M., ed.: Der Liquor Cerebrospinalis. Berlin, Verlag Volk und Gesundheit, 1968.
14. Spriggs, A. I., and Boddington, M. M.: The Cytology of Effusions and of Cerebrospinal Fluid. 2nd Ed., London, William Heineman, 1968.
15. Wassermann, A., Neisser, A., and Bruck, C.: Eine serodiagnostische Reaktion bei Syphilis. Deutsch. Med. Wschr., 32:745, 1906.
16. Widal, F., Sicard, J., and Ravaut, P.: Cytologie du liquide céphalorachidien. Au cours de quelques processus méningés chroniques (paralysie generale et tables). Bull. Soc. Méd. Hôp. Paris (S. 3) *18*:31, 1901.
17. Wynter, W. E.: Four cases of tubercular meningitis in which paracentesis of the theca vertebralis was performed for the relief of fluid pressure. Lancet, *1*:981, 1891.

Indications, Technique, Complications

18. Adams, R. D., Fisher, C. M., Hakim, S., et al.: Symptomatic occult-hydrocephalus with "normal" cerebrospinal-fluid pressure. A treatable syndrome. N. Eng. J. Med., *273*:117, 1965.
19. Baker, A. H.: Lesions of the intervertebral disc caused by lumbar puncture. Brit. J. Surg., *34*:385, 1947.
20. Bradshaw, P.: Benign intracranial hypertension. J. Neurol. Neurosurg. Psychiat., *19*:28, 1956.
21. Brocher, R. J.: Technique to avoid spinal puncture headache. J.A.M.A., *168*:261, 1958.
22. Bronsky, D., Schrifter, H., De La Huerga, J., et al.: Cerebrospinal fluid proteins in myxedema with special reference to electrophoretic partition. J. Clin. Endocr., *18*:470, 1958.
23. D'Angio, G. J., French, L., Stadlan, E. M., et al.: Intrathecal radioisotopes for the treatment of brain tumors. Clin. Neurosurg., *15*:288, 1968.
24. Dottner, B., and Thomas, E. W.: Bilateral ab-

ducens palsy following lumbar puncture. New York J. Med., *41*:1660, 1941.

25. Elsberg, C. A., and Hare, C. C.: A new and simplified manometric test for the determination of spinal subarachnoid block by means of inhalation of nitrite of amyl. Bull. Neurol. Inst. N. Y., *2*:347, 1932.

26. Fishman, R. A.: Cerebrospinal fluid. *In* Baker, A. B., ed.: Clinical Neurology. New York, Hoeber Medical Div., Harper & Row, 1962, pp. 350–384.

27. Gellman, M.: Injury to intervertebral discs during spinal puncture. J. Bone Joint Surg., *22*:980, 1940.

28. Goodman, J. L., Baumoel, S., Frankel, L., et al.: The Diabetic Neuropathies. Springfield, Ill., Charles C Thomas, 1953.

29. Grant, W. T., and Cone, W. V.: Graduated jugular compression in the lumbar manometric test for spinal subarachnoid block. Arch. Neurol. Psychiat., *32*:1194, 1934.

30. Grinker, R. R., and Sahs, A. L.: Neurology. 6th Ed. Springfield, Ill., Charles C Thomas, 1966.

31. Hill, M. E., Lougheed, W. M., and Barnett, H. J. M.: A treatable form of dementia due to normal-pressure communicating hydrocephalus. Canad. Med. Ass. J., *97*:1309, 1967.

32. Howland, W. J., and Curry, J. L.: Pantopaque arachnoiditis. Experimental study of blood as a potentiating agent and corticosteroids as an ameliorating agent. Acta Radiol., *5*(special suppl. Seventh Symp. Neuroradiol.)1032, 1966.

33. Ives, R.: Protein content of the cerebrospinal fluid in diabetic patients. Bull. Los Angeles Neurol. Soc., *22*:95, 1957.

34. Kaplan, L., and Kennedy, F.: The effect of head posture on the manometrics of cerebrospinal fluid in cervical lesions: A new diagnostic test. Brain, *73*:337, 1950.

35. Katzman, R., and Hussey, F.: A simple constant-infusion manometric test for measurement of CSF absorption. I. Rationale and method. Neurology, *20*:534, 1970.

36. Kempe, H., and Yeager, A.: Modified from Silver, H., Kempe, H., and Bruyn, H., eds.: Handbook of Pediatrics. 8th Ed. Los Altos, Calif., Lange Medical Pubs., 1969.

37. Kerr, F. W. L., Schwartz, H. G., and Seaman, W. B.: Experimental effects of radioactive colloidal gold in the subarachnoid space: Clinical applications in treating brain tumor. Arch. Surg., *69*:694, 1954.

38. Kieffer, S. A., Stadlan, E. M., and D'Angio, G. J.: Anatomic studies of the distribution and effects of intrathecal radioactive gold. Acta Radiol., *8*:27, 1969.

39. Korein, J., Cravioto, H., and Leicach, M.: Reevaluation of lumbar puncture: A study of 129 patients with papilledema or intracranial hypertension. Neurology, *9*:290, 1959.

40. LaLonde, A. A., and Gardner, W. J.: Chronic subdural hematoma. Expansion of compressed cerebral hemisphere and relief of hypotension by spinal injection of physiologic saline solution. New Eng. J. Med., *239*:493, 1948.

41. Lubic, L. G., and Marotta, J. T.: Brain tumor and lumbar puncture. Arch. Neurol. Psychiat., *72*:568, 1954.

42. Maher, R. M.: Further experience with intrathecal and subdural phenol. Lancet, *1*:805, 1960.

43. Manno, N. J., Uihlein, A., and Kernohan, J. W.: Intraspinal epidermoids. J. Neurosurg., *19*: 754, 1962.

44. Mark, V. H., White, J. C., Zervas, N. T., et al.: Intrathecal use of phenol for the relief of chronic severe pain. New Eng. J. Med., *267*: 589, 1962.

45. Meredith, J. M.: The inefficacy of lumbar puncture for the removal of red blood cells from the cerebrospinal fluid. Surgery, *9*:524, 1941.

46. Nathan, P. W.: Intrathecal phenol to relieve spasticity in paraplegia. Lancet, *2*:1099, 1959.

47. Nathan, P. W., and Scott, T. G.: Intrathecal phenol for intractable pain: Safety and dangers of the method. Lancet, *1*:78, 1958.

48. Newton, W. A., Jr., Sayers, M. P., and Samuels, L. D.: Intrathecal methotrexate (NSC-740) therapy for brain tumors in children. Cancer Chemother. Rep., *52*:257, 1968.

49. Robinson, H. M., Jr.: Abducens palsy (with subsequent recovery) following lumbar puncture. Amer. J. Syph., *29*:422, 1945.

50. Rose, H. D.: Pneumococcal meningitis following intrathecal injections. Arch. Neurol., *14*:597, 1966.

51. Sayers, M. P.: Intrathecal methotrexate therapy of brain tumors of childhood. Ohio Med. J., *65*:383, 1969.

52. Sprong, W.: The disappearance of blood from the cerebrospinal fluid in traumatic subarachnoid hemorrhage. The ineffectiveness of repeated lumbar punctures. Surg. Gynec. Obstet., *58*:705, 1934.

53. Stookey, B., Merwarth, H. R., and Frantz, A. M.: A manometric study of the cerebrospinal fluid in suspected spinal cord tumors. Ass. Res. Nerv. Ment. Dis. Proc., IV. The Human Cerebrospinal Fluid. New York, Hoeber, 1926, p. 185.

54. Tobey, G. L., and Ayer, J. B.: Dynamic studies on the cerebrospinal fluid in the differential diagnosis of lateral sinus thrombosis. Arch. Otolaryng., *2*:50, 1925.

55. Wetchler, B. V., and Brace, D. E.: A technique to minimize the occurrence of headache after lumbar puncture by the use of small bore spinal needles. Anesthesiology, *16*:270, 1955.

Properties and Composition of Cerebrospinal Fluid

56. Arnhold, R. G., and Zetterström, R.: Proteins in the cerebrospinal fluid in the newborn. Pediatrics, *21*:279, 1958.

57. Ayala, G.: Ueber den diagnostischen Wert des Liquordruckes und Einer Apparat zu Seiner Messung. Z. Ges. Neurol. Psychiat., *84*:42, 1923.

58. Bauer, H.: Cerebrospinal fluid findings in panencephalitis. *In* Boegaert, L., et al., eds.: Encephalitides. Amsterdam, Elsevier, 1961, pp. 675–680.

59. Bauer, C. H., New, I., and Miller, J. M.: Cerebrospinal fluid protein values of premature infants. J. Pediat., *66*:1017, 1965.

60. Berg, L.: Hypoglycorrhacia of non-infectious origin: Diffuse meningeal neoplasia. Neurology, *3*:811, 1953.

61. Bergmann, L., Gilland, O., Olanders, S., et al.: Clinical profile and paper electrophoresis in multiple sclerosis. Acta Neurol. Scand., *40*: suppl. 10:33, 1964.

62. Bering, E. A., Jr.: Choroid plexus and arterial pulsation of cerebrospinal fluid. Demonstration of the choroid plexuses as a cerebrospinal fluid pump. Arch. Neurol. Psychiat., *73*:165, 1955.

63. Bering, E. A., Jr.: Circulation of the cerebrospinal fluid. Demonstration of the choroid plexuses as the generator of the force for flow of fluid and ventricular enlargement. J. Neurosurg., *19*:405, 1962.

64. Bito, L. Z., and Davson, H.: Local variations in cerebrospinal fluid composition and its relationship to the composition of the extracellular fluid of the cortex. Exp. Neurol., *14*:264, 1966.

65. Bradshaw, P.: The relation between clinical activity and the level of gamma globulin in the cerebrospinal fluid in patients with multiple sclerosis. J. Neurol. Sci., *1*:347, 1964.

66. Crone, C.: Facilitated transfer of glucose from blood into brain tissue. J. Physiol. (London), *181*:103, 1965.

67. Cutler, R. W. P., Watter, G. V., Hammerstad, J. P., et al.: Origin of cerebrospinal fluid gamma globulin in subacute sclerosing leukoencephalitis. Arch. Neurol., *17*:620, 1967.

68. Dunbar, H. S., Guthrie, T. C., and Karpell, B.: A study of the cerebrospinal fluid pulse wave. Arch. Neurol., *14*:624, 1966.

69. Eidelberg, E., Fishman, J., and Hams, M. L.: Penetration of sugars across the blood–brain barrier. J. Physiol. (London), *191*:47, 1967.

70. Fishman, R. A.: Carrier transport of glucose between blood and cerebrospinal fluid. Amer. J. Physiol., *206*:836, 1964.

71. Foster, J. B., and Horn, D. B.: Multiple sclerosis and spinal-fluid gamma globulin. Brit. Med. J., *1*:1527, 1962.

72. Geiger, A.: Correlation of brain metabolism and function by the use of a brain perfusion method in situ. Physiol. Rev., *38*:1, 1958.

73. Geiger, A., Magnes, J., Taylor, R. M., et al.: Effect of blood constituents on uptake of glucose and on metabolic rate of the brain in perfusion experiments. Amer. J. Physiol., *177*:138, 1954.

74. Goldring, S., and Harford, C. G.: Effects of leucocytes and bacteria on glucose content of cerebrospinal fluid in meningitis. Proc. Soc. Exp. Biol. Med., *75*:669, 1950.

75. Gyllens--ward, Å., and Malmström, S.: The cerebrospinal fluid of newborn infants. Acta Paediat., *135*:suppl., 54, 1962.

76. Harter, D. H., Yahr, M. D., and Kabat, E. A.: Neurological diseases with elevation of cerebrospinal fluid gamma globulin: A critical review. Trans. Amer. Neurol. Ass., *87*:120, 1962.

77. Hartley, T. F., Merrill, D. A., and Claman,

H. N.: Quantitation of immunoglobulins in cerebrospinal fluid. Arch. Neurol., *15*:472, 1966.

78. Herndon, R., and Johnson, M.: A method for the electron microscopic study of cerebrospinal fluid sediment. J. Neuropath. Exper. Neurol., *29*:320, 1970.

79. Hoepffner, L., and Wolf, H.: Liquordiagnostik bei Neu- and Frühegeborenen. Mschr. Kinderheilk., *107*:435, 1959.

80. Ivers, R. R., McKenzie, B. F., McGuckin, W. F., et al.: Spinal fluid gamma globulin in multiple sclerosis and other neurologic diseases: Electrophoretic patterns in 606 patients. J.A.M.A., *176*:515, 1961.

81. Kabat, E. A., Freedman, D. A., Murray, J. P., et al.: A study of the crystalline albumin, gamma globulin, and total protein in the cerebrospinal fluid of one hundred cases of multiple sclerosis and in other diseases. Amer. J. Med. Sci., *219*:55, 1950.

82. Kabat, E. A., Glusman, M., and Knaub, V.: Quantitative estimation of the albumin and gamma-globulin in normal and pathologic cerebrospinal fluid by immunochemical methods. Amer. J. Med., *4*:653, 1948.

83. Kabat, E. A., Moore, D. H., and Landow, H.: An electrophoretic study of the protein components in cerebrospinal fluid and their relationship to the serum proteins. J. Clin. Invest., *21*:571, 1942.

84. Klein, J. R., Hurwitz, R., and Olsen, N. S.: Distribution of intravenously injected fructose and glucose between blood and brain. J. Biol. Chem., *164*:509, 1946.

85. Kolar, O., and Zeman, W.: Spinal fluid cytomorphology. Arch. Neurol., *18*:44, 1968.

86. Laterre, E. C.: Les gammaglobulines du liquide céphalorachidiene dans la sclérose en plaques. Acta Neurol., *66*:305, 1966.

87. LeFevre, P. G., and Peters, A. A.: Evidence of mediated transfer of monosaccharides from blood to brain in rodents. J. Neurochem., *13*:35, 1966.

88. Lemmen, L. J., Newman, N. A., and DeJong, R. N.: Study of cerebrospinal fluid proteins with paper electrophoresis: I. A review of the literature. Univ. Mich. Med. Bull., *23*:3, 1957.

89. Madonick, M. J., and Saviosky, N.: Spinal fluid sugar in subarachnoid hemorrhage. J. Nerv. Ment. Dis., *108*:45, 1948.

90. Marks, V., and Marrack, D.: Tumor cells in the cerebrospinal fluid. J. Neurol. Neurosurg. Psychiat., *23*:194, 1960.

91. Masserman, J. H.: Cerebrospinal fluid hydrodynamics. IV. Clinical experimental studies. Arch. Neurol. Psychiat., *32*:523, 1934.

92. Menkes, J. H.: The causes for low spinal fluid sugar in bacterial meningitis: Another look. Pediatrics, *44*:1, 1969.

93. Merritt, H., and Fremont-Smith, F.: The Cerebrospinal Fluid. Philadelphia, W. B. Saunders Co., 1937.

94. Nellhaus, G.: Personal communication. December, 1969.

95. Park, C. R., Johnson, L. H., Wright, J. H., Jr.,

et al.: Effect of insulin on transport of several hexoses and pentoses into cells of muscle and brain. Amer. J. Physiol., *191*:13, 1957.

96. Petersdorf, R. G., and Harter, D. H.: The fall in cerebrospinal fluid sugar in meningitis. Arch. Neurol., *4*:21, 1961.

97. Prineas, J., Teasdale, G., Latner, A. L., et al.: Spinal-fluid gamma-globulin and multiple sclerosis. Brit. Med. J., *2*:922, 1966.

98. Prockop, L. D., and Fishman, R. A.: Experimental pneumococcal meningitis. Arch. Neurol., *19*:449, 1968.

99. Rogers, D. E., and McDermott, W.: Neoplastic involvement of the meninges with low cerebrospinal fluid glucose concentrations simulating tuberculous meningitis. Amer. Rev. Tuberc., *69*:1029, 1954.

100. Sadler, K., and Welch, K.: Concentration of glucose in new choroidal cerebrospinal fluid of the rabbit. Nature (London), *215*:884, 1967.

101. Schaltenbrand, G., and Wolff H.: Die Produktion und Zirkulation des Liquors und Ihre Störungen. *In* Olivecrona, H., and Tönnis, W., eds.: Handbuch der Neurochirurgie. Berlin, Springer-Verlag, 1959, pp. 91–207.

102. Schapira, K., and Park, D. C.: Gamma globulin studies in multiple sclerosis and their application to the problem of diagnosis. J. Neurol. Nurosurg. Psychiat., *24*:121, 1961.

103. Schneck, S. A., and Claman, H. N.: CSF immunoglobulins in multiple sclerosis and other neurological diseases. Arch. Neurol., *20*:132, 1969.

104. Spriggs, A. I., and Boddington, M. M.: The Cytology of Effusions and of Cerebrospinal Fluid. 2nd Ed. London, William Heinemann, Ltd., 1968.

105. Tourtellotte, W. W.: A selected review of reactions of the cerebrospinal fluid to disease. *In* Fields, W. S., ed.: Neurological Diagnostic Techniques. Thirteenth Annual Houston Neurological Scientific Symposium. Springfield, Ill., Charles C Thomas, 1965, pp. 25–50.

106. Tourtellotte, W. W., Haerer, A. F., Heller, G. L., et al.: Post-Lumbar Puncture Headaches. Springfield, Ill., Charles C Thomas, 1964, p. 50.

107. Tourtellotte, W. W., and Parker, J. A.: Multiple sclerosis: Correlation between immunoglobulin-G in cerebrospinal fluid and brain. Science, *154*:1044, 1966.

108. Troost, B. T., Walker, J. E., and Cherington, M.: Hypoglycorrhachia associated with subarachnoid hemorrhage. Arch. Neurol., *19*:437, 1968.

109. Widell, S.: On the cerebrospinal fluid in normal children and in patients with acute abacterial meningo-encephalitis. Acta Paediat., *115*: suppl., 5, 1958.

110. Wolf, H., and Hoepffner, L.: The cerebrospinal fluid in the newborn and premature infant. World Neurol., *2*:871, 1961.

111. Yahr, M. D., Goldensohn, S. S., and Kabat, E. A.: Further studies on the gamma globulin content of cerebrospinal fluid in multiple sclerosis and other neurological diseases. Ann. N.Y. Acad. Sci., *58*:613, 1954.

112. Ziegler, D. K., and Ross, G.: Cerebrospinal fluid gamma globulin as a diagnostic test for multiple sclerosis. Neurology, *5*:573, 1955.

11

ECHOENCEPHALOGRAPHY

The use of ultrasound to extend our perception is not limited to neurological surgery or to man. It is used extensively in the communication, transportation, and metallurgic industries. The ability of bats, whales, and dolphins to generate and discriminate subtle variations in this mode is among the great wonders of nature; man's efforts in this area are comparatively crude.

DEFINITION

Sound is classified by its frequency. The range of audible sound is from 16 to 18,000 cycles per second. Infrasound has a frequency below this. Ultrasound spans a frequency of 18,000 cps to 100,000 megacycles per second. The lower spectrum of ultrasound is transmitted in air (e.g., Galton's whistle), but in this discussion ultrasound is considered only in the higher frequencies at which the waves are confined to liquids and solids. Diagnostic ultrasound utilizes a frequency range of 1 to 10 megacycles per second. One megacycle per second is one million cycles per second or one megahertz (MHz). The most commonly used echoencephalographic unit transducer houses a crystal that vibrates at 2.25 MHz. This sound is not transmissible in air but travels only in liquids and solids. Consequently a concerted effort is made to exclude air as the transducer is applied to the structure under examination.

HISTORICAL SURVEY

In 1917, Langevien was commissioned by the French Government to design a method of ultrasonic submarine detection.[17] With the end of World War I the interest in this investigation ceased. World War II revived the interest, and by 1943 the sonar system had been developed in several countries. In the early 1940's Sokolov in the USSR and Firestone in the United States developed their pulse-echo techniques using very short pulses of energy.[17] The first attempts to adapt ultrasound for medical purposes dates back to 1937. The brothers Dussik in Vienna, utilizing direct transmission (nonpulsed) ultrasound, attempted to outline the cerebral ventricular system. They called it a "hyperphonogram" and continued to develop this technique for over a decade until Guettner showed that the variations in attenuation were largely caused by the skull, which obscured any variations due to the brain.[2, 7]

Although the use of direct transmission ultrasound in medical diagnosis was abandoned, reflection techniques were being developed. French, Wild and Neal, in 1950, demonstrated at autopsy that "echoes" were detectable from brain tumors.[4] In 1951 they recorded similar "tumor echoes" from the brain of a living patient at the time of craniotomy.[5]

In 1956 Leksell published a monograph that opened extensive investigation into the clinical application of diagnostic reflected ultrasound.[10] He demonstrated that the midline structure of the brain reflected ultrasound and that its lateral displacement could be demonstrated in craniocerebral trauma.[11] He coined the term "echo-encephalography" to describe his technique.

The clinical importance of echoencephalography is well documented by now, but experience indicates that its reliability depends entirely upon the skill of the personnel using it. Its conventional use is to demonstrate the diencephalic midline or

P. DYCK
T. KURZE

third ventricle within the skull. Ventricular dilatation can be measured, particularly in the pediatric age group. This has various applications in the management of the child with hydrocephalus. Transcalvarial sonography for detection of neoplasm or intracranial bleeding is possible in some cases. Echo-ranging of the operative site transdurally or on exposed brain is harmless, is expeditious, and yields invaluable information.

PHYSICAL PRINCIPLES OF ULTRASOUND

In 1880, J. Currie and P. Currie discovered that when quartz, a natural piezoelectric crystal, was compressed, an electrical potential was generated.[6] In 1881, Lippman reasoned that if stress applied to a piezoelectric crystal produced an electrical potential, the converse must also be true.[6] That is, if one applied a potential to such a crystal, it should result in deformation of its surface, changing its shape.

It followed, therefore, that if one applied high-frequency alternating electric current, the crystal would vibrate, arranging and rearranging its molecular lattice in response to polarity change. The frequency of vibration would vary with the frequency of the alternating current applied and the natural resonant frequency of the crystal.

If such a vibrating crystal were placed in an appropriate conducting medium, a disturbance would be created. At megacycle frequency this disturbance is termed ultrasound. Such ultrasound has three types of electric waves: (1) surface or Rayleigh waves (e.g., like surface water waves); (2) longitudinal waves, i.e., compressional or dilatational waves propagated by compression and expansion of molecules moving parallel to the direction of the wave impulse; and (3) transverse or shear waves, which have an up and down motion of particles at right angles to the direction setting up shear stresses. It is the longitudinal waves that can be directionally beamed when the transducer dimensions are large compared with its wavelengths, making it the energy source of diagnostic ultrasound.[6]

Although natural minerals such as quartz are still used as piezoelectric oscillators, medical diagnostic units employ almost exclusively man-made crystals that are composed of oxides of various metals. These materials, of which barium titanate ($BaTiO_3$) is the most widely used polycrystalline ceramic, are baked and polarized by the application of a static potential difference (e.g., 50,000 v direct current per inch). Such a crystal is now capable of converting electrical energy into mechanical energy and vice versa. It has piezoelectric properties.

The block diagram indicates that the piezoelectric crystal housed in the transducer is connected to a sender and receiver system (Fig. 11–1). The received information is displayed on the screen of a cathode ray tube. An attached polaroid camera is provided to photograph and permanently record the data displayed.

In 1/1000 of a second the high-frequency oscillation activates the crystals in the transducer and produces a pulse of ultrasound. This pulse is transmitted to the surrounding medium, in which it travels at a constant speed. When it encounters a medium of a differing molecular density (e.g., brain–third ventricle interface), it is partially reflected and returned to strike

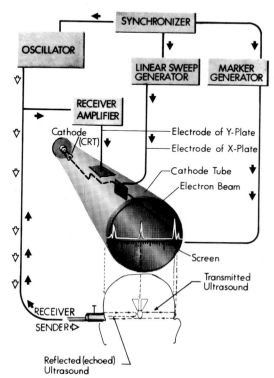

FIGURE 11–1 Block diagram of an echo-ranging system.

the crystal, which is now at rest. The stress thus created against the crystal produces deformation and piezoelectricity, which is amplified and displayed on the y-axis of the cathode ray tube. This reflected ultrasound is said to have echoed and forms the basis of one-dimensional sonography or A-scanning.

PROPERTIES OF ULTRASOUND

Most American diagnostic units employ a 2.25-MHz transducer. This frequency sound will generally penetrate 17 to 18 cm of soft tissue and return recordable echoes.

Higher-frequency ultrasound, having a shorter wavelength, gives better resolution of detail but poorer penetrance of tissues. For example, a 5-MHz crystal produces sound that will travel only 4 to 5 cm in soft tissues and still return recordable echoes.

The human skull is a major obstacle to ultrasound; approximately 90 per cent of the sound energy is reflected, absorbed, and deflected from this structure, never entering the cranial cavity when a transducer is applied to the head. For this reason it is at times technically impossible to obtain satisfactory echoes with the conventional 2.25-MHz transducer. A 1-MHz crystal will usually overcome this difficulty since it has greater penetrance.

A simple equation relates the velocity (v), the wavelength (λ), and frequency (f) in the following manner:

$$\lambda = \frac{v}{f} \text{ or } v = \lambda f.$$

For example, at 1 MHz (f) sound would travel at a velocity (v) of 1.5 km per second in water. Consequently the wavelength (l) would be 1/1,000,000 of 1.5 km or 1.5 mm.

TABLE 11–1   *VELOCITY OF ULTRASOUND IN VARIOUS MEDIA AT 37°C*

MEDIUM	METERS PER SECOND
Water	1526
Cerebrospinal fluid	1538
Blood	1548
Brain	1571
Bone	3265

Such sound velocity is transmitted poorly in air and not at all in a vacuum, but is well transmitted through liquid and solid media. Its velocity also increases with temperature rise. At 37° C ultrasound travels at velocities that differ according to the media in which it is transmitted (Table 11–1).[8]

DIAGNOSTIC TECHNIQUE

Although there are a number of diagnostic units on the market, the Echoline-20 (Smith-Kline Instrument Company) is used in this discussion to illustrate the technique and data. The unit is not portable, but is transportable to the bedside of a patient (Fig. 11–2). A bed patient is best examined in the supine position.

Aquasonic, a commercially available water-soluble medium, is applied to the crystal to provide good contact between the transducer and the scalp. This maneuver

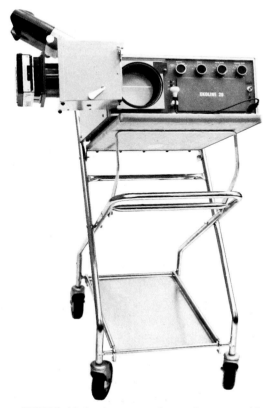

FIGURE 11–2   A commonly used sonographic unit.

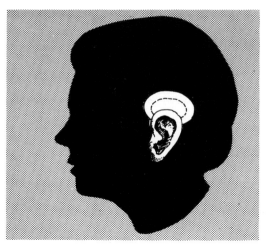

FIGURE 11–3 Area from which most satisfactory midline and far-wall echoes can be obtained simultaneously.

THE NORMAL AND ABNORMAL ECHOENCEPHALOGRAM

The normal echoencephalogram is illustrated in Figure 11–4. The "initial echo" represents reflections from the immediately underlying soft tissues and skull. Occasionally the reflections from the skull can be distinguished from the "crystal noise."

The "end-echo" represents reflections from the brain–inner table interface as well as the scalp. Often a "scalp echo" may be identified and separated from the end-echo. These far-wall echoes should line up or measure equal distances in order to evaluate the "M-echo" or midline complex properly.

Scalp contusion or subgaleal bleeding will result in a separation of the inner table and the scalp reflections. In this situation alignment of the inner table skull echoes is sought. This is the most prominent and reliable deflection of the end-echo complex.

The following midline structures of the brain have been identified as the source of the M-echo complex: the pineal gland, the septum pellucidum, the falx, and the interhemispheric fissure. The third ventricle has also been suggested by experience and convincing data. All these structures can be the source of the M-echo, but when the transducer is conventionally positioned just above the root of the ear, the posterior

must exclude air. Figure 11–3 shows the site where midline echoes are most easily obtained. The transducer may have to be tilted in various directions or moved back and forth before the desired midline reflection is obtained. The smallest possible amount of ultrasound should be used to obtain the desired information. A satisfactory echogram can usually be obtained in from one to three minutes.

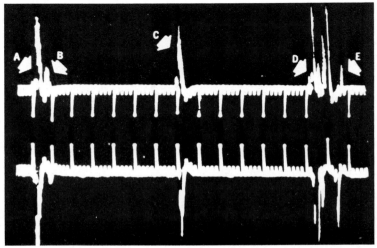

FIGURE 11–4 A normal echoencephalogram. A, initial echo; B, skull echo occasionally obtained; C, midline or diencephalic echo; D, echo reflection from inner table of skull; E, scalp-air interface.

third ventricle has been demonstrated to be the most consistent and likely source.

A displacement of the M-echo in excess of 3 mm from the midline is considered pathological. In children a shift of 2 mm is probably outside the normal range.

Midline distortion is sometimes so massive that it is impossible to obtain reflections from it. This has been observed in extensive capsular hemorrhage, massive subdural collections, or ventricular casting with blood. Under these circumstances, the third ventricle is so distorted it cannot reflect enough appropriately directed ultrasound to record an M-echo. In spite of this, in over 90 per cent of patients the M-echo can be obtained with the standard 2.25 MHz transducer.

The authors and Zuelch have emphasized that extensive frontopolar and occipital distortion may not necessarily result in an M-echo shift.[1, 18] Likewise bilateral mass lesions of equal size, e.g., subdural hematoma, will not produce a midline shift. The absence of midline shift does not mean there is no intracranial mass. This is an important dictum to be remembered.

When echo-ranging the third ventricle a very prominent double reflection can be obtained. In such a situation it is possible to measure the width of this structure. In health the third ventricle reaches a maximum width of 7 mm as confirmed by air contrast studies. Measurements in excess of this indicate ventricular dilatation. If the third ventricle is dilated, such a patient's papilledema would be attributed to ventricular obstruction and not to pseudotumor cerebri, since the ventricles are usually "small" in the latter situation.

An M-echo shift can result from any supratentorial mass lesions, the largest shifts being documented in patients with chronic subdural hematomas.

In the evaluation of craniocerebral trauma, the determination of the position of this diencephalic midline is invaluable.

During management of a rapidly expanding intracranial lesion without localizing neurological deficit when there is no time or facility for contrast studies, the direction of the midline shift will indicate the side of the potentially operable lesion.

Postoperatively, particularly in the management of subarachnoid hemorrhage due to rupture of an aneurysm, echo-ranging may help separate vasospasm from postoperative hematoma by determining the position of the third ventricle. However, postoperative unilateral frontotemporal cerebral edema may cause a significant midline shift of the third ventricle and provide a false suggestion of postoperative hemorrhage. An arteriogram is therefore more reliable but more hazardous than echoencephalography in distinguishing between brain swelling and postoperative hemorrhage.

It is unnecessary to continue listing examples in medical and surgical neurology in which it is beneficial to know of the presence or absence of distortion of the diencephalic midline. Echo-ranging provides this information expeditiously and without harm to the patient. A shift of the diencephalic midline is illustrated in Figure 11–5.

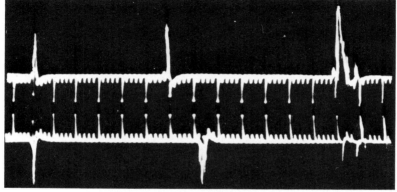

FIGURE 11–5 This illustration demonstrates an approximate 6-mm left to right shift. In the upper trace the transducer is applied to the right side of the head, in the lower trace to the left.

HYDROCEPHALUS AND SONOGRAPHY

The human cerebral ventricles have a very complex contour, and precise ultrasonic documentation of their shape is probably not possible. Some information, however, can be obtained. In the adult the width of the third ventricle may be measured; as previously mentioned, if it exceeds 7 mm it is probably abnormal.

Schiefer and co-authors have described a brain mantle index that measures the distance between the temporal horn and the end-echoes.[14] Under normal circumstances this index should be 2 to 2.2. That is, the thickness of the cerebral mantle in the region of the temporal horns measures about one half the hemisphere's cross-section. With ventricular enlargement the cerebral mantle thins and the brain mantle index consequently increases (Fig. 11–6).

Ford has shown that it is feasible to measure the gross width of the anterior ventricular system by echo-ranging across the frontal horns with the transducer placed 4 cm above and in front of the ear.[9]

All these methods have been utilized in the evaluation of the infant with hydrocephalus. The transfrontal measurements and the Schiefer index, as well as the determination of the dimensions of the third ventricle, add invaluable information about the dimensions of the ventricular system.

This information is more easily obtained from the child's skull, since it is thin and absorbs less energy. Marked ventricular enlargement adds to the ease with which information is obtained. Because of interfering crystal noise on the side of the "near echo," a cerebral mantle of less than 1 cm is difficult to map. It may, however, be more easily measured on the "far side" in respect to the transducer.

The foregoing technique will never replace ventricular contrast studies, but has quite accurately demonstrated the cerebral mantle in the infant. It has shown progressive ventricular enlargement and cerebral mantle thinning due to ventriculoatrial shunt failure in the absence of the classic signs of progressive hydrocephalus.

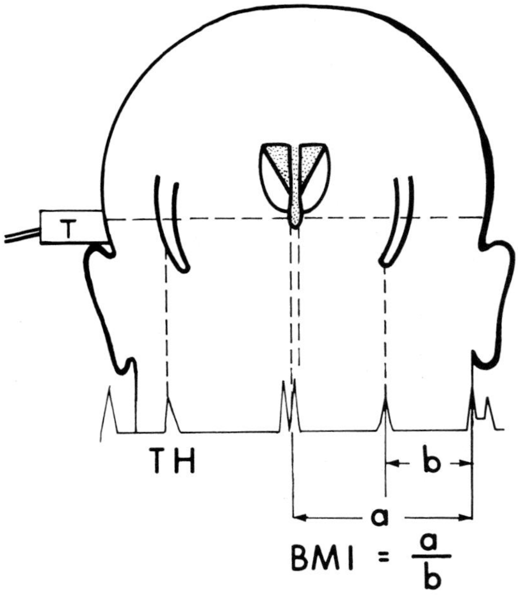

FIGURE 11–6 The schematic demonstration of the brain mantle index (BMI). Normally the value is 2 to 2.2 It increases with progressive hydrocephalus. T, transducer; TH, temporal horn. (After Schiefer, W., and Kazner, E.: Klinische Echo-Encephalographie. Berlin, Heidelberg, New York, Springer-Verlag, 1967, p. 56.)

INTRAOPERATIVE SONOGRAPHY

In spite of sophistication in diagnostic procedures, the surgical neurologist occasionally encounters situations that lead to an intraoperative search for a mass lesion. An echoencephalographic search would appear less traumatic than repeated needling or incisions in the cerebral or cerebellar hemispheres.

In most cerebral neoplasms ultrasonic velocities differ slightly from those in surrounding brain. Although this difference is very slight (e.g., normal brain, 1530 m per second; meningioma, 1550 m per second), an interface is provided that serves to reflect ultrasound and create a tumor echo. Because of necrosis, hemorrhage, cavitation, and variable cellular density within a tumor, multiple interfaces are created; therefore, the "tumor echo complex" (Fig. 11–7).

Tanaka and his pupils probably have the most extensive experience with this technique.[16] The authors and others have confirmed its usefulness and have modified the

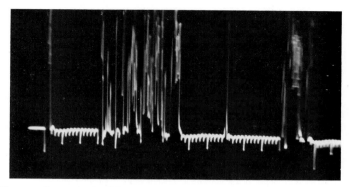

FIGURE 11–7 Tumor echoes obtained from a temporal lobe metastatic mass. Note the tumor echo indicates the subcortical depth, diameter, and medial extent of the lesion.

method so it can be used expeditiously without contamination of the operative field or elaborate sterilization (Fig. 11–8).[3] Müller has ingeniously improved the transdural technique so that a grid maps the operative site and multiple recordings on the same film result in a tomographic section through the tumor mass.[13]

Intraoperative sonography is extremely reliable, and with it, tumor echoes can be obtained in almost all cerebral neoplasms. With extra-axial lesions it defines the medial extent of the mass, often not visualized by angiography. In the case of an infiltrating tumor it locates the area most severely in-

volved or points to cystic degeneration. An intracerebral hemorrhage is easily located by the same technique. The characteristics of the tumor echo are determined by the consistency of the tumor.

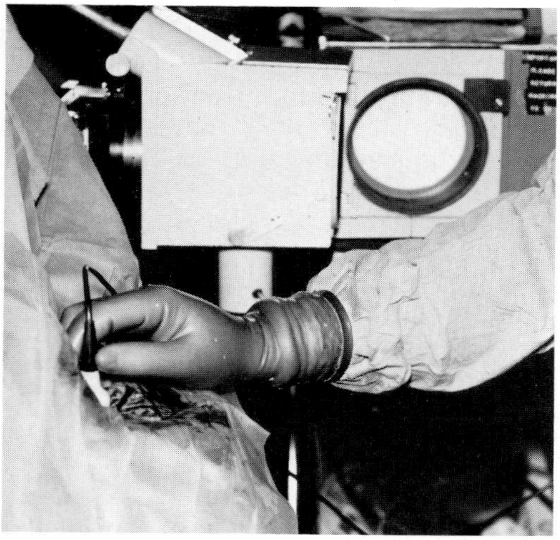

TRANSCALVARIAL SONOGRAPHY

As has been repeatedly emphasized, the human skull is the major deterrent to diagnostic sonography of supratentorial intracranial bleeding and neoplasm. The reported success rate ranges from 5 to 78 per

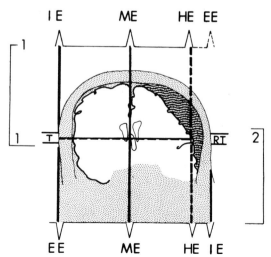

FIGURE 11–9 One method by which a hematoma echo (HE) is obtained. With the transducer placed on the right side (1) no end-echo was obtained. All reflecting energy was spent at the hematoma-brain interface. With the transducer on the left (2), one obtains both a hematoma echo and an initial echo (IE) on some occasions. ME, midline echo; EE, end-echo; T and RT, site of transducer applied to skull.

FIGURE 11–8 Transdural sonographic technique. The operative field remains sterile by its exclusion by a self-adhering surgical drape (Steri-Drape). The transducer is not sterilized. At completion, the operator changes gown and gloves after he removes the draping and continues with the operation.

cent in the detection of supratentorial neoplasms.

The technique is generally more reliable in the detection of the so-called hematoma echo reflected from the interface between the brain and subdural membranes. This hematoma echo may be obtained from the ipsilateral or the contralateral side. In chronic subdural hematoma most of the abnormal echoes have been obtained proximal to the end-echo.

It is important to realize that the intracranial sound energy may be completely spent at the hematoma-brain interface, and consequently the hematoma echo may manifest itself as a one-sided foreshortening of the biparietal diameter rather than a deflection medial to the end-echo (Fig. 11–9).

The principles just outlined apply to the detection of epidural hematoma as well. In fact, the dural membrane is a better reflector of ultrasound than the brain-subdural interface.

ULTRASONIC TOMOGRAPHY (B-SCANNING)

The A-scan depicts a reflected sound beam on the y-axis of the cathode ray tube. The B-mode records the returning echoes as a "dot" on the oscilloscopic screen rather than as a vertical deflection. The intensity or brightness of this dot then represents the strength of the echo signal, and the distance between two dots, the distance it has traveled. It is possible to obtain tomographic representation of anatomical structures by mounting a transducer on a linear synchronized scanning device. In actuality such a tomograph is a composite of a large number of one-dimensional pictures. The method is known as intensity modulation or B-scanning. Although various modifications in techniques have been published, B-scanning is still experimental at this point.

ULTRASONIC BLOOD FLOW MONITORS

In 1963 Watson and Rushner made potentially important contributions to the diagnostic armamentarium by developing an ultrasonic method by which venous and arterial blood flow could be studied.[17] The technique involves the Doppler effect. A change in frequency can be recorded when ultrasound is reflected from moving red blood cells and converted to an audible signal.

Such a "Doppler flowmeter" transducer houses a sending and a receiving crystal. The transmitting crystal generates a 5-MHz frequency signal and beams it at an angle through the vessel. It is reflected from the moving red blood cells to the receiving crystal. These sound waves, changed in frequency by the moving blood cells, are amplified to drive the loudspeaker.

A stenotic vessel lesion (e.g., atheromatous carotid plaque) produces a more high-pitched sound than does the patent vessel, since the velocity of blood flow increases.

This technique has been applied to the evaluation of carotid flow in extracranial vascular disease. More recently Müller has studied the flow in the ophthalmic artery and has produced encouraging results.[12] It must be kept in mind, however, that the ophthalmic artery is an important anastomotic channel between the internal and external carotid systems. Ultrasonic blood flow monitoring remains an encouraging but experimental method that warrants clinical trials.

SUMMARY

The diagnostic concepts of echoencephalography as described by Leksell in 1955 have been tremendously modified in the decade that followed.[17] It now includes not only the determination of diencephalic midline displacement but also the detection of interval intracranial bleeding, preoperative and intraoperative localization of brain tumors or blood clots, and the evaluation of the patient with hydrocephalus.

Linear scanning (A-scan) is in extensive clinical use. Ultrasonic tomography (B-scan) remains experimental to date.

Results of application of the principles of the "Doppler flowmeter" to the evaluation of extracranial occlusive vascular disease are highly encouraging, particularly if flow through the ophthalmic artery is studied. This technique, however, has not yet stood the test of time.

Improvements in instrumentation may result in further refinements of ultrasound as a diagnostic tool.

In general, if echoencephalography is looked upon as "another reflex hammer" of the neurological examination, useful information can be gained about the patient's neurological status. This information is expeditiously and harmlessly obtained at the patient's bedside or in the operating room.

Familiarity with the basic principles of ultrasound and realistic knowledge of the expectations, limitations, and artifacts of contemporary instrumentation is the basis for a useful clinical application of echoencephalography to neurosurgery and neurology. Its contribution to the improvement of patient care is ultimately related to the skill and ingenuity of the physician applying this information to clinical problems.

REFERENCES

1. Barrows, H. S., Dyck, P., and Kurze, T.: The diagnostic applications of ultrasound in neurological disease: The intracerebral midline. Neurology, *15*:361–365, 1965.
2. Dussik, K. T., Dussik, F., and Wyt, L.: Auf dem Wege zur Hyperphonographie des Gehirnes. Wien. Med. Wschr., *97*:425–429, 1947.
3. Dyck, P., Kurze, T., and Barrows, H.: Intraoperative ultrasonic encephalography of cerebral mass lesions. Bull. Los Angeles Neurol. Soc., *31*:114–124, 1966.
4. French, L. A., Wild, J. J., and Neal, D.: Detection of cerebral tumors by ultrasonic pulses: Pilot studies on postmortem material. Cancer, *3*: 705–708, 1950.
5. French, L. A., Wild, J. J., and Neal, D.: The experimental application of ultrasonics to localization of brain tumors: Preliminary report. J. Neurosurg., *8*:198–203, 1951.
6. Gordon, D.: Ultrasound as a Diagnostic and Surgical Tool. Baltimore, Md., Williams & Wilkins Co., 1964.
7. Guettner, W., Fielder, G., and Paetzold, J.: Ueber Ultraschallabbildungen am menschlichen Schadel. Acustica, *2*:148–156, 1952.
8. Iizuke, J. H.: Correlation between neuroradiological and echoencephalographical findings. Symposium Neuroradiol., Paris, 1967.
9. Kazner, E., Schiefer, W., and Zuelch, K. J.: Proceedings of International Symposium in Echo-Encephalography. New York, Springer-Verlag, 1968.
10. Leksell, L.: Echo-encephalography. I. Detection of intracranial complications following head injury. Acta Chir. Scand., *110*:301–315, 1955–56.
11. Leksell, L.: Echo-encephalography. II. Midline echo from the pineal body as an index of pineal displacement. Acta Chir. Scand., *115*:255–259, 1958.
12. Müller, H. R.: Personal communication, 1970.
13. Müller. H. R., Lévy, A., Klingler, M., and Blauenstein. U.: 4. Zur Technik der transduralen Echoenzephalographie. Schweiz. Arch. Neurol. Neurochir., Psychiat., *102*:313–319, 1968.
14. Schiefer, W., and Kazner, E.: Klinische Echo-Encephalographie. Berlin, Heidelberg, New York, Springer-Verlag, 1967, pp. 56–63.
15. Tanaka, K.: Diagnosis of Brain Disease by Ultrasound. Tokyo, Shindan-To-Chiryo Sha Co. Ltd., 1969.
16. Tanaka, K., Ito, K., and Wagai, T.: The localization of brain tumors by ultrasonic techniques: A clinical review of 111 cases. J. Neurosurg., *23*:135–147, 1965.
17. White, D. N.: Ultrasonic Encephalography. Kingston, Ont., Hanson and Edgar Ltd., 1970.
18. Zuelch, K. J.: The morphologic basis of the abnormal echoencephalogram. *In* Proceedings of International Symposium on Echo-Encephalography, Erlangen, 1967. New York, Springer-Verlag, 1968.

12

ELECTROENCEPHALOGRAPHY

Electroencephalograms were clearly recorded from animals nearly a hundred years ago by Caton in England, but the father of human electroencephalography was Hans Berger of Jena, Germany, who began his pioneering work less than 50 years ago.[3, 6] Berger's writings on electroencephalography were in German, but in 1969 a complete English translation of his 14 most essential papers was published.[15] Within 10 years of Berger's first paper, the electroencephalogram was known all over the world. World War II and the growth of electronic technology increased the availability of the necessary apparatus so that at the end of the war, electroencephalography was no longer a laboratory curiosity; it had been firmly accepted as a useful diagnostic aid in neurology and neurosurgery. Subsequently, the electroencephalograph has proved to be a harmless and painless, if time consuming, diagnostic tool. As will be seen later, the techniques involved in making satisfactory recordings are painstaking ones. Therefore, because of the time and effort involved, they are relatively expensive in both personal and financial terms.

TECHNIQUE AND ROUTINE PROCEDURES

The commercial apparatus available for recording electroencephalograms is, on the whole, quite reliable. These machines usually contain 8 or 16 channels of equipment capable of recording from 8 or 16 different areas over the head. Each channel has an amplifying system that detects and magnifies the voltage difference between two electrodes. The current produced is then used to drive pens beneath which the paper moves at a constant and accurately determined rate. The inked line on the paper, therefore, plots out a "voltage versus time" graph that is called the electroencephalogram.[7]

Computer techniques are just beginning to be applied to electroencephalography, primarily for the purpose of averaging small cerebral responses produced by peripheral stimuli (such as a flash of light, a brief tone, or an electrical stimulus to one of the peripheral nerves).[10] The cerebral responses produced by these stimuli are much smaller than the on-going electroencephalographic activity and so are, in a sense, lost in the noise of a routine study. If, however, one averages these responses in a time-locked fashion, they superimpose one upon the other, whereas the on-going cerebral activity, which is not locked in time to the stimulus, tends, with sufficient repetition, to average out, leaving a relatively flat baseline upon which the "evoked response" is superimposed. At this time, these averaging techniques are useful clinically for the evaluation of hearing in infancy and, occasionally, for studies of vision.[10] Otherwise, computer techniques are now of research interest only and cannot be used to interpret electroencephalograms or to record low-voltage "spontaneous" activity.

Electrodes

Usually the recordings are made with metal electrodes applied to the surface of the scalp, and occasionally, with needles positioned subcutaneously over the head.

R. S. SCHWAB

R. R. YOUNG

The latter technique is unpleasant and requires repeated sterilization of the electrodes, but it is particularly useful in the operating room, when recording from comatose patients, or when speed of application is very important. The electrodes routinely placed over the calvarium detect electrical activity from the cerebrum several centimeters below and hence record only from the convexity of the hemispheres. Therefore, techniques have been devised for placing electrodes nearer to the under surface of the brain, particularly to the inferior and medial surfaces of the temporal lobes.[35] These utilize long metal probes that can be applied through the nostrils to reach the nasopharyngeal mucosa or needles that can be directed percutaneously under the zygoma to reach the parasphenoidal regions. Such techniques are rarely necessary for the diagnosis of temporal lobe epilepsy. In the evaluation of a patient for possible operation for epilepsy, however, unless a single focus is unequivocally seen with routine surface leads, "nasopharyngeal" or "sphenoidal" leads may be useful in demonstrating such a focus. It is also possible now under even more specialized circumstances to record, on either a short-term or long-term basis, from the depth of the cerebral hemispheres by using metal multiple electrode arrays, positioned by the neurosurgeon through small trephine holes.

The routine surface electrodes are placed with great care in certain positions over the skull, which, for purposes of standardization, have been specified by international convention.[19] Not only must they be positioned accurately, but the electrical conductivity between them and the scalp must be good enough so that the resistance or impedance is lower than 5,000 ohms. The electrodes must also be fixed securely so that their positions on the scalp do not shift if the patient moves his head.

After the electrodes have been applied, recordings are made from certain pairs of them in a routine and repeatable fashion; these "montages" or associations of electrodes vary from laboratory to laboratory. "Bipolar recordings" are made of the voltage difference between two electrodes on the scalp and "reference (or so-called 'monopolar') recordings" between one electrode on the scalp and an "indifferent" electrode elsewhere (e.g., neck, chest, chin, nose, or ear).[7]

Activation Procedures

Routine recordings are made with the patient awake but resting quietly with his eyes closed. In addition to this, certain "activation procedures" are employed:

1. The patient is asked to hyperventilate at the rate of 20 respirations per minute for three or four minutes. The resulting hypocapnia, alkalosis, increased cerebrovascular resistance, and decreased cerebral blood flow increase the likelihood of abnormal electroencephalographic activity. This is particularly true of patients with petit mal epilepsy, as seen in Figure 12–1. Hyperventilation also tends to produce slow-wave activity, especially in children and in normal adults who haven't eaten in the two to three hours before the test.

2. A bright stroboscopic light is flashed at various frequencies (1 to 20 per second) into the patient's eyes. The cerebral response normally produced posteriorly in the hemispheres by each flash ("photic driving") can be seen on the routine recording of many patients (Fig. 12–2). In some normal subjects, however, averaging techniques, as described earlier, may be necessary to show it. Asymmetries of driving have the same significance as other asymmetries to be described later. More useful diagnostically are the grossly exaggerated responses, sometimes to the point of being epileptic, that are recorded from photosensitive subjects whose studies may otherwise be normal (Fig. 12–3).

3. Sleep is one of the most important "activation procedures." This is true especially for patients in whom temporal lobe epilepsy is suspected. Figures from various laboratories show that only 35 to 50 per cent of patients with clear-cut temporal lobe epilepsy have diagnostic abnormalities when awake, whereas 80 to 90 per cent have them while asleep (Fig. 12–4). In addition, abnormalities that were diffuse or bilateral with the patient awake may lateralize or localize during sleep. Ordinary sleep studies are done with patients in light sleep (Stages I or II); however, recordings

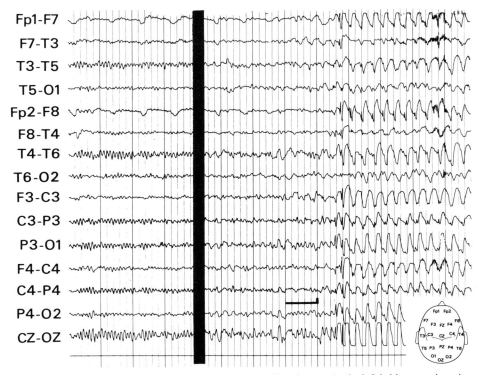

FIGURE 12–1 The electroencephalogram of a young man with seizures. At the left is his normal resting record; at the right of the vertical line is his record during the third minute of hyperventilation. Note that hyperventilation produced increased slowing in the theta frequency range and attenuation of the alpha activity as it usually does in younger people. The diffuse spike-wave discharge occurring at the far right is superimposed upon these changes normally produced by hyperventilation. Calibration marks in this and subsequent figures, unless specified, represent 1 second and 50 μv. The electrode placements and linkages are depicted.

during all-night sleep may show focal activity only during rapid eye movement sleep, a stage of sleep that is associated with dreaming and is almost never reached during routine recordings.[9, 32] The night before a routine "sleep electroencephalogram" the patient should be kept awake for all but four hours and then allowed to fall asleep in the laboratory after the electrodes have been applied. Sedation may be necessary for some patients. As will be seen later, sleep is associated with slowing of the cerebral rhythms and sleep studies are *not* particularly useful in the evaluation of patients with head injuries, tumors, or cerebrovascular disease.

4. It is also possible to elicit abnormal activity by the systemic injection of certain pharmacological substances. Intravenous pentylenetetrazol (Metrazol) has been used to activate seizure foci, and the resultant focal abnormality may be useful if a seizure is produced that exactly reproduces the patient's spontaneous spells.[27] More often, however, a generalized abnormality, or even convulsion, is produced. This can also happen in persons who do not suffer from seizures, and pentylenetetrazol activation is rarely used now. Barbiturates produce excessive fast activity, and the absence of this activity over a certain area may be the only evidence of an underlying lesion (such as a tumor). Phenothiazines, administered parenterally, are said to increase electroencephalographic activity.[22, 38] However, they do not appear to cause seizures when administered by the oral route as they are routinely given and are *not* contraindicated in patients with epilepsy. Chlordiazepoxide (Librium) may abolish diffuse seizure activity on the recording and leave only that of the primary focus. These latter agents are less widely used, and their general applicability remains to be proved.

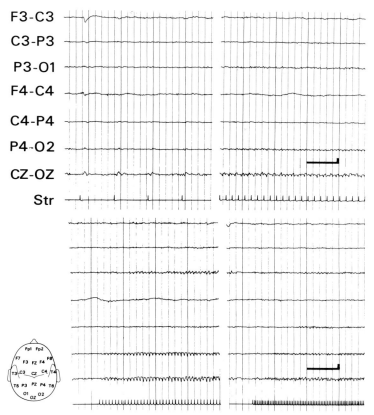

F3-C3
C3-P3
P3-O1
F4-C4
C4-P4
P4-O2
CZ-OZ
Str

FIGURE 12–2 These normal cerebral responses to stroboscopic stimulation are readily visible in the posterior leads, especially CZ–OZ. The stroboscope flashes (Str) at 1, 5, 10, and 20 per second are marked on the bottom line of each record. The electrode linkages are the same in all four records.

Artifacts

The electrical activity of the cerebrum, as recorded from the scalp, is roughly in the $50\text{-}\mu v$ range (0.00005 v), and many other electrical activities than those of cerebral origin are of this same or greater amplitude. These other activities tend to obscure the electroencephalogram and are referred to as "artifacts" (Fig. 12–5). For example, electromyographic impulses from muscular activity are recorded on the electroencephalogram if the patient has not relaxed his facial, temporal, and scalp muscles. Electrocardiographic activity from contractions of the heart, which is of much greater amplitude, can also be recorded on the electroencephalogram, particularly on reference runs in which the two electrodes being recorded from are not equidistant from the heart. With each blink, the superior rectus muscle involuntarily contracts, and the eyeball moves up (Bell's phenomenon). There is a steady direct current potential between retina and cornea, the latter being positive, and as this dipole moves with each movement of the eye during blinking or other eye movements, an electromotive force is induced that produces quite a sizable artifact on the electroencephalogram. Tongue movement also produces this sort of artifact, and movements of the patient's head or body produce static and capacitative changes in leads that introduce still other artifacts. To minimize these artifacts, the patient must be quiet and reasonably cooperative. Sweating is associated with large, very slow waves, and faulty contact of electrode to scalp produces other artifacts. High electrode impedances also increase the likelihood of nonbiological artifacts, which include airborne interference

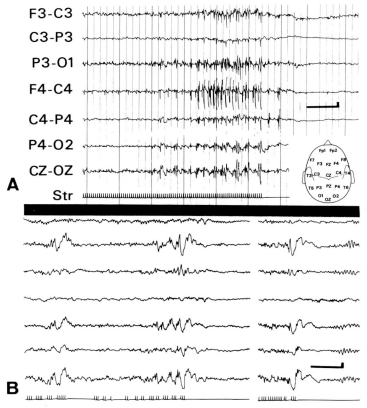

FIGURE 12–3 Photomyoclonic activity in *A* and photoconvulsive activity in *B* represent unusual responses to stroboscopic stimulation. The photomyoclonic discharges arise in muscle and are much more common than the photically evoked paroxysmal cerebral activity recorded in the lower half of the figure.

associated with 60-cycle current and radio-frequency emissions from x-ray equipment, electrocoagulators, radio and electronic call systems, and so forth. Most of the latter can be eliminated by using good technique, superior equipment, and suitable positioning of the electroencephalographic rooms except, of course, when "portable" units are used in the operating or recovery room or the intensive care unit. Screening of the recording rooms is rarely necessary these days.

Limiting Factors

There are limitations on the electroencephalogram that are imposed by the recording system. The recordings are done under rather restricted conditions, with the patient at rest, during 30 to 45 minutes—an infinitesimal portion of his life span. There-fore, cerebral activity that is of infrequent occurrence or is associated with some unusual activity may not be seen during the routine recording. Furthermore, the recording is made at a distance from the cerebral surface, and both the passive electrical properties of the skull and scalp, and the frequency characteristics of the recording equipment impose certain limitations on what is actually seen on the paper. For example, the recordings consist only of frequencies between approximately $\frac{1}{2}$ and 30 cycles per second. Cerebral activity at much higher frequencies, even though of considerable amplitude, may not be conducted through the skull and therefore cannot be recorded adequately on the routine study. For these reasons, negative results (the absence of a certain electrical activity that might be expected during a focal seizure, for example) do not rule out the possibility that abnormalities might actually be

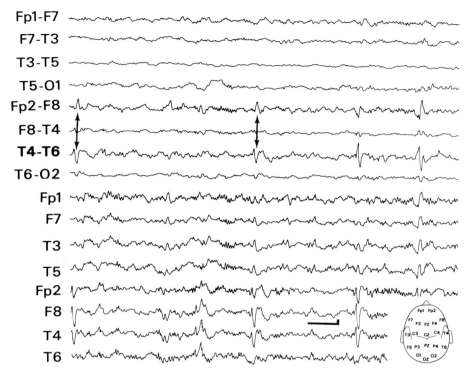

FIGURE 12–4 This recording from a patient with temporal lobe epilepsy shows focal spike discharges during sleep—all studies with this patient awake were normal. In the bipolar linkages at the top, "phase reversals" can be seen around electrodes F8 and T4 (*arrows*), while simultaneously, in the reference linkages at the bottom, the spikes are seen with highest amplitude at these same electrodes. The indifferent electrode in this and other reference or "monopolar" runs is a combined neck-chest linkage.

recorded if it were possible to sample the electrical activity of the cerebrum more directly with different techniques. Hunger or sedation also produce certain changes (slowing with or without hyperventilation) and, therefore, should be avoided.

It will be appreciated that a well-trained technician is absolutely essential. The skill with which the recording was made is most important. Once the patient has left the laboratory, it may be very difficult for the electroencephalographer to get the necessary information from the ink-tracing unless the proper sort of testing has been done by the technician. Not only must the patient be connected most fastidiously and precisely to the recording apparatus, but the entire test must be carefully performed in a routine fashion but yet with sufficient imagination so that when indicated, the routine can be varied.

Ideally, every neurosurgeon and neurolo-

gist could be trained to interpret the recordings from his patients and to correlate what this test has to offer with the patient's clinical status. This is, of course, what the physician does with the results of his clinical examination, x-rays, scans, and other laboratory data. However, many neurosurgeons and neurologists are not sufficiently trained in interpreting the electroencephalogram and must rely upon the routine reports that both the technician and electroencephalographer should make after each recording. Although the electroencephalographer's report should describe in an objective way his analysis of the frequencies, amplitudes, asymmetries, and presence or absence of abnormal activity, he usually has little or no knowledge of the patient's clinical situation. Only the primary physician can weave the results of the study into the patient's entire clinical picture in a meaningful way. Studies that are

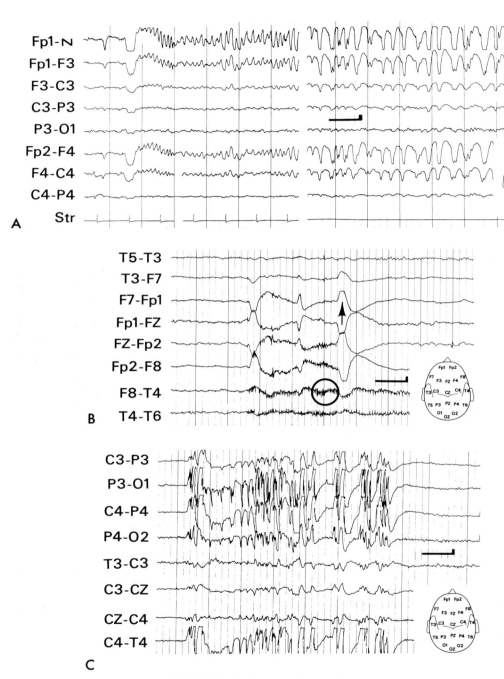

FIGURE 12–5 *See opposite page for legend.*

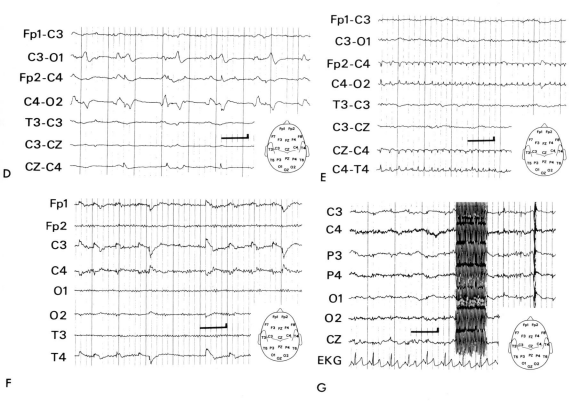

Figure 12–5 *Continued*

FIGURE 12–5 These are various artifacts. *A.* The results of rapid eye blink in response to stroboscopic light are seen on the left; those of voluntary eye blink on the right. N refers to an electrode on the bridge of the nose. In *B* one may see both eye movements (*arrow*) and muscle (*circle*) artifacts. Movement artifacts are seen in *C.* Note that these artifacts and those in *A* may appear to the unwary to represent seizure activity. In *D* the only activity seen is artifactually produced by the patient's respirator; no encephalographic activity was recorded from this patient with electrocerebral silence. In *E,* artifacts from a malfunctioning electrode (C4) are seen. The artifacts in *F* are caused by a "bell-boy" radiofrequency call system and those in *G* by the telephone.

completely normal or clearly abnormal because they do or do not contain focal or
local or generalized slowing, absence of
electrical activity, or the abnormal activity
detailed in the following section are easily
interpreted and present little problem, even
to the relatively inexperienced electroencephalographer. However, records that are
on the borderline between clearly normal
and clearly abnormal are very difficult indeed. Slight degrees of slowing (perhaps
related to drowsiness), mild asymmetry of
activity, the presence of a rare unusual
wave, and so forth, are difficult to interpret;
in fact, it is sometimes impossible for the
electroencephalographer to state honestly
and categorically that a record is normal or
abnormal. Except in emergency situations,
the electroencephalogram should follow the
routine collection of clinical information.
Ideally, it is taken to obtain certain data
that are otherwise unavailable and that will
then serve to corroborate or refute the
physician's clinical impression. All too
often, they are requested automatically
without a clear formulation of the question
they are meant to answer.

THE NORMAL ELECTROENCEPHALOGRAM

The activity recorded from normal subjects varies considerably with age. The normal newborn has low voltage with irregular,
poorly organized activity. The normal infant begins to show some rhythmic activity,
first in the 5- to 7-per-second range and

eventually in the 8- to 13-per-second range,
by the time the child is between 6 and 12
years of age. In the normal adult, there is
usually rhythmic, sinusoidal activity over
the parieto-occipital regions in the 8- to
13-per-second (particularly the 10-per-
second) frequency range, which is referred
to as "alpha rhythm." It is more or less
symmetrical on the two sides, disappears
when the eyes are opened, as shown in Figure 12–6, or when the patient is anxious,
and is the prototype of normal activity.
However, there are many normal patients
who have very little, if any, alpha rhythm.
As a person ages, particularly in the 70- to
90-year range, the alpha activity may slow
to six to seven per second, and activity in
the four- to seven-per-second range may
appear in the temporal leads. In other abnormal situations, such as hypothyroidism,
an alpha-like rhythm of five to seven per
second may be recorded; it behaves physiologically like the normal alpha rhythm, and
its frequency gradually increases to the
normal range as the person becomes euthyroid. It is, therefore, important to note that
alpha activity has certain biological characteristics and cannot be defined simply by
frequency in other than a most arbitrary
fashion. In addition, the normal adult has
lower-voltage, faster rhythms, which are
called "beta" and which tend to predominate over the anterior portion of the
scalp (Fig. 12–7; cf. Fig. 12–9 D). Slower
activity in the four- to seven-per-second
range is also quite common, and a certain
amount of this so-called "theta rhythm" ap-

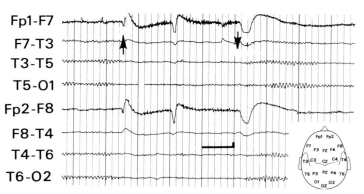

FIGURE 12–6 Normal alpha activity is seen posteriorly in both hemispheres. It is markedly reduced when the patient opens his eyes (↑) and reappears after they are closed (↓). Note the frontal artifacts produced by eye movement and by muscle activity.

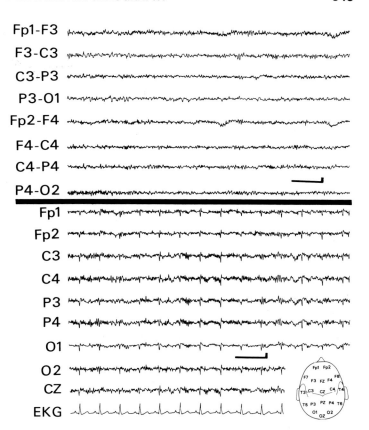

FIGURE 12–7 The predominant fast activity seen in both records here should be contrasted with the alpha activity shown in Figure 12–6. The excessive fast activity in the bottom record is caused, in part at least, by diazepam that the patient is receiving. Note the electrocardiographic artifacts in the lower record.

pears to be normal (cf. Fig. 12–19 *B*). Seizure patterns or slower activity in the range from one half to four per second ("delta rhythm") is not seen in the normal alert adult (cf. Figs. 12–10 and 12–16).

The pattern also varies with levels of alertness.[9,32] When the subject is unusually alert or concentrating, the alpha activity disappears, and the record is relatively flat and "desynchronized." During sleep, normal subjects do not have alpha or beta activity, but instead they have a mixture of slower rhythms that, in light sleep (Stage II), is interspersed with higher-voltage ver-

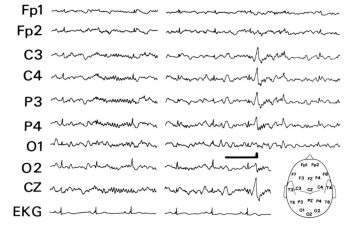

FIGURE 12–8 This is the normal electroencephalographic activity during light sleep. Spindles are seen on the left and vertex sharp waves ("biparietal humps") followed by spindles on the right.

tex sharp waves (so-called "biparietal humps") and "sleep spindles" (Fig. 12–8). Because infants and young children are too restless to allow satisfactory recordings to be obtained with them awake, most are made with them asleep. The patterns of the normal sleeping and waking infant, child, and adult must be thoroughly familiar to the electroencephalographer.[14]

The records of 10 to 20 per cent of apparently normal subjects contain some activity (usually generalized excessive theta, rare delta, or an asymmetry of some type) that would ordinarily be called abnormal. Apart from the semantic problem raised, it is important to remember this because the same percentage of patients being evaluated for head injuries, tumors, and so forth, have these constitutional "abnormalities" that are unrelated to any acquired disease.[14, 17]

THE ABNORMAL ELECTROENCEPHALOGRAM*

The worst of all electroencephalographic abnormalities is the absence of electrical activity from the cerebrum (Fig. 12–9 *A* and *B*). This may, on rare occasions, be seen focally in association with a very large tumor, infarction (Fig. 12–9 *C*), or hemorrhage; the normal rhythms are then said to be completely "suppressed" over this region. Such a localized total absence of electrical activity is, however, a very uncommon finding, and in routine clinical practice the most frequent association of electrocerebral silence is with "irreversible coma."[36]

With modern techniques, mechanical respiration may sustain ventilation in the absence of central nervous system activity; it is then possible for a patient to have suffered total and irreversible cerebral necrosis ("brain death") and yet to be maintained with artificially supported cardiac activity, temperature, and blood pressure. In such a situation, it is of obvious importance to be able to make a diagnosis of irreversible coma so that the fruitless supportive measures can be discontinued. The diagnosis, brain death, is made on the basis of the following criteria: (1) absolute unresponsivity to all stimuli and absence of reflex activity in response to stimuli such as

*See references 20 and 21.

pain, light shone into the eye, and nasopharyngeal stimulation; (2) absence of all spontaneous muscle activity, including respiration, decerebration, shivering, and so forth; and (3) the presence of all these findings for 6 to 24 hours in the absence of severe hypothermia or sedative medication.[2, 37] As demonstrated in Figure 12–9 *A* and *B,* the electroencephalogram fails to show cerebral activity in these patients. Currently it is being used to facilitate the diagnosis of irreversible coma.

During deep anesthesia, such as that following an overdose of barbiturates, all reflex and spontaneous motor and electrical activity of the central nervous system may be absent (Fig. 12–9 *E*). In such a case, if the patient's vital functions (respiration and cardiovascular status) are maintained artificially, recovery should be complete. Otherwise, however, if the criteria for irreversible coma are fulfilled in patients who have suffered cardiac arrest, respiratory collapse, massive head trauma, intracranial hemorrhage, and so forth, a diagnosis of brain death can be made.[1] There has been no evidence of any return of cerebral function in more than 200 consecutive cases in the authors' experience nor in any of the smaller series that have been reported. Neuropathological findings of total cerebral necrosis also support the conclusion that the concept of irreversible coma is eminently sound. Taking a somewhat more restricted view, a committee of the American Electroencephalographic Society ascertained that, except for those who were anesthetized, there was no recovery in more than 3,000 patients who demonstrated "electrocerebral silence" (flatness or absence of electroencephalographic activity) without reference to the neurological examination. The technical details and specifications required for the demonstration of electrocerebral silence should be studied by those who are interested.[37]

Lesser degrees of suppression are quite common. Normal activity, such as alpha or beta rhythm, is usually absent or markedly reduced in the presence of local delta and excessive theta activity caused by lesions of various kinds (cf. Figs. 12–10, 12–16, 12–17, and 12–18). At times the opposite occurs; alpha or fast activity may be greatly increased over an old gliotic area of brain

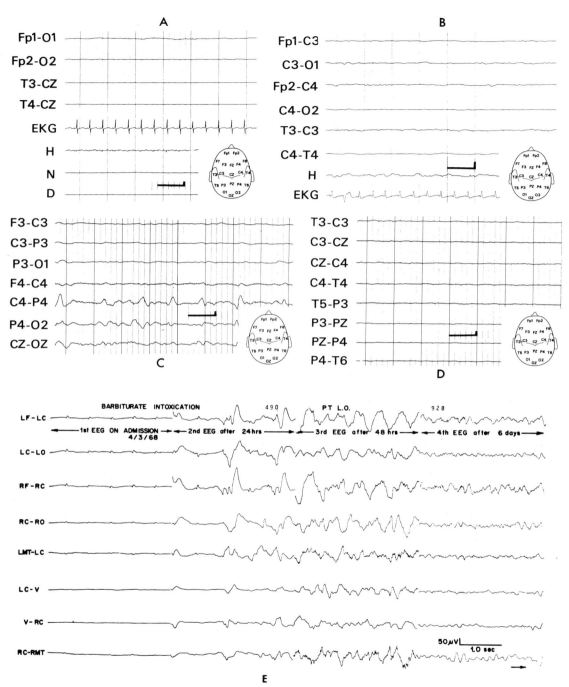

FIGURE 12–9 In *A* the patient with irreversible coma shows electrocerebral silence. H, N, and D refer to pairs of electrodes placed on the hand and neck of the patient and on a dummy patient respectively to monitor various artifacts. *B* is the record of another patient with proved total cerebral necrosis and irreversible coma. The activity recorded here, though artifactually produced, looks somewhat like an electroencephalogram. Note that it is of higher amplitude on the hand (H) than on the scalp. The vertical calibration mark signals $10\,\mu v$ in *A* and *B*. In the upper half of *C* very little electroencephalographic activity is seen over the left hemisphere, which was almost totally infarcted, whereas highly abnormal slow activity is seen over the right. *D* is the normal study of a normal patient — note how low the voltage of normal activity may be. The records in *E* were made over a six-day period in a patient who attempted suicide by ingestion of barbiturates. Note the electrocerebral silence the first day followed by burst-suppression activity and eventual recovery toward normal.

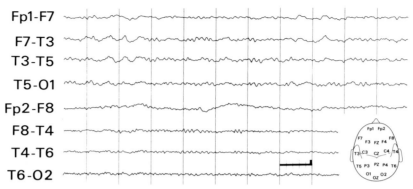

FIGURE 12–10 Slow activity, much of it in the delta range, is seen in the upper four channels over the left hemisphere of a patient with a unilateral cerebral infarction secondary to carotid artery disease.

(or, artifactually, if a skull defect is present beneath the electrodes).

Other more frequently encountered abnormalities include excessive slow-wave activity, either local or generalized. Delta activity (frequency of one half to four per second) in the alert adult is abnormal in and of itself; it may either be irregular or, more rarely, rhythmic. Excessive theta activity is also abnormal. It is important to remember

that these abnormal slow rhythms, as well as the paroxysmal activity to be described later, all arise from viable and at least partially functional cerebral tissue that surrounds the tumor, blood clot, or necrotic brain. None of the activity comes from tumor, blood clot, or dead brain itself. In other words, the pathophysiology of the various electrical abnormalities is more or less the same for all types of lesions, and it

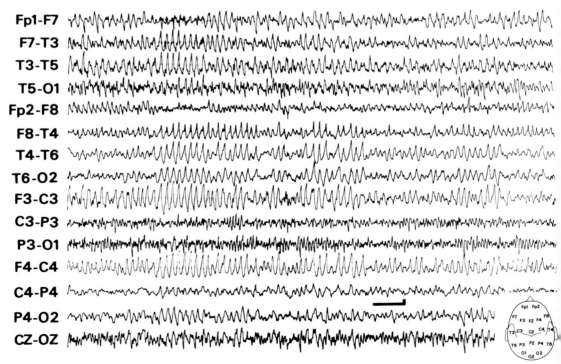

FIGURE 12–11 This is diffuse seizure activity from a patient during a generalized convulsion. Some of the smaller spikes may represent muscle activity.

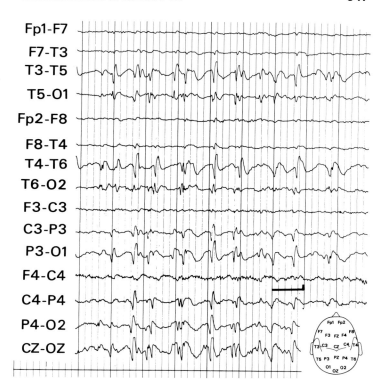

FIGURE 12–12 Bilaterally synchronous posterior hemisphere spike and sharp wave activity is evident.

is not possible to make etiological diagnoses on the basis of the abnormal activity itself. However, the temporal profiles of various lesions differ, and sequential recordings that show a subsidence of delta activity favor the diagnosis of stroke as opposed to tumor and vice versa (Fig. 12–10).

No anatomical abnormality may be recognizable to account for the pathophysiology of seizure activity or generalized abnormalities, and indeed, it is not reasonable to expect that even the most modern anatomical techniques can reveal a morphological abnormality underlying every physiological

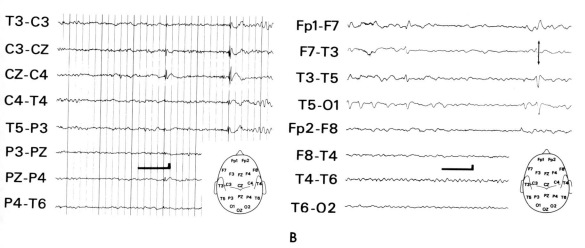

FIGURE 12–13 *A.* Spike-wave complexes reverse phase over the vertex (CZ) in a patient with posthypoxic intention myoclonus. *B.* Seizure activity is seen with phase reversal over leads F7 and T3 (*arrows*).

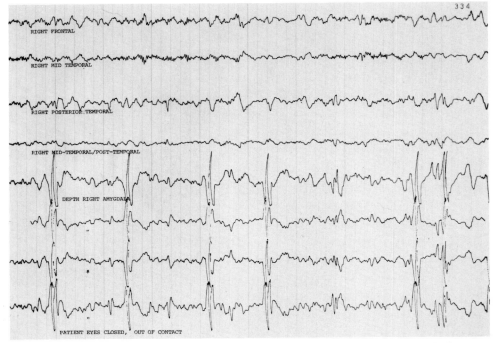

334

RIGHT FRONTAL

RIGHT MID TEMPORAL

RIGHT POSTERIOR TEMPORAL

RIGHT MID-TEMPORAL/POST-TEMPORAL

DEPTH RIGHT AMYGDALA

PATIENT EYES CLOSED, OUT OF CONTACT

FIGURE 12–14 Activity is recorded simultaneously from the scalp over the right temporal lobe (upper four channels) and from depth electrodes in the right amygdala. Note that seizure activity can, at times, be recorded from the depth of the temporal lobe when it cannot be on the routine recording from the scalp.

disorder. However, focal delta activity usually *is* associated with a gross neuropathological lesion.

Spikes are defined as brief transients less than 80 msec in duration while sharp waves are similar in configuration but longer in duration than 80 msec (Figs. 12–11 to 12–14). Spikes may be multiple ("polyspikes") or single, and various slow-wave complexes are often associated with spikes; this is referred to then as spike-wave activity (see Fig. 12–1). It is important to note that all spikes are not abnormal; certain highly specific patterns such as "14- and 6-per-second positive spikes" and "small sharp spikes" (both seen primarily in sleep) have been found quite frequently in normal control groups and, therefore, cannot be considered abnormal in and of themselves.[33] There are other kinds of paroxysmal activity, including occasional rhythmic "hypersynchronous" 10-per-second alpha-like activity, paroxysmal slowing, and so forth.

The physiology underlying the genesis of both normal and abnormal electrical activity is of great interest but remains poorly understood. It would appear that the activ-

ity arises from the geometrical and temporal summation of many graded postsynaptic potentials on dendrites of cortical neurons and not from the spike activity of individual neurons themselves.[8] The problem of bilateral synchrony, as with simultaneous three-per-second spike and wave activity throughout the hemisphere is also of great interest. It was initially suggested that a "centrencephalic" pacemaker was responsible for these discharges. Evidence of such a pacemaker, however, has been lacking, and the term "centrencephalic" should not be considered to refer to an anatomically or physiologically localized region.

EPILEPSY AND SURGERY

The electroencephalogram is *always* abnormal, and characteristically so, during generalized seizures, whether petit or grand mal (see Figs. 12–1 and 12–11). Following a petit mal seizure, the record immediately returns to the normal preictal state. Immediately following a grand mal seizure, postictal flattening with subsequent slow activity may be seen. This is sometimes useful diagnostically if one is uncertain whether a seizure occurred just before the recording. On the other hand, if the patient clearly has had a seizure, this study probably should not be requested for several days because one done sooner will show postictal slowing and be of little diagnostic help. (This is obviously a very different situation from the evaluation of cardiac dysrhythmias, in which an immediate electrocardiogram is of crucial importance.) Generalized convulsions can be well treated clinically without electroencephalographic monitoring.

During the more restricted spells, such as focal seizures of psychomotor, myoclonic, or jacksonian variety, the electroencephalogram *usually* is abnormal, with spikes or sharp waves or both (see Figs. 12–4 and 12–12). It certainly is *not always* abnormal, even during these spells. It may be that the discharge responsible for the clinical spell is too poorly localized, too deep, or of too high frequency to be recorded by the ordinary methods. Therefore, the fact that the electroencephalogram fails to show seizure activity during one of these focal epileptic attacks should not be considered evidence that the seizure is functional or hysterical in nature.

The interictal electroencephalogram, that is, the one between seizures, is normal in perhaps 20 per cent of patients with epilepsy. In another 40 per cent of epileptics, it is abnormal between seizures, but in a nonspecific fashion (excessive bilateral slowing, for example), so that a diagnosis of epilepsy cannot be made from it alone. These findings stimulated the search for the various activation procedures that were discussed earlier. In the remaining 40 per cent of patients, characteristic epileptic discharges, such as are shown in Figure 12–13, are seen even between seizures. The percentage of diagnostic records during the interictal period varies with different types of seizures. It is much more common for patients with petit mal attacks to have an abnormal cerebral rhythm than for those with a rare generalized or focal seizure. Patients undergoing abrupt withdrawal from alcohol, barbiturates, or other sedatives, or with hypocalcemia, hypoglycemia, or other metabolic bases for isolated seizures have, once the acute aberration

has disappeared, a normal record. It is important to remember, therefore, that a diagnosis of epilepsy cannot be excluded by a normal interictal electroencephalogram. If the patient is already receiving anticonvulsant medication, the probability of obtaining a diagnostic abnormality is increased somewhat if the medication is discontinued for 24 hours before the test. This has its obvious drawbacks, however, and the authors do not routinely change the medication before the study.

The electroencephalogram (especially an abnormal one) is nevertheless useful in the diagnosis of epilepsy and in the evaluation of syncope or other spells, particularly in children or in situations in which the history may be difficult to obtain. It appears to be less useful in the follow-up evaluation of therapy in seizures. However, it may be helpful in evaluating the patient who is well controlled over a long period of time when there is a question of stopping the medication. If such a patient has paroxysmal activity while receiving medication, then the medication should be continued. If the record is normal, there is no guarantee that the patient will remain seizure-free when anticonvulsant therapy is discontinued. In either case, whether to discontinue the medication remains a clinical decision.

Electroencephalography has also proved useful in the surgery of epilepsy, and repeated preoperative studies may be necessary to be certain of a focal discharge in which "phase reversal" may be seen (see Figs. 12–4 and 12–13).[34] Morrell and others have shown that an experimentally induced chronic epileptic focus, particularly in the temporal lobe, can give rise to a "mirror focus" in the other temporal lobe, and that if sufficient time is allowed to elapse before the initial focus is removed, the secondary or mirror focus may continue to discharge.[28] This affords a theoretical argument for the early removal of seizure foci, and certain patients with intractable temporal lobe (or other) seizures have been markedly improved by removal of the primary focus in one temporal lobe or elsewhere.[30, 31] Localization of such an offending focus is of obvious neurosurgical importance. In temporal lobe epilepsy especially, bilateral discharges are very common, and this makes evaluation of patients prior to surgery particularly difficult. In this situation, although intracarotid pentylenetetrazol (Metrazol) and amobarbital (Amytal) techniques have sometimes proved useful, it may at times be necessary to implant electrodes into the depth of the temporal lobe for recording purposes.[13] This seems justified only when operation is planned and, even then, only rarely. Numerous recordings of this type have been done and interesting comparisons can be made between the activity recorded from the depth of the temporal lobe, the activity recorded by electrocorticography over the surface, and routine recording either from the surface of the scalp or from nasopharyngeal or sphenoidal electrodes. Often, seizure discharges may be seen in all three locations, but there are many examples in which the epileptic electrical activity may only be recorded from the depths of the temporal lobe (Fig. 12–14). In these patients, it may not be possible to record the abnormal rhythm with any technique that does not require entry into the calvarium.

During an operation, the recording from electrodes placed on the cortex (electrocorticogram) and the stimulation of and subsequent recording from the exposed cortex have proved to be useful.[29] By these means, it may be possible to distinguish the areas of morphological change from other areas that are, in fact, the main source of epileptic activity and also to delineate primary from secondary epileptic foci.

There are other examples of the usefulness of the electroencephalogram during an operation. Continuous monitoring during cardiac operations as well as operations on the large vessels of the chest and neck, is very useful. For example, if during the monitoring of cerebral activity in this way there is evidence of cerebral dysfunction, occlusions of vessels may be corrected or bypass grafts may be repositioned before large areas of cerebral necrosis result. Also, although not commonly used in clinical practice, it has long been possible to monitor the level of anesthesia by its influence on the electroencephalogram.[11]

INTRACRANIAL SPACE-OCCUPYING LESIONS

Any impairment of consciousness is associated with diffuse electrical abnormalities that are characterized by the decrease or absence of normal rhythms and the appearance of slow-wave activity.[16, 23] If the pathological process that is responsible for the disturbance of consciousness affects the cerebrum diffusely (severe trauma, hypoxia, and the like), generalized abnormalities will result from primary dysfunction of cerebral neurons. Certain of these processes (and also some general anesthetics), however, have their effect primarily on brain stem structures responsible for consciousness (the "reticular activating system" of Magoun[24]). These include posterior fossa mass lesions and transtentorial herniations with brain stem compression as well as contusion of brain stem following trauma. The generalized abnormalities associated with these lesions will present as so-called "projected rhythms" (Fig. 12–15). The abnormalities may be bilateral because of primary dysfunction either supratentorially or in the posterior fossa, and it may be seen that any significant intracranial space-occupying lesion may produce an abnormal study by virtue of its effect on mechanisms underlying the patient's consciousness. In addition, there may be more focal changes relating to the lesion itself, if it is in the cerebrum; these are described later.

The nature of the changes produced in either a diffuse or specific fashion by space-occupying lesions depends in large part upon the nature of the lesion. Rapidly enlarging processes, such as intracerebral hemorrhage, temporal lobe herpes simplex encephalitis, abscess, glioblastoma, or metastatic tumor, tend to produce abnormal recordings in at least 95 per cent of patients. In the case of abscess, temporal lobe encephalitis, or intracerebral hemorrhage, the recording is for practical purposes, always abnormal. On the other hand, meningiomas *may* grow to enormous size and produce quite striking clinical signs without affecting electrical activity in any way. Pituitary and other parasellar tumors do not cause any affect unless the extrasellar mass is large. Then medial temporal lobe compression may produce bitemporal theta activity, or if consciousness is affected by compression of brain stem or hydrocephalus, diffuse changes may be seen. The more classic and diagnostically

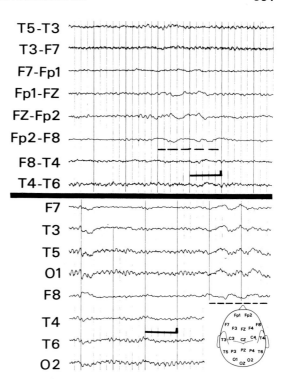

FIGURE 12–15 These are studies of two patients with small brain stem infarcts. Note that above the dotted lines the episodic slow activity is superimposed on a normal background.

helpful abnormalities relating to space-occupying lesions consist of focal or localized decrease of normal rhythms and their replacement by slow activity, especially in the delta range (Fig. 12–16). This gives the correct lateralization in at least 80 per cent of supratentorial tumors, but it is useful for exact preoperative localization in less than 50 per cent.

It must be remembered that the electroencephalogram is a physiological test that is related to function, whereas neuroradiological tests are essentially anatomical in type and are to be preferred for exact preoperative localization. The evolution of abnormal electrical activity is important. If it worsens sequentially, it is likely that an expanding space-occupying lesion is present. The same rule applies in following the clinical course of a cerebral abscess under treatment. A change in electrical activity may be helpful since it can occur before clinical signs of expansion of the abscess are present.

Tumors, abscesses, and hematomas may produce clinical or electroencephalo-

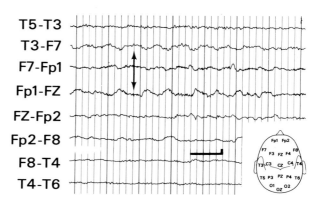

FIGURE 12–16 This record is from a patient with a left frontal meningioma and shows focal slowing (*arrows*) in the delta range over electrodes Fp1 and F7.

graphic evidence of seizure activity. In this context, it should be stressed that the typical three-per-second spike and wave activity of petit mal epilepsy is never produced by space-occupying lesions whether they be deep in central structures or located elsewhere and that there is nothing unique about the electroencephalographic aspects of "symptomatic epilepsy." It is not possible to differentiate the seizure activity caused by space-occupying lesions from that discussed in the preceding section.

HEAD INJURY AND COMA

Animal experiments have shown that during the period of concussion, the electroencephalogram is abnormal with generalized flattening of the wave forms.[12] However, humans are practically never tested before concussive changes have disappeared. Therefore, characteristically after a simple concussion, their records are normal. In patients with more severe head injuries involving cerebral contusion, laceration, edema, and subdural or epidural and intracerebral hemorrhage, it may be either focally or asymmetrically abnormal (reduction of normal rhythms and presence of slow activity) or generally and diffusely slow if the patient has a depressed level of consciousness. Patients with slight injuries may show only a marked reduction of alpha activity over one hemisphere. In patients with increasingly severe injuries, first local and then generalized delta and theta activity may be seen.[4] Extremely severe head injuries may, because of direct trauma to cerebrum or brain stem or both and resulting respiratory failure, produce irreversible coma with electrocerebral silence (see Fig. 12–9 A and B). Patients with lesser injuries who have persistent headache, dizziness, irritability, inability to concentrate, and difficulty with memory, sleep, and balance following head injury (the "post-traumatic syndrome") rarely, early in their course, have slowing of the cerebral rhythms that may help to delineate this syndrome from compensation neurosis.

When patients with serious head injuries are followed sequentially, and recovery

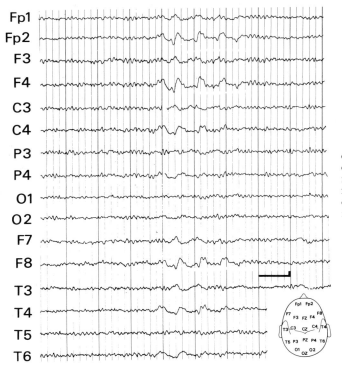

FIGURE 12–17 This record shows episodic slowing in the delta range with occasional sharp waves and decreased normal rhythms particularly over the right frontotemporal regions from which a subdural hematoma was subsequently removed.

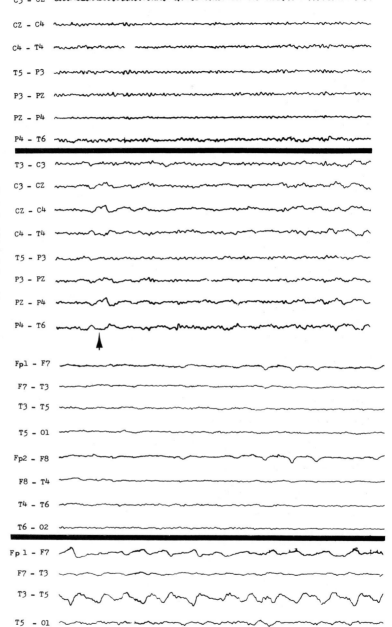

FIGURE 12–18 In each of these records of two different patients, the top half was made before removal of a small subdural hematoma and the bottom half postoperatively. Note the appearance in both patients, postoperatively, of considerable slow activity on the operative side—right centrotemporal in *A* and left frontotemporal in *B*.

ensues, the diffuse, nonspecific, slow-wave changes associated with the initial altered state of consciousness often disappear, and more focal abnormalities may be seen, usually in the form of delta or theta activity. Depending on the nature and severity of the underlying neuropathological process, these changes may or may not subsequently disappear or, in the event that post-traumatic epilepsy develops, may eventually be replaced by spikes or sharp-wave activity. These latter abnormalities are rather characteristic and may be helpful in determining the prognosis and in deciding when to begin medical therapy either to prevent or to relieve epilepsy. It should be remembered, however, that 40 to 50 per cent of patients with clear-cut post-traumatic epilepsy have normal or minimally (and nondiagnostically) abnormal electroencephalograms.[26] Also, an unknown number of these patients have seizure activity shown on their records without clinical evidence of epilepsy.

In many instances, the electroencephalograph is used to evaluate patients for possible subdural hematoma after a head injury. In two thirds of patients with a proved subdural hematoma, it is of localizing value. There will be slight to moderate or marked slowing of the rhythm. Less commonly, there may be a decrease of the alpha rhythm or an asymmetry of the voltage with the affected hemisphere being significantly lower (Fig. 12–17). With sequential recordings, these changes may increase, and this serves to distinguish the subdural collection from cerebral laceration or contusion, which should improve with time. In about one third of patients, therefore, the recording is either bilaterally abnormal or entirely normal. Patients who are poorly responsive will, as discussed earlier, have bilateral abnormalities, but the presence of bilateral subdural hematomas should also then be considered. In the patients who are normal preoperatively, a focal abnormality (delta focus) may be seen only after operation for the removal of the subdural hematoma (Fig. 12–18). It is important to recognize this fact since, if the patient is doing well clinically, a postoperative worsening of the electrical pattern does not necessarily mean that another exploration should be performed for a reaccumulation of the he-

matoma. In the evaluation of asymmetries of rhythm following head trauma or operation, one must consider the effects produced by cranial defects. If bone is missing beneath the electrodes, the amplitude will be larger on that side than on the normal one. If, however, an acrylic or tantalum plate is in place, the amplitude should be symmetrical.

In the evaluation of a comatose patient when an adequate history is unavailable, electroencephalography may be useful in the following ways. Barbiturates and most sedatives produce excessive fast activity, and when this is seen, intoxication with one of these agents should be suspected (see Fig. 12–7). In hepatic and certain of the metabolic comas, rather characteristic bilateral large "triphasic" waves are seen, especially frontally, and the presence of these may aid in diagnosis. Seizure activity or postictal extreme flattening and slowing may be seen if the patient is in "subclinical status epilepticus" or a postictal coma. Focal delta waves may be present if a rapidly expanding space-occupying lesion is responsible for the coma.

VASCULAR DISEASE

Typical electroencephalographic findings in the various cerebrovascular syndromes are as yet poorly worked out. However, electroencephalography has been useful in the differential diagnosis of vascular hemiplegia. That produced by large-vessel disease, in which arteriography and carotid surgery may at least be considered, is always associated with a focal or lateralized slow-wave abnormality (Figs. 12–10 and 12–19 B), whereas the hemiplegia produced by deep, small-vessel disease associated with hypertension ("lacunes") and not amenable to surgery usually produces no abnormality (Fig. 12–19 A). With certain pontine strokes, the patient may appear to be comatose while having a normal electrical rhythm. Most of these patients, however, if examined closely will show evidence of higher cerebral function even though they may only be able to communicate by movements of the eyes when all other functions are paralyzed.

The electroencephalogram has long been used in patients with subarachnoid hemor-

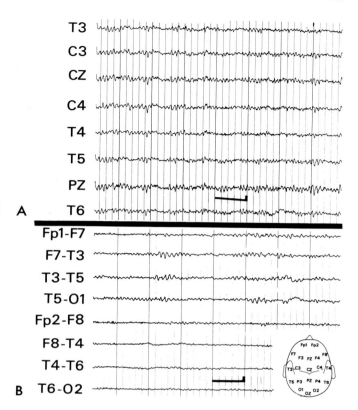

FIGURE 12–19 These are the records of two patients with acute hemiplegia. *A*. The record from a patient with lacunar hemiplegia is normal. *B*. In this record, left temporal slow-wave activity is visible throughout — this patient's hemiplegia was the result of carotid artery disease.

rhage in an attempt to localize or lateralize the aneurysm that has bled. In a recent study of 70 patients with ruptured aneurysms, correct localization was possible in more than 80 per cent when the study was done shortly after the ictus.[5] The accuracy of localization was 97 per cent in those in whom the abnormality (delta and theta slowing with reduction of normal activity) was especially clear-cut. If these findings are confirmed, this test may be increasingly useful in the evaluation of subarachnoid hemorrhage.

Vascular headaches (migraine and others) are very common, and many patients who have them are evaluated for possible tumors or arteriovenous malformations. In a clinical study of 560 patients with migraine, Hockaday and Whitty found the interictal electroencephalogram to be abnormal in 61 per cent.[18] The abnormalities were nonspecific (unilateral or bilateral theta or delta — sometimes occurring in paroxysms — and sharp or spike and spike-wave activity), but of those patients with a lateralized nonvisual aura, 47 per cent had an asymmetrical abnormality and of these, the abnormality was on the appropriate side in 88 per cent. They made the point, however, that a permanently abnormal recording, even if the abnormality and the clinical localization are on the same side, does not *in itself* indicate the need for further neuroradiological evaluation of patients with migraine.

PSYCHIATRIC DISEASE

The incidence of electroencephalographic abnormalities is no greater in a population of psychiatric patients than in a group of normal controls, nor are there any abnormalities peculiar to psychiatric disease, level of intelligence, motivation, and so forth. Therefore, this test is a useful screening measure in patients with suspected psychiatric disease. If it is abnormal, there is an 80 per cent chance that the patient has some neurological or neurosurgical disease affecting his cerebrum as well. If a slow-wave focus, seizure activity (see Fig. 12–4), excessive fast activity, or others of the abnormalities already mentioned are found, the patient should be evaluated further. One must bear in mind, of course, that drugs used in the treatment of psychiatric patients can produce excessive fast activity and, if they make the patient drowsy, slowing of the rhythm as well (see Fig. 12–7 *B*). Also, both electroconvulsive therapy and lobotomy produce long-lasting slow-wave activity.

Automatic, and sometimes combative, behavior during the "psychomotor attacks" of temporal lobe epilepsy has long been recognized. Most exciting for psychiatrists, neurologists, and neurosurgeons alike are the studies showing that temporal lobe epilepsy may be a more frequent association of episodic violence in the community than was heretofore recognized.[25] Attempts are being made in a number of centers to treat selected persons with this disorder with neurosurgical operative techniques.

NEGATIVE VALUE OF THE ELECTROENCEPHALOGRAM

Some of the characteristic abnormalities to be expected in neurosurgical patients with various types of lesion have just been described. As noted, this test is not particularly useful for localization of tumors, and with the advent of reliable brain scans and contrast neuroradiology, a *normal* study may have become more useful to the neurosurgeon than an abnormal one. For example, in the evaluation of a patient with headache and a normal neurological examination, it is extremely valuable when normal, since the chance of the patient having a brain tumor is less than 10 per cent. If both the electroencephalogram and brain scan are normal, the likelihood that such a patient has a cerebral tumor is on the order of 1 per cent or less. A normal recording is also useful in ruling out subdural empyema, cerebral abscess, or significant cerebral disease shortly following a head injury.

Acknowledgement: We would like to thank Mr. Lawrence Cherkas for preparing the figures for this chapter.

REFERENCES

1. Alderete, J. F., Jeri, F. R., Richardson, E. P., Jr., Sament, S., Schwab, R. S., and Young, R. R.: Irreversible coma: A clinical, electroencephalographic and neuropathological study. Trans. Amer. Neurol. Ass., *93*:16–20, 1968.
2. Beecher, H. K. (Chairman): A definition of irreversible coma. J.A.M.A., *205*:337–340, 1968.
3. Berger, H.: Über das Elektrenkephalogramm des Menschen. Arch. Psychiat. Nervenkr., *87*: 527–570, 1929.
4. Bickford, R. G., and Klass, D. W.: Acute and chronic EEG findings after head injury. *In* Caveness, W. F., and Walker, A. E., eds.: Head Injury. Philadelphia, J. B. Lippincott Co., 1966, pp. 63–88.
5. Binnie, C. D., Margerison, J. H., and McCaul, I. R.: Electroencephalographic localization of ruptured intracranial aneurysms. Brain, *92*:679–690, 1969.
6. Caton, R.: The electrical currents of the brain. Brit. Med. J., *2*:278, 1875.
7. Cooper, R., Osselton, J. W., and Shaw, J. C.: EEG Technology. London, Butterworth & Co., Ltd., 1969.
8. Creutzfeldt, O. D.: Nueronal mechanisms underlying the EEG. *In* Jasper, H. A., Ward, A. A., Jr., and Pope, A.: Basic Mechanisms of the Epilepsies. Boston, Little, Brown and Co., 1969, pp. 397–410.
9. Dement, W., and Kleitman, N.: Cyclic variations in EEG during sleep and their relation to eye movements, body motility and dreaming. Electroenceph. Clin. Neurophysiol., *9*:673–690, 1957.
10. Donchin, E., and Lindsley, D. B., eds.: Average Evoked Potentials: Methods, Results and Evaluations. Washington, D.C., Scientific and Technical Information Division, National Aeronautics and Space Administration, 1969.
11. Faulconer, A., Jr., and Bickford, R. G.: Electroencephalography in Anesthesiology. Springfield, Ill., Charles C Thomas, 1960.
12. Foltz, E. L., Jenkner, F. L., and Ward, A. A., Jr.: Experimental cerebral concussion. J. Neurosurg., *10*:342–352, 1953.
13. Garretson, H., Gloor, P., and Rasmussen, T.: Intra-carotid amobarbital and Metrazol test for the study of epileptiform discharges in man: a note on its technique. Electroenceph. Clin. Neurophysiol., *21*:607–610, 1966.
14. Gibbs, F. A., and Gibbs, E. L.: Atlas of Electroencephalography, 2nd Ed. Reading, Mass., Addison-Wesley Pub. Co., Inc., 1950–1964.
15. Gloor, P.: Hans Berger—on the electroencephalogram of man. Electroenceph. Clin. Neurophysiol., suppl. 28, 1969.
16. Hess, R.: Significance of EEG—signs for location of cerebral tumours. pp. 75–110. *In* Magnus O., Storm van Leeuwen, W., and Cobb, W. A., eds.: Electroencephalography and Cerebral Tumours. Electroenceph. Clin. Neurophysiol., suppl. 19, 1961.
17. Hill, D., and Parr, G., eds.: Electroencephalography: A Symposium on its Various

Aspects. 2nd Ed. New York, The Macmillan Co., 1963.

18. Hockaday, J. M., and Whitty, C. W. M.: Factors determining the electroencephalogram in migraine: A study of 560 patients, according to clinical type of migraine. Brain, *92*:769–788, 1969.

19. Jasper, H. H.: The ten twenty electrode system of the international federation. Electroenceph. Clin. Neurophysiol., *10*:371–375, 1958.

20. Kiloh, L. G., and Osselton, J. W.: Clinical Electroencephalography. 2nd Ed. London, Butterworth and Co., Ltd., 1966.

21. Kooi, K. A.: Fundamentals of Electroencephalography. New York, Harper & Row, 1971.

22. Lyberi, G., and Last, S. L.: The use of chlorpromazine as an activating agent. Electroenceph. Clin. Neurophysiol., *8*:711–712, 1956.

23. Magnus, O., Storm van Leeuwen, W., and Cobb, W. A.: Electroencephalography and Cerebral Tumours. Electroenceph. Clin. Neurophysiol., suppl. 19, 1961.

24. Magoun, H. W.: The Waking Brain. Springfield, Ill., Charles C Thomas, 1958.

25. Mark, V. H., and Ervin, F. R.: Violence and the Brain. New York, Harper & Row, 1970.

26. Marshall, C., and Walker, A. E.: The value of electroencephalography in the prognostication and prognosis of post-traumatic epilepsy. Epilepsia, *2*:138–143, 1961.

27. Merlis, J. K., Henriksen, G. F., and Grossman, C.: Metrazol activation of seizure discharges in epileptics with normal routine electroencephalograms. Electroenceph. Clin. Neurophysiol., *2*:17–22, 1950.

28. Morrell, F.: Physiology and histochemistry of the mirror focus. *In* Jasper, H. H., Ward, A. A., Jr., and Pope, A., eds.: Basic Mechanisms of the Epilepsies. Boston, Little, Brown and Co., 1969, pp. 357–370.

29. Penfield, W., and Jasper, H.: Epilepsy and the Functional Anatomy of the Human Brain. Boston, Little, Brown and Co., 1954.

30. Rasmussen, T.: Surgical therapy of post-traumatic epilepsy. *In* Walker, A. E., Caveness, W. F., and Critchley, M.: The Late Effects of Head Injury. Springfield, Ill., Charles C Thomas, 1969, pp. 277–305.

31. Rasmussen, T.: The neurosurgical treatment of focal epilepsy. Epilepsy, Mod. Probl. Pharmaco-psychiat. vol. 4, pp. 306–325, Karger, New York, 1970. (ed. by E. Niedermeyer)

32. Rechtschaffen, A., and Kales, A.: A Manual of Standardized Terminology, Techniques and Scoring System for Sleep Stages of Human Subjects. Bethesda, Md., U.S. Public Health Service, National Institute of Neurological Diseases and Stroke, 1968. (N.I.H. Publication No. 204.)

33. Reiher, J., and Klass, D. W.: Two common EEG patterns of doubtful clinical significance. Med. Clin. N. Amer., *52*:933–940, 1968.

34. Rovit, R. L., Gloor, P., and Henderson, L. R.: Temporal lobe epilepsy—a study using multiple basal electrodes. Neurochirurgia, *3*:6–19, 1960.

35. Rovit, R. L., Gloor, P., and Rasmussen, T.: Sphenoidal electrodes in the electrographic study of patients with temporal lobe epilepsy—an evaluation. J. Neurosurg., *18*:151–158, 1961.

36. Schwab, R. S., Potts, F., and Bonazzi, A.: EEG as an aid in determining death in the presence of cardiac activity (ethical, legal and medical aspects). Electroenceph. Clin. Neurophysiol., *15*:147–148, 1963.

37. Silverman, D., Masland, R. L., Saunders, M. G., and Schwab, R. S.: Irreversible coma associated with electrocerebral silence. Neurology (Minneap.), *20*:525–533, 1970.

38. Stewart, L. F.: Chlorpromazine: Use to activate electroencephalographic seizure patterns. Electroenceph. Clin. Neurophysiol., *9*:427–440, 1957.

13

ELECTROMYOGRAPHY

In clinical electromyography, the electrical activity of muscle and peripheral nerve (electroneurography) is recorded. The purpose is to detect abnormalities that may indicate the presence and the nature of a neuromuscular disorder. The examination is concerned chiefly with the diagnosis of conditions that affect the lower motor neuron, the neuromuscular junctions and skeletal muscle fibers, the primary sensory neuron, and the volitional and reflex activity of muscles. Several electrophysiological techniques are employed: (1) the classic electromyographic examination in which a needle electrode is inserted into the muscle to record its electrical activity at rest and during voluntary contraction; (2) the measurement of the compound action potential that is evoked in a muscle by maximal stimulation of its motor nerve and estimation of the conduction velocity of the nerve; (3) the observation of transient changes in the muscle action potential during repetitive electrical stimulation, and (4) the measurement of the compound action potential that is evoked in a nerve by electrical stimulation and estimation of its conduction velocity in the nerve.

In neurological surgery, the electromyograph has its greatest value in providing evidence of damage to the lower motor neuron. It can detect minimal denervation of a muscle when the clinical evidence is equivocal or absent and it can do so in the presence of such conditions as pain, an upper motor neuron lesion, or hysteria that make the neurological examination of muscle strength unreliable. Furthermore, muscles whose weakness may be obscured by the action of synergists can be tested individually with the needle electrode. The more complete picture of the distribution of affected neurons that it provides is an aid in establishing whether the pattern of denervation is diffuse or is consistent with a lesion of nerve root, plexus, peripheral nerve, or segment of the spinal cord. Study of responses to nerve stimulation aids in detecting and locating peripheral lesions affecting motor or afferent fibers of nerves by the block of conduction or slowing of conduction that they produce.

The electromyogram is of little value in determining the nature of the lesion affecting the nerve. There is no reliable difference in electrical signs, for example, between damage to a nerve root by a protruded disc, a neurofibroma, or a diabetic radiculitis. In the latter case there may be electromyographic evidence of more diffuse neuropathy, but this is not helpful in excluding the possibility that the diabetic patient has a protruded disc.

In addition to its use in the study of nerve lesions, the electromyogram is helpful in differentiating primarily neuropathic from myopathic disorders and in demonstrating defects of neuromuscular transmission, myotonia, and other phenomena.

A preliminary neurological examination is essential for planning and interpreting the electromyographic examination. The nerves and muscles to be tested must be selected according to the problem that is presented by the patient. Skill is required to elicit and identify meaningful patterns of abnormality in the study. In contrast to the electroencephalogram and the electrocardiogram, the procedure must be modified and the results interpreted as the examination proceeds. The usefulness of an electromyogram depends largely on the training, experience, and knowledge of

E. H. LAMBERT

neurological problems of the person who performs the examination.

THE ELECTROMYOGRAPH

The basic electromyographic equipment consists of an electrode system, an amplifier, a cathode-ray oscilloscope and a camera with provision for calibration of both voltage and time, a loud speaker (which aids in identification of wave forms and patterns of activity by the sounds they produce), and a nerve stimulator. In several commercial electromyographs these components have been integrated in a single instrument that is relatively simple to operate. The technical requirements of the instrumentation have been outlined by the Committee on EMG Instrumentation of the International Federation of Societies for EEG and Clinical Neurophysiology. The prospective user of an electromyograph should be aware of these requirements.

THE NEEDLE ELECTRODE EXAMINATION

Examination of the electrical activity of muscle with a needle electrode provides information about the integrity and function of the motor units. A motor unit consists of a single lower motor neuron and the muscle fibers that are innervated by its branches. The number of muscle fibers innervated by a single neuron varies from a few in extraocular muscles to over 1,000 in large limb muscles. A muscle such as the biceps

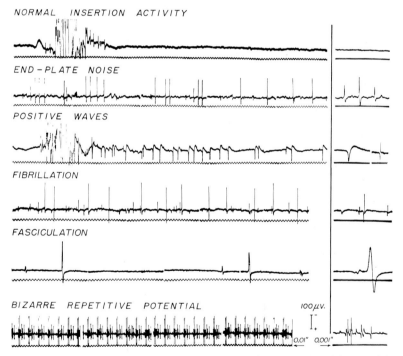

FIGURE 13–1 Example of insertion activity and spontaneous activity recorded with a coaxial needle electrode from voluntarily relaxed muscle. In all records negativity of the central core of the electrode causes an upward deflection. "Normal insertion activity," a brief discharge of potentials lasting little longer than the movement of the needle. "End-plate noise," low-voltage negative potentials (irregular baseline) and negative-positive spikes recorded when the needle is in contact with motor end-plates and injures nerve terminals. This activity occurs in normal muscle and should not be confused with fibrillation potentials. "Positive waves," activity evoked by movement of the electrode in denervated muscle. This form of potential results when the needle electrode records from denervated muscle fibers it has injured. Note the initial sharp positive phase followed by a long negative phase in the potentials following the brief burst of activity associated with movement of the electrode. Positive waves are often accompanied by brief fibrillation potentials (*far right*). "Fibrillation," spontaneous occurrence of fibrillation potentials in denervated muscle. Note the initial negative phase. "Fasciculation," sporadic occurrence of motor unit potentials, often with an associated visible twitch. "Bizarre repetitive potential," a form that may occur in some myopathies as well as in motor neuron disorders.

brachii has 400 to 500 motor units. The *motor unit action potential* is the electrical sign of the activity of the motor unit. It is the summation of the action potentials of the muscle fibers of the unit. Those fibers closest to the electrode contribute the greatest share to the action potential of the motor unit.

Insertion or movement of a needle electrode in normal muscle evokes a brief burst of sharp potentials as a result of mechanical stimulation of muscle and nerve fibers (insertion activity) (Fig. 13-1). The activity ceases when the needle comes to rest, except in occasional minute areas where the needle injures nerve terminals and lies in contact with motor end-plates. In the latter instance unique low-voltage negative potentials (end-plate noise) and irregularly occurring diphasic spikes continue to occur when the needle is at rest. In all other areas in relaxed muscle, with the needle undisturbed, no electrical activity is detected (electrical silence). During a very weak voluntary or postural contraction a single motor unit may be active in the vicinity of the electrode. Its action potential recurs at a rate of 4 to 10 times per second. As the strength of contraction increases, the rate at which the unit fires increases, and other motor units are recruited. Each unit fires rhythmically and independently. During a strong contraction so many units are active that single motor unit action potentials can no longer be identified (interference pattern).

In a systematic examination the needle electrode is inserted into the muscle and advanced by steps to several depths of the muscle. Observations are made of the electric activity on insertion or movement of the needle, while the muscle is at rest with the needle undisturbed, and while the muscle is voluntarily contracted. During a weak contraction, action potentials of single motor units are characterized as to their amplitude, duration, shape, rhythm, and rate. During strong volition, the number of units recruited and their rate of discharge are observed in relation to the strength of contraction. A thorough examination of a single muscle may require three or more insertions of the electrode with movement to several positions in each area of the muscle after each insertion.

Abnormal Insertion Activity

Either prolonged activity or the absence of activity upon insertion or movement of the needle is abnormal. In a denervated muscle, prolonged repetitive activity of denervated muscle fibers follows needle movement. The action potentials are usually "positive waves" ("positive sharp waves"), a form that results when the action potential of the muscle fiber is recorded from a portion of the muscle fiber injured by the needle electrode. Similar activity may occur in muscle in which degeneration or regeneration of muscle fibers is occurring. In the myotonias, prolonged trains of positive waves and spikes that wax and wane in amplitude and frequency produce a characteristic "dive-bomber sound" over the loudspeaker. Similar "myotonic discharges" may occur in myopathy with acid maltase deficiency, in hyperkalemic periodic paralysis, and occasionally in inflammatory myopathies. Potentials that occur repetitively at a very regular rate without significant variation in shape or size, changing or stopping abruptly, have been called pseudomyotonic discharges. Those with a complex wave form, called bizarre repetitive potentials or bizarre high-frequency potentials, occur occasionally in anterior horn cell disorders, including segmental lesions as well as progressive muscular atrophies, but are also seen in myopathies, such as polymyositis and progressive muscular dystrophy. Their origin is not known. They may result from repetitive firing of abnormal nerve terminals.

Insertional activity is reduced or absent when muscle fibers are incapable of being excited. Examples of this condition are a severe attack of periodic paralysis, or severe disintergration of the muscle fibers and their replacement by fat or connective tissue. Increased resistance to insertion of the needle suggests an increase in relative amount of collagen in the muscle.

Spontaneous Activity

Fibrillation

Classically, the term "fibrillation" refers to the spontaneous, rhythmic contractions of muscle fibers that have been denervated. These contractions can be observed as a delicate flickering of light reflected from the surface of an exposed muscle, but they are not visible through the intact skin. Fibrillation can be detected by recording the electrical activity of the fibrillating muscle fibers with a needle electrode. The action potentials are brief diphasic or triphasic spikes (most commonly, 2 to 3 msec in duration and 25 to 250 μv in amplitude). The action potential of a single fiber usually occurs with a regular rhythm at a rate of from 2 to 10 per second. Many fibers firing independently of one another produce a profusion of action potentials and a sound over the loudspeaker like rain on a tin roof. Particularly just after needle insertion many of the action potentials of fibrillating muscle fibers may be the positive waves described in the section on abnormal insertion activity. The clinical significance of the two forms of potential, the spike and the positive wave, is the same. They usually occur together and can be referred to collectively as fibrillation potentials.

Care must be taken not to confuse the brief diphasic potentials associated with end-plate noise in normal muscle with the fibrillation potentials of denervated muscle. The former can be identified by their irregular, "sputtering" rhythm, initial negative phase, frequent association with the low-voltage component of end-plate noise, and their occurrence in very localized areas (often with a complaint by the patient of more acute pain). This is in contrast to the more regular rhythm, usually initial positive phase and more diffuse occurrence of fibrillation potentials in denervated muscle. End-plate noise is encountered more frequently in small muscles of the hands and feet than it is in larger muscles of the extremities, and complicates the examination of the small muscles.

Although fibrillation potentials occur in denervated muscle, they are not pathognomonic of a nerve lesion in the usual sense. Similar potentials are found in some myopathic disorders. They are common in the inflammatory myopathies (polymyositis) and occasionally are seen in muscular dystrophy. Their occurrence by itself, cannot be used to differentiate neuropathic from myopathic disorders in the classic sense. The clinical history and the associated abnormalities of motor unit activity are important in making this differentiation.

Fasciculation

Fasciculation potentials resemble the action potentials of motor units, but they occur sporadically at relatively low rates. They are associated with spontaneous contraction of a motor unit or bundle of muscle fibers. The twitch may be visible through the skin. Although fasciculation occurs almost invariably in amyotrophic lateral sclerosis, it also may occur in patients with relatively benign conditions and in otherwise healthy persons. Consequently, the diagnosis of a degenerative disease of lower motor neurons should not be based on the presence of fasciculation alone.

Activity of motor units resembling that seen in voluntary contraction occurs in reflex muscle spasm and in spasticity, rigidity and other involuntary contractions associated with diseases of the central nervous system. The frequency and pattern of the motor unit activity reflects the frequency and pattern of discharge of lower motor neurons. The activity is periodic in tremors. The electromyogram can provide an objective record of tremor for quantitative studies. In muscle cramp, large numbers of motor units discharge at relatively high frequency. Although nerve block prevents the voluntary induction of a cramp, cramp can still be produced by repetitive electrical stimulation of the nerve below the block. This indicates that cramps, like most fasciculations, originate in the periphery, probably in nerve terminals. Tetany, associated with hyperventilation or hypocalcemia is associated with spontaneous firing of motor units that originates in the axon. Many of the discharges are double or multiple ("doublets" or "multiplets").

ELECTRICAL STIMULATION OF NERVES

Conduction in motor Fibers.

The excitability of a motor nerve can be tested by electrical stimulation. The response of a muscle is observed visually or by palpation to determine whether the peripheral motor innervation is intact. When there is paralysis of voluntary contraction, a good response to electrical stimulation suggests that the paralysis is due to a block of conduction proximal to the point of stimulation or to an upper motor neuron lesion, hysteria, or malingering. By noting the response to stimulation at several points along the length of the nerve, the site of a local block of conduction may be located by the difference in response to stimulation above and below the block. A routine technique in electromyography is to record the compound action potential of the muscle as a measure of its response to nerve stimulation. This recording provides not only a measure of the magnitude of the response, but also allows precise timing of the response so that a measurement of the conduction velocity of the nerve can be made.

To record the muscle response, small disc electrodes on the skin surface or small bare needle electrodes placed just under the skin are fixed over the belly and tendon of the muscle. A stimulus to the motor nerve evokes a compound muscle action potential whose size is roughly proportional to the number of muscle fibers that respond. However, the size of the action potential is also affected by other factors, such as the position of the recording electrodes, the position of the muscle, the bulk of tissue around the muscle, and the muscle temperature. The amplitude of the action potential varies widely among individuals. The range of amplitude of the negative spike varies from 5 to 15 mv.

If a standard technique is used, the size of the action potential can be used as a crude measure of the degree of involvement of the muscle in neuromuscular disorders. It can be used as an indication of differences in magnitude of the response to stimulation at different points along the nerve in locating a block of conduction, in comparison of responses of muscles of the two extremities to detect unilateral lesions, or in serial examinations of the same muscle when following progress of a lesion or reinnervation in a patient.

The latency of the response, which is measured from the beginning of the stimulus to the beginning of the action potential, is a measure of the time required for excitation of the nerve, the conduction of the nerve impulse from the point of stimulation to the nerve ending, transmission across the neuromuscular junction, and excitation of the muscle fibers. When the nerve is stimulated successively at two points along its length, "conduction velocity" of motor fibers over the distance between the points can be determined from the difference in the latency of the action potential that is evoked in the muscle. Usually the stimulus to the nerve is supramaximal for the motor response, and all the alpha motor fibers to the muscle are excited. The conduction velocity calculated from these values is the conduction velocity of the "fastest" fibers or the "maximal" conduction velocity. The latency of the response to stimulation at the distal point along the nerve, which is a standard distance from the muscle, is called the "distal latency" or "terminal conduction time." The duration of the muscle action potential is related to the differences in latency of response of various fibers of the muscle, which, in part, are the result of differences in conduction time in the various axons of the nerve.

Conduction in Afferent Fibers

Conduction in large afferent fibers is studied by recording the action potential that is evoked in a cutaneous nerve by a maximal electrical stimulus. A small triphasic action potential, usually less than 50 μv in amplitude, can be detected by electrodes at standard positions on the skin surface over the nerve or by a needle electrode inserted to the vicinity of the nerve. This is the action potential of the large myelinated fibers. Components representing the small delta fibers and the unmyelinated C fibers are not demonstrated by this technique.

In cutaneous nerves such as the digital, radial, and sural nerves the nerve action potential can be recorded almost invariably in healthy persons by relatively simple techniques. An action potential can also be recorded easily from mixed nerves such as the ulnar, median, and peroneal nerves. The major component of the action potential in these nerves consists of impulses of large afferent fibers, which conduct at a velocity slightly higher than that of motor fibers. By special techniques, including the averaging of many responses to reduce the noise in the recording, action potentials of as few as one or two nerve fibers can be detected.

Abnormalities of Conduction

Conduction velocity of the nerve is reduced in some diseases that affect peripheral nerves and is an aid in diagnosis of neuropathies. Slowing of conduction may be evident as a reduction in conduction velocity between two points along the nerve or as an increase either in distal latency or in duration of the nerve or muscle action potential or in both. Conduction velocity of myelinated axons is determined principally by their diameter and the insulating properties of the myelin sheath. Little or no change in conduction velocity occurs during acute degeneration of axons after nerve section or administration of axonal poisons

such as thallium or acrylamide. However, conduction velocity is markedly low in sparsely myelinated, small-diameter, regenerating axons and increases in direct proportion to the increase in axon diameter during maturation. Conduction velocity often is markedly low (5 to 60 per cent of the normal mean) in nerves with segmental demyelination, especially in disorders such as the Guillain-Barré syndrome and diphtheritic neuropathy. The conduction velocity is slowed in hypertrophic neuropathies in which there is a primary disorder of the myelin sheath. In neuropathies such as uremic neuropathy that have primarily axonal degeneration, a slight or moderate reduction of conduction velocity may result from attenuation of axon diameter and secondary changes in myelin in degenerating fibers or from selective loss of the large-diameter, fast-conducting fibers.

In anterior horn cell disorders, such as amyotrophic lateral sclerosis, conduction velocity of motor fibers is usually within the normal range, but in rare instances is as low as 60 per cent of the normal mean in se-

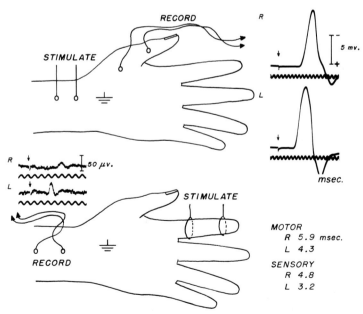

FIGURE 13–2 Latency of muscle and nerve action potentials in right carpal tunnel syndrome. Nerve action potentials evoked by stimulation of digital nerves in index finger are detected by surface electrodes over median nerve at wrist. The action potentials of thenar muscles evoked by stimulation of the median nerve at the wrist are recorded by surface electrodes over the belly and tendon of the abductor pollicis brevis. Latency of both responses (to start of muscle action potential and peak of nerve action potential) is prolonged on the right. Small arrows indicate the shock artifact. (From Electromyography and electric stimulation of peripheral nerves and muscle. *In* Mayo Clinic Clinical Examinations in Neurology. Philadelphia, W. B. Saunders Co., 1971.)

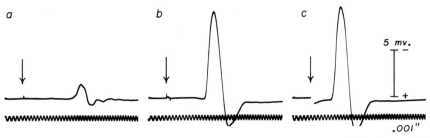

FIGURE 13–3 Compound action potential of extensor digitorum brevis muscle following maximal electrical stimulus to the peroneal nerve (*a*) just above head of fibula, (*b*) just below head of fibula and (*c*) at ankle. Action potential was detected by electrodes on the skin surface over the belly and tendons of the muscle. Arrow indicates the shock artifact. Low response to stimulation in (*a*) indicates block of conduction in many motor fibers at the head of the fibula.

verely affected nerves. Even then, conduction in afferent nerve fibers is normal. In myopathies, there is no slowing of conduction in motor or afferent fibers.

The site of compression or an entrapment lesion of a nerve often can be located by the slowing of conduction or the block of conduction that the lesion produces (Figs. 13-2 and 13-3). A decrease in diameter and demyelination of nerve fibers occurs in the compressed area. Although some fibers degenerate, a "physiological block" of conduction may persist in other fibers for many weeks and permit precise localization of the lesion. In the absence of blocked fibers, slowing of conduction through the affected area is an aid to localization. Some slowing of conduction also may occur proximally, as well as distally to the lesion.

Often in neuropathies and particularly in entrapment neuropathies, abnormalities of conduction may be detected in large afferent fibers even though abnormalities of conduction in motor fibers are absent or equivocal. The electromyographer should not limit his studies to the motor nerve. The cutaneous nerve action potential may be delayed, small, or not detectable by routine procedures, even though the neurological examination reveals little or no sensory deficit. On the other hand, the cutaneous nerve action potential is preserved in the presence of lesions proximal to the dorsal root ganglion; for example, it may be preserved despite loss of sensation after avulsion of the roots.

Errors in estimation of nerve length and latency cause proportional errors in the calculation of conduction velocity. Over a segment of nerve 25 cm in length duplicate

measurements of velocity on different days may differ by as much as 10 to 15 per cent. The error may be greater in measurements made over shorter lengths of nerve. Variations in temperature of the nerve contribute to the error. Conduction velocity decreases about 3 to 4 per cent with each degree centigrade decrease in nerve temperature. Knowledge of the temperature of the nerve is particularly important when assigning significance to slight prolongation of distal latency in diagnosis of such conditions as carpal tunnel syndrome. To minimize error, the extremity may be warmed to a standard temperature or the latency measurement can be corrected on the basis of temperature measurements at standard positions near the nerve. Age is another factor to be considered in the interpretation of conduction velocity measurements. Conduction velocity of peripheral nerves at birth is about half of the adult values. It reaches adult values between 3 and 5 years of age. After age 30 the velocity begins to decrease, and by the age of 80 years, conduction is 5 to 10 meters per second slower.

SEQUENCE OF ABNORMALITIES AFTER ACUTE NERVE DAMAGE

Immediately after a nerve injury, the only abnormality in the electromyogram is a reduction in the number of motor units that can be activated by maximal volition. Unfortunately, only gross reductions in number of motor units can be recognized with any degree of reliability in the electromyographic examination. If only a few motor units are active, a rapid rate of firing is evidence that the patient is using maximal effort to contract the muscle. If the units fire at a slow rate, as in a weak contraction of normal muscle, limitation of the contraction may be the result of pain, an upper motor neuron lesion, or malingering. After a severe nerve lesion, electromyography is useful for detecting minimal residual innervation that is not evident on clinical examination. Provided innervation of the muscle by an anomalous or accessory nerve can be excluded, the presence of a few motor unit potentials indicates that at least a few nerve fibers are intact and are conducting through the lesion.

During the first two to four days after a nerve injury, the muscle responds normally to a maximal electrical stimulus to its nerve distal to the site of injury. However, the response to stimulation of the nerve proximal to the injury is reduced in proportion to the number of motor fibers in which conduction is blocked either temporarily or permanently.

After three to four days the axons that have been irreversibly damaged begin to degenerate and the response of the muscle to a maximal nerve stimulus distal to the lesion is reduced. Gross reductions in the response serve as objective evidence of loss of axons. On the other hand, a good response to nerve stimulation at a time when maximal volition activates only a few motor units that fire at a rapid rate is evidence that, in large part, the weakness is the result of a reversible block of conduction proximal to the site of nerve stimulation.

Strength-duration curves as a measure of excitability of muscle to stimulation at its motor point may begin to demonstrate abnormalities at this time, but minimal loss of innervation cannot be detected by such curves and they are not widely used.

After 8 to 21 days, abnormal irritability of denervated muscle fibers becomes evident. Insertion or movement of the needle electrode is followed by transient trains of positive waves that persist longer than the insertion activity usually observed in normal muscle. Because occasional healthy persons may demonstrate slightly prolonged insertion activity, use of this criterion of abnormality is controversial. However, when the unusual insertion activity is clearly limited in distribution to a segmental or nerve innervation pattern and the history is consistent with a recent lesion, it may be helpful confirmatory evidence of nerve damage.

Prolonged insertion activity and persistent, "spontaneous" fibrillation appear 14 to 35 days after nerve injury. The long time required for the appearance of fibrillation in a muscle after nerve injury seriously limits the usefulness of this sign in the diagnosis of acute nerve lesions. In fact, if there has not been a direct injury to the muscle, the presence of fibrillation in an electromyogram that is performed within a few days after nerve injury suggests that there was a pre-existing lesion. This information may be of value in some cases, and examination for fibrillation early after injury may be justified even at a time when electromyographic criteria of the recent nerve damage would not be fully developed. However, it should be remembered that the focal injury to muscle and nerve fibers by the needle electrode can be the cause of minor abnormalities that may be detected in later studies.

The time required for the appearance of fibrillation is related inversely to the metabolic rate and temperature of the muscle. The time is also dependent on the length of the nerve between the lesion and the muscle. Fibrillation appears earlier in muscles closer to the lesion than in muscles more distal to the lesion. Following acute nerve root compression, fibrillation may appear in paraspinal muscles one to three weeks before it appears in the distal extremity muscles. It is essential that the electromyographer examine the paraspinal muscles even though an examination of the extremity muscles has not revealed a significant abnormality. The presence of fibrillation in the paraspinal muscles is an indication that the lesion may be intraspinal rather than in the plexus or peripheral nerve. However, the location and extent of the lesion cannot be adequately determined without evidence of the distribution of its effects in the extremity. Furthermore, metastatic lesions may occasionally affect the posterior rami of spinal nerves alone.

Fibrillation persists for many months until reinnervation occurs or until the muscle fibers become severely atrophic or degenerate. The earliest evidence of reinnervation is the appearance during voluntary effort of low-amplitude motor unit action potentials, many of which are highly polyphasic. These may be present for several weeks before there is clinical evidence of recovery of function.

LOCATION OF NERVE LESIONS

Electromyography aids in the location of a lesion by determining whether evidence of denervation is distributed widely or is confined to muscles innervated by a particular segment of the spinal cord, a root, plexus, or peripheral nerve (Fig. 13-4).

Although the electrical activity associated with the fibrillation of denervated muscle fibers is the most useful and most easily recognized evidence of damage to lower motor neurons, other abnormalities of the electromyogram are helpful in the investigation of nerve lesions. An integrated examination that takes advantage of all techniques of electromyography is essential.

Motor unit action potentials of large size may be found when there is involvement of anterior horn cells. They may occur in a segmental distribution, often without fibrillation, when there is involvement of the anterior part of the cervical spinal cord by spondylosis. They occur more frequently with cervical than with lumbar radicular lesions, possibly because of the proximity of the spinal cord to the lesion in the cervical region.

An increase in proportion of polyphasic or complex motor unit potentials may occur in a segmental distribution in patients with cervical radicular syndromes. It has been suggested that they are a more sensitive criterion of abnormality than fibrillation, but a quantitative evaluation remains to be made.

The occurrence of fasciculation in a segmental distribution has been used to localize root or spinal cord lesions, but it is not observed often enough to be of great value.

Misinterpretation of Incidental Lesions

Incidental lesions cause confusion in interpretation of the electromyogram. Fibrillation may result from injury to muscle and

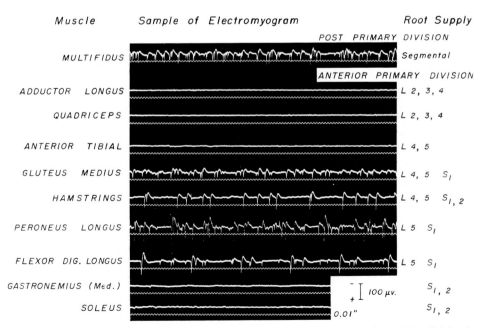

FIGURE 13–4 Electrical activity after needle insertion in relaxed muscles of patient with a fifth lumbar root lesion. Fibrillation, predominantly positive waves, occurred in muscles innervated by this root. The anterior tibial muscle may in some persons be innervated exclusively by the fourth root.

nerve by intramuscular injections. Isolated abnormalities in the glutei, deltoid, or triceps brachii should be questioned from this point of view. The needle electrode in the electromyographic examination damages nerve and muscle fibers and can cause abnormalities that, on a subsequent examination, might be considered the result of progression of a lesion. Sites of previous electromyographic examination should be avoided in biopsy of muscle for diagnostic purposes.

Especially disturbing to the electromyographic examination are the effects of a previous laminectomy. Following laminectomy there may be extensive denervation of paraspinal muscles, which results from an unavoidable damage to dorsal rami of spinal nerves. Fibrillation may be found for many months and perhaps years thereafter. Subsequent electromyographic examination of these muscles for evidence of recurrence of a lesion or for localization of another lesion is of little value. If an operation is contemplated in a patient with atypical symptoms, it is advisable that an electromyogram with examination of the paraspinal muscles be performed before the operation. After operation, the usefulness of the examination for localization is lost.

REFERENCES

1. Guld, C., Rosenflack, H., and Willison, R. G.: Report of the committee on EMG instrumentation. Electroenceph. Clin. Neurophysiol., 28:399-413, 1970.
2. Knutsson, B.: Comparative value of electromyographic, myelographic, and clinical-neurological examinations in diagnosis of lumbar root compression syndrome. Acta Orthop. Scand., Suppl. 49:108-135, 1961.
3. Licht, S.: Electrodiagnosis and Electromyography. 3rd Ed. New Haven, Conn., Elizabeth Licht, Publisher, 1971.
4. Weddell, S., Feinstein, B., and Pattle, R. E.: The electrical activity of voluntary muscles in man under normal and pathological conditions. Brain, 67:178-257, 1944.

III

Special Tests and Evaluation

14

NEURO-OPHTHALMOLOGICAL EVALUATION OF THE NEUROSURGICAL PATIENT

The eye and the structures associated with it are supplied by one half of the cranial nerves. Any careful evaluation of a neurosurgical patient should, therefore, include investigation for the ocular signs of neural damage. Although the ophthalmologist is best prepared to evaluate the eyes, a good examination can be made by anyone willing to spend a few additional minutes. The items needed for the examination are shown in Figure 14–1. With practice in the use of these instruments and in the interpretation of the findings, there are few major diagnostic eye signs that the neurosurgeon could overlook.

No matter how carefully the examination is performed, it is worth little if a detailed history is not included. Although physicians are trained as medical students to take good quality histories, the press of a busy practice may tend to interfere with detailed history-taking. It bears repeating that difficult diagnostic problems are more often solved by additional history than by further laboratory tests. The astute clinician distinguishes himself from the average clinician by taking a better than average history.

NEURO-OPHTHALMOLOGICAL HISTORY

The neurosurgical patient is often incapable of giving a concise detailed account of the events that led to his present state of affairs. He may be dysphasic from a dominant hemisphere lesion or obtunded following seizures or a rise in intracranial pressure. One may have to rely on members of the family, friends, or total strangers for some historical clues to the nature of the patient's disorder. This is particularly true in children. One must rely on the parents for information about the patient's growth, development, behavior, and habits. Specific questions should be asked concerning difficulties during the pregnancy, labor, or delivery. The history of skin rash and low-grade fever during the first trimester of the pregnancy may explain retardation, nystagmus, and peculiar retinal pigmentation in an infant as being due to maternal rubella.

Old photographs are an important part of any history. They are especially helpful in those patients who have recently noticed the drooping of one upper eyelid, a small difference in pupil size, or the sudden onset of diplopia. A good look at several old photographs under bright light with a magnifier may save the patient needless hospitalization for evaluation of a congenital ptosis, or aniscoria (unequal pupil size), or an old strabismus. A modest head-tilt in an old photograph may be all that is needed to explain the onset of vertical diplopia.

It is not sufficient merely to obtain the history of diplopia. It is equally important to know if it was of sudden onset (vascular) or slow (increased intracranial pressure), transient (myasthenia gravis), or progres-

J. A. McCRARY III
J. L. SMITH

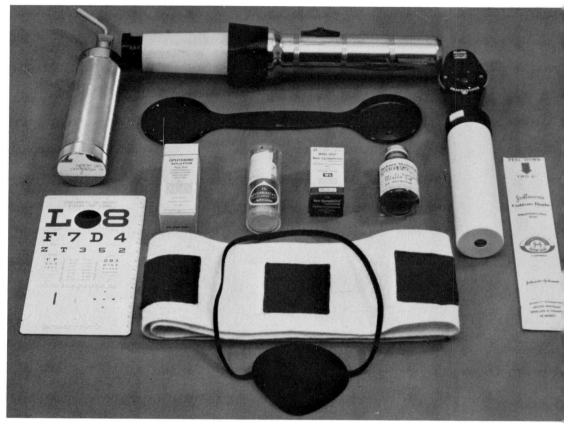

FIGURE 14–1 Examination materials. *Left to right, top row:* hand light, projector light, Maddox rod-occluder, and direct ophthalmoscope. *Middle row:* ophthalmic solutions. *Bottom row:* near card, optokinetic tape, occluder patch, and cotton-tipped applicators.

sive. If it is horizontal and worse at distance, a sixth nerve paresis or internuclear ophthalmoplegia is suggested. If the diplopia is vertical, it is usually worse when looking into the distance with disorders of the vertical rectus muscles and worse at near with disorders of the oblique muscles. It is also helpful to know if the diplopia increases when the patient looks to the right or left, up or down. The symptomatic correlate of acquired nystagmus is oscillopsia, or the apparent to and fro movement of the environment. The patient with vertical oscillopsia may describe it as though the vertical hold of a television picture were out of adjustment. Oscillopsia does not occur in congenital nystagmus.

Transient loss of vision may occur in one or both eyes. Transient obscurations of vision are bilateral and generally last 5 to 15 seconds. They are associated with chronic papilledema and are described as brief "gray-outs" or "brown-outs" or occasionally as complete loss of vision in both eyes. There may be hundreds of such episodes per day, but *they always last seconds, not minutes.* Transient ischemic attacks (TIA's) may be unilateral (carotid artery disease) or bilateral (basilar artery disease) and consist of sudden loss of vision, often preceded and followed by a "curtain" or "shade ' moving across the visual field. If the carotid circulation is involved, the attacks occur in one visual field (eye), and the shade may approach either horizontally or vertically. If the basilar arterial circulation is involved, the attack occurs in both visual fields. Often the lower half is involved more than the upper half, and in both types the attacks last 5 to 15 minutes. Occasional episodes may last up to 20 minutes. If an attack lasts over 20 minutes, there is usually some permanent impairment of visual field function. The major exception is the hemianopia associated with migraine.

Migraine is the most common cause for homonymous hemianopia. Migraine attacks may affect the visual field for more than 20 minutes without permanent damage. These hemianopias may occur without headache, nausea, emesis, scintillating scotomas, or any of the other usual stigmata of migraine. Migraine may affect the vascular supply of a s ngle eye, rather than of the hemisphere, in which case a unilateral visual field disturbance is found. Migraine is worsened by the use of oral contraceptives. Many of the patients who develop vascular complications while using progestational agents have a previous history of migraine.

Photophobia is not uncommon in the history of neurosurgical patients. The causes for discomfort or headache brought on by exposure to light of even moderate intensity has many causes. Photophobia is most often related to primary ocular disease, such as glaucoma or uveitis, but it may be found in diseases of the central nervous system (Table 14-1).

Less than 5 per cent of all headache is due to disorders of the eye primarily. Certainly errors of refraction, ocular muscle imbalance, and glaucoma can cause discomfort about the eyes (asthenopia) or headache. Headache so related is usually noted later in the day, with increased use of the eyes, and is often frontal. The simple question regarding the relationship of headache to increased use of the eyes may help in deciding whether there may be an ocular cause for the headache. Three common causes for frequent changes in glasses prescription are: glaucoma, cataract, and diabetes mellitus. Any patient who com-

TABLE 14-1 *DISEASES OF THE CENTRAL NERVOUS SYSTEM WITH PHOTOPHOBIA AS A RELATED COMPLAINT*

Migraine
Subarachnoid hemorrhage
Aura preceding seizure or in the postictal state
Mass lesion
Arachnoiditis (viral, bacterial, chemical)
Postconcussion state
Encephalitis
Acromegaly
Trigeminal neuralgia

plains of variation in visual acuity from day to day or hour to hour should have a formal three-hour glucose tolerance test. Intraocular pressure should be measured.

The past history and family history must also be carefully reviewed. The patient presenting a history of blepharospasm may also have a history of previous encephalitis several years before. One would thus be attuned to a possible diagnosis of postencephalitic Parkinson's disease with blepharospasm as one of its features. A careful review of the patient's medications should always be included. It is wise not to ask what drugs the patient is taking, but instead to ask what medications are used. Some patients equate drugs with narcotics, to the exclusion of all other medications. The family history should include specific details concerning the ages of the patient's parents, and the cause of their death, if they are deceased. Also, it is helpful to know how many siblings were produced, how many are living, their medical histories (if pertinent), how many are deceased, and the exact causes of death. Other details of the medical and ocular history in close relatives may be important.

NEURO-OPHTHALMOLOGICAL EXAMINATION

Visual Acuity Determination

Accurate determination of the visual acuity is the foundation upon which the entire eye examination rests. Only the best vision for each eye should be recorded. Ideally, the eye that is not being tested should be completely occluded. Some type of patch is required for children. A black occluder with an elastic band works well and is inexpensive. When testing vision in a patient with glasses, a cleansing tissue may be placed between the lens and the closed eyelids. The best test of visual acuity consists in measurement at distance and near, if a distance (20-foot) Snellen chart is available. This should include the vision with and without glasses. The addition of a pinhole before the tested eye with poor vision will generally increase its visual acuity if the cause for decreased vision is refractive. It will reduce the acuity if the decrease in vision is due to opacities of the media (cornea, lens, vitreous) or a central scotoma. The patient should be encouraged to demonstrate the best possible acuity. Many times better visual acuity can be recorded if the examiner allows sufficient time for the patient to find the best head position and encourages an occasional guess.

If facilities do not allow the distance vision to be tested, the near card (reduced Snellen) should be used. The ideal near card should have letters, numbers, and sentences. A dysphasic patient may be capable of identifying numbers but not letters, letters but not numbers, or both letters and numbers when shown in an isolated manner, but be unable to read them accurately as used in sentences. The patient should be asked to move the card into the best reading position. An alert observer can detect a visual field defect by watching the position of the near card. A card held slightly off center often means that a central scotoma is present. The card held in the nasal field of each eye suggests chiasmal disease with a bitemporal hemianopia. Similarly, other positions may be the clues to a homonymous hemianopia or an altitudinal visual field loss. In patients over the age of 50, the acuity at near will be reduced simply because of the effects of presbyopia. The patient will tend to hold the card at an excessively long reading distance. The near vision should be tested with the patient's glasses in place. Presbyopia is the most common cause of visual complaints concerning near visual tasks in patients over the age of 50. Repeat testing of vision should be done in light similar to that used for the initial test. A near card held far from one eye and near to the other may imply: (1) anisometropia (unequal refractive error between the two eyes), (2) accommodative weakness in one eye — the card would be held further away than usual — suggesting impairment of cranial nerve III, or (3) increased depth of accommodation — common with Horner's syndrome — in which the card would be held closer than usual.

It may not be possible to test vision with the near card in some patients, especially if they are dysphasic, and one may have to rely on finger counting techniques in order to assess vision. The extended fingers are about the equivalent of the letters or numbers on the Snellen distance chart, which should be visible to the normal eye at 200 feet. In the ophthalmologist's office, the patient who can just see these letters at 20 feet is given a vision of 20/200. A patient who must walk to within 5 feet of the letters before recognizing them is given a vision of 5/200. Using his fingers alone, the examiner can obtain a good estimate of the patient's vision by having him count the number of fingers presented at increasing distances from the bedside until the patient no longer responds correctly. In the dysphasic patient, one may have to communicate with sign language until he understands that he should hold up the same number of fingers as the examiner for a correct response. This can be time-consuming but really worth the effort; however, even this may be impossible, and the examiner may have to be content with a very gross estimate of visual acuity made by evaluating the patient's response to moving targets, such as a pen or handlight, his response to optokinetic targets, or finally the pupillary response to light.

A special problem is encountered in testing the vision in children. The average visual acuity of children with increasing age is as follows:

Birth	10/400 (or 5/200)
1 year	20/200
2 years	20/40
3 years	20/30
4 years	20/25
5 years	20/20

It is possible to determine whether or not vision is present *even in the newborn infant* with the use of optokinetic targets and pupillary responses to light. One should be able to elicit some ocular movement by using an optokinetic tape. The child must be fully awake and not crying. The optokinetic tape will produce responses in patients who have 5/200 or better visual acuity. A normal child will be able to fix and follow a handlight or another rather large target by the age of 3 months. Formal testing of visual acuity is not usually possible before the age of 3 years. The child must be learning some verbal skills. Sometime between the ages of 3 and 4 years, most children are capable of learning to play the "E game." They are asked to point one finger in the direction of the "legs" on the E. This can be taught at home by the parents, using a letter E cut from a piece of cardboard. When the parents have not been successful in teaching a child of 5 or 6 years to play the game, three possible causes of their failure are mental retardation, a parietal lobe lesion, or poor vision. After the age of 9 years, most children will be able to respond accurately to the adult vision test. In very young children, it is often best to test them with both eyes open initially, and later to test each eye individually.

External Examination

General inspection is important in the external examination. The subtle flattening of the nasolabial fold on one side of the face may be the clue to a central facial paralysis. Acne rosacea of the facial skin may point to chronic alcoholism as the cause for tremor and ataxia. It may also explain a sudden loss of vision from nutritional amblyopia. Careful attention to the color, quality, and texture of the skin are of great importance.

The eyelids should next be considered. The width of the lid fissures (maximum diameter between the edges of the upper and lower lids) should be measured or estimated. The average width of the lid fissure is 11 mm in the adult. A range of 8 to 12 mm is certainly within the limits of normal. The upper lid margin usually lies at or just about 1 mm below the upper limbus (junction of the cornea and sclera). In small children, especially under the age of 2 years, the upper lid usually rests at the upper limbus. The lower lid margin is usually at the limbus in children and adults. Knowing these simple landmarks, one can estimate very accurately whether the fissures are abnormally wide or narrow.

The fissures may be abnormally wide owing to extreme concentration, fear, sympathomimetic drugs, thyroid eye disease, or the pathological lid retraction seen with lesions of the posterior commisure (Collier's sign). Thyroid eye disease with its lid retraction and lid lag is usually easy to diagnose. Collier's sign is one of the very important external ocular findings in mesencephalic disease. Whereas the lid retraction of thyroid disease is often bilateral but asymmetrical, the lid retraction in Collier's sign is generally quite symmetrical unless there is a superimposed Horner's syndrome or involvement of the nucleus of the third cranial nerve that is causing ptosis. Another common cause of unilateral widening of the lid fissure is a peripheral palsy of nerve VII. Supranuclear damage to the facial nerve complex causes paralysis of the lower side of the face, sparing the upper face, contralateral to the lesion. The lids are little involved except for some slight weakness of closure. The eyelids are little affected compared to the peripheral seventh nerve palsy because of the bilateral representation of the upper face in the supranuclear pathways. A handy clinical guide to the level of a lesion in the stem is: (1) a lesion above the nucleus of nerve VII causes a contralateral paralysis of the *central* face, arm, and leg; (2) the lesion at the level of the nucleus of nerve VII causes an *ipsilateral peripheral* facial palsy and *contralateral* hemiparesis; and (3) with one below the nucleus a contralateral hemiparesis occurs that spares the face. The lid fissure is widened not only by the weakness of closure of the upper lid and unopposed force of the levator, but also from the slight sagging downward of the lower lid (lagophthalmos). Because exposure of the cornea to drying and foreign bodies invites corneal ulcer formation, the eye should be kept moist with artificial tear solutions (Liquifilm, Isopto tears) or ointments (0.5 per cent boric acid, ophthalmic). If it is not desirable to use these measures, the eyelids may be closed with tape or a minor surgical procedure, the lateral tarsorrhaphy (Fig. 14–2). Either of these protects the cornea. The tarsorrhaphy can be released at any time.

Narrowing of the lid fissure (ptosis) may occur in the following circumstances: (1) fatigue, (2) loss of sympathetic innervation of the smooth muscle of the upper lid (Müller's muscle), (3) lesions of the third cranial nerve (levator), (4) neuromyopathic diseases such as myasthenia gravis, (5) direct myopathic disease (Kiloh-Nevin syndrome), and (6) pseudoptosis due to inflammatory or infiltrative lesions of the upper lid that increase its weight and produce an apparent ptosis. Congenital ptosis may be separated from acquired ptosis by

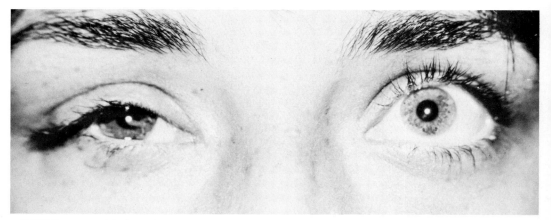

FIGURE 14–2   Right lateral tarsorrhaphy for exposure keratitis from facial palsy in postoperative angle tumor case.

the history, old photographs, and its stability (acquired forms are often variable).

The most profound ptosis occurs with lesions of the oculomotor nerve. More common, but less impressive, is the ptosis seen with lesions of the sympathetic system. The amount of ptosis is often small (0.5 mm). It is variable, depending on the degree of alertness of the patient, the level of the lesion, and the length of time it has been present. The signs of oculosympathetic paralysis are listed in Table 14–2. Other less frequent eyelid signs of neurological disease are myokymia, myoclonic lid movements, lid nystagmus, lid "flutter" in myasthenia gravis, fasciculations, blepharospasm, and apraxia of lid opening.

Exophthalmos is best discussed by classification according to the age of the patient, the presence or absence of pulsation of the globe, and the presence or absence of a bruit. The most common cause of pulsating exophthalmos without a bruit in childhood is neurofibromatosis with a defect in the orbital roof. In adults, the most common cause for pulsating exophthalmos without a

TABLE 14–2   CLINICAL SIGNS OF OCULOSYMPATHETIC PARESIS

Ptosis—may be minimal
Miosis—may be minimal
Enophthalmos—more relative than real
Anhydrosis—variable, depends on level
Increased depth of accommodation
Transient increase facial skin temperature
Ocular hypotony
Heterochromia iridis—if damage occurs before age 2 years.

bruit is a defect in the orbital roof (traumatic) and the most common cause with a bruit is the carotid-cavernous fistula. The most common cause of nonpulsatile exophthalmos in children under the age of 2 years is metastatic adrenal neuroblastoma; over the age of 2 the common causes are orbital hemangioma, lymphoma, dermoid, and glioma of the optic nerve. The optic nerve glioma should be suspected when the eye is displaced down and outward, the optic nerve is undergoing progressive atrophy, and the optic foramen is enlarged on x-ray. These occur most often in the first decade of life. They grow slowly and cause enlargement of the optic foramen by pressure from the expanding nerve substance and the proliferation of the overlying meningeal coverings. Gliomas should be suspected in children with evidence of neurofibromatosis who develop proptosis. Approximately 10 per cent of these gliomas are associated with cafe-au-lait spots or other signs of neurofibromatosis. Rhabdomyosarcoma is the most common primary malignant tumor of the orbit in children. It is also the third most common tumor in children. Only leukemia and neuroblastoma precede it in frequency. This tumor presents as a rapidly enlarging mass in the orbit, often palpable through the lid, and usually located in the upper nasal quadrant of the orbit. It may cause papilledema, optic atrophy, and even enlargement of the optic canal. It requires radical surgical removal.

In adults, exophthalmos is usually due to thyroid eye disease (Fig. 14–3). With proptosis the eye may be markedly injected or may appear completely normal in every respect. It is common to have bilateral protrusion of the globes, but this may be quite asymmetrical. The patient may be hyperthyroid, euthyroid, or hypothyroid by laboratory studies. Proptosis associated with a history of previous treatment with thyroid preparations, swelling of the upper eyelids, difficulty with vertical gaze, vertical diplopia, congestion of the conjunctiva, and retraction of the upper lids is thyroid eye disease, regardless of the laboratory results. *Thyroid eye disease is a clinical diagnosis.* It often advances more rapidly after treatment with radioactive iodine or subtotal thyroidectomy. The major complications are drying of the eye from exposure and corneal ulcer formation. A helpful aid to diagnosis is the Werner thyroid suppression test. This is performed by determining the baseline radioactive iodine (RAI) uptake, following which the patient takes T_3 (Cytomel, 25-μg tablets) three times per day for 7 to 10 days, and the RAI uptake is retested. In the normal person, the uptake is depressed, but in the thyrotoxic patient it is not. This test will be positive in approximately 50 per cent of persons with thyroid eye disease.

Other causes of nonpulsating exophthalmos in adults are lymphoma, hemangioma, pseudotumor of the orbit, metastatic tumor from the breast or lung, lacrimal gland tumor, and meningioma either arising de novo in the orbit or as an orbital extension of a sphenoid wing meningioma. Lymphoma, hemangioma, pseudotumor, and meningioma are the most frequent causes of proptosis in adults with the exception of thyroid eye disease.

The presence of exophthalmos is best determined with the Krahn exophthalmometer. Serial measurements are the best method for following the progress of a patient under treatment for exophthalmos. Over 2 mm difference in the measurements between the two eyes is suggestive of proptosis; over 3 mm. is pathological. It should be noted that the range of normal ocular protrusion is 12 to 21 mm with a mean of 16 mm.

Every medical student knows that the three common causes for a "red" eye are glaucoma, infection, and uveitis. The neurosurgeon should know that a red eye may be the clue to unilateral carotid insufficiency, Sturge-Weber syndrome, ataxia-telangectasia, Wyburn-Mason syndrome, sickle cell anemia, beginning carotid-cavernous fistula, or polycythemia vera. The presence of isolated elevated injected patches of episcleral tissue (nodular episcleritis) is common in severe collagen disease, as is the conjunctival injection and furrow ulcer formation at the limbus in the diffuse arteritis of collagen disease. This may be of value diagnostically in certain

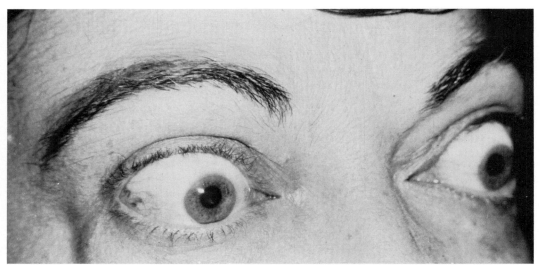

FIGURE 14–3 Thyroid eye disease.

patients with a history of seizures, syncopal episodes, transient ischemic attacks, or multisystem complaints and nervous system signs.

The Pupil

The pupil has three major functions: to control the volume of light entering the eye, to increase the depth of focus (as it contracts), and to decrease spherical and chromatic aberration. The normal pupillary diameter varies between 2 and 6 mm with an average diameter of 3.5 mm. The pupils tend to be small and resistant to dilation in infants and the elderly, large and easy to dilate in the teens and early adult life. The pupil is larger in women than in men, larger in myopes than in hyperopes, and larger in blue-eyed than in brown-eyed persons. In 17 per cent of normal persons there is a slight but perceptible anisocoria (unequal pupil size), and in 4 per cent the difference is pronounced (over 1 mm).

Anatomy of the Pupillary Pathways

Afferent Pathway

This begins in the retina at the rod and cone layer, and fibers concerned with the pupillary function proceed to the optic nerve. The fibers are scattered in a random distribution throughout the substance of the optic nerve. Whether the afferent pupillomotor fibers are the small or large fibers seen on careful histological analys s of the optic nerve is still open to debate.

After crossing in the chiasm, in equal proportions, the afferent fibers then enter the optic tract, the brachium of the superior colliculus (but not the colliculus proper), and the pretectum. From the pretectum, an equal number of fibers pass to the right and left sides of the commissure (partial decussation). They then proceed around the aqueduct in the periaqueductal gray matter until they enter the Edinger-Wesphal nucleus. At this point another synapse occurs. *This is the beginning of the efferent limb of the pupillary reflex arc.*

Efferent Pathway

After synapsis, the parasympathetic fibers pass ventrally with the fibers of cranial nerve III through the substance of the midbrain. The pupillary fibers occupy the superior aspect of the nerve as it passes through the middle cranial fossa. They are in close relation to the tentorial margin and the hippocampal gyrus. The nerve then passes through the cavernous sinus and then to the superior orbital fissure. It divides into an upper and lower division. The upper division supplies innervation to the levator of the upper lid and the superior rectus muscle. The lower division supplies the medial rectus, inferior rectus, and inferior oblique muscles and the intrinsic muscles of the eye. Those fibers in the lower division that subserve the pupil and accommodation leave the inferior division at the lateral border of the inferior rectus. They then turn upward to enter the ciliary ganglion as the short or motor root. At this juncture, another synapse occurs, and finally the postganglionic fibers pass from the ciliary ganglion to the globe by the short ciliary nerves. They enter the posterior aspect of the globe and pass into the suprachoroidal space. They then proceed to the musculature of the pupil and the ciliary body. These pupillary fibers are parasympathetic and are the most important factor determining the size of the pupil. They affect the sphincter of the pupil and secrete acetylcholine at the myoneural junction.

Sympathetic Influence on the Pupil

The fibers of the sympathetic pupillary pathway arise in the hypothalamus and pass downward in the substance of the midbrain tegmentum. Gradually, they assume a more lateral position. In the pons, they lie in the reticular substance and in the cervical cord, in the superficial layers of the cord just under the dentate ligaments. From C7 to T2, three cord segments, the first neuron sympathetic fibers synapse with the second neuron fibers at the ciliospinal center of Budge. The second neuron fibers pass out of the cord through the white rami to form the cervical sympathetic chain.

The pupillary fibers pass through the inferior and middle cervical sympathetic ganglia without synapsing. These fibers synapse only at the superior cervical ganglion. The fibers leaving this synaptic junction (third neuron) are the final pathway for sympathetic influence on the pupil.

They pass upward wrapped about the sheath of the internal carotid artery, enter the cavernous sinus, then join with the first division of the fifth nerve to enter the orbit through the superior orbital fissure. The sympathetic fibers are then concentrated in the nasociliary division of nerve V. They enter the globe in the two long ciliary nerves and pass forward through the suprachoroidal space to form a plexus at the ciliary body. Finally, fibers from the ciliary plexus proceed to the dilator muscle of the iris. Norepinephrine is secreted at the myoneural junction.

Other intracranial fibers of sympathetic origin form the cavernous sympathetic plexus. Before it is formed, however, some of the fibers loop posteriorly over the petrous portion of the temporal bone and then course anteriorly. These enter the orbit with the two divisions of the oculomotor nerve to supply the Müller's muscle of the upper and lower lids. Those fibers of the sympathetic plexus that follow the course of the external carotid artery supply the innervation for facial sweating.

Reactions and Reflexes in Normal Pupils

Direct Light Reflex

In the normal person, the direct reaction of the pupil to light is at least as good, and usually better, than the reaction to a *near* stimulus. If the direct light reflex of the pupil is poorer than the contraction to near, the term "light-near dissociation of the pupil" is used. When testing the direct light reflex, the patient's gaze must be fixed on a distant object and a bright light must be used. The most common cause for a misdiagnosis of light-near dissociation is a weak light source. The Welch-Allyn battery powered handle with the Finoff transilluminator is the best light source for this purpose. The direct light reflex is graded from 1+ to 4+. If the response is less than 1+, it is recorded as *nil* or 0.

Consensual Reflex

In the normal person, when a strong light is placed before one eye, the pupil of the opposite eye responds by contracting as promptly and as forcefully as the pupil of the stimulated eye.

Near Pupillary Reflex

When the normal person makes an effort to focus the eye on an object near the face, the pupils promptly become miotic. By using the patient's finger as the object, this reflex can be tested even in a person who is totally blind. This may be of importance in separating blindness of ocular origin from that of cerebral origin.

Westphal-Piltz Reaction

When one tests a patient for Bell's phenomenon by holding apart the upper and lower lids of one eye—the correct way to perform this test is monocularly, not binocularly—and asking him to forcefully close the eye, pupillary miosis may be noted as the eye moves upward. This occurs only on the *homolateral side*. It is seen in 35 per cent of normal individuals. When it is present, despite loss of other pupillary reactions, one may assume a supranuclear interruption of pupillary function, *not a peripheral one*. This is the pupillary correlate of the Bell's phenomenon.

Pathological Pupillary Reactions and Reflexes

Oculosympathetic Paresis (Horner's Syndrome)

This is the most common cause of pupillary inequality in neurosurgical practice. Careful observation will reveal that most patients who undergo direct carotid angiography develop a transient pupillary miosis. Bilateral decrease of sympathetic innervation to the pupil is difficult to prove without the aid of pupillography. Denervation of the sympathetic pathways may produce the signs listed in Table 14–2. The number of signs produced depends on the age of the patient and the level and magnitude of involvement of the pathways. Discovery of a Horner's syndrome when and where expected is very helpful in localizing neurological lesions.

Much has been made of the value of chemical testing to determine the level of involvement (first, second, or third neuron) of sympathetic damage. Recent evidence obtained in patients with lesions of the first, second, and third neurons demonstrated the

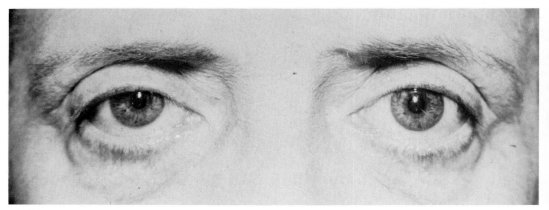

FIGURE 14–4 Right Horner's syndrome before cocaine instillation. Note the minimal miosis and ptosis, which could be easily overlooked.

value of hydroxyamphetamine (Paredrine) in accurately localizing the level of the lesion.[8] The chemical test of most value is the cocaine test. It will be positive in lesions at all levels, but the degree of anisocoria produced by the instillation of 10 per cent cocaine increases progressively as lesions become closer to the third neuron.

The cocaine test should be performed in the following manner. Since it is not reliable if the corneas have been manipulated, the cocaine should be the first drops instilled, and the testing of the corneal reflexes should be reserved for later. One drop of cocaine 10 per cent solution should be instilled in the lower cul-de-sac *in each eye*— this test depends on the comparison of the dilation of the normal versus the sympa-

thectomized pupil. In 10 minutes, if the pupils have not begun to dilate, two more drops should be instilled. The response to cocaine is evaluated 30 to 45 minutes after the last instillation. The authors regard a positive test as one in which the sympathectomized pupil remains at least 2 mm smaller than the normal one at the end of 30 minutes. The belief that a "central Horner's syndrome," a first neuron neuron lesion, cannot have a positive cocaine test has been disproved. Positive cocaine tests do occur if the criteria for a positive test will allow for some dilation of the sympathetically denervated pupil (Figs. 14–4 and 14–5).

A few of the causes of oculosympathetic paresis that should be included in differ-

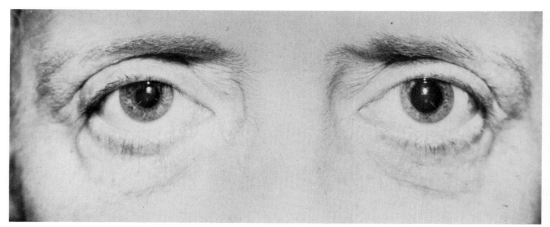

FIGURE 14–5 Right Horner's syndrome after cocaine instillation. Note the obvious value of the cocaine test in detecting a subtle sympathetic underaction.

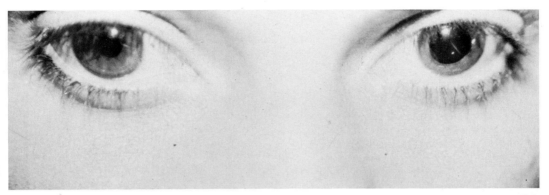

FIGURE 14-6 Left Adie's tonic pupil. Photograph taken in standard room illumination. The left pupil is widely dilated and responds poorly to light and near stimuli.

ential diagnosis are: (1) first neuron lesions —vascular accidents of the brain stem, syringomyelia, syringobulbia, tumors of the brain stem or cervical cord, meningitis, and meningomyelitis; (2) second neuron lesions —cervical rib, cervical trauma, infection or metastatic tumor to cervical nodes, and Pancoast's tumor; and (3) third neuron lesions—carotid aneurysm, carotid angiography, carotid inflammatory disease as with cranial arteritis or periarteritis nodosa, tumor at the base of the skull, otitis media (severe), cholesteatoma, temporal lobe abscess or tumor, Raeder's paratrigeminal syndrome, and skull fracture.

Tonic Pupil (Adie's Syndrome)

This pupillary abnormality results from the postganglionic denervation of the parasympathetic supply to the pupil (Fig. 14-6). Although it may follow a viral infection such as varicella or mumps, most often no cause is established. There are two common causes for the sudden onset of a dilated pupil, responding poorly to light, in an otherwise healthy young person: accidental instillation of atropine or some other cycloplegic medication into the eye (common in medical students, nurses, or young mothers who have children under treatment with cycloplegics) and Adie's tonic pupil. The clinical features of the tonic pupil are summarized in Table 14-3. It is incorrect to apply the term Adie's pupil to a pupil that responds poorly to light and near stimulus in a person with diabetes mellitus, lues, alcoholic polyneuritis, or pineal tumors.

Argyll Robertson Pupil

This pupillary abnormality is the most conclusive ocular sign of neurosyphilis. Approximately 13 per cent of patients with tabes dorsalis and 8 per cent of those with general paresis have Argyll Robertson pupils. Over 70 per cent of patients with neurosyphilis will have some abnormality of pupillary function during the course of the disease. The Argyll Robertson pupil has very strict criteria, which include the following: (1) some vision must be present; (2) miosis, which may be unilateral; (3) dilates poorly to atropine, cocaine, and similar agents; (4) has irregular shape; (5) *does not react to light regardless of its intensity;* but (6) does react to accommodation.

The Argyll Robertson–like pupil is more often seen in patients with neurosyphilis

TABLE 14-3 CLINICAL FEATURES OF ADIE'S TONIC PUPIL

Unilateral in 80 per cent of patients
Affected pupil usually larger (dilated)
Direct light reflex almost abolished
Pupil dilates slowly in dark
Pupil contracts slowly on prolonged light exposure
During accommodation miosis occurs, may exceed that of normal pupil
Pupil dilates slowly when accommodation discontinued
Reacts normally to mydriatics
More common in females (20–30 age group)
Bilateral tonic pupils occur
Patient should be neurologically intact except for absence of knee and ankle jerks
Prompt miosis occurs with instillation of 2.5 per cent methacholine (Mecholyl)—this does not occur in normal eye

TABLE 14-4 *POSITIVE MECHOLYL TEST IN PUPILLARY DISORDERS*

Argyll Robertson pupil
Myotonic dystrophy
Primary amyloidosis
Riley-Day syndrome (familial dysautonomia)

and is a pupil that does respond to light but not as well as to the near stimulus (light-near dissociation). These pupils may be large or small, may be round or irregular in shape, and respond normally to mydriatics and cycloplegics. The differential diagnosis of the Argyll Robertson–like pupil is as follows: (1) lues—especially juvenile paresis; (2) diabetes mellitus (diabetic pseudotabes); (3) pituitary tumors (tabes pituitaria); (4) lesions of the periaqueductal gray matter (midbrain); (5) primary amyloidosis; (6) myotonic dystrophy; and (7) misdirection in regeneration of nerve III (called the pseudo–Argyll Robertson pupil here because its size often varies with different directions of gaze). A positive test with 2.5 per cent methacholine (Mecholyl) can be found in the conditions listed in Table 14–4.

Miotic Pupils

The three most common causes for pupillary miosis are miotics, morphine, and pontine miosis. The latter is found usually in patients who have large pontine hemorrhages, and the pronounced miosis is a grave prognostic sign. It may result from destruction of the sympathetic and disruption of the inhibitory pathways to the Edinger-Westphal nucleus arising in the lower stem and the spinal cord.

Traumatic Mydriasis or Miosis

Direct ocular trauma may lead to either a dilated or miotic pupil. Dilation is usually the result of paralysis of the sphincter because of local damage to the nerve endings supplying it. It may also result from one or more tears of the sphincter muscle, in which case the pupil is often irregular in outline. Miosis after direct ocular injury is most often due to the associated intraocular inflammation.

Closed head trauma with increased intracranial pressure frequently produces a dilated pupil that responds poorly to light and near stimulus, the so-called Hutchinson's pupil. Most often this results from cerebral edema; subdural or intracerebral hematoma forces the uncus of the hippocampus downward, thus pressing on the superior aspect of the adjacent third nerve. The nerve is trapped between the uncus and the tentorium. At other times there may be horizontal shifting of the intracranial contents so that the mesencephalic pyramidal tract will press the third nerve against the tentorial edge. With a more or less unilateral increase in intracranial pressure, as with a rapidly expanding mass, one expects to see a contralateral hemiparesis and ipsilateral Hutchinson's pupil. In some patients, because of the horizontal shifting due to pressure, the patient may develop a hemiparesis ipsilateral to the lesion with a contralateral dilated and fixed pupil (Kernohan's notch)[5] Compression of the posterior cerebral artery may occur, causing a homonymous hemianopia. With sufficiently increased intracranial pressure, all parameters of third nerve function can be affected either unilaterally or bilaterally. Bilateral dilation of the pupils with increased intracranial pressure is a grave prognostic sign.

The Amaurotic Pupil

The five pupillary signs of the blind eye are: (1) no *direct* pupillary response with light on blind eye, (2) no *consensual* response with light on blind eye, (3) intact *direct* pupillary response with light on normal eye, (4) intact consensual response in blind eye with light on normal eye, and (5) the near pupillary response normal in both eyes.

The Marcus Gunn pupillary phenomenon (swinging flashlight sign) indicates a defect in the afferent arc of the pupillary light reflex. It is invaluable as an aid to confirmation of visual loss resulting from a lesion anterior to the chiasm and is found in optic nerve disease even when the reduction in visual acuity is minimal (Figs. 14–7, 14–8, and 14–9). It is also present when visual loss is the result of retinal dysfunction, but the retina must be severely damaged. With the patient fixing at distance, a strong light is placed before the intact eye. A crisp con-

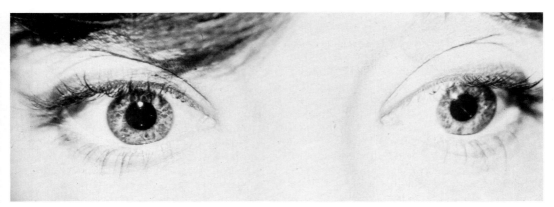

FIGURE 14-7 Patient with conduction defect of the left optic nerve in standard room illumination before testing for Marcus Gunn pupil.

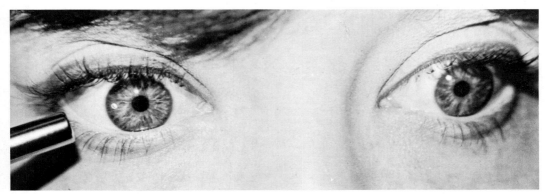

FIGURE 14-8 Conduction defect of left optic nerve. Light before right eye, both pupils constrict.

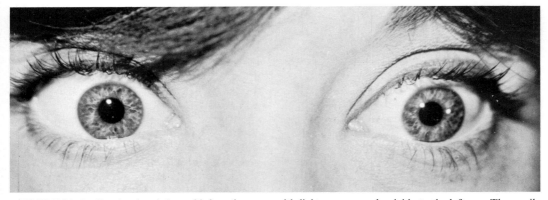

FIGURE 14-9 Conduction defect of left optic nerve with light now moved quickly to the left eye. The pupils dilate under the light for a short time before constriction occurs.

traction of the pupil is noted bilaterally, assuming no other lesions are affecting pupillary diameter. When the light is then moved quickly to the affected eye, the pupils will dilate slightly. This dilation continues for a short period while light is pouring into the eye. The pupils may then begin to contract. The light is then quickly moved to the sound eye and the pupils contract promptly. Unless vision is severely reduced, the direct pupil response may appear normal in the poorer eye. The swinging flashlight test is a very sensitive guide to minimal damage of the optic nerve.

The Pupils in Epilepsy

During the aura, the pupils are often miotic. As convulsions begin, they are usually dilated and often fixed to light. This is helpful in differentiating true from hysterical seizures. It is unusual for the pupils to become fixed to light in petit mal seizures.

DISORDERS OF OCULAR MOTILITY

Definition of Terms

Versions — both eyes turned to the right, left, up, or down; this is also a "conjugate deviation" of the eyes because they are moving in the same direction.

Ductions — movements of one eye.

Vergence — movement of both eyes in different directions. Convergence is the movement of each eye toward the midline. Divergence is the reverse of convergence. These are also called dysjugate or non-conjugate movements.

Eso — inward deviation of the eye (toward the midline).

Exo — outward deviation of the eye.

Hyper — upward deviation of the eye.

Phoria — a latent tendency for the eye to deviate. It is manifest when binocular fixation is disrupted by any means. When the disrupting "cover" is removed, the eye turns to pick up fixation again. With or without the cover, the opposite fixing eye never moves. In the cover-uncover test to determine the presence or absence of a phoria, one eye is allowed to fix on an object at all times while an occluder is placed before the other eye. When the cover is removed, if a phoria is present the eye

moves to pick up fixation. Normally a small esophoria is present when fixing on distant objects, and a small exophoria when fixing at near. If the eye does not move when the cover is removed, there is no phoria.

Tropia — a manifest deviation of the eye. This may be alternating (either eye can fix accurately and hold fixation), and the fixing eye may have good visual acuity. It may be monocular with only one eye used constantly for fixation while the deviating eye has poor visual acuity (amblyopia). In either case, when the cover-uncover test is performed and the cover is placed before the eye preferred for fixation, removal of the cover results in movement of *both* eyes. This is the method of separating phorias from tropias.

Comitancy — a tropia with the same amount of deviation in all fields of gaze. A noncomitant deviation is characteristically found in recent palsies of nerves III, IV, and VI. They are easily recognized by the presence of "secondary deviation." When the alternate cover test is performed, the ocular deviation is greater when the eye with the paretic muscle fixes than when the nonparetic eye fixes (primary deviation). This same characteristic serves as the basis for the red-glass diplopia test.

Suppression amblyopia — the loss of usable vision in an eye that has not maintained a visual direction compatible with the other eye. This is due to central inhibition of the visual field of the deviating eye. It occurs as the result of inability to superimpose disparate retinal images simultaneously. This is found with constant ocular deviation occurring before the age of 6 years. After that age, the patient rarely develops dense amblyopia. The usual result is the onset of diplopia. An ocular deviation in a child should prompt a careful ophthalmological examination. An unsuspected intraocular tumor may produce such a deviation.

Most of the ocular deviations occurring shortly after birth, or noted at birth, are the result of anatomical defects in the orbit. Those arising between the ages of 1 and 2 years are usually the result of an accommodation-convergence derangement. Most children with acquired unilateral visual loss will develop an esotropia; whereas most adults will develop an exotropia.

Childhood esotropias may decrease in amount as the patient ages, although the vision in the deviating eye is poor. This is the reason some physicians make the error of telling the parents of children with strabismus that "they will grow out of it." The child may look cosmetically better as the esodeviation decreases, but the chance for treatment is usually lost. Severe bilateral loss of vision in childhood or adult life will infrequently produce strabismus.

Head Tilt, Face Turn, and Chin Position

It is vital to note the presence of any of these signs of motility dysfunction. Face turn in the horizontal plane is most pronounced in defects involving the horizontal rectus muscles. The face turns *toward* the paretic muscle. Minimal face turn may be present in patients with weakness of the vertically acting muscles. A face turn as the result of horizontal muscle dysfunction would be suggested by horizontal diplopia coupled with little tendency for head tilt or elevation or depression of the chin. The reverse would suggest a defect in vertical muscle action. The patient thus adapts himself to horizontal deviations with the face turn, to vertical deviations by elevating or depressing the chin, and to torsional defects by tilting the head. The position of head, face, and chin should be written down to be analyzed later. It is always worthwhile to compare old photographs with the present head position.

Action of the Ocular Muscles

The horizontal recti (1) (lateral recti)— abduct the eye and are more effective in upward gaze; and (2) (medial recti)—adduct the eye and are more effective in downward gaze.

The superior recti are primarily elevators but also adduct and intort.

The inferior recti are primarily depressors but also adduct and extort.

The superior obliques are primarily depressors but also abduct and intort.

The inferior obliques are primarily elevators but also abduct and extort.

One can better understand the actions of the vertically acting muscles by a study of the anatomy. The vertical rectus muscles insert on the globe at an angle of 23 degrees from the anteroposterior plane of the globe and anterior and lateral to the sagittal plane of the globe. Their unique position produces essentially pure vertical movement of the eye, when it is ABducted to an angle of 23 degrees. When the eye is in the ADducted position, at an angle of 67 degrees, the action of the vertical recti is almost exclusively torsional. Conversely, the obliques insert at an angle of 51 degrees and thus are most effective in vertical movement of the eye when the globe is in the ADducted position. The vertical function of the obliques is almost pure when the eye is adducted to 51 degrees. When the eye is in the divergence position, the obliques become more efficient in torsion. This effect is greatest when the eye is abducted to 39 degrees.

When these facts are kept in mind, it is obvious that with complete paralysis of nerve III the only sign of an intact nerve IV would be some torsional movement of the eye. The eye is in the ABducted position when nerve III is paralyzed. This is the favorable position for the torsional effect of the obliques. This also explains why the vertical recti are most important in control of the vertical position of the eye at distance, whereas the obliques are most important at near.

Tests for Weakness of an Ocular Muscle

The subjective red-glass test (cover-uncover) and the objective cover test (alternate cover) are adequate to identify any motility problem. The motility examination is best carried out with the patient wearing his glasses. It is good practice to obtain both the subjective and objective measurement of the patient's ocular deviation.

Subjective Red-Glass Test

By convention, the patient usually has the red glass placed before the right eye (Fig. 14–10). He is then asked to look at a light at distance with both eyes open. If no ocular deviation exists, he will see the red

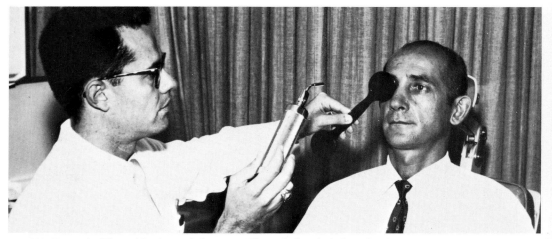

FIGURE 14–10   The subjective red-glass test. The red glass is before the right eye as the patient observes the hand light.

and white images superimposed as a single pink image. If the patient has an exophoric or exotropic deviation, he will see the red image to his left and the white image to his right (crossed diplopia). It may be helpful to assign a color to each hand and then have the patient show with his hands the relationship of the two images in space. For example, if the right hand is "red" and the left hand is "white," a patient with an exo-deviation will cross his hands when asked to show the relationship of the lights to each other in space. (A useful mnemonic: There is an *x* in exo and an *x* is also a cross-crossed diplopia.) If the patient has an esodeviation, the red image is to the right and the white image to the left (uncrossed or homonymous diplopia). A hyper-deviation will be manifest as a vertical displacement of the images. This may occur alone or in combination with a horizontal deviation. If the right eye is deflected upward, the image is displaced downward or "the red light is lower than the white light."

The test light is then moved to about 33 cm from the patient with the red glass before the right eye. The light is moved into the cardinal fields of gaze and the patient is asked to comment on the relative separation of the red and white images. Again his hands may indicate the amount of separation. After the field of greatest separation is located, a cover test will make final determination of the paretic muscle. The amount of deviation can be measured by inserting prisms of the proper amount and direction before the eyes until the images are superimposed.

The Cover Test

This may be done with the eyes fixing at any distance, but for most neurosurgical examinations it is best done with the patient fixing at near (33 cm). The patient is asked to follow the movements of a handlight into the cardinal fields. The light is then held steady, and the patient's eyes are alternately covered by any convenient object (i.e., a hand or cardboard). The alternate cover test will disclose any tendency for the eyes to deviate when fixation with both eyes is disrupted. The cover-uncover test will determine if the deviation is a phoria or a tropia. It then remains to decide in which of the cardinal fields the deviation is maximal. One must also note whether the deviation is greater with the right or left eye fixing. It is usually abnormal to find hyperdeviations at near. Once the decision is made as to the cardinal field with the greatest deviation, and the amount of deviation with the right and left eye fixing is settled, the paretic muscle is identified (Table 14–5).

Confirmation of a superior oblique palsy can be made with the Bielschowsky head tilt test. Because the superior oblique muscle has a significant torsional effect even in straight ahead gaze, weakness of a superior

TABLE 14–5 *IDENTIFICATION OF A PARETIC EXTRAOCULAR MUSCLE*

POSITION OF GAZE	MUSCLES INVOLVED	GREATEST DEVIATION
Right gaze	Right lateral rectus	Right eye fixing
	Left medial rectus	Left eye fixing
Up-right	Right superior rectus	Right eye fixing
	Left inferior oblique	Left eye fixing
Down-right	Right inferior rectus	Right eye fixing
	Left superior oblique	Left eye fixing
Left gaze	Left lateral rectus	Left eye fixing
	Right medial rectus	Right eye fixing
Up-left	Left superior rectus	Left eye fixing
	Right inferior oblique	Right eye fixing
Down-left	Left inferior rectus	Left eye fixing
	Right superior oblique	Right eye fixing

oblique will allow the eye to extort. To compensate for this, the patient learns to tilt his head *away from the side with the paretic muscle.* Thus, one has a left head tilt with a right fourth nerve palsy. To prove the right fourth nerve is underacting, the patient is asked to tilt his head to the right. When this is done, the right eye shows further hyperdeviation. When the red glass is used, the patient notes improvement of diplopia when the head is tilted to the left. If an inferior oblique is involved, the patient tilts the head to the same side as the paretic muscle. This is also true for the superior and inferior rectus muscles. The chin is elevated if an elevator is involved (superior rectus or inferior oblique) and depressed if a depressor is at fault. Using the outlined approach, a reasonable conclusion can be made as to which muscle is underacting.

Supranuclear Gaze Palsies

Supranuclear gaze palsies are differentiated from nuclear and infranuclear palsies primarily by loss of voluntary movement with retention of following ocular movement. Also, supranuclear gaze palsies are conjugate gaze problems. The patient often has great difficulty in moving the eyes on command, but can move them much better when following a moving target. The Bell's phenomenon is typically intact in supranuclear lesions.

Ocular Motor Apraxia

In this disturbance of ocular motility, the patient has full random movement capacity of the eyes. If he attempts to move the eyes purposefully toward a specific object, he experiences more difficulty than if random movements are used. The condition may be either congenital or acquired.

In congenital ocular motor apraxia there is loss of willed movements of the eyes with full movement in random gaze. Horizontal movement is selectively involved. Vertical movements are usually full on willed gaze. There is also a characteristic compensatory movement of the head to change the direction of gaze. The patient moves the head toward the object of regard, and this quick turn of the head produces a contraversive movement of the eyes away from the object. The head must then be turned past the object sufficiently far so that the eyes will eventually be brought about to fix on it. Once fixation is established, the head is then rotated until it is straight with the eyes. This movement of the head and eyes is not seen in any other abnormal state of gaze. Cogan suggested that this form of conjugate gaze disturbance implied no associated significant neurological defect. Yet this entity has been seen with significant intracranial defects such as porencephaly, hamartoma of the third ventricle, and agenesis of the corpus callosum. A child with this gaze disorder deserves evaluation. Pneumography may be in order before one can assure the parents that no neurological defect exists.

In acquired ocular motor apraxia the patient can turn neither eyes nor head voluntarily. Random movements may be somewhat restricted. There may be preferential loss of vertical rather than horizontal movements, as in the sylvian aqueduct syndrome. Lesions of the hemisphere commonly produce this type of motility disorder affecting horizontal gaze. Tumors, intracranial hemorrhage, and direct damage to the surface of the brain (contusion, laceration) are common causes. The findings in other supranuclear gaze palsies are listed in Table 14–6.

TABLE 14–6　OCULAR SIGNS IN DISEASES AFFECTING SUPRANUCLEAR GAZE MECHANISMS

Sylvian aqueduct syndrome
　Retraction nystagmus
　Vertical nystagmus
　Difficult voluntary vertical gaze (especially upgaze)
　Vertical gaze better following or doll's head than on command. Bell's phenomenon intact
　Adduction movements with attempted vertical gaze
　Defective convergence
　Retraction movements of eyes with downgoing optokinetic targets
　Pupillary anomalies
　Collier's sign (pathological lid retraction)
Parkinsonism
　P = paresis of vertical gaze, pupillary changes
　A = accommodative paresis (drug and/or disease related)
　R = reflex blepharospasm, retraction upper lids (Collier's sign)
　K = keratitis from drying, cogwheeling ocular movements
　I = infrequent blinking
　N = nystagmus, vertical
　S = seborrheic dermatitis of lids and face
　O = oculogyric crises, optokinetic dissociation, vertical
　N = no bifocals, no hemianopias
　I = impossible tonometry
　S = styes, Wilson's sign (inability to change direction of gaze without a blink)
　M = Myerson's sign (inability to suppress blinking when examiner taps on lateral orbital margin)
Progressive supranuclear palsy
　Early onset of downgaze weakness
　Horizontal gaze often affected but less than vertical gaze
　Following movements and doll's head ocular movements much better than ocular movements on command
　Dystonic neck rigidity
　Decreased mentation
　Dysarthria
　Occasional cerebellar and pyramidal tract signs
Pseudobulbar palsy
　Inappropriate affect
　Thickened speech
　Moderate dementia
　Exaggeration of jaw jerk
　Appearance of snout, suck, and palmarmental reflexes
　Eye movements slow, possible cogwheeling
　Conjugate gaze restricted in all fields, especially on command
　Corneomandibular reflex often present (lateral movement of jaw away from cornea stroked with cotton wisp)
　Usually due to bilateral destruction of corticobulbar pathways by vascular disease in the elderly or severe head trauma or demyelinizing disease in young adults

Internuclear Ophthalmoplegia

The medial longitudinal fasciculus extends from the thalamus superiorly to the anterior horn cells of the spinal cord inferiorly. It functions in part by connecting the homolateral oculomotor nerve nucleus to the contralateral vestibular nuclei. A lesion in this fasciculus between the pons and mesencephalon produces a characteristic ocular motility disorder, the internuclear ophthalmoplegia. Recent neuropathological studies have proved that the lesion responsible for this gaze disorder is in the fasciculus ipsilateral to the paretic medial rectus. The clinical signs of internuclear ophthalmoplegia are defective adduction of the ipsilateral eye and dissociated nystagmus, with the nystagmus more pronounced in the abducting eye. Convergence may be intact or absent depending on the level of involvement of the brain stem. In anterior internuclear ophthalmoplegia, convergence is lost. This is found with lesions at the level of the upper stem, at or near the oculomotor nuclei. In posterior internuclear ophthalmoplegia, convergence is intact. This implies a lesion at the pontine level. With the posterior type, there may be an associated conjugate gaze palsy. Most internuclear palsies are of the posterior type. It is possible to have a lesion of the medial longitudinal fasciculus in the region of the oculomotor nuclei with intact convergence if the lesion is dorsal to the nuclei.

Other clinical signs of subtle internuclear ophthalmoplegias are dysmetria and dissociation of horizontal optokinetic responses. With minimal damage to the fasciculus, an internuclear ophthalmoplegia may be difficult to recognize. This can sometimes be made more apparent by using horizontal optokinetic targets and looking for dissociation of the responses between the two eyes. The same phenomenon may be seen if the patient is tested for ocular dysmetria by having him shift fixation of the eyes on command from the examiner's finger to his nose. A dysmetric overshoot of the abducting eye is often found.[7]

Unilateral internuclear palsies are of vascular etiology in 75 per cent of patients, and bilateral ones are related to disseminated sclerosis in over 90 per cent of patients. Bilateral internuclear palsies have been described in brain stem vascular accidents, brain stem encephalitis, Wernicke's encephalopathy, syringobulbia, and a pseudointernuclear palsy has been reported with the ocular signs of myasthenia gravis.[3] Bilateral internuclear palsy is the most common sign in disseminated sclerosis, and retrobulbar neuritis is the most common ocular sensory manifestation. They usually occur separately.

Skew Deviation

The four ocular signs of cerebellar disease are: nystagmus, ocular dysmetria, flutter-like oscillations, and skew deviation. The latter is also called the Hertwig-Magendie vertical divergence ocular position. Skew deviations may be classified as comitant, noncomitant, or laterally comitant.

Comitant Skew Deviation

When a patient experiences the onset of vertical diplopia that is comitant in all fields of gaze, there are only two possibilities. Either the patient has a previously unrecognized vertical muscle underaction with sudden loss of fusional amplitude, or a comitant skew deviation is present. The presence of a head tilt or face turn suggests the former. Patients with long-standing vertical muscle underactions also have the capacity to fuse large amounts of vertical prism power. Normal is 2 prism diopters; some of these patients can fuse as much as 10 prism diopters.

Noncomitant Skew Deviation

This mimics an isolated overaction or underaction of a vertical rectus or oblique muscle of recent onset. The vertical disparity is definitely greater in one field of gaze and greater with either the right or left eye fixing. Orbital disease must be ruled out prior to making the diagnosis of a noncomitant skew deviation.

Laterally Comitant Skew Deviation

This is the least difficult type of skew deviation to diagnose as it presents with the sudden onset of vertical diplopia and a comitant hypertropia only in gaze right or left. A patient with this type of skew deviation will show little or no vertical separation in one field of gaze and a comitant deviation in the opposite field. It will measure the same with either eye fixing.

Many patients with skew deviations can be satisfactorily managed with vertical prism correction in their glasses. This may require frequent changes of glasses, and the patient must be so advised. Surgery is rarely indicated and should not usually be done until more than six months have elapsed and at least three successive sets of measurements of the vertical imbalance are in agreement. Occasional patients are found with evidence of dysfunction at the midbrain level who also have vertical diplopia. The differential diagnosis is between a nuclear third nerve palsy or a midbrain skew deviation.

Isolated Cranial Nerve Palsies

Abducens Palsy

The most common cause for paresis of the sixth nerve is brain tumor. This is not usually the result of direct involvement of

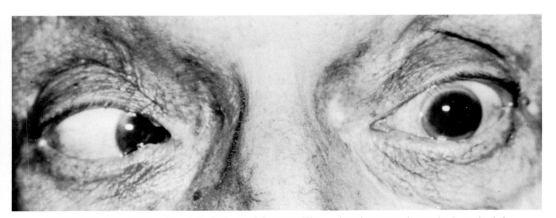

FIGURE 14–11 Palsy of the left sixth cranial nerve. The patient is attempting to look to the left.

the nerve by tumor, but the result of increased intracranial pressure and stretching of the nerve over the crest of the temporal bone. It has the longest intracranial course of any cranial nerve and innervates only the lateral rectus muscle. Underaction produces esotropia. It is especially vulnerable in basilar skull fracture. It is also commonly affected in patients with Wernicke's encephalopathy, but responds quickly to thiamine.[2]

Other less common causes of underaction of nerve VI are: demyelinizing disease; otitis media; purulent meningitis; tumor, sarcoid, or amyloid at the orbital apex; painful ophthalmoplegia; diabetes mellitus (Fig. 14–11); herpes zoster; and cerebellopontine angle tumor or intrapontine neoplasm.

Spasm of the near reflex is commonly confused with unilateral or bilateral abducens weakness. The patient frequently complains of blurring of vision at near or occasionally of diplopia, but no neurological signs are elicited except the apparent underaction of nerve VI. The apparent underaction of the abducens nerve is explained when one observes the pupillary contraction in lateral gaze when the patient begins to complain of diplopia. It is the result of convergence in lateral gaze. Voluntary nystagmus may be superimposed. These patients are managed with weak cycloplegic solutions or by increasing the minus sphere in their glasses prescription.

Oculomotor Palsy

The eight anatomical types of third nerve palsy are listed in Table 14–7. The two most common causes for paralysis of nerve III are trauma and aneurysm. Trauma may or may not be associated with an identifiable skull fracture. Exact localization of the site at which the nerve is damaged may be difficult. One should look diligently for a fracture line at the base of the skull. Aneurysms causing complete paralysis of the oculomotor nerve are usually located at the junction of the internal carotid artery and the posterior communicating artery. Two less common causes for paralysis are tumor and lues; others are listed in Table 14–8. Diabetes mellitus as a cause for third nerve

TABLE 14–7 EIGHT ANATOMICAL TYPES OF OCULOMOTOR NERVE PALSIES*

Nuclear	Isolated involvement of an ocular muscle innervated by III, due to disease in the orbit in 99% and the nucleus 1% of the time
Dorsal fascicular	Homolateral paralysis of III with a contralateral hemitremor
Ventral fascicular	Homolateral paralysis of III with contralateral hemiplegia
Root type	Same as ventral fascicular but due to lesion extrinsic to the mesencephalon May be operable
Basal type	Very common type of paralysis of III related to fractures at the base of the skull, tumor, herniation of the uncus with increased intracranial pressure, and aneurysms of the internal carotid artery and posterior communicating artery
Cavernous sinus type	Dysfunction of III usually accompanied by underaction of IV and VI. If the anterior portion of the sinus is involved, the first division of V is commonly affected In disease of the posterior or middle cavernous sinus both the first and second divisions of V are affected Proptosis frequent
Superior orbital fissure	Same as anterior cavernous sinus If lesion is at the fissue, VI cannot be spared when there is total paralysis of III
Orbital apex	Usually have simultaneous involvement of IV, VI, first division of V, and optic nerve with paralysis of III Proptosis common

*After Kestenbaum, A.: Clinical Methods of Neuro-ophthalmologic Examination, 2nd Ed. New York, Grune & Stratton, 1961.

palsy most often presents in the elderly patient who has had the disease for years. It is distinctly rare in the young diabetic. The paralysis starts suddenly and is often accompanied by headache. The pupil is usually spared. The exact cause of these paralyses is not known, but most writers believe they have a vascular etiology. The course is one of gradual clearing to com-

TABLE 14–8 ADDITIONAL CAUSES OF OCULOMOTOR PALSY

Diabetes mellitus
Sphenoid ridge meningioma
Nasopharyngeal carcinoma
Metastatic carcinoma to base of skull
Vascular insufficiency to mesencephalon
Syphilitic and tuberculous meningitis (basilar)
Viral diseases
Sarcoid or amyloid
Herpes zoster
Heavy metal intoxication

TABLE 14–9 *CAUSES OF ISOLATED INTERNAL OPHTHALMOPLEGIA*

Cycloplegic ocular medications (most common cause)
Adie's syndrome
Nasopharyngeal carcinoma (early)
Diphtheria
Botulism
Viral diseases (mumps, chickenpox)
Increased intracranial pressure

TABLE 14–10 *ADDITIONAL CAUSES OF TROCHLEAR NERVE PALSY*

Postinfectious — diphtheria or Guillain-Barré
Vascular — especially upper stem ischemia
Intracavernous carotid aneurysm
Migraine
Diabetes mellitus
Mesencephalic neoplastic — pinealoma, glioma
Postoperative temporal lobectomy or temporal lobe intra-
    cerebral hematoma

plete recovery in 2 to 3 months. The causes of isolated internal ophthalmoplegias are listed in Table 14–9.

Trochlear Nerve Palsy

Severe head trauma is the most common cause of paralysis of the fourth nerve (Fig. 14–12). It may be a bilateral palsy. This is the only cranial nerve that shows complete decussation, as the nucleus is located opposite the exposed portion of the nerve exiting the midbrain. It is also the most commonly congenitally affected cranial nerve and is often responsible for torticollis in early life. Such patients are not infrequently subjected to myotomy of the sternocleidomastoid, only to have no benefit because a congenital paralysis of the trochlear nerve was overlooked. Other causes of fourth nerve palsy are listed in Table 14–10.

Diseases That Affect the Myoneural Junction

Another important group of diseases affects ocular motility directly at the muscle or the neuromuscular junction. Three diseases are of importance: myasthenia gravis, thyroid myopathy, and progressive ocular myopathy of Kiloh-Nevin.

The eye is often the first organ affected by myasthenia gravis. The patient generally has intermittent ptosis, characteristically better in the morning when he is rested and worse at night. This is usually the first ocular sign of the disease. Later there is diplopia that is usually worse in the evening. Any of the external muscles of the eye may be affected, but the pupillary and accommodative functions are left intact. The patient may have other systemic signs of myasthenia or it may affect the eyes alone, in which case the term ocular myasthenia is used. In either case, the edrophonium chloride (Tensilon) test will be positive. Fresh Tensilon must be used. For best results, the patient should look upward until upper lid fatigue is at the maximum and then 1 ml of Tensilon should be given rapidly intravenously. The eyes should be maintained in up gaze for at least two minutes after the drug is given in order to evaluate its effect. A significant number of

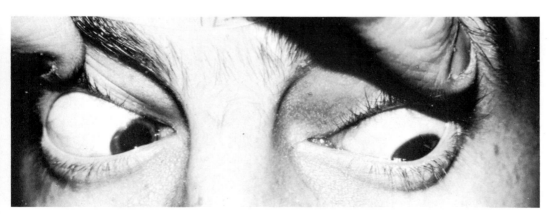

FIGURE 14–12 Right fourth nerve palsy following severe closed head trauma. Note the higher position of the right eye in gaze down and to the left. The deviation was greatest with the right eye fixing.

patients will have other endocrine disturbances associated with myasthenia. Every patient with myasthenia should be evaluated for thyroid disease and diabetes mellitus. The Tensilon tonogram is helpful in diagnosis of difficult cases. It remains axiomatic that any patient who has significant ocular muscle imbalance should have this test. Ocular myasthenia deserves a trial of medical management, as does systemic myasthenia.

Thyroid ocular disease is described in part in the section on external diseases of the eye. Regardless of whether the patient has laboratory confirmation of thyroid disease, the diagnosis of ocular disease related to disturbed thyroid metabolism is clinical. Monocular limitation of up gaze is the hallmark of thyroid ocular myopathy. This is due to chronic inflammation of the orbital tissue. An outpouring of mucopolysaccharides is followed by infiltration of all orbital tissues with lymphocytes and plasma cells. Increased orbital fat is said to be the cause of proptosis; inflammatory changes in the region of the inferior rectus and inferior oblique muscles result in severe limitation of upward gaze. It may be bilateral, and usually is, but is often asymmetrical. Motility is much the same as that seen in the patient with an orbital floor fracture. The eye does not move up well, but moves down almost fully. The horizontal excursions are often normal. The patient appears to have an underaction of

the superior rectus muscle. Surgery on the ocular muscles can be of help in managing patients with diplopia on this basis.

Another form of severe, progressive damage to the ocular muscles is progressive dystrophy of the external ocular muscles described by Kiloh and Nevin.[6] The main clinical features are: (1) it usually begins before age 30, (2) frequency is the same in males and females, (3) there is a family history of either ptosis or ophthalmoplegia or both in over 50 per cent of patients (Fig. 14–13), (4) diplopia is the earliest symptom and ptosis the earliest sign, (5) onset is progressive and insidious, (6) exacerbations and remissions are not common, (7) advance of the disease may be halted temporarily or permanently at any stage, (8) pupils are normal unlike those in myotonic dystrophy with light-near dissociation of the pupils, (9) an expressionless facies is present, and (10) the temporalis and masseter muscles are often involved as are those of the upper spinal segments (10 per cent of cases). There is no associated baldness, cataract, or testicular atrophy with this disease. The basic change is fibrillary degeneration of the striated muscle fibers with some inflammatory cell infiltration and fat deposition in a patchy arrangement. A few patients with progressive external ophthalmoplegia will have retinitis pigmentosa–like retinal changes and fit the diagnostic group of Refsum's syndrome. A very few may also have signif-

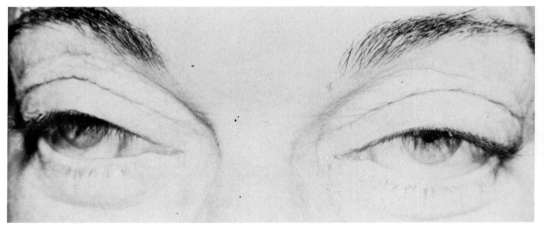

FIGURE 14–13 Bilateral ptosis in patient with advanced Kiloh-Nevin syndrome. Previously thought due to degeneration of the cranial nerve nuclei, the disease is now considered muscular degenerative.

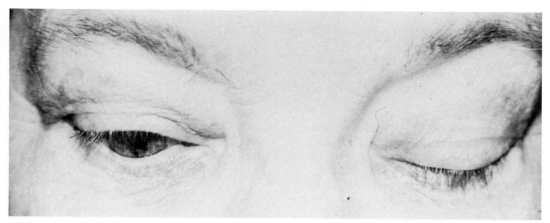

FIGURE 14–14 The pseudo-Graefe sign in misdirection of oculomotor nerve. The right upper lid retracts in downgaze.

icant difficulty with an associated heart block and should have an electrocardiogram.

Cranial Nerve Regeneration

Significant damage to the peripheral segments of a cranial nerve may produce initial degeneration of nerve fibers followed by haphazard regrowth, so that muscles of the face and eyes are incorrectly innervated (Fig. 14–14). The ocular signs found in the misdirection syndrome of nerve III, listed in Table 14–11, are explained by the mass firing effect of misdirected nerve fibers.[1] For example, the eye is unable to move up or down fully because the nerve fibers originally destined for the superior rectus and levator are partly supplying the inferior rectus and medial rectus and inferior oblique muscles. When the patient attempts to look up, the superior rectus and inferior oblique and inferior rectus muscles are all fired simultaneously, and the eye is unable to move. The signs of misdirection of the third nerve are important to recognize as they imply old disease. Over three months are required to obtain significant signs of misdirection. Diabetes alone never causes misdirection of nerve III.

Misdirection of the motor division of the fifth cranial nerve produces the Marcus Gunn jaw winking phenomenon. It is characterized by ptosis of the ipsilateral eye, which changes to lid retraction as the patient opens the mouth or moves the jaw to the opposite side. It is a unilateral process and is usually more of a cosmetic detriment than a functional one. The pathways implicated by the clinical findings are afferent ones beginning with the external pterygoid muscle supplied by the motor division of nerve V. The mesencephalic root of the trigeminal nerve, which supplies the external pterygoid, is linked to the muscles of the oculomotor nerve and finally to the levator of the upper eyelid, forming the efferent arc.

Misdirection in regeneration of the seventh cranial nerve may involve the motor and secretory pathway for lacrimation. Peripheral damage to the facial nerve due to any cause will produce misdirection

TABLE 14–11 OCULAR SIGNS OF MISDIRECTION OF CRANIAL NERVE III

Pseudo-Graefe lid sign	As eye attempts to move downward, upper lid retracts (Fig. 14–15)
Pseudo-Argyll Robertson pupil	Minimal or no response to light, but diameter may vary with direction of gaze
Horizontal gaze lid dyskinesis	Diameter of lid fissure varies with direction of gaze
	As eye is adducted the fissure widens, and the fissure narrows as eye is abducted
	This sometimes best seen in downgaze if misdirection is minimal
Difficult vertical gaze	Eye moves poorly in vertical plane
	Adduction on attempted vertical gaze
Monocular optokinetic responses	As vertical optokinetic targets are presented, the eye with misdirection moves little if at all

if it is severe. If only the motor function is involved in misdirection, an interfacial synkinesis is produced. When the patient attempts to close the eye, synchronous movements of the upper and lower face occur. This is often quite subtle and may be missed unless specifically sought for in the examination. Paroxysmal lacrimation (crocodile tears) is the secretory correlate of regeneration of nerve VII. It may be congenital and bilateral. In the adult it usually follows Bell's palsy and is often unilateral. It is rather common in the Möbius syndrome of childhood with bilateral paresis of nerves VI and VII as the major findings.

Optokinetic Nystagmus

The value of optokinetic nystagmus (ON) in the investigation of patients with disease of the hemisphere or brain stem is generally underestimated. To evaluate optokinetic nystagmus carefully only two simple pieces of equipment are required— an optokinetic tape having 12 to 14 2-by-2-inch squares of red felt sewed to a strip of white felt and a drum, which is advantageous in subtle optokinetic dissociation. A cloth tape measure can be useful but requires a vision of at least 20/70 in order to elicit responses.

In lesions involving the cerebral hemispheres, the optokinetic response is positive in deep parietal lobe disease and negative with lesions elsewhere. Poor optokinetic nystagmus is found with deep parietal lobe lesions when targets are moved toward the side of the lesions. By comparison, moving targets away from the side of the lesion should produce crisp optokinetic nystagmus. Although a hemianopia (homonymous) should be present with parietal lobe damage that is sufficiently deep to produce a positive optokinetic nystagmus sign, this sign must not be considered a test for hemianopic visual field loss.

The vertical optokinetic nystagmus response is useful in localizing certain brain stem lesions. In the normal patient, a crisp sustained vertical response can be elicited with ease. With aging, the vertical responses may be slightly depressed, as compared to the horizontal responses. Adequate responses are never produced without encouragement. The patient should count the targets to himself as they are presented. It is necessary to test a large number of patients to become familiar with the limits of the normal optokinetic response.

Abnormal Vertical Responses

Vertical Optokinetic Nystagmus Dissociation

Horizontal responses are symmetrical, but a gross asymmetry exists between the responses obtained with targets moving vertically (up better than down or vice versa). This is found with regularity in Parkinson's disease, brain stem and cerebellar neoplasms, familial nystagmus, multiple sclerosis, and postoperative stereotaxic lesions. The responses to vertical targets are better in one direction. Spontaneous vertical nystagmus is often present or can be elicited with vertical gaze in patients who have vertical optokinetic nystagmus dissociation.

In brain stem disease, some patients will show poor horizontal responses, but excellent responses to vertical targets. This suggests a lesion at the pontine level. One would expect other neurological signs consistent with pontine damage. These would include slowing or loss of conjugate gaze movements, internuclear ophthalmoplegia, spontaneous nystagmus, Horner's syndrome, and underaction of nerves VI or VII or both. In children, optokinetic testing can be helpful in differentiating congenital from acquired nystagmus. It can also serve to distinguish whether the patient's vision is severely reduced when congenital nystagmus is present. Cogan classified nystagmus in children as of two types. Type I patients have absence of horizontal ON responses, but vertical ones are intact and the reading vision and ocular fundi are usually normal. Type II children have either no ON responses in any direction, or very poor ones, and these children often have significant ocular disease with a poor visual prognosis. Congenital nystagmus can be further differentiated from acquired nystagmus in that vertical optokinetic targets often produce horizontal movements of the eyes. This is excellent evidence for congenital nystagmus. Any patient who has horizontal nystagmus on vertical gaze should be immediately suspected of having congenital nystagmus.

Loss of Rapid Phase

This is sometimes found in vertical optokinetic testing. It is due to the same mechanism in any case — destruction of the corticifugal pathways from the cerebrum to the nuclear masses of the stem. The cause is the same as that for loss of the rapid phase in any form of acquired nystagmus. Sustained slow phase is called the Roth-Bielschowsky deviation.

Monocular Vertical Responses

This is found in the syndrome of misdirection of nerve III as previously described. For practical purposes, this is the only condition causing such responses. It occurs because of mass firing of the vertically acting muscles innervated by the oculomotor nerve when vertical movements are attempted.[1]

Poor Vertical and Intact Horizontal Responses

This dissociation of optokinetic responses is particularly common in patients with disease at the mesencephalic level. This is because the locus for vertical ocular movements is at this level. The selective depression or complete absence of vertical responses with intact horizontal responses strongly suggests the upper brain stem as the site of involvement. It can be produced with lesions outside the stem from simple pressure effects as with pinealomas or meningiomas. It can also be seen with intrinsic stem disorders such as gliomas, hemorrhage, arteriovenous malformation, infarction, inflammatory or degenerative disease. Retraction nystagmus is also found with lesions in this area.

Nystagmoid Movements of the Eyes

Opsoclonus

This dramatic neurological disorder consists of ataxic conjugate movements of the eyes. It has a sudden onset generally following an episode of low-grade fever and upper respiratory disease. Approximately seven days later, the ocular signs of ataxic chaotic conjugate movements begin. The movements are rapid and of large amplitude. There is no diplopia because the movements are conjugate. The patient may close one eye or cover an eye with his hand in an attempt to reduce the amplitude of movement. The movements persist during sleep, but are less violent. Myoclonic jerks of the extremities, face, neck, and trunk are often present. The sensorium is generally clear, and the neurological examination is usually negative except for the myoclonus. The cerebrospinal fluid is normal or shows a slight pleocytosis. The majority of patients have normal hearing, yet cold caloric testing produces no nystagmus. The prognosis is good with complete recovery occurring within four months.

Oculopalatopharyngeal Myoclonus

This unusual ocular movement disorder appears much like nystagmus, but the movement, though rhythmic, lacks a definite slow phase. It is also synchronous with movements of the palate, pharynx, tongue, face, larynx, and the eustachian tube orifice, which may cause the patient to complain of clicking in the ear. It may also be associated with arrhythmic movements of the diaphragm, abdomen, and extremities. These movements are thought to be related to a disturbance of the myoclonic triangle (dentate nucleus of the cerebellum, inferior olive, and red nucleus). The common antecedent causes are multiple sclerosis, trauma, vascular accident of the stem, degenerative disease (olivopontocerebellar degeneration), and severe inflammatory disease of the brain stem. Once developed, it does not remit.

THE VISUAL FIELDS

Several techniques are available for evaluation of the visual fields. The most commonly employed is the confrontation method. The neurosurgeon should, however, be capable of using techniques other than confrontation in the diagnosis of visual field defects.

Confrontation Testing

The usual confrontation test is performed by having the patient cover one eye and look into the examiner's open eye. The patient is then asked to tell the examiner when an object is in motion and when it is not. This method of testing the visual field leaves much to be desired in both accuracy and sensitivity. A much better method is the "three-stage confrontation technique." One must be certain that the covered eye is completely occluded. The patient is then asked to fix his gaze on the examiner's nose. The examiner then presents the extended fingers of one hand in the various quadrants of the visual field, asking the patient to count the number of extended fingers. The number of fingers presented on each occasion is varied. This requires that the patient remain alert. The speed of presentation will vary according to the patient's ability to respond, and great care must be exercised in visual field testing not to exceed his reaction time. Visual field testing is particularly difficult in a patient with dysphasia. If he is encouraged to mimic responses, rather than to verbalize, some useful information may be gained about visual field function. The most useful numbers are one, two, five, and none.

In the second stage of the confrontation test, fingers are presented simultaneously in the two half-fields (Fig. 14–15). The patient is asked to count the total number of fingers he sees. This "double simultaneous stimulation" of the right and left half-fields is particularly helpful in detecting subtle parietal lobe hemianopias and is a manifestation of the extinction phenomenon found with lesions of the parietal lobe.

In the third stage, the examiner's hands are waved in the two half-fields and the patient is asked to "point to the clearest hand." If the patient is unable to recognize any difference in the clarity of the examiner's hands, the visual field is judged normal.

Projector Light Testing

This method has two major advantages over the confrontation and standard tangent screen examination: The presentation of the test target can be fully randomized, and the target size and intensity can be varied at will. The field can be quickly screened in less than five minutes. The examiner stands behind the patient during the test and repeatedly checks fixation by localization of the blind spot (Fig. 14–16). This method is adequate for neurosurgical diagnosis. If more detailed quantitation is needed, an opthalmologist is usually consulted.

The visual field of each eye is recorded as the patient sees it with the fixation point

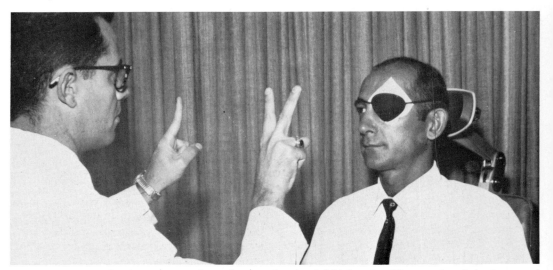

FIGURE 14–15 The three-stage confrontation test for visual field function. The examiner is in the second stage of the method — double simultaneous stimulation of the half-fields.

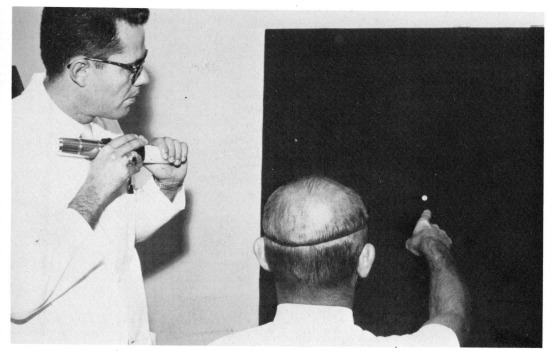

FIGURE 14–16 The projector light in visual field examination. The patient points to the light as a check on his responses.

represented anatomically by the macula and the field reversed relative to the visual pathways. Thus, the nasal retina sees the temporal field and the upper retina the lower field. The blind spot represents the visual field projection of the optic disc. The visual field can be divided into four quadrants by drawing an imaginary line vertically through the macula to divide the field into a right and left half (Fig. 14–17). A horizontal line through the macula then divides the field into four quadrants. The same anatomical relationship of reversal of field to neural pathways (upper retina represents lower field) holds from the retina to the occipital lobe of the brain. In the occipital lobe, the major part of the cortex is devoted to representation of the macula.

Definition of Terms

Full field—the normal extent of the field of vision is: nasal = 60 degrees, temporal = 100+ degrees, superior = 60 degrees, and inferior = 70 to 75 degrees (Fig. 14–17). Tested at the tangent screen, with the patient 1 m from the screen, the blind spot is 15 degrees temporal to fixation and meas-

ures 132 by 96 mm with the 6/1000 white target.

Scotoma—a defect in the visual field, which is surrounded by normal or relatively normal functioning field. The best example of a scotoma is the blind spot. It is a dense scotoma because it may be found even with large-diameter test objects, so long as they do not exceed the visual angle of the blind spot. Scotomas may be dense or relative (subtle).

Hemianopia—a defect in function of one half of the visual field. This includes those types of visual field defects that involve the upper or lower half of the field of each eye, the so-called altitudinal hemianopias (Fig. 14–18). If the field loss is homonymous, the lesion must be posterior to the chiasm. Bitemporal or binasal field loss is characteristic of lesions of the chiasm. The bitemporal type is most common.

Depression—the most common form of visual field dysfunction. It may be dense or relative, generalized or localized. Generalized depression of field function is commonly due to opacities of the ocular media (corneal scar, cataract) or weak stimulus intensity.

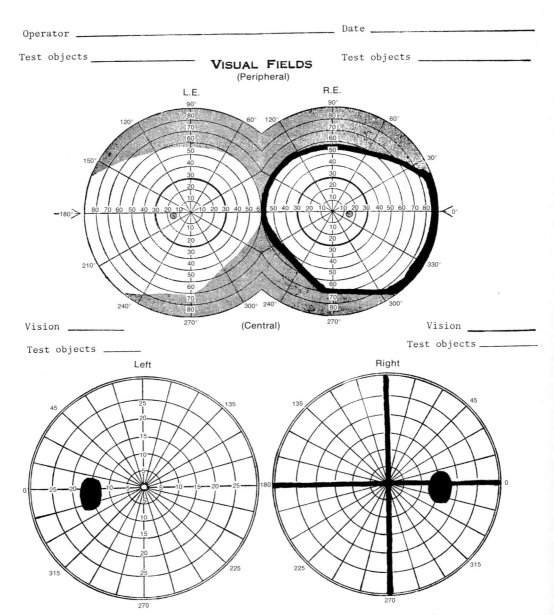

FIGURE 14–17 *Top,* Outline for peripheral (perimetric) visual field study. *Bottom,* The visual field may be divided into four quadrants as shown on the right. Normal blind spot size is shown also on central field plot (tangent screen).

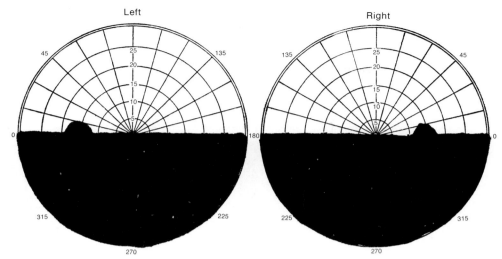

FIGURE 14-18   Bilateral altitudinal hemianopias.

Congruous—a visual field defect that is essentially a carbon copy of another in the same half of visual space. The defects are called congruous in contradistinction to the defect seen in bitemporal hemianopia in which the field defects are "mirror images." Homonymous hemianopias tend to become more congruous as the lesion producing the defect moves toward the occipital cortex. Occipital lobe hemianopias tend to be extremely congruous. Congruity cannot be judged if the defect is a full hemianopia; some part of the half-field must be spared for the assessment of congruity.

Macular sparing—a much overrated sign for localization of the lesion producing the field defect. Classic teaching states that the further posterior a lesion is placed in the visual radiations, the more likely the chance that the field defect will spare fixation. In our experience, even most occipital lobe hemianopias split fixation.

Field Loss as Related to Anatomical Location

Retina and Optic Nerve

Unilateral lesions of the retina and optic nerve produce disturbances of visual field only in the field of vision of the involved eye. If the contralateral visual field is also involved there must be more than one le-

sion or the lesion, if only one exists, is posterior to the optic nerve. An altitudinal field defect in one eye often suggests retinal detachment or vascular optic nerve damage. Retinal detachment is usually preceded by subjective manifestations of flashing lights, a shower of dark spots, and finally the onset of a shade or veil before the involved eye. This may occur suddenly or over a matter of days. A common ocular manifestation of carotid ischemic disease is the transient ischemic attack. The patient complains of sudden loss of vision in the ipsilateral eye. The onset of the visual loss is often altitudinal, as is the recovery. The episode lasts only 5 to 15 minutes, and the patient may or may not note the simultaneous occurrence of crossed motor or sensory signs with the attack. Ophthalmic migraine and ischemic optic neuritis may also produce altitudinal visual field impairment.

The visual field defects produced by glaucoma are common, usually accompanied by significant glaucomatous optic atrophy, and when they are advanced, should be followed with the perimeter rather than the tangent screen.

Congenital anomalies of the optic disc may produce visual field disturbances. These lesions include tilting of the optic disc, coloboma, myopic temporal crescent, myelinated nerve fibers, and hyaline bodies of the optic nerve. Tilting of the disc and coloboma of the optic nerve and choroid

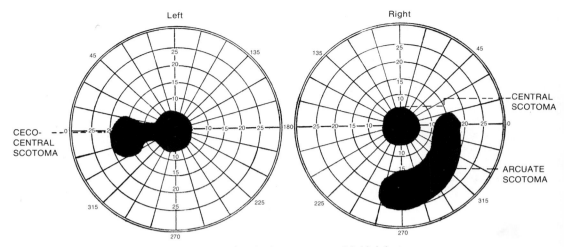

FIGURE 14-19 Optic nerve type of field defects.

are important as they can produce bitemporal hemianopias on visual field examination. Hyaline bodies of the optic nerve head are a frequent cause of pseudopapilledema and often are associated with a defect in the inferior nasal field and enlargement of the blind spot (Fig. 14-19).

Several important causes for visual field loss are the nontoxic causes of optic nerve dysfunction. Disseminated sclerosis frequently gives rise to optic neuritis. This typically presents as a retrobulbar neuritis with a tendency for rapid spontaneous remission and a central scotoma as the characteristic visual field defect (Fig. 14-19). Papilledema commonly causes enlargement of the blind spot and on rare occasions may have an associated central scotoma. This is seen only in severe choking when edema fluid leaks into the macular area and the central scotoma occurs. More commonly, a central scotoma follows papilledema when secondary optic atrophy is severe. When serial measurements of the blind spot diameter are used to follow the course of papilledema, at least a 6/1000 white target must be used. Ischemic optic neuritis usually leaves visual acuity relatively spared, as compared to other forms of optic neuritis, and the common visual field defect is the inferior altitudinal type that is connected to the blind spot. Neuromyelitis optica generally presents as an acute bilateral papillitis with dense large-diameter central scotomas. Visual acuity is often reduced to bare light perception. Full re-

missions are not so common as in the retrobulbar neuritis of disseminated sclerosis. Schilder's disease is a demyelinizing neurological process of children and young adults who have progressive visual loss, deterioration of mentation, and spastic paraplegia. Visual field loss, due to progressive optic atrophy or papilledema followed by atrophy, is often generalized with more profound effects seen at the central field early. Total blindness occurs late in the disease and most patients do not live over two years. The hereditary optic atrophy of Leber is a disease of young males that begins in the 15- to 20-year age group with sudden loss of central vision in one or both eyes. Central or cecocentral scotomas are found. Complete blindness may occur.

Syphilitic optic neuritis is a frequent cause of optic nerve disease and consequent visual field loss. Visual field defects may be produced as follows: (1) concentric peripheral contraction, (2) localized peripheral field wedge-shaped scotomas, (3) central and cecocentral scotomas (Fig. 14-19), (4) central scotomas combined with peripheral defects, (5) altitudinal defects, and (6) field changes arising in the absence of any ophthalmoscopic evidence of optic nerve disease with defects arising at the blind spot. Peripheral damage to the optic nerve fibers is histologically more common than axial involvement, but central scotomas are seen in 53 per cent of patients with optic nerve injury of this etiology.

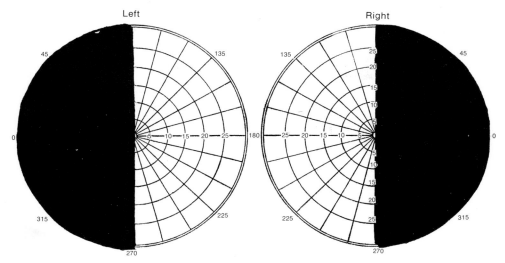

FIGURE 14-20 Full bitemporal hemianopia, dense.

Optic Chiasm

The classic visual field defect found in diseases affecting the chiasm is the bitemporal hemianopia (Fig. 14–20). Bitemporal hemianopias may be scotomatous or non-scotomatous. The former are more common with lesions in the area of the posterior chiasm; there may be a bitemporal paracentral scotoma. Kearns and Rucker described nerve fiber bundle defects and peripheral midzonal arcuate defects with chromophobe adenomas.[4] In the non-scotomatous type of defect only the periph-

eral field is influenced. Bitemporal field loss tends to progress clockwise in the right field and counterclockwise in the left field. Altitudinal deficits are rarely seen in chiasmal lesions. Unexplained optic atrophy should always arouse suspicion of disease in or about the chiasm.

Optic Tract

Primary lesions of the tract are rare. Visual field defects associated with tract dysfunction are most often the result of encroachment upon the tract by disease in

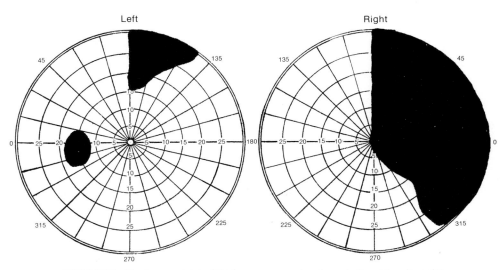

FIGURE 14-21 Incongruous right homonymous hemianopia (tract hemianopia).

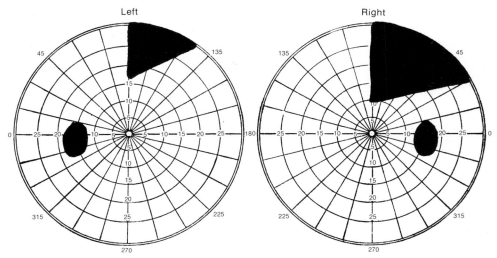

FIGURE 14-22 Incongruous right homonymous hemianopia upper quadrant defect of the temporal lobe type.

surrounding structures. The close relationship of the circle of Willis, pituitary gland, and temporal lobe of the brain account for the majority of tract-induced visual field loss. These visual field defects are characterized by homonymous hemianopia, incongruity, variable density, and some macular sparing, and finally a complete loss of tract function results in a full hemianopia with splitting of fixation (Fig. 14–21).

Temporal Lobe

Because the temporal lobe carries the lower fibers of the visual radiations in its anterior segment, the Meyer's loop, an early lesion of the temporal lobe usually produces an upper quadrantic visual field defect opposite the side of the lesion. This may progress to full hemianopia. The main features of field defects associated with lesions of the temporal lobe are: homonymous hemianopia, incongruity, variable density, early defect starting along the vertical meridian, and early fixation encroachment (Fig. 14–22). Temporal lobe disease producing defect in visual field function is often associated with symptoms of formed visual hallucinations, auditory or olfactory hallucinations, and teleopsia.

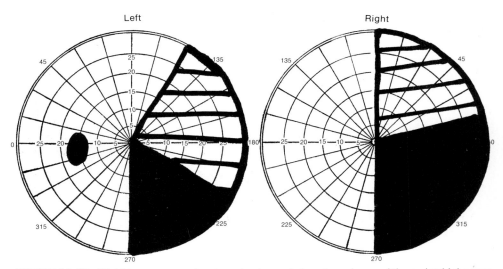

FIGURE 14-23 Right homonymous hemianopia, denser below than above, of the parietal lobe type.

Parietal Lobe

The parietal lobe carries the majority of the visual radiations coming from the upper portion of the lateral geniculate body. An early lesion of the parietal lobe tends to produce a homonymous hemianopic visual field loss that is denser below than above. This may progress to a full hemianopia, just as can occur with extensive damage to the temporal lobe, lateral geniculate body, or optic tract. Parietal lobe field loss is more congruous than that of temporal lobe origin (Fig. 14–23). It is less so than that due to disease in the occipital lobe.

Occipital Lobe

The usual occipital lobe type of visual field defect is homonymous hemianopic and congruous, and splits fixation (Fig. 14–24). Density varies markedly in these visual field disorders. Because the calcarine cortex is divided into an upper and lower bank, the visual field deficit may occupy only a quadrant. Ischemia of the upper bank of the left occipital lobe produces a right lower quadrant hemianopia. If the lesion is located very near the tip of the occipital pole, the visual field defect will tend toward a paracentral hemianopia. Lesions placed anteriorly in the occipital cortex classically produce the "monocular temporal crescent" type of field loss. The most anterior part of the occipital cortex receives the visual fibers from the peripheral retinae. The right anterior occipital lobe cortex, for example, takes the fibers from the temporal periphery of the right eye and the nasal periphery of the left eye. A lesion in that area of the occipital lobe would cause early loss of the temporal field of the left eye, which would be impossible to find without the perimeter because only the extreme temporal field is lost. In fact, this type of visual field defect is rare with lesions of the occipital lobe.

If bilateral damage to the occipital lobe cortex occurs, the patient may develop cortical blindness. This is seen with severe ischemia due to saddle emboli of the basilar artery, most often, or with trauma to the occiput. Such blindness has been described in children with relatively minor trauma, but then it is generally of short duration. Cortical blindness has the following clinical characteristics: (1) bilateral homonymous hemianopias, (2) total blindness with intact pupillary responses, (3) denial of blindness, (4) visual hallucination, (5) confabulation as in Korsakoff's psychosis, (6) amnestic amnesia—loss of recent memory, (7) often no other localizing neurological signs, and (8) allochiria in which sensation from stimuli applied to one limb is localized by the patient in the opposite limb. Such blindness may follow ventriculography, but in these instances there is a much better prognosis for return of visual function than

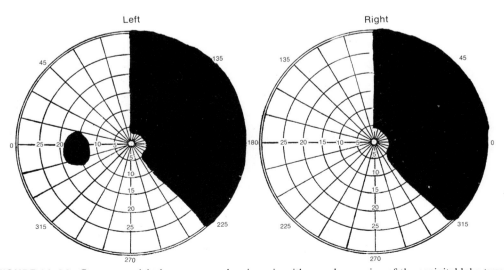

FIGURE 14–24 Congruous right homonymous hemianopia with macular sparing of the occipital lobe type.

in the usual patient with cortical blindness. Homonymous hemianopias may follow arteriography, especially with direct carotid punctures. This also has a good prognosis for functional recovery.

OPHTHALMOSCOPY

The appearance of the optic disc is of major concern to the neurosurgeon and this section confines itself entirely to discussion of that structure.

The normal optic nerve head usually appears larger in the myopic eye and smaller in the hyperopic eye. The myopic disc is often rather pale on the temporal side suggesting optic atrophy. The hyperopic disc, especially in eyes with refractive errors of more than 4 diopters, may mimic papilledema. It is helpful to look at the patient's glasses to decide whether he is myopic or hyperopic. Myopic lenses minify objects viewed through them and hyperopic lenses magnify.

Papilledema, Pseudopapilledema and Papillitis

Papilledema is the swelling of the tissues of the optic disc, usually because of an increase in intracranial pressure. The rise in pressure within the cranial vault is transmitted to the subarachnoid space around the optic nerves as this space is continuous with the intracranial subarachnoid cavity. A rise in pressure within this space causes the venous outflow from the disc to slow. This allows fluid to exude from the capillaries of the disc into the tissues of the area. Although other mechanisms have been suggested for the production of papilledema, this one is the most generally accepted. The clinical signs of papilledema are (1) loss of a previously seen spontaneous venous pulse; (2) elevation of the disc; (3) blurring of the disc margins (especially temporally as slight nasal blurring is normal); (4) overfilling of the retinal veins; (5) hemorrhages on the surface of the disc and later in surrounding retina; (6) concentric folds surrounding the disc, owing to edema fluid leaking from the disc; and (7) cystic elevation of the macula in chronic papilledema.

Papilledema requires several hours to develop. When it is well developed, it requires weeks to clear. Papilledema usually occurs in both eyes except in special circumstances. Pre-existing optic atrophy may mask the onset of disc swelling. Greatly increased spinal fluid pressure without papilledema means that there has been a false reading, not enough time for papilledema to develop, pre-existing optic atrophy, or a spinal subarachnoid block. Loss of the previously seen spontaneous venous pulse on the central retinal vein is the *earliest ophthalmoscopic sign of papilledema*. It is the first to return when intracranial pressure becomes normal. Transient obscurations of vision are common in patients with papilledema. They describe them as brief periods (seconds) of blurred, fuzzy, or hazy vision followed by instantaneous complete clearing of vision. Transient obscurations may occur hundreds of times per day and they are bilateral with rare exceptions. Chronic papilledema may occur in patients with increased intracranial pressure over long periods of time. The ophthalmoscopic picture differs in this circumstance from that seen in the more typical onset of papilledema. Hemorrhages are less conspicuous, the surface of the disc appears dry, and the degree of elevation is often exceptional—4 diopters plus with the direct ophthalmoscope (Fig. 14–25).

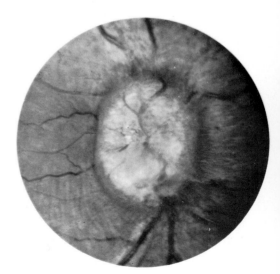

FIGURE 14–25 Chronic papilledema. Note the crenated surface of the disc, the marked elevation, and the concentric folds in the peripapillary retina.

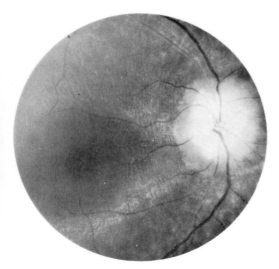

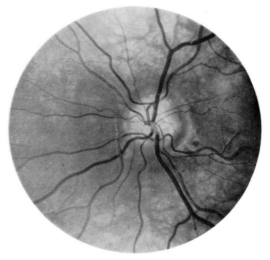

FIGURE 14–26 Hyaline bodies of the optic nerve. Note the irregular surface of the disc and the small cup.

FIGURE 14–27 Hyaline bodies of the optic nerve located deeper in the substance of the disc.

The causes of pseudopapilledema include high hyperopic refractive errors, hyaline bodies of the optic nerve head, myelinated nerve fibers, and ischemic optic neuritis. In patients with hyperopia of more than 4 diopters, the disc is often elevated with some blurring of both the nasal and temporal margins. This is thought to be the result of crowding of nerve fibers, as they enter the optic nerve, in a small eye. The elevation of the disc is usually rather symmetrical between the two eyes, the physiological cup is small to nonexistent, a spontaneous venous pulse is usually present, and there are no hemorrhages on the surface of the disc. The blind spot is small.

Hyaline bodies (drusen) of the optic nerve are developmental lesions and are often familial (50 per cent). They are round laminated translucent structures. They usually occur bilaterally, but may be very asymmetrical (Figs. 14–26 and 14–27). They are known to increase slowly in size, but even though they may produce visual field defects, the patient rarely loses significant visual acuity. Although hyaline bodies are said to occur with increasing frequency in patients with tuberous sclerosis and neurofibromatosis, evidence now suggests that the hyaline masses seen at or near the disc in these diseases are astrocytic hamartomas and not simple products of secretion from the neuroglial structure in

the nerve. Differentiation from papilledema may be difficult at times.

Myelinated nerve fibers usually occur at the margin of the disc (Fig. 14–28). Myelination normally ends at the cribiform plate of the optic nerve. Occasionally it continues into the eye for variable distances producing a patch of white on the surface of the retina. Its configuration is characteristic in that the patch has a "feathered edge" especially noticeable in the peripheral portion of the lesion. It may obscure parts of the retinal vessels, and vice versa,

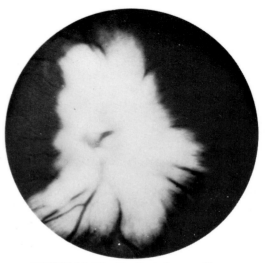

FIGURE 14–28 Myelinated nerve fibers.

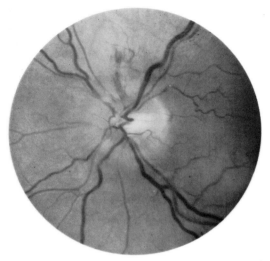

FIGURE 14–29 Ischemic optic neuritis. Blurred disc margins and flame hemorrhage at the edge of the disc mimic papilledema.

proving its superficial location. These are essentially stable deposits; they may be found in the peripheral retina also. They rarely produce a field defect except for a very relative scotoma. They may regress if the patient develops optic atrophy for any reason. These lesions are most often confused with exudates at the margin of the disc and are occasionally mistaken for evidence of papilledema.

Ischemic optic neuritis is sometimes confused with papilledema (Fig. 14–29). It occurs in patients of 50 to 60 years. They often have pre-existing vascular disease (angina, claudication, myocardial infarction). The common complaint is sudden loss of visual field. Visual acuity is often good. The ophthalmoscopic findings are elevation of the disc, some degree of pallor, and one or more small flame hemorrhages at the edge of the blurred disc margin. The visual field deficit is characteristically inferior altitudinal. The process tends to be bilateral, but the attacks are usually separated by months or years. A patient who has had a previous bout of ischemic optic neuritis will have primary optic atrophy as the residual. The eye with a fresh ischemic lesion of the nerve will show a picture much like papilledema. This has caused confusion in the past with the Foster Kennedy syndrome (primary optic atrophy ipsilateral to sphenoid wing meningioma with contralateral papilledema) (Fig. 14–30). The

Foster Kennedy syndrome is very rare, whereas ischemic optic neuritis is common. These patients deserve a careful work-up to identify diabetes mellitus, hypertensive cardiovascular disease, collagen vascular disease, lues, and cranial arteritis. Repeated measurement of the blood pressure in *both arms,* a carefully done three- to four-hour glucose tolerance test, erythrocyte sedimentation rate determination, and ophthalmodynamometry are indicated. If the sedimentation rate is over 30 mm per hour, a temporal artery biopsy should be obtained. Large amounts of systemic steroids or anticoagulation or both may be of value in gaining some return of visual function or preventing further ischemia. Women with a past history of migraine or other vascular disease should avoid using conjugated estrogens as there is evidence that use of these medications may predispose the patient to ischemic disease of the optic nerve.

Papillitis is an ophthalmoscopic classification for optic neuritis in which the optic nerve involvement is located relatively far anteriorly, producing elevation of the disc. The disc is usually more pink than normal owing to increased circulation through the capillaries on the surface. The physiological cup may be smaller than normal. The central retinal vessels are generally normal to somewhat full. There may be frank hemorrhage, and the surrounding retina is not in-

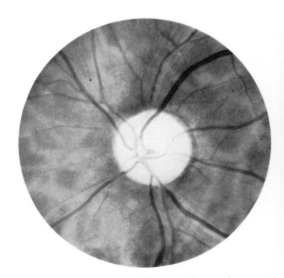

FIGURE 14–30 Primary optic atrophy.

TABLE 14–12 CAUSES OF OPTIC NEURITIS (PARTIAL LIST)

Post-traumatic—direct ocular trauma or orbital trauma
Intraocular inflammatory—uveitis with bacterial, viral, fungal, or idiopathic etiology
Meningitis—due to any cause
Metabolic—diabetes mellitus, thyroid disease, nutrition (alcohol, tobacco, diet) related
Familial—Leber's optic neuritis
Toxic—drugs or heavy metals (Chloramphenicol, lead)
Demyelinating disease—disseminated sclerosis, Schilder's disease, Devic's disease
Postinfectious—viral
"Septic foci"—teeth, sinuses, etc.
Idiopathic

frequently involved. The process is then called neuroretinitis. It is more often unilateral than bilateral and may look like papilledema. The major distinguishing features are: (1) unilaterality, (2) marked loss of vision and visual field function, (3) "cells" in the vitreous, and (4) Marcus Gunn pupil. A partial list of the causes of optic neuritis is seen in Table 14–12.

Retrobulbar optic neuritis is another ophthalmoscopic class of optic neuritis in which the disc appears perfectly normal in the acute stage of the disease and often the only residual is some pallor of the temporal disc. There is often a profound loss of visual acuity in an eye that is ophthalmoscopically normal. It has the same causes as papillitis, but tends to suggest a diagnosis of demyelinating disease when it is unilateral. Pain on motion of the eye is common. The attacks of retrobulbar optic neuritis associated with disseminated sclerosis are generally unilateral, rarely bilateral, and almost never bilateral and simultaneous. The visual prognosis for the first attack is good in disseminated sclerosis, which rarely occurs under the age of 10 years. Neuromyelitis optica, however, usually presents a bilateral simultaneous optic neuritis, and the visual prognosis is much less satisfactory.

Optic Atrophy

Four ophthalmoscopic classes of optic atrophy are: primary, secondary, glaucomatous, and consecutive. No etiology is implied except in the case of glaucomatous atrophy.

Primary optic atrophy is, except for glaucomatous atrophy, the most common.

It leaves the margins of the disc sharp, the central retinal vessels in their normal position, and the color of the disc "bone white." Loss of the exact outline of the physiological cup is frequent. Primary optic atrophy has causes as listed in Table 14–13.

Secondary optic atrophy is characterized by a generalized change of color of the disc from pink to a dirty gray. There is an associated proliferation of glial elements over the surface, often obscuring the physiological cup and making the margins of the disc difficult to outline. This type of atrophy follows on the heels of papilledema, regardless of cause, or papillitis.

Glaucomatous optic atrophy is recognized by enlargement and undercutting of the edge of the physiological cup, shifting of the central retinal vessels to the nasal side of the cup, and progressive loss of nerve substance at the temporal edge of the cup. Such changes are usually seen in those persons who have a definite increase in the intraocular pressure above normal limits (12 to 22 mm of mercury). In some the intraocular pressure may be normal or low, and yet a progressive loss of visual field and steady increase in atrophy occurs. These are the so-called "low-tension glaucoma" patients and they should be suspected of having carotid arterial insufficiency if the intraocular pressure is normal when measured repeatedly by applanation and if the atrophy is unilateral.

Consecutive optic atrophy follows disease of the retina or the choroid and retina. Extensive damage to the retina is needed to produce significant consecutive atrophy.

TABLE 14–13 SOME CAUSES OF PRIMARY OPTIC ATROPHY

Intoxication (alcohol, tobacco, diet)
Intracranial mass lesions (aneurysm, sphenoid wing meningioma, pituitary tumor, suprasellar mass, dilated third ventricle with internal hydrocephalus)
Compression from intraorbital mass lesion (meningioma, dermoid, pseudotumor, thyroid orbital disease, severe orbital hemorrhage)
Direct invasion (glioma of optic nerve)
Trauma (contusion, laceration associated with fracture of optic canal)
Demyelinating disease
Vascular accidents of the optic nerve
Inflammatory disease of the nerve (tuberculosis, lues) may produce this type of atrophy rather than the usual form of postinflammatory atrophy

Central retinal artery occlusion causes consecutive optic atrophy because of degeneration of the internal layers of the retina following the occlusion. It is also common in retinitis pigmentosa.

REFERENCES

1. Bender, M. B., and Fulton, J. F.: Factors in functional recovery following section of the oculomotor nerve in monkeys. J. Neurol. Psychiat., 2:285, 1939.
2. Cogan, D. G., and Victor, M.: Ocular signs of Wernicke's disease. A.M.A. Arch. Ophthal., 51:204–211, 1954.
3. Glaser, J. S.: Myasthenic pseudo-internuclear ophthalmoplegia. Arch. Ophthal. (Chicago), 75:363–366, 1966.
4. Kearns, T. P., and Rucker, C. W.: Arcuate defects in the visual fields due to chromophobe adenoma of the pituitary gland. Amer. J. Ophthal., 45:505–507, 1958.
5. Kernohan, J. W., and Woltman, H. W.: Incisura of the crus due to contralateral brain tumor. Arch. Neurol. Psychiat., 21:274, 1929.
5a. Kestenbaum, A.: Clinical Methods of Neuro-ophthalmologic Examination. 2nd Ed., New York, Grune & Stratton, 1961.
6. Kiloh, L. G., and Nevin, S.: Progressive dystrophy of the external ocular muscles. Brain, 74:115–143, 1951.
7. Smith, J. L., and David, N. J.: Internuclear ophthalmoplegia. Two new clinical signs. Neurology (Minneap.), 14:307–309, 1964.
8. Thompson, H. S., and Mensher, J. H.: Adrenergic mydriasis in Horner's syndrome. The hydroxy-amphetamine test for diagnosis of postganglionic defects. Amer. J. Ophthal., 72:472–480, 1971.

15

NEURO-OTOLOGY

Because of a fine, constant, muscular tonus, man is able to strike and maintain a posture and carry out many precise coordinated activities such as swimming, writing, and ice skating. This muscle tonus is kept in a delicate state of balance by a constant barrage of electrical impulses arising in the central nervous system and passing to the peripheral musculature. Before the brain can dispense such orders it must be oriented with regard to man's position with respect to his environment. Such intelligence is gained through a number of informer systems such as the touch receptors in the soles of the feet, the visual sense, the proprioceptive receptors in the muscles and tendons and joints, and the neural receptors in the inner ear. When something goes wrong with one of these informer organs it may make itself known to the patient in the form of vertigo or unsteadiness of gait. When the patient presents with such a complaint it then becomes incumbent upon the physician to proceed with an evaluation of the vestibulocerebellar complex. Before this is possible it is essential to possess some knowledge of the anatomical principles of this intricate system. Only a brief outline of the pathways is presented here, and standard publication on the subject should be consulted.[3, 9]

ANATOMY

The internal auditory meatus provides a good point of departure, for within it is housed the vestibular ganglion (ganglion of Scarpa), the cells of which are bipolar. The peripheral fibers pass to the cristae am-

pullares of the semicircular canals and the maculae of the utricle and saccule. The primary function of the static labyrinth is to put out a constant rhythmic volley of electrical discharges to the central nervous system, even when the body is completely at rest. This has been named the resting discharge. When the body is in movement, an alteration in this electrical discharge is produced, and the central nervous system is thereby informed of such motion. It has not been determined whether the otic fluid actually moves or whether the electrical impulse is generated by simple motion of the structures attached to the receptors. In any event, the semicircular canals inform the brain of angular acceleration, and the utricle provides information concerning linear acceleration. The function of the saccule is, for the most part, unknown although it has been said to be a receptor of vibratory stimuli. The central fibers (first neurons) enter the brain stem between the pons and the medulla and plunge into the floor of the fourth ventricle where they end in the vestibular nuclei. The latter are four in number: the superior nucleus of Bechterew, the lateral nucleus of Deiters, the medial nucleus of Schwalbe, and the inferior nucleus of Roller. A fifth nucleus in the cerebellum has been postulated. It has been shown that a number of fibers pass directly from the ganglion of Scarpa to the cerebellum. These are known as the vestibulocerebellar interrelation. The second neurons from the nuclei of Deiters and Schwalbe enter into the median longitudinal fasciculus, and it is probable that those from Roller's nucleus do the same. Once they have entered the median longitudinal fasciculus, some fibers remain ipsilateral, whereas some cross. Either group may ascend or descend, and with the

G. O. PROUD

latter we are not concerned. The ascending fibers pass to the nucleus of the sixth cranial nerve, and this is the pathway for horizontal nystagmus. The second neurons, from the nucleus of Bechterew, also enter the median longitudinal fasciculus, but neither cross nor descend. They are simple ascending ipsilateral fibers, and proceed to the nucleus of the fourth and third cranial nerves providing the pathway for vertical nystagmus.

Above the level of the oculomotor nuclei the vertigo pathways are actually unknown. Most observers feel that the termination of the vertigo pathway is in the contralateral temporal lobe. In the roof of the fourth ventricle the fastigial nucleus is found, and through the hook bundle it exerts an inhibitory effect upon the vestibular nuclei of the opposite side and a stimulatory effect upon the ipsilateral vestibular nuclei. It should be borne in mind that the entire vestibulocerebellar complex is under the control of the corticopontinecerebellar fibers.

THE PHYSICAL EXAMINATION

A complete examination of the ears, nose, and throat is carried out first; during this standard procedure, if one is alert, many of the cranial nerves can be tested at the same time. This is a great time-saving device. For example, the gag reflex can be tested while examining the pharynx, nasopharynx, and larynx. Paralysis of the vocal cords should be noted and the sense of smell tested. The patient should be quizzed concerning his vision, and a complete audiological evaluation including pure tone air and bone conduction, speech discrimination scores, binaural loudness balance tests, and tonal decay test should be performed. All the cranial nerves are checked, and particular attention is given to the corneal reflex on both sides.

The patient is then given the Romberg test. It should be noticed whether, with his eyes closed and standing erect with feet together, the subject is steady or has a tendency to fall consistently to one side or the other. In the presence of a recent peripheral lesion on the right, there will be a tendency to fall toward the right. The reason becomes apparent when one realizes that the resting discharge of the labyrinth on that side has been interrupted, and this results in a subsequent lack of muscle tonus on the same side. The patient falls, or rather feels as if he is pushed, toward the side of the lesion. If the labyrinthine paralysis is temporary, or if labyrinthine destruction is complete, the resting discharge is taken over by the vestibular nuclei and the muscle tonus will return; the patient will fall only if the paralysis is a recent one. If the lesion is in the cerebellum, the patient will usually fall to the side of a hemisphere lesion; however, in cerebellar lesions the direction of fall is not as localizing as it is in peripheral involvement. When the difficulty is in the vermis, the subject is more apt to fall forward or backward. Although the direction of fall in central disease is not too significant, it should be mentioned that patients with cerebellar disorders will very frequently exhibit unsteadiness. The patient's gait is tested with and without the blindfold. Wandering from a straight line is not significant, but the individual who has a peripheral lesion will tend to fall again toward the side on which there is interruption of the resting discharge. A wide gait indicates difficulty in the vermis.

The Heath rail test is of great value in estimating the equilibrium for it will bring out balance difficulties that are not apparent on the ordinary gait test. It is of special value in children who are terrified by caloric or spinning tests.

In evaluating the cerebellum it is well to recall that cerebellar disease does not produce loss of movement, for no muscular effort stems from this area. With cerebellar involvement one is able, however, to observe *alteration in the character of the movement.* With the patient sitting, arms extended and eyes closed, and with the fingers spread wide apart for 15 seconds, there is a tendency for the arms to drift toward the side of a recent labyrinthine lesion. If the lesion is in the cerebellar hemisphere there may be homolateral asthenia, but no drift. If the lesion is in the vermis there may be bilateral asthenia. The past-pointing test is merely a refinement of the extended arm test. It is performed with the subject in the sitting position with the eyes closed, the arm and index finger of one side is fully extended and placed on top of the examiner's finger. He is then commanded to raise the arm high in the air and bring it down slowly and into contact with the examiner's finger once more. If the lesion is peripheral and recent, there will be past-pointing toward the side of the difficulty. At the same time, one may look for tremor or asthenia. The finger-to-nose test is performed with the subject's eyes closed and the arms extended to the side. He is then instructed to bring each index finger into contact with the tip of the nose. Overshooting indicates trouble in the cerebellar hemisphere, and at the same time one may again observe for intention tremor. Alternate fine-skill movements should be performed by the subject, for the cerebellar hemisphere is responsible for the smoothness of such acts. It is the vermis that is responsible for the individual's ability to strike a posture, whereas fine, coordinated muscular movements are controlled by the cerebellar hemisphere. It is interesting to note that hypotonia results in constant attention in order to accomplish fine movements. The latter results in physical and mental fatigue, which in turn causes the patient to be irritable. This may well explain why most patients with cerebellar difficulty are easily irritated.

NYSTAGMUS

Nystagmus is a rhythmic, involuntary, usually rapid movement of the eyes. Pendular nystagmus is characterized by equal speed in both directions. In other words, there is no quick component. The patient may move his head in the plane of the nystagmus in order to prevent visual disturbance. In most individuals with pendular nystagmus the vision is nearly normal. When the condition is very advanced, however, the distant vision may be poor. It is present in the primary position with the eyes looking straight ahead at the examiner, but it may change to the jerk variety when looking out of the primary position. Pendular nystagmus is usually of congenital origin, and the gene may be dominant or recessive. On occasions it is caused by ocular albinism. Rarely, one sees a patient with spasmus nutans. Such an individual exhibits a wild pendular nystagmus with rotation of the head in the plane of the eye motion. It may be confused with labyrinthine disease; its organic cause is unknown.

Jerk nystagmus features both a quick and a slow component, and the direction of the nystagmus is named by the direction of the quick component.

Optokinetic nystagmus is one variety of jerk nystagmus. It is also known as railroad, picket fence, or train nystagmus, and it is present in the normal individual. When one is riding in a train and looking out the window his eyes pick up an object in the environment and follow it until it is out of the field of vision. The eyes then jerk back to the original position and pick out another object and follow it until it in turn is invisible. The examiner may test for it by having the subject watch a carpenter's tape while it is pulled from its spool; the quick component will be in the direction opposite to the motion of the tape. It is normally present, but its absence is localizing. If the tape is moved to the right, and the quick component to the left is absent, it indicates, according to Smith and Cogan, that the disease is in the right parietal lobe. The test is also of value in differentiating between vestibular and ocular nystagmus. If the tape is moved in the direction of the quick component, the speed and crispness of the nystagmus will be increased if the disease is of vestibular origin, but it will not be affected if the nystagmus stems from ocular difficulty.

Spontaneous Nystagmus

Spontaneous nystagmus may be of peripheral (labyrinthine), intermediate (vestibular nerve), or central origin. The subject is instructed to follow the examiner's finger, which is kept about 2 feet from the patient's eyes. The finger is moved, slowly in order to avoid saccadic movements, to the limit of peripheral vision, first to the right, then to the left, then up and down. If nystagmus is seen it should be noted whether it is unidirectional or multidirectional, and the direction of the quick component should be noted. The afferent reflex arc extends from the cristae through the vestibulo-oculomotor pathways to the oculomotor nuclei. The efferent arc extends through the oculomotor nerves to the eye muscle nuclei. When spontaneous nystagmus is of peripheral origin, the slow component is probably of central origin. Peripheral nystagmus is nearly always unidirectional, and the quick component beats toward the healthy side. It is transient and will ordinarily be seen only when the vestibular lesion is recent. If the disease is reversible it will disappear, or if labyrinthine death occurs, the vestibular nuclei take over the resting discharge and the nystagmus will disappear. Vestibular nystagmus may be caused by trauma, toxic drugs (streptomycin), extension of middle ear disease into the inner ear, Ménière's disease, tumors, and nonspecific virus infections. It will usually be attended by a diminished or absent caloric response.

When unidirectional nystagmus is of central origin it may be caused by difficulty located anywhere in the brain, for the entire vestibulocerebellar complex is under control of the corticopontinecerebellar fibers. Under these circumstances, the caloric response may be normal. Multidirectional nystagmus is ordinarily of central or intermediate origin, and the quick component beats toward the diseased side. It is usually due to a posterior fossa lesion, but it also exists when there is involvement of the vestibular nerve. If, during the course of acute mastoiditis with labyrinthitis, one observes a change in the direction of the nystagmus, intracranial complications should be suspected.

Positional Nystagmus

Positional nystagmus may exist in the absence of spontaneous nystagmus, and it has an entirely different significance from the latter. The test is performed by having the patient suddenly assume the supine position with the head hanging over the end of the table. The head is first turned to the right, and the patient is ordered to look to the right for a period of 15 seconds. If no nystagmus appears, the head is turned to the left, and the direction of gaze reversed for 15 seconds. Two types of positional nystagmus may be provoked. The first is not immediately apparent, but comes on only after a latent period of 10 to 15 seconds, is associated with vertigo, and disappears after 15 or 20 seconds. Sometimes the vertigo is so intense that it will be difficult to hold the patient on the table. Such a patient is suffering from a condition known as benign paroxysmal postural vertigo, the origin of which is unknown. The caloric response in such a case will usually be normal, as will the audiological tests. Arguments have been proposed in favor of both central and peripheral origin; the latest theory suggests that arterial compression, due to the head twisting, is the cause. Occasionally, it is seen in patients who have undergone stapes operations, but whatever its origin, the condition is seldom to be feared, for it is ordinarily self-limited, although the patient may experience several attacks before it disappears entirely.

The second type of positional nystagmus appears immediately when the patient assumes a new position, is not fatiguable, and is not associated with vertigo. Present evidence seems to indicate that the difficulty is in the floor of the fourth ventricle where the vestibular nuclei are irritated but not destroyed.[1] Cawthorne reported a series of patients with this physical finding as the only evidence of disease. It indicated central metastasis in patients with bronchogenic carcinoma when there were no other symptoms. The lesion need not necessarily be caused by tumor. For example, a head injury with microhemorrhage can produce the same picture.

One observer endeavored to ascribe a localizing value to change of direction of the positional nystagmus upon change of position of the head.[6] He referred to the direction-changing type as type I, and the nonchanging type as type II. Others have indicated, however, that such change is of no value in localization.

Nystagmoid Phenomenon

It is not too unusual to see a senseless wandering motion of the eyes, particularly in the vertical plane, and without a quick component. Actually, this is merely the absence of the stamp of cerebellar smoothness on the eye muscle activity, and may be referred to as oculomotor asthenia.

Some observers classify ocular nystagmus as true nystagmus, although it is absent in the neutral zone. When there is an eye muscle weakness, there is a tendency for the eye to return to the side on which the muscle is strongest. In general, it should be said that nystagmus will be enhanced in both amplitude and crispness when the eyes are gazing in the direction of the quick component.

Postcaloric Nystagmus

The static labyrinth may be tested by rotational, electric, or thermal means. The rotational test is of limited value because it is not possible to selectively stimulate one labyrinth. The electrical tests, by galvanic current, may lead to confusion because one cannot predict the depth of the stimulus. It may not stop with the static labyrinth; the current may actually reach the median longitudinal fasciculus, or even the vertigo center. The thermal tests are the most popular of the day, and although they remain crude, they do yield a considerable amount of valuable information. The horizontal semicircular canal is the easiest to test because it is closest to the surface. The patient is placed in the supine position, and the head is elevated to a point 30 degrees from the horizontal. Three milliliters of ice water are delivered to the surface of the tympanic membrane under visualization with a head mirror and ear speculum. The nystagmus is timed from the beginning of douching until the cessation of nystagmus. As soon as the water has remained in the ear canal for three seconds, it is allowed to run out of the ear. The timing is done with a stop clock, and although the tests are largely qualitative, considerable quantitation becomes possible with diligent practice.

Whether the fluid in the semicircular canals actually moves when the temperature is changed is subject to considerable debate. Some authorities feel that there is simply a gliding of the cupula owing to the convection current. In any event, if the test is performed on the right ear, the cupula glides downward and the eyes are pulled to the right. The quick component will be toward the left and will persist from 50 seconds to three minutes after the onset of douching. This is probably the normal response. While the nystagmus is going on the observer notes something of its speed and briskness, for labyrinthine hypoactivity may exist even when the postcaloric reaction time is equal on the two sides. The reason that nystagmus does not cease immediately after the cold stimulus has been discontinued is that it takes a certain time for the cupula to return to its rest position on the summit of the crista. The test is usually performed with the eyes in the primary position because if the patient has a spontaneous nystagmus, it would be difficult to estimate the end point. On occasion the nystagmus is so minimal that it becomes necessary to have the patient gaze in the direction of the quick component in order to see it.

There is considerable debate whether cold stimulates or paralyzes the labyrinth. In answer to this, it can be said that if 3 ml of ice water are delivered to the right and left tympanic membranes syncronously and for the same period of time, no nystagmus will appear, nor will the patient complain of vertigo. Furthermore, he is able to assume the standing position and remain steady. Obviously, if both labyrinths are thereby paralyzed, the subject would be ataxic. Therefore, one might assume that the thermal stimulus is indeed a stimulus. Perhaps it is simpler to think that the thermal change is responsible for an alteration in the electrical discharge of peripheral origin. During the period of postcaloric response the individual will sometimes complain bitterly of vertigo. On other occasions the vertigo is very mild, and one will know of its presence only if the patient is quizzed concerning it. After the ice water has been delivered to the drumhead and has been emptied out of the ear, the head is returned to the midline; the nystagmus, with a quick component toward the left (if the water is delivered to the right ear), will be apparent shortly thereafter. If there is a latent period of over 30 seconds, it perhaps indicates supratentorial disease, but the reason for this remains obscure.

A diminished or absent postcaloric response usually indicates a peripheral or intermediate (nerve trunk) lesion. Examples of this are Ménière's disease, streptomycin intoxication (bilateral response), or vestibular neuronitis. Eighth nerve tumor will produce the same alteration. Hallpike has described the phenomenon of directional preponderance.[4] This observer performs the caloric test using water at 30° C and

44° C on each ear. He feels that a tendency for nystagmus to be prolonged to the left by a cold stimulus delivered to the right ear and by a hot stimulus applied to the left (directional preponderance to the left), indicates localization to the posterior portion of the left temporal lobe. Riesco, however, is not convinced of the localizing value of directional preponderance. Hot and cold disassociation in the postcaloric response unquestionably exists, but its exact significance remains unknown. Riesco observed that failure of the static labyrinth to respond to cold water, in cases of streptomycin intoxication, held a promising prognosis for return of function if the hot water reaction was not ablated.

Hyperexcitability to cold stimulus, in the form of a prolonged erratic postcaloric response, is said to be indicative of disease of the fastigial nucleus in the roof of the fourth ventricle of the opposite side. The fastigial nucleus exerts, through the hook bundle, an inhibitory effect upon the vestibular nuclei of the same side. Destruction of the fastigial nucleus of the left would, therefore, result in hyperexcitability of the right static labyrinth on caloric testing. Other observers feel that hyperexcitability may be demonstrated in the very earliest phase of Ménière's disease.

Another abnormal postcaloric response is that of perversion of nystagmus. This is evidenced by the appearance of a vertical nystagmus after stimulation of the horizontal canal. A lesion in the floor of the fourth ventricle, which destroys the lower vestibular nuclei (Deiters, Schwalbe, and Roller) and leaves the superior nucleus of Bechterew undisturbed, could be responsible for such an abnormal postcaloric response. Since the second neurons from the lateral and medial nuclei ascend only as far as the sixth nucleus, a lesion that destroyed these nuclei would erase the horizontal nystagmus after stimulation of the horizontal canal. If the stimulus were strong enough, however, and ice water would provide a sufficiently strong stimulus, the second neuron would carry the information from the nucleus of Bechterew to the fourth and third nuclei, and a vertical nystagmus would be apparent.

ELECTRONYSTAGMOGRAPHY

At this time, the technique by which one may investigate the vestibulocerebellar complex by electronystagmography is in the process of transference from the experimental laboratory to the clinician's office. The method entails electrical measurement and paper recording of potentials developed by eye movements of spontaneous, positional, or calorically evoked nystagmus. Leads are taken from the skin just lateral to the outer canthus of each eye and the indifferent electrode is placed in the midline at the root of the nose. Thus a graphic recording of the characteristics of the nystagmus may be obtained.

Whether or not the actual timing of the duration of the postcaloric response by electronystagmography is more accurate than that obtained by the observer's eye and stop-clock technique is debatable, but other factors such as frequency, intensity, and maximum speed of the slow component may be evaluated. These are used as criteria for assessing the activity of one labyrinth as compared with its fellow. Furthermore, such a graphic recording is of value in the event of litigation.

REFERENCES

1. Cawthorne, T.: Positional nystagmus. Ann. Otol., 63:481–490, 1954.
2. Crosby, E. C.: Nystagmus as a sign of central nervous system involvement. Ann. Otol., 62: 1117, 1953.
3. Crosby, E. C., Humphrey, T., and Lauer, E. W.: Correlative Anatomy of the Nervous System. New York, Macmillan, 1962, pp. 149–158.
4. Hallpike, C. S.: The caloric tests. J. Laryng. Otol., 70:15–28, 1956.
5. Heath, S. R.: Rail-walking performance as related to mental age and etiological type among the mentally retarded. Amer. J. Psychol., 55:240–247.
6. Nylen, C. O.: The posture test. Acta Otolaryng., 109:suppl.: 125–130, 1953.
7. Scala, N. P., and Spiegel, E. A.: The mechanism of optokinetic nystagmus. Trans. Amer. Acad. Ophthal. Otolaryng., 43:277–299, 1938.
8. Smith, J. L., and Cogan, D. G.: Optokinetic nystagmus: A test for parietal lobe lesions. Amer. J. Ophthal., 48:187–193, 1959.
9. Spiegel, E. A., and Sommer, I.: Neurology of the Eye, Ear, Nose and Throat. New York, Grune & Stratton, 1944.

16

HEARING TESTS IN OTONEUROLOGICAL DIAGNOSIS

Time-honored tests of hearing such as the whispered voice, tuning forks, and the watch tick are inherently too variable in stimulus control for precise auditory measurement. Precision in the measurement of hearing did not become an eventuality until the introduction of the pure tone vacuum tube audiometer in 1922. It was not until after the Beasley study of 1935–1936 that a standard for normal hearing was developed in the United States.

The outbreak of World War II provided the impetus for a vast amount of research in the field of communications. In general, two types of test emerged from the research. Tests were developed to determine quantitatively the auditory threshold for speech, and to evaluate how clearly speech is understood after hearing loss has been overcome, either through raising the voice or through amplification. In 1948 the classic study of Dix, Hallpike, and Hood was published in England.[2] This study demonstrated the use of the alternate binaural loudness balance test in the differential diagnosis of cochlear and retrocochlear lesions. Briefly, they demonstrated that cochlear hair cell deafness, as in Ménière's disease, was characterized by marked recruitment in contrast to a lack of recruitment in retrocochlear deafness as demonstrated in verified cases of acoustic tumor.

About this same time, Luscher and Zwislocki, in Europe, reported the difference limen (DL) of intensity test as a method to differentiate cochlear from other types of deafness.[21] A difference limen is the increment in a stimulus that is just noticed in a specified fraction of trials. The relative difference limen is the ratio of the difference limen to the absolute magnitude of the stimulus to which is is related. Patients with cochlear deafness were found to recognize smaller changes in the intensity of pure tones at a 40-db sensation level than either normal hearers or patients with either conductive or eighth nerve deafness did at 40-db sensation levels. In this context, sensation level is the pressure level of the sound in decibels above its threshold of audibility for the individual observer.[10]

In the early part of the fifties, Bocca, in Italy, was the first to demonstrate the efficacy of distorted speech tests as adjuncts in the diagnosis of temporal lobe lesions.[1] Matzker, Jerger, and others were quick to follow with other tests designed to provide information at the various levels of the auditory system.[12a, 21a] About this same time, Carhart proposed the tone decay test as a method to assess retrocochlear lesions.[1c] Finally, Jerger in 1960 proposed the four types of Békésy tracings as differential diagnostic indices associated with cochlear, retrocochlear, and conductive deafness.[10a]

In the light of the preceding background review, a description of audiological tests and their contribution to the diagnosis of lesions affecting the auditory system is presented. Rather than just central tests alone, tests for all levels of the auditory system are discussed in order to provide a better understanding for test interpretations.

Pathological conditions affecting the au-

C. P. GOETZINGER

ditory mechanism may be classified as follows: lesions of the outer and middle ear, of the inner ear or cochlea, of the eighth nerve from the spiral ganglion up to and including the cochlear nucleus, and central lesions including the cortex.

OUTER AND MIDDLE EAR DISEASE

Disorders of the outer ear or external auditory canal, such as blockage of the orifice or a reduction in its size due to foreign bodies, impacted wax, strictures from accident, or congenital atresia of the external canal as in the Treacher Collins syndrome, induce a conductive hearing loss of greater or lesser degree depending upon the extent of closure. For example, ear wax rarely causes a socially handicapping hearing impairment unless it is impacted. Strictures of the ear canal resulting from burns and other injuries will induce hearing loss in accordance with the amount of blockage. However, even if only a small

opening remains, sound is transmitted, and hearing is socially adequate. In the case in which middle ear ossicles are deformed and nonfunctional, the hearing loss is usually 50 to 70 db by air conduction throughout the frequency range. Bone conduction is normal or near normal, thereby indicating a conductive deafness.

It should be noted that conductive deafness of the outer and middle ear, regardless of its degree, does not preclude the development of language. In short, other things being equal, such as normal intelligence, a child with a congenital atresia will eventually develop speech and language, although it may be greatly limited. Clinical observations of such children indicate that if early habilitation measures are not taken, their language, as indirectly measured by vocabulary tests and verbal tests of intelligence, shows about a 2½- to 3-year retardation at age 7 years despite normal intelligence as measured by performance intelligence quotient tests.

Disorders that are primarily of middle ear

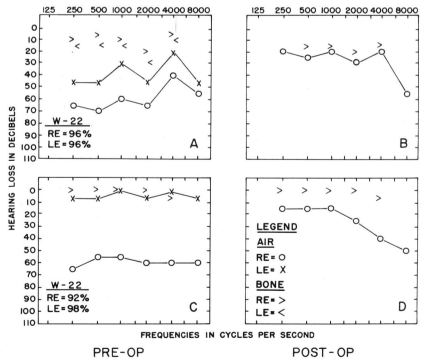

PRE-OP   POST-OP

FIGURE 16--1 *A* and *B*. Preoperative and postoperative audiograms of the right ear for a patient with otosclerosis. After stapedectomy, the hearing in the right ear is now within normal limits. *C* and *D*. Preoperative and postoperative audiograms of a patient with congenital incudostapedial discontinuity of the right ear. The stapes was mobile. A House wire prosthesis was used to articulate the incus with the stapes.

origin are otitis media, middle ear effusion, clinical otosclerosis, cholesteotoma, and glomus jugulare. The hearing losses by air conduction range over the same magnitude as those previously discussed in connection with the external canal, with the exception that the incidence of socially handicapping loss is substantially higher. The primary audiological characteristics of conductive deafness, whether as a result of external or of middle ear lesions, are: hearing loss by air conduction with normal or near normal bone conduction, hearing loss by air conduction that does not exceed about 70 db, good to excellent auditory discrimination for speech either by air or bone conduction, a lack of tone decay, absence of recruitment, and low small increment sensorineural index (SISI) scores.

Operative treatment is highly successful in alleviating deafness due to outer and middle ear disease. Procedures that are in extensive use are tympanoplasty for reconstruction of the middle ear, stapedectomy for otosclerosis, and myringotomy for drainage of the middle ear. Figure 16–1 shows the preoperative and postoperative audiograms of two patients with conductive hearing loss. Note the near normal bone conduction and the excellent auditory discrimination.

The small increment sensorineural index is determined by having the patient identify 1-db increments in sound superimposed upon a discrete continuous tone presented 20 db above threshold.[13] The increments are spaced five seconds apart with 20 constituting a test run. The test frequencies are usually 500–1000–2000–4000 Hz. The score at each test frequency is the percentage of 1-db increments correctly heard by the subject. Normal-hearing persons, as well as those with conductive impairment (outer or middle ear deafness or both) and those with retrocochlear deafness, are found to have small increment sensorineural index scores that range usually between 0 and 20 per cent. In short, very few of the increments are heard. Conversely, scores of 65 per cent and higher are found in cochlear deafness.

INNER EAR DEAFNESS

Hearing losses of cochlear etiology range from slight to total deafness. They may be hereditary, or a result of disease or trauma. Many children in schools for the deaf are afflicted with severe bilateral cochlear deafness. Schiebe's type of deafness, which involves the saccule and the cochlea, accounts for about 70 per cent of the hereditarily deaf children in schools for the deaf. Hearing loss in Schiebe's deafness is usually severe to extreme (70 to 90 db = severe; 90 db plus = extreme). Nevertheless, locomotor ability, as in walking the Heath rails, is often normal, as are the caloric test results. The explanation is that the utricle and the semicircular canals, which control the sense of balance, are not infrequently normal in Schiebe's deafness, particularly in cases with less than a 90-db hearing loss.[26] Hearing impairment stemming from insults to the cochlea may be induced by Ménière's disease, maternal rubella, viral labyrinthitis, measles, mumps, noise exposure, acoustic trauma, and the like.

In contrast to outer and middle ear conductive hearing loss, the audiological manifestations of inner ear impairment are as follows: (1) the threshold of bone conduction is superimposed on air conduction or there is an absence of bone conduction in extreme deafness; (2) auditory discrimination is frequently reduced or may be absent in extreme congenital deafness; (3) recruitment is complete or incomplete; (4) small increment sensorineural index scores are high, 65 to 100 per cent; and (5) Békésy tracings are Type II. However, in common with outer and middle ear conductive deafness, there is an absence of severe tone decay. Audiograms A and B of Figure 16–2 compare unilateral conductive deafness with unilateral cochlear deafness. Audiograms C and D illustrate complete and incomplete recruitment, respectively, in high-tone deafness. In addition, audiograms A and B of Figure 16–3 contrast low and high SISI scores.

EIGHTH NERVE DEAFNESS

During the last 15 years there have been many reports concerned with the contribution of the audiological tests to the diagnosis of acoustic tumors. The cardinal audiological signs of lesions of the eighth nerve are progressive unilateral perceptive

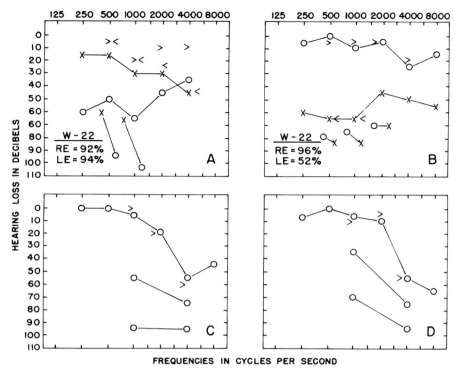

FIGURE 16–2 *A* and *B*. Audiograms comparing a unilateral middle ear conductive hearing loss with a unilateral cochlear deafness due to Ménière's disease. Auditory discrimination is normal (94 per cent) in the conductively deafened ear and there is an absence of recruitment at 500 and 1000 Hz by the alternate binaural loudness balance test (ABLB). Conversely, auditory discrimination is poor (52 per cent) in the ear deafened by Ménière's disease, and there is severe recruitment at 500, 1000, and 2000 Hz by ABLB. *C* and *D*. Audiograms illustrating complete and incomplete recruitment, respectively, by MLB. The left ears of these patients were were similar to the right ears and therefore, their audiograms are not shown. In each case the diagnosis was noise-induced hearing loss.

hearing loss, abnormally poor auditory discrimination, lack of recruitment by the balance tests, rapid and severe tonal decay by the Carhart test, Type III or IV Békésy tracings, and low small increment sensori-neural index.

Tumors of the eighth nerve are, in general, unilateral. Loss of hearing sensitivity is usually the initial auditory sign. At times, however, a severe decrease in auditory discrimination has been observed to precede the pure tone deficit.[5] The audiological tests per se cannot be used as the sole index for diagnosis. They must be considered in conjunction with the otoneurological, radiological, and other findings.

The tone decay test is a measure of eighth nerve function. The patient is presented with a steady pure tone that is 5 db above, or louder than, his threshold. The purpose of the test is to determine whether

he is able to hear the tone for a full minute. If the tone is heard for the full minute, the test is terminated at that frequency and another tone is selected for evaluation. However, if the tone fades away, the intensity is raised by 5 db so that it is again heard, and timing continues in order to ascertain whether the tone can be perceived at this new level for a full minute. The tone is raised as indicated until it is heard for a full minute or until the limits of the hearing loss dial on the audiometer have been reached.

Scoring consists of the amount of tone decay in decibels and the rapidity of decay. In general, 15 db of decay is regarded as being within normal limits. Tone decay in excess of 15 db is usually regarded as significant. However, factors such as age, degree of loss, rapidity of decay, and the test frequency at which there is decay should be taken into consideration in diagnosis. For example, tumors of the eighth nerve frequently are characterized by exceedingly rapid decay, which may reach the limits of the audiometer within a minute even though there is only slight hearing loss. In addition, significant decay is usually found at all or several frequencies. By contrast, in presbycusis, extensive but very slow tone decay (40 db in five minutes) may occur at 4000 Hz, but at no other frequency. In general, it might be said that the amount of tone decay is an index of the extent of eighth nerve dysfunction (Fig. 16–3).

Békésy tracings also contribute to the differential diagnostic battery of tests in audiology. The Békésy audiometer is an automatic instrument by which an individual is able to trace his threshold of hearing for either interrupted or continuous tones over the frequency range of 100 to 10,000 Hz. A control switch in the hands of the patient regulates a motor-driven attenuator through which he is able to keep the tonal stimuli varying above and below his threshold of hearing. The patient is instructed to press the switch until the sound disappears, and to release the switch to bring the sound back again. He continues to press and release the switch so that he alternately does and does not hear the tone. The attenuator or hearing-loss dial is geared to a vertically moving pen that leaves an up and down tracing, over time, on an audiogram chart that is fixed to a table moving horizontally and synchronized to the continuously variable oscillator of the audiometer.

Jerger, after extensive testing of diseased ears with Békésy interrupted and continuous sweep frequency tones, identified the four basic patterns as shown in Figure 16–4. The Type I Békésy tracing,

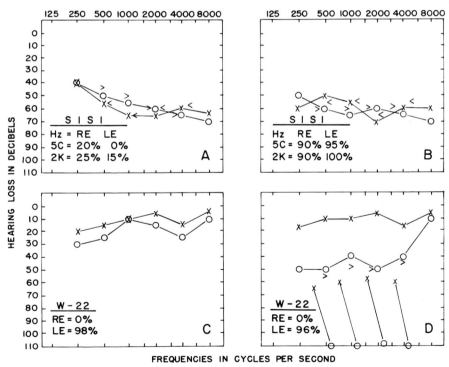

FIGURE 16–3 *A* and *B*. Audiograms illustrating the application of the SISI test in two patients with bilaterally symmetrical hearing losses, not appropriate for the ABLB and MLB tests. Patient A was a presbyacusic and patient B was an adolescent with congenital hearing loss. *C* and *D*. Audiograms of a patient with a verified acoustic tumor, taken about a month apart. Audiogram C demonstrates that a profound auditory discrimination deficit can precede hearing loss. This patient, one month later, had complete and rapid tone decay, a Type III Békésy tracing, and no recruitment by ABLB.

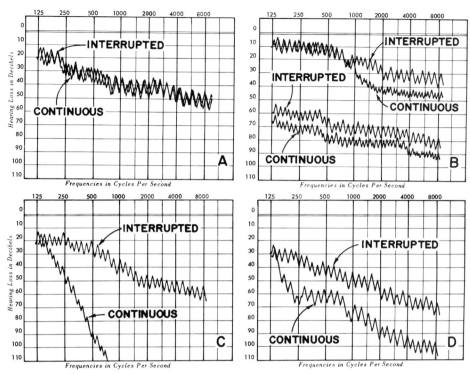

FIGURE 16–4 Békésy tracings showing the four types of pattern. Type I is associated with normal hearing and conductive deafness, Type II with cochlear hearing impairment, Type III and Type IV with eighth nerve lesions.

typical of normal persons and those with conductive deafness, is characterized by the superimposition of the continuous on the interrupted threshold. The Type II Békésy tracing, most often obtained in inner ear or cochlear deafness, is identified either by the superimposition of the interrupted and continuous tracings up to about 1000 Hz with a slight separation occurring above that frequency, or by a separation of less than 20 db for all frequencies. In the Type III pattern, the continuous tracing breaks away immediately from the interrupted tracing and fades rapidly until the limits of the equipment are reached. Type III is characteristic of eighth nerve lesions. Finally, the Type IV Békésy tracing is indicated by substantial separation (more than 20 db) between the tracings. The Type IV tracing is found primarily in retrocochlear lesions. Many cases of acoustic tumor present the Type IV pattern.

Although eighth nerve lesions are fre- quently associated with acoustic tumors, nevertheless, it must be emphasized that any type of lesion of the eighth nerve can produce the same audiological picture. The caloric test results are particularly definitive in this respect. To be more explicit, the indications of an acoustic tumor are strengthened when an absence of response to the caloric test accompanies the audiological signs.

CENTRAL LESIONS

In recent years, tests to differentiate central nervous system dysfunction have been developed. Routine pure tone and speech tests are inadequate for the assessment of the integrity of the central pathways and cortex. Bocca and his associates have devised sensitized speech tests that afford promise.[1a] Tests of this nature may be grouped under three distinct classifications, namely, monaural, binaural, and dichotic (competing message) tests.

Monaural Tests

These tests usually consist of words of reduced redundancy as, for example, filtered, accelerated, slow, interrupted, and distorted speech. Unless otherwise noted, central tests are discussed with reference to patients who have normal auditory sensitivity. Hence, performance as such is uncontaminated with hearing loss.

One version of a filtered speech test involves the presentation of standard phonetically balanced words through a low pass filter condition. Such distorted speech causes poorer auditory discrimination for normal listeners, but the reduction is the same for each ear. When the words are presented to individuals with temporal lobe lesions, these patients frequently manifest greater than normal reduction in auditory discrimination in the ear contralateral to the lesion. Jerger's study showed that patients with clinical signs of lesions in the "posterolateral regions of the brain stem either at or above cranial VIII," and those who "had lesions involving the superior temporal convolution, with possible involvement of the area known as Heschl's gyrus," had reduced auditory discrimination for phonetically balanced words in the ear contralateral to the site of the lesion as compared to the homolateral ear.[12a]

Binaural Tests

In one of these tests monosyllabic phonetically balanced words are presented simultaneously to the two ears while a white noise 20 db above speech level is alternated between ears. A white noise is a sound whose frequency spectrum is continuous (no gaps or frequencies missing in the included frequency range) and uniform (all frequencies occurring with the same average intensity). A white noise is not necessarily the same as random noise.[4] With these tests, poor scores are obtained with either the one or the other ear in monaural listening. Under binaural listening, subjects with normal hearing obtain very high or nearly perfect scores. However, individuals with central nervous system lesions show poorer scores than normal subjects. This test has had only limited use.

Dichotic or Competing Message Tests

The most common attribute of all tests of this type is that each ear receives a different message. In addition, speech reaches the ears simultaneously. One version of this type of test is the staggered spondaic word test of Katz.[14, 15] The test requires that the patient attend to the information in one ear, in both ears simultaneously, and finally in the other ear. For example, the right and left ears might receive respectively, "playground" and "batboy," with "play" being heard alone in the right ear (noncompeting right ear condition), "ground" and "bat" simultaneously ("ground" to the right ear and "bat" to the left ear, competing right and left ear conditions) and finally, "boy" to the left ear (left ear noncompeting condition). The test therefore includes a monaural monosyllabic auditory discrimination test for each ear plus a monosyllabic competing message condition. Test results are considered in terms of the number of errors in the noncompeting and competing conditions. A standard phonetically balanced word test is also administered to each ear, and scores from this test are taken into consideration in the scoring of the staggered spondaic word test.

This particular test is perhaps being utilized more widely than many of the other central tests and, as a consequence, is likely to provide some informative patterns relative to the site of the lesion in central disorders of the auditory mechanism. Patients with temporal lobe lesions have been found to give poorer scores in the competing message condition in the ear contralateral to the injury.

In addition to the speech tests as discussed, there have been a number of attempts to develop localization tests using pure tones. At the present time, however, there is no one method that is used widely in a number of clinics.

Finally, evoked response audiometry has reached a point in development at which it is now feasible as a clinical tool. The method essentially involves the sampling of cortical potentials evoked by sound. The potentials are picked up by an averaging computer, summed, and stored, while the random background noise is canceled out. Evoked response audiometry is of particular value in assessing the hearing sensitivity of infants and of uncooperative children and adults.

1. Bocca, E.: Clinical aspects of cortical deafness. (Special issue — International Conference on Audiology, St. Louis, Mo., U.S.A.) Laryngoscope, 68:301–309, 1958.

1a. Bocca, E., and Calearo, C.: Central hearing processes. In Jerger, J., ed.: Modern Developments in Audiology. New York and London, Academic Press, 1963.

1b. Bordley, J. E., Hardy, W. G., and Richter, C. P.: Audiometry with the use of galvanic skin resistance response: A preliminary report. Johns Hopkins Hosp. Bull., 82:569, 1948.

1c. Carhart, R.: Clinical determination of abnormal auditory adaptation. Arch. Otol., 65:32–39, 1957.

2. Dix, M. R., Hallpike, C. S., and Hood, J. D.: Observations upon the loudness recruitment phenomenon with especial reference to the differential diagnosis of disorders of the internal ear and eighth nerve. Proc. Roy. Soc. Med., 41:516–525, 1948.

3. Fields, W. S., and Alford, B. R.: Neurological Aspects of auditory and vestibular disorders. Springfield, Ill., Charles C Thomas, 1964.

4. Glorig, A.: Audiometry: Principles and Practices. Baltimore, Williams & Wilkins Co., 1965.

5. Goetzinger, C. P., and Angell, S. N.: Audiological assessment in acoustic tumors and cortical lesions. Eye Ear Nose Throat Monthly, 44:39–49, 1965.

6. Goetzinger, C. P., and Rousey, C. L.: Hearing problems in later life. Med. Times, 87:771–780, 1959.

7. Goetzinger, C. P., Dirks, D. D., and Baer, C. J.: Auditory discrimination and visual perception in good and poor readers. Ann. Otol. 69:121–137, 1960.

8. Goetzinger, C. P., Proud, G. O., Dirks, D. D., and Embrey, J.: A study of hearing in advanced age. Arch. Otolaryngology, 73:662–674, 1961.

9. Goldstein, R., Goodman, A. C., and King, R. B.: Hearing and speech in infantile hemiplegia before and after hemespherectomy. Neurology, 6:869–875, 1956.

10. Hirsh, I.: The Measurement of Hearing. New York, McGraw-Hill Book Co., 1952.

10a. Jerger, J.: Békésy audiometry in analysis of auditory disorders. J. Speech Hearing Res., 3:275–287, 1960.

11. Jerger, J.: Hearing tests in otologic diagnosis. A.S.H.A., 4:139–145, 1962.

12. Jerger, J.: Modern Developments in Audiology. New York and London, Academic Press, 1963.

12a. Jerger, J.: Auditory tests for disorders of the central auditory mechanism. In Fields, W. S., and Alford, B. R., eds.: Neurological Aspects of Auditory and Vestibular Disorders. Springfield, Ill., Charles C Thomas, 1964.

13. Jerger, J., Shedd, J., and Harford, E.: On the detection of extremely small changes in sound intensity. Arch. Otolaryng., 69:200–211, 1959.

14. Katz, J.: The use of staggered spondaic words for assessing the integrity of the central auditory nervous system. J. Auditory Research, 2:327–337, 1962.

15. Katz, J.: A staggered spondaic word test for detecting central auditory lesions. Ann. Otol., 72:908–917, 1963.

16. Katz, J.: The SSW Test: An interim report. J. Speech Hearing Dis., 33:132–146, 1968.

17. Kimura, D.: Some effects of temporal lobe damage on auditory perception. Canad. J. Psychol., 15:156–165, 1961.

18. Kimura, D.: Cerebral dominance and the perception of verbal stimuli. Canad. J. Psychology, 15:166–171, 1961.

19. Kimura, D.: A note on cerebral dominance in hearing. Acta Otolaryng., 56:617–618, 1963.

20. Kimura, D.: Speech lateralization in young children as determined by an auditory test. J. Comp. Physiol. Psychol., 56:899–902, 1963.

21. Luscher, E., and Zwislocki, J.: A simple method for indirect monaural determination of the recruitment phenomenon (difference limen in intensity in different types of deafness). Acta Otolaryng., Suppl. 78, 156–168, 1949.

21a. Matzker, J.: Two new methods for the assessment of central auditory function in cases of brain damage. Ann. Otol., 68:1185–1197, 1959.

22. Newby, H. A.: Audiology. New York, Appleton-Century-Crofts, 1964.

23. O'Neill, J., and Oyer, H.: Applied Audiometry. New York and London, Dodd, Mead & Co., 1966.

24. Shambaugh, G. E.: Surgery of the Ear. 2nd Ed. Philadelphia and London, W. B. Saunders Co., 1967.

25. Watson, L. A., and Tolan, T.: Hearing Tests and Hearing Instruments. Baltimore, Md., Williams & Wilkins Co., 1949.

26. Whetnall, E., and Fry, D. B.: The Deaf Child. London, William Heinemann Medical Books Ltd., 1964.

17

PSYCHOLOGICAL TESTING IN NEUROLOGICAL DIAGNOSIS

CONCEPTUALIZATION OF THE PROBLEM

While the brain has long been recognized as the organ of behavior, subserving intelligence, cognition, and emotional responses, specific attempts to elucidate brain-behavior relationships by formal psychological testing are relatively recent. Until recently these efforts had not made great contributions, principally because so many factors over and beyond recognized brain damage are significant determinants of psychological status. Consequently it has been difficult to devise an approach for psychological evaluation that would have specific significance with regard to the condition of the human brain. The problems in this area have related principally to the complexity of human behavior on the one hand and the complexity of the pathological conditions that involve the human brain on the other hand. Finally, procedural requirements in correlating brain and behavioral findings constitute another problem.

The Behavioral Model

Most investigation in this area has tended to oversimplify the behavioral model. Many inquiries have used only a single test for evaluation of the possible consequences of brain lesions, or at most a very limited number of psychological tests. Thus, sampling of the complex ability structures of human beings has often been severely restricted. If, indeed, the brain is the organ of adaptive behavior, such limited sampling of behavior could scarcely be sufficient to represent the behavioral aspect of brain functions. In many instances this tendency toward oversimplification has resulted from the investigator's desire to identify a score or index that would help to distinguish between subjects with and without brain damage.[9] This approach has not been especially helpful in elucidating the basic aspects of brain-behavior relationships. It is clear that the fundamental frame of reference within which the effects of brain lesions should be studied is related to a comprehensive description of human ability structure. The field of psychology does not yet have a clear grasp of this entity (total human ability structure) or its parts (discrete abilities). As a result it is difficult to design an adequate battery of psychological tests for describing human ability structure as it relates to the condition of the brain. Further, it is difficult to understand particular deficits within the frame of reference of overall ability. Thus, the significance of particular types of deficit is not at present subject to full understanding.

In spite of these problems, it is clear at present that a broad battery of psychological tests is necessary if we are to make an even partially adequate assessment of individual human abilities subserved by the cerebral hemispheres. It would appear that such a battery of tests should measure simple sensory-perceptual functions (uti-

R. M. REITAN

lizing at least the sensory modalities of vision, hearing, and touch) as well as the speed and strength of motor functions. Further, more complex tests of psycho-motor functions should also be included, measuring the ability of the subject to organize and integrate sensory information with the motor output necessary to solve relatively complex problems. The tests obviously must assess language and communication skills because of the extent to which these functions are subserved by the brain. Evidence has also indicated that visuospatial, manipulatory, and perform-ance abilities of various kinds are also closely related to the integrity of the cerebral hemispheres. Finally, the areas of abstraction, analytical reasoning, and concept formation represent fundamental abilities, important not only as indicators of brain function but also in adapting to problems of everyday living.

Evaluation of Brain Disorders

As in any area of developing knowledge, the original concepts and criteria prove inadequate with respect to the knowledge eventually needed. A great majority of the investigations into the effects of brain-behavior relationships have concerned themselves only with the effects of "brain damage" on selected abilities, without any further attempt to specify the nature of the damage. While it is clear that difficult problems are inherent in the attempt to describe in detail the precise condition of any living individual's brain, available diagnostic methods in the neurological sciences permit good approximations in many instances of the areas of principal damage, the type of lesion present, the age at which the lesion was sustained, and the length of time since the lesion was sus-tained. Despite the basic difficulty that brain lesions in human beings occur as "accidents of nature," a good deal of in-formation is potentially available to relate them to differential aspects of psycholog-ical deficits. At first glance it would appear that the critical information could routinely be obtained from autopsy findings and that psychological measurements could be related to this information. In practice this procedure becomes difficult because of the frequency with which changes in the con-dition of the brain have intervened be-tween the last valid psychological examina-tion and the time of the patient's death. During this interval the lesion, provided that it has been the cause of death, has certainly advanced, and it is difficult to correlate precisely the condition of the brain at the time of examination with the results of psychological testing.

Among the major requirements for addi-tional progress in understanding the effects of brain lesions on behavior are the mean-ingful and rational subdivision of the gross concept of "brain damage" and the relation of the subdivisions to their behavioral correlates. It is apparent that the con-ceptual approach in this area must address itself to the broad range of disorders in-volving the brain on the one hand, and on the other, to the rich and varied behavioral repertoire of human beings that may be altered by brain disease or damage.

APPROACHES TO EVALUATING BRAIN-BEHAVIOR RELATIONSHIPS

Three major procedural requirements should be observed in evaluating brain-behavior relationships in human beings: (1) The range of behavioral functions measured should be sufficiently broad to sample the major areas of human ability and thus to permit a psychologically mean-ingful expression of the effects of brain lesions. (2) The battery of psychological tests should be composed of measures that controlled investigations have previously indicated are valid with respect to the effects of cerebral lesions. This require-ment has the advantage of providing data of known relevance with regard to brain functions rather than measurements that may be tangentially related to the imme-diate biological condition of the brain. (3) The battery of psychological tests should be so composed that the integrated and complementary use of various principles of inference of psychological deficit be-comes possible. Most prior investigations of human brain-behavior relationships have exploited only a single inferential approach and thus have frequently failed to reflect the variety of ways in which the psychological effects of brain damage may be expressed in individual subjects. Essentially, the methodological deficiency in many investigations has been that of presuming that the behavioral effects of brain lesions, variable as they are, will produce a standard type of deficit. As already mentioned, this approach has underestimated the complexity of the pathology of the human brain. Because the methodological approaches to brain-behavior relationships reflect essentially the conceptual models involved, a brief description of these approaches is given.

Level of Performance

The level of performance (or how well a subject does) on one or more psychological tests, as compared with some type of normative standard, has frequently been used to characterize the nature and degree of deficit resulting from cerebral damage. In fact, most of the research reports in the literature have been oriented specifically toward identifying deficiencies in level of performance. Thus, this approach has dominated the literature in this area, and a considerable number of studies have appeared in which striking and highly significant intergroup mean differences between patients with and without cerebral damage have been reported.[1, 3, 5, 8] It is perfectly clear that cerebral damage reduces many abilities, but the generalizations derived from group comparisons are difficult to apply in evaluating an individual subject. Three factors are principally responsible for this difficulty: (1) A great number of variables other than brain damage also have a clear and unequivocal effect on level of psychological performance (e.g., genetic variables, cultural deprivation, educational disadvantages, psychotic and other emotional conditions, normal aging, and many others that overlap only partially if at all with what is usually meant by cerebral damage). It is entirely possible that a person who performs poorly on any particular psychological test may do so for a number of reasons other than brain damage. (2) Persons who sustain cerebral lesions have varying premorbid ability levels. A person of very superior initial ability, for example, may have sustained a pronounced psychological deficit but still be in the average range for persons without evidence of cerebral damage. This deficit may be of great significance for the individual involved, even though his actual ability still continues to be at the average level with respect to normative data. (3) Psychological deficits resulting from cerebral damage, while frequently having long-term residual consequences, are not necessarily constant in individual subjects but may show striking changes in time. Such changes may be in the direction of improvement or in the direction of deterioration of abilities, depending upon the nature of the underlying brain lesion. Conditions of disease that are progressive may lead to corresponding progressive deterioration of psychological functions. Conversely, insults to the brain may cause deficits, but these deficiencies frequently show improvement in time as the brain has an opportunity to reorganize itself in a biological sense. Because of differing criteria with respect to diagnostic conclusions, the psychological improvement in some instances may occur even though no change in the neurological diagnosis per se is indicated. For example, the author recently examined a 32-year-old woman who had suffered a dissecting aneurysm of the left internal carotid artery. Angiography shortly after the incident demonstrated complete occlusion of the artery. Psychological testing at this time indicated very poor levels of performance on many tests, illustrated by the fact that the patient had a verbal IQ of 52 and a performance IQ of 80. Three months later, even though angiograms still showed complete occlusion of the vessel (but also evidence of developing collateral circulation), the patient's verbal and performance IQ values were 105 and 110, respectively. The patient had not been given any formal rehabilitation program during the three-month interval and, in all probability, the dramatic improvement was mainly a reflection of biological recovery and improvement of brain function. It is apparent that reference to psychological test scores for individual subjects, in terms of level of performance alone, is not an adequate basis for relating the findings to known variables regarding the condition of the brain. Realization of this has led some investigators to devise other approaches to the question of brain-behavior relationships in human beings.

Specific or Pathognomonic Signs of Cerebral Damage

Discrete deficiencies in performance that supposedly specifically indicate the presence of a brain lesion have been described in the literature.[2,9] These specific deficits may be thought of in the behavioral area much as positive signs are considered in the neurological area. Among these manifestations of psychological deficit can be included organic language losses that fall in the category of aphasia as well as specific difficulties in copying simple spatial configurations. Further, specific perceptual disorders, such as impairment of tactile finger localization or inability to perceive double simultaneous sensory stimulation, may also be considered in this category.

The same types of difficulties accompany the attempt to use neurological signs as indications of cerebral damage in the behavioral areas as in other areas. First, many of the signs must be identified through gross observation by the examiner, a matter of clinical judgment. A certain degree of unreliability in identification of the signs is inevitable, and difficulties in communicating the definition of the sign also occur. A second difficulty relates to the specificity of the sign with respect to its diagnostic significance. While some signs may relate quite definitely to impairment of the condition of the cerebral hemispheres, considerable validational data is necessary for such interpretation. Obtaining such validational results, in turn, is hampered by the judgmental or permissive nature of identification and classification of the sign.[6] Nevertheless, the occurrence of certain signs of psychological deficit may very possibly prove of great value in supplementing the findings obtained on quantified and continuous scales of psychological measurement. The third difficulty in using the sign approach relates to the requirement that the sign have pathogno-monic significance—which leads to overly rigid definition. In order to avoid identification of the sign in patients without cerebral disease, it is apparent that it must be identified as present only when it occurs in a very pronounced and definite manner. Thus, if the deficit is sufficiently pronounced to be reliably classified as a positive "sign," additional instances will occur in which the "sign" is not perfectly obvious even though present. Under these conditions many persons with proved cerebral disease or damage, but who demonstrate the sign in a mild form, will fail to give sufficient evidence of the sign. This problem stems in part from the primitive nature of "signs" as a form of psychological scaling.

While it is apparent that this method has clear difficulties, it may be of definite value in instances in which specific signs occur in a pronounced form. In these instances the sign may serve as a definite positive finding, around which other psychological measurements may be oriented.

Comparisons Before and After Brain Damage

A few reports in the literature have made direct comparisons between psychological test results obtained before brain damage had been sustained or early in the course of progressive brain disease and results obtained after definite brain damage had occurred. At first sight this approach may seem to be the most obvious and direct method of validating indications of cerebral damage. However, the difficulties in applying this method are inherent in the reports in the literature.[6] First, few reports of this kind exist, indicating that very rarely do persons with cerebral lesions become available for examination who have had adequate evaluation before the injury or disease was present. Thus, in a practical sense, the method is not generally applicable. This in turn limits the range of neurological conditions of disease and damage that may be studied. The question of localization or the effects of lesions involving one area or another can scarcely be addressed using this approach. The advantages in comparing pre– and post–

brain damage findings are obvious, but the limited number of available subjects restricts the use of this method essentially to illustrations with individual patients. Sometimes anamnestic information or quasiquantitative data such as school grades have been used in this context, but the variable and uncontrolled conditions that determine school grades, parental reports, and other such information have made it difficult to establish firm relationships to the neurological disorders that are present.

Differential Score Comparisons

This approach presumes that certain types of psychological test data are relatively unaffected by cerebral damage, whereas other types of measurement are subject to severe impairment. The method usually calls for establishing a ratio between these two types of tests, with deviations in the direction of poorer performance on the especially sensitive tests reflecting cerebral damage. Since the work of Babcock in 1930, this concept has been utilized in tests devised by Shipley, Hunt, Wechsler, and Graham and Kendall. The various tests that have been proposed for comparison, and the resulting ratios, have, in many instances, yielded conflicting results, with earlier investigations not being substantiated by later findings. Initially, such conflicting results were explained by postulating sampling variability. Later evaluations, however, have suggested that the method was not adequate to reflect brain-behavior relationships. Brain lesions vary greatly from one individual to another and psychological deficits are correspondingly diversified. Therefore, it can hardly be expected that certain abilities would consistently be spared and others would consistently be impaired. As an illustration of these difficulties, the Block Design subtest of the Wechsler Scale (which requires the subject to duplicate visuospatial designs using colored blocks) had been suggested as one of the most sensitive tests for brain damage. This certainly is true for subjects with right hemisphere lesions; however, a group of patients with left hemisphere lesions performed better on this test than they did on most others.[5] It is apparent from current findings that differential scores may have value, but the method must be applied in terms of hypotheses concerning brain-behavior relationships rather than in a framework that presumes that a single simple relationship will hold in all patients with cerebral damage. An inferential method that has no flexibility in evaluating the many ways in which psychological deficit may be produced by cerebral lesions can hardly do justice to an adequate concept of the brain as the organ of adaptive behavior.[7] As illustrated in a later part of this chapter, differential levels of performance may contribute significantly to understanding brain-behavior relationships and the effects of brain lesions in individual patients.

Functional Efficiency of the Two Sides of the Body

This method is concerned with tests that reflect the efficiency of functioning of the two sides of the body, from both a motor and a sensory point of view. The method presumes that persons with cerebral damage will demonstrate particular types of deficiencies more frequently than will normal subjects and, further, that disparities may exist within the same individual on the two sides. An advantage of this method is that it is based on intraindividual comparisons and thus escapes many of the problems implicit in certain of the other methods of inference. For example, if a subject consistently performs poorly on the left side of the body as compared with his own performance on the right side, the findings would appear to have a biological reference point open to evaluation within the known structure of the nervous system. It is unlikely that such lateralized findings could be caused by lack of cooperation, emotional disturbance of the patient, or malingering. However, this conceptual model must contend with the many orthopedic, neuromuscular, spinal, and brain stem disorders that may cause lateralized functional deficiencies even though cerebral involvement is not necessarily present. For example, impairment of motor strength or finger tapping speed in one upper extremity as compared with the other could readily result from a recent joint sprain, muscle strain, or peripheral nerve injury. The approach in problems of this type is to develop tests that measure not only motor functions but also psychomotor performances, and tests that require sensory perception alone. If deficiencies occur on the same side of the body, across this broad range of measurements, the likelihood that the limiting lesion is at a cerebral level rather than lower in the nervous system or neuromuscular apparatus is greatly increased. The major disadvantage of this approach is that some subjects with diffuse or generalized cerebral lesions fail to show any clear differences on the two sides of the body. However, available data suggest that significant deviations of performance on the two sides frequently do occur in persons who are classified neurologically as having diffuse or generalized cerebral dysfunction.

CURRENT PSYCHOMETRIC MODELS OF BRAIN-BEHAVIOR RELATIONSHIPS

It is apparent that each of the foregoing approaches is valid to a degree in spite of its equally obvious limitations. The practical approach at the present time, therefore, is an attempt to exploit the major strengths of the various methods in a way that will enhance their complementary aspects and permit their conjoint application to research and clinical problems. The first step toward implementing such an aim is the selection and design of a battery of tests. The first full-time laboratory for the study of human brain-behavior relationships was developed by Halstead at the University of Chicago in 1935. Many of the principles just described were implicitly recognized in the tests that he described.[1] The field, nevertheless, is at present in a state of rapid development, and individual psychologists demonstrate broadly varying degrees of sophistication with relation to the nature of the problem. A battery of tests, including Halstead's neuropsychological test battery as well as additional measures, was composed to meet the requirements just described and has given evidence of excellent validity both from a research point of view and in terms of clinical evaluation of individual patients.[8]

The Wechsler scales of intelligence are the most widely used tests for individual (as opposed to group) evaluation of adult intelligence. The Wechsler-Bellevue Scale was superseded in recent years by the Wechsler Adult Intelligence Scale, but both sets of tests are similar in content, scoring, and interpretation. Six verbal subtests are included and five performance subtests. The verbal subtests include Information (a test of general information), Comprehension (understanding of statements that have a certain degree of complexity or social significance), Digit Span (repetition of series of digits, both forward and backward), Arithmetic (solution of arithmetical problems presented orally and in written form), Similarities (requiring knowledge of the common category or meaning of pairs of words), Vocabulary (definition of words). Among the performance tests the Picture Arrangement test requires the subject to arrange pictures in a proper sequence in order to tell a meaningful story (much like arranging comic strip squares that were put in improper sequence). The Picture Completion test requires the subject to identify missing parts of a series of pictures. Block Design requires the subject to duplicate spatial configurations shown on cards using a set of colored blocks. The Object Assembly test is similar to a jigsaw puzzle in which the subject is required to put parts together to complete a whole figure. The Digit Symbol test requires the subject to substitute symbols for numbers, using a code that is presented with the test. These particular tests constitute the Wechsler scales and presently provide the best basis for individual evaluation of general intelligence. Both a verbal and a performance IQ may be obtained, as well as a full-scale IQ. Previous results have shown that these measures are impaired to some extent in persons with cerebral damage as compared with comparable subjects without brain damage. Further, a good deal of evidence suggests that the verbal subtest scores tend to be lowered with lesions of the left cerebral hemisphere (especially in the presence of aphasic difficulties), whereas the performance subtest scores generally tend to be lowered with lesions of the right cerebral hemisphere. It should be noted, however, that the Wechsler scales were not developed specifically to assess the psychological consequences of cerebral lesions, and other tests have been developed that are considerably more sensitive to the presence of cerebral lesions.

Among these more sensitive tests are those developed by Halstead.[1] This battery, called the Halstead Neuropsychological Test Battery for Adults, consists of a number of tests that form the basis for the Halstead Impairment Index. Probably the most sensitive of these tests is the Category Test, and for this reason in addition to the fact that it illustrates a significant supplementation of the general IQ test, it is described in some detail. This test utilizes a projection apparatus for presenting 208 stimulus figures on a screen in front of the patient. After viewing each stimulus figure, the patient selects an answer by depressing any one of four levers labeled 1, 2, 3, and 4. A harsh buzzer sounds if the "wrong" lever is depressed; a pleasant bell sounds if the answer is correct. Before the test begins the subject is informed that the test is divided into several groups of items and that in each group a single principle underlies the correct response for each item. On the first item in a group, the subject can only guess at the right answer; but, as he progresses through the items, the bell or buzzer accompanying each response permits testing of one possible principle after another until the solution is found.

Since the Category Test employs the kind of mental processes that are among the most vulnerable to impairment by cerebral damage, an illustration (not based on the actual principles used in the test) is presented in Figure 17–1. Begin with column A. Remember that a single principle governs the "correct" answer for each item in the column. Answers should be given by selection of items 1, 2, 3, or 4

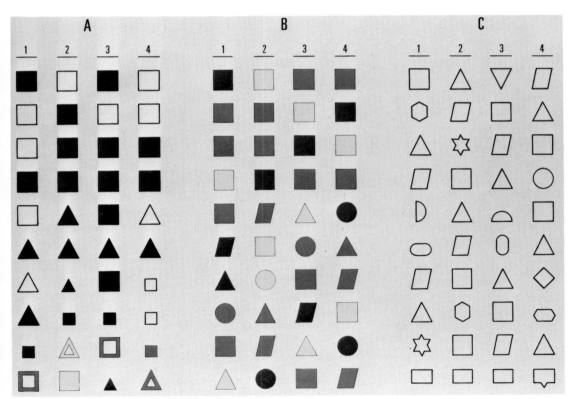

FIGURE 17–1 Illustration of the types of problem included in the Halstead Category Test (see text for explanation).

for each figure. It is possible to derive information from "wrong" as well as "right" answers, since a "wrong" answer provides evidence for eliminating irrelevant or incorrect principles. A "correct" answer is more helpful in a positive way, however, because it may offer substantiation of the correct principle. Beware of the possibility of "correct" answers given for the wrong reason, since these can be very costly in one's attempt to solve the problem.

Expose the correct answers for the first column, given at the end of this sentence, one at a time and only after having first responded to each item: 2, 1, 3, 4, 2, 4, 2, 3, 2, 2. Even though you may have gotten more than a "chance" number correct, the principle may not be entirely clear. This frequently happens in persons with normal brain function and, in its own right, serves to illustrate the relatively loose coupling that may exist between rational behavior and one's ability to explain verbally why the behavior was rational. The principle governing correct choices in the first column is quite simple—the correct answer for each item was the number of solid, as contrasted with outlined, figures.

The type of reasoning, abstraction, or concept-formation processes needed for this test are further illustrated in column B, but now the principle governing correct choices has changed. The answers for the 10 items in column B are: 1, 4, 3, 2, 4, 1, 1, 3, 4, 2. The principle again is simple, even though the diversity of the stimulus material may have confused the issue. One of the basic characteristics of this test is to identify those persons who can recognize and then ignore extraneous aspects of the stimulus material and thereby get to the essential nature of the problem. This type of intelligence, which Halstead has called one of the factors of *biological intelligence,* is related to, but rather different from, formal educational training or IQ and differentiates between persons with normal and those with damaged brains. The principle was to select the answer corresponding to the position of the *darkest* figure in each item. Column C presents a more difficult set of items. Again, one can only guess on the first item. This is unimportant, because the test results are principally a function of how much one can learn from

his mistakes as well as from his successes. The answers for the third column are as follows: 3, 1, 2, 4, 1, 3, 4, 2, 1, 4. The principle is to select the number of the figure in each item that did not have a horizontal base.

The Halstead Category Test requires the use of mental processes that are fundamental to practical intelligence. The subject must observe similarities and differences of the stimulus material, both within single items and between successive items. In other words, the first requirement is for careful observation and discerning description of the elements of the problem. Next, the subject must postulate a reasonable principle for organization of the similarities and differences in the stimulus material. He must be ready to reject or modify this principle according to new facts as they appear in successive items. Finally, he must face up to the consequences of his decisions as represented by the bell and buzzer for right and wrong answers. If his answers are wrong, he must have the adaptability, flexibility, and patience to go on searching for the right answer.

Technically, this test is described as measuring abstraction, concept formation, and organizational ability. When one considers the nature of the task, it is not surprising that the results on the Category Test are highly effective in showing the significant but subtle and sometimes elusive kinds of deficit that are frequently present in persons with cerebral lesions. Interestingly, the ability to perform well on this test also drops off with advancing age more rapidly than does performance on most psychological tests.

A number of additional tests included in Halstead's battery have been found to be highly valid in reflecting various types of psychological deficit caused by cerebral damage. These include performance measures of various types as well as tests that are principally perceptual in nature. The Seashore Rhythm Test, which requires the subject to perceive similarities and differences in pairs of rhythmic beats, reflects a significant difference between persons with and without brain lesions. Another perceptual test, the Speech-sounds Perception Test, requires the subject to respond to an auditory stimulus and match it with alternative printed speech sounds on his answer form. Measurement of finger tapping speed (Finger Oscillation Test) represents a basic aspect of fine motor function that is frequently impaired by brain damage. Comparison of the performance with each hand (right versus left) is even more helpful than measurement of speed by itself. Research with normal adults has shown that the tapping speed attained in a 10-second period with the preferred hand is customarily four to six taps more than that with the nonpreferred hand. Any significant deviation from this relationship may indicate impaired function of the cerebral hemisphere contralateral to the slow hand. Such findings, of course, should be considered within the context of other inferential methods as described earlier. A more complex type of task that involves problem-solving elements as well as integration of sensory and motor functions (and is therefore called a psychomotor test) is represented by the Halstead Tactual Performance Test. This test utilizes a form board and blocks, and the task requires the subject to place the blocks in their proper spaces as quickly as possible. Two aspects of the procedure used in this test make it especially valuable for assessing the effects of brain lesions. First, the subject is blindfolded without being permitted to see the board or blocks. He is thus required to forego visual cues that ordinarily guide this type of performance and to depend instead upon tactile and kinesthetic input. The test thus becomes, in part, a measure of the subject's ability to adapt successfully to a novel type of approach. Second, the subject is required to perform the task three times— first using his preferred hand, then his nonpreferred hand, and finally both hands. Since the subject is never given any warning that successive trials will be required, the test provides an opportunity to assess how much the subject has learned by practice. After the task is completed, a further reflection of incidental learning is obtained by asking the subject to draw the board and fill in as many of the shapes as he possibly can. Scores, based on the number of correct shapes in the drawing and the number placed approximately in their correct positions, reflect consistent and highly significant differences between groups of subjects with and without cerebral lesions. The results obtained with procedures of this kind suggest that one of the important deficits resulting from cerebral lesions relates to incidental learning, the ability to profit from experience even though specific attention has not been directed to the learning aspect of the task.

A relatively simple paper-and-pencil test called the Trail Making Test has proved highly effective in revealing the effects of cerebral damage. In Part A of this test the subject is merely required to connect circles on a page as quickly as possible, taking them in order of their numbers from 1 to 25. Part B of the test, however, is more complicated. Both numbers and letters are included, and the subject is required to alternate between them following the sequence of 1, A, 2, B, 3, C, 4, D, and so on. While he is searching the page to find the next number or letter, the subject must also face the unusual task of integrating the numerical and alphabetical series. The problem of simultaneous organization of these various dimensions of the task, under pressure to complete the test as quickly as possible, is relatively easy for the normal subject but extremely difficult for many subjects with cerebral lesions.

In spite of the apparent necessity for rather detailed study in evaluating human brain-behavior relationships, many psychologists still use a simplified approach that underestimates the complexity of the problem. The customary psychological evaluation of the neurological patient may include only tests such as the Wechsler Scale, the Bender Gestalt test, the Draw-a-Person test, and perhaps the Rorschach Test. The Wechsler Scale was described briefly earlier. The Bender Gestalt test requires the subject to copy some designs; he is instructed to draw human figures (usually a man, a woman, and himself) in the Draw-a-Person test. The Rorschach Test requires the subject to report his associations with a standard set of inkblots. While these tests may reveal certain deficits in persons with cerebral lesions, they do not reflect an adequate sampling of behavior subserved by the brain, are oriented only toward dichotomous classification of subjects into those with brain damage and those without brain damage (as contrasted with exploration of brain-behavior relationships), and do not permit an organized and complementary use of the various methods of inference that have been described.

The psychologist may also evaluate the emotional status of the patient and his affective integrity. Various types of instruments are available for this purpose, including some objective and standardized tests as well as some of the projective testing techniques. The Minnesota Multiphasic Personality Inventory provides quantitative scores for individual subjects on the basis of their answers to a large number of questions. The test can be scored with respect to normative data on a series of scales, which include Hypochondriasis, Depression, Hysteria, Psychopathic Deviate, Paranoia, Psychasthenia, Schizophrenia, and Hypomania. In addition to a number of other experimental scales, the test also includes validational scales, which provide some assistance in judging whether the answers of the subject are consistent and reasonable and therefore open to valid interpretation. Additional tests for assessment of emotional stability include the Rorschach Test (mentioned earlier), the Thematic Apperception Test (based on the subject's verbalizations in response to a series of ambiguous pictures), and tests based on human figure drawings and other types of drawings that might provide clues to his emotional tensions. Little work in evaluating the validity of emotional changes as they relate to the condition of the brain has been done. This latter area, therefore, has much less of value to offer in terms of psychological assessment than the area of intellectual and cognitive functions.

SIMPLE TESTING PROCEDURES IN THE NEUROLOGICAL EXAMINATION

A number of simple tests that involve fundamental aspects of language, drawing ability, and perception within the tactile, auditory, and visual modalities frequently provide information useful in assessing the condition of the brain. Many of the tests described in this section may well be thought of as part of the physical neurological examination although they often are not routinely included. When simple behavioral examinations are included the stimulus material used and the specific requirements of the tests often vary from one examiner to another. A major drawback in developing examining techniques in this area has been the lack of sufficient emphasis on standardization of procedure. While it is entirely possible to use whatever objects one has at hand in examining the patient's ability to name common objects, for example, using exactly the same stimulus material for one subject after another is a great advantage in developing the examiner's skill in evaluating the finer aspects of the subject's responses. For this reason, it is clearly desirable to use an instrument such as the Halstead-Wepman Aphasia Screening Test. We have devised a modification of this test, abbreviating it somewhat, that provides significant evidence of both left and right hemisphere dysfunction. The test uses standard stimulus figures on flip-over cards to test the subject's ability to name common objects, spell, identify individual numbers and letters, read, write, calculate, ennunciate, understand spoken language, identify body parts, and differentiate between right and left. Further, the test requires the subject to copy simple figures in order to demonstrate ability in visuospatial performance.

The subject is first shown a picture of a square and is asked to draw a figure like it, name the figure, and spell the name of the figure. Essentially the same instructions are given using a Greek cross and a triangle as stimulus figures. The subject is asked to name a picture of a baby, to write (but not say aloud) the proper name for a picture of a clock, to read individual numbers and letters, to read simple material at approximately the second and fourth grade levels, to comprehend verbal instructions through audition, and so on. In addition to such examinations, certain other tests have proved extremely valuable in indicating impairment of sensory perception. Particularly recommended are tests of sensory imperception, tactile finger recognition, and fingertip number writing perception. A standard procedure for administering such tests follows.

Sensory Imperception

This test, following a prior determination that the subject is able to perceive unilateral stimulation on each side, attempts to determine whether he can perceive bilateral simultaneous sensory stimulation. The procedure is applied through tactile, auditory, and visual sensory modalities in separate tests. For routine clinical purposes only a rough control of stimulus intensity is attempted. Our procedure calls for use of a stimulus of the minimal intensity necessary to achieve consistently correct responses to unilateral stimulation.

To test tactile function, each hand is first touched separately in order to determine that the subject is able to respond with accuracy to unilateral stimulation on each side. Following this a series of trials using unilateral stimulation, interspersed with bilateral simultaneous stimulation, is performed. The normal response is for the subject to respond accurately with the following alternatives: right hand, left hand, or both hands, depending upon the stimulus delivered. Subjects with lateralized cerebral lesions are usually able to identify unilateral stimulation correctly but sometimes fail to respond, under bilateral simultaneous stimulation, to the hand contralateral to the damaged hemisphere. Contralateral face-hand combinations are also used with a single or double simultaneous stimulation as part of our standard procedure.

Testing for auditory imperception makes use of an auditory stimulus produced by rubbing the fingers lightly together very quickly and sharply. Essentially a similar procedure is applied in visual examination with the examiner executing discrete movements of the fingers while the subject focuses on the examiner's nose. If the patient has a serious lateralized tactile, auditory, or visual loss, the test for bilateral simultaneous stimulation is, of course, obviated.

Tactile Finger Recognition

This procedure tests the ability of the subject to identify individual fingers on both hands as a result of tactile stimulation of each finger. Before the examination begins, the examiner must work out a system with the patient for reporting which finger was touched. Customarily, the patient reports by number, but some patients prefer to identify their fingers in other verbal terms. Although the test itself is given without the subject's use of vision as a basis for his response (and therefore depends upon tactile input alone), it is sometimes necessary to give certain patients practice with their eyes open in order to be sure that the report is reliable. When the patient is not able to give a reliable verbal report, he is asked to point to the finger touched using his other hand. Four trials are used routinely for each finger on each hand, yielding a total of 20 trials on each hand. The score is recorded as the number of errors for each hand.

Fingertip Number Writing Perception

This procedure requires the subject to report numbers written on the fingertips of each hand, without the use of vision. Standard numbers are used and written on the fingertips in a standard sequence. We have found the numbers 3, 4, 5, and 6 to be least subject to confusion, and while these numbers are used on each finger, the order of their presentation is varied. A total of four trials is given for each finger, yielding 20 responses for each hand. This test is sometimes difficult for young children, and in such instances, we use X's and O's as the stimulus figures rather than numbers.

While the tests described do not require any particular apparatus, additional simple testing procedures that do require apparatus may also be used to supplement the physical neurological examination. For example, measurement of finger tapping speed (described earlier) often provides useful information with respect to the differential function of the two hands even though such differences may be so small that they are difficult to perceive reliably through gross observation.

ILLUSTRATIVE CASES OF PSYCHOLOGICAL DEFICIT

Intrinsic Tumor of the Left Cerebral Hemisphere

This patient was a 45-year-old left-handed man who was working as a painter. He entered the hospital with complaints of headache on the left side, numbness of the right arm and leg, some hearing loss on the right side, occasional episodes of difficulty with speech, and exhaustion after only brief periods of work. Psychological examination revealed a full-scale Wechsler-Bellevue (Form I) IQ of 119 with a verbal IQ of 114 and a performance IQ of 122. Results for the 11 subtests of this scale showed some differential levels of performance, but these did not seem to have any particular significance with respect to possible cerebral damage. The examination for aphasia indicated no evidence of organic language deficits in spite of the fact that the patient had complained of occasional episodes of difficulty with speech. The complete battery of psychological tests showed no highly specific deficits. The results were interpreted as indicating mild and diffuse involvement of the cerebral hemispheres and corresponding mild impairment of adaptive abilities.

Neurological diagnostic procedures were performed concurrently with the psychological testing. Although the patient was hospitalized for several weeks and studied thoroughly, no definite neurological diagnosis was reached. He was discharged and, the evidence from neurological evaluation indicating some generalized disorder of the cerebral hemispheres of an unspecified type, was instructed to report on a scheduled basis for outpatient evaluation.

The patient was readmitted three and one half months later. His behavioral deficits at this time had become much more specific and pronounced. The Wechsler-Bellevue Scale (Form I) now yielded a full-scale IQ of 87 as compared with the previous score of 119. The impairment of the patient was particularly marked on the verbal subtests, the current verbal IQ being only 67 as compared with the original verbal IQ of 114. The performance IQ had also declined, but only from 122 to 112.

Although the initial examination had shown no evidence of dysphasia, many such symptoms were now present. The patient had severe deficiencies in receptive as well as expressive language functions. Auditory receptive difficulties (auditory-verbal dysgnosia) were manifested by the patient's great difficulty in understanding spoken language. This difficulty probably was responsible for the impression of several neurologists that the patient had suffered mental deterioration since the time of the first hospitalization. Actually, he had not deteriorated as grossly as appeared, but he was unable to grasp the full symbolic significance of verbal communication and therefore was unable to respond appropriately to it. In addition, he was not able to monitor his own voice with

respect to appreciating "feedback" information regarding his own verbalizations. Difficulties of this type can frequently make a patient appear to be extremely bewildered and confused even though his general understanding is relatively intact. The patient had profound receptive difficulties along the visual avenue also, not only being impaired in reading ability but also in ability to recognize individual numbers and letters of the alphabet.

Typical expressive aphasic difficulties were also present. When shown a triangle, the patient identified it by saying something that sounded like "cryan." His response to a picture of a baby was, "paby — paby — right?" His spelling ability varied, in some instances being nearly correct but in others not even coming close. When asked to spell the word triangle, he responded, "c-r-a-n-t-i-n-i, that right?" He was able to copy written words and to write an occasional word from dictation correctly, but he failed nearly completely in attempts to write simple sentences. His ability to perform simple arithmetical computations was markedly impaired; occasionally he had great difficulty enunciating even simple words. He showed some right-left confusion. In spite of this evidence of profound impairment in using language symbols for communicational purposes, he continued to be able to copy simple spatial configurations as well as he had at the time of the first examination (Fig. 17–2).

The patient also showed some progression of deficits on the rest of the tests in our battery as compared with the results obtained on the first examination, but the area of major impairment related to the use of language and verbal symbols. Results of this kind are quite characteristic of a seriously destructive lesion of the left cerebral hemisphere. The pronounced evidence of both expressive and receptive difficulties tends to implicate the entire language area, extending generally from the posteroinferior frontal area to the posterior part of the temporal lobe. A "blind" interpretation of the psychological test results at this time indicated that they were entirely consistent with an hypothesis of an intrinsic tumor in the left temporoparietal area.

Left carotid angiography indicated the presence of a large lesion located principally in the left posterior temporoparietal area. The lesion was identified histologically as a glioblastoma multiforme. The comparison of results obtained from this

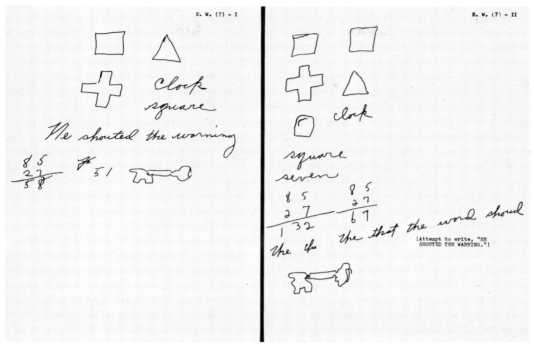

FIGURE 17–2 Simple performances of drawing and writing of a 45-year-old man before and after serious impairment caused by development of a left temporoparietal glioblastoma multiforme. Note the deterioration of ability in writing the sentence, "He shouted the warning."

patient on the two examinations illustrates the most typical and outstanding types of deficits that are associated with a seriously destructive lesion of the left cerebral hemisphere. The deficits contrast sharply with those shown by patients who sustain damage of the right cerebral hemisphere, as indicated by the results on the following patient.

Meningioma and Surgical Damage of the Right Cerebral Hemisphere

This patient was a 52-year-old right-handed man who had been employed as a radio news editor and announcer. He was reported to have had three complete "nervous break-downs" several years prior to his current complaints and had undergone psychotherapy in connection with each of these episodes. During the one and one half years prior to admission, however, he had experienced a number of convulsions, which began with tingling in the left lower arm and hand and progressed into major generalized convulsions. Five days before psychological evaluation he had experienced two such

generalized convulsions. Psychological test results indicated that the patient was quite intelligent with a full-scale Wechsler-Bellevue (Form I) IQ of 135. His verbal IQ was 130 and his performance IQ was 136. The examination for aphasia and sensory-perceptual deficits failed to reveal any striking disabilities. The general level of performance shown by this patient was well within the normal range. On many tasks, in fact, he did outstandingly well. Nevertheless, certain of his performances with the left hand as compared with the right hand were markedly deficient, and these results raised a definite question regarding possible impairment of function of the right cerebral hemisphere. A "blind" analysis of the psychological test results was interpreted as suggesting the presence of an irritative focus in the right parietal area. The area of involvement appeared to be discrete in nature, since the subject performed very poorly with his left hand on the Tactual Performance Test (a test that requires integration of haptic input in a general sense) whereas his finger tapping speed with the left hand was almost in the expected relationship to the speed achieved with the right hand. Since the parietal area seems to be involved in somaesthetic functions, whereas the posterior frontal area (motor strip) is involved in motor functions, a dissociation of deficits suggested that the parietal area was definitely involved while the adjacent frontal area was minimally affected.

Neurological evaluation identified the presence of a meningioma in the right parietal area. Great difficulty in controlling bleeding was encountered during the attempt to remove the lesion surgically. In order to preserve the patient's life under these circumstances, a good deal of damage was done to the posterior part of the right cerebral hemisphere. Postoperative examination results, in comparison with those obtained in the initial examination, reflect the pronounced effects of serious damage to the posterior part of the right cerebral hemisphere and illustrate the extent to which this area subserves abilities in dealing with visuospatial relationships.

The postoperative psychological test results were obtained one month and eight days following the first examination. At this time the patient was ambulatory and feeling well in a general sense. His verbal IQ had decreased 15 points, from a preoperative value of 130 to 115. The performance IQ, however, had decreased 57 points, from a value of 136 to 79. Inspection of the weighted scores for the individual performance subtests indicated that he was scarcely

able to make any progress on them. The patient also performed more poorly on a number of additional tests, demonstrating severe impairment in his ability to deal with visuospatial problems of various types.

Examination for aphasia indicated that the patient had no specific language difficulties. However, Figure 17–3 demonstrates very clearly the great difficulty he had in reproducing spatial configurations. In repeated attempts to copy simple figures, such as a Greek cross, he made very little progress. He was able to form letters correctly either in copying words or in writing from dictation, but he was not able to go back and cross *t*'s or dot *i*'s because of his difficulty in finding them. Thus, his limitation in writing was also essentially a problem in adapting to spatial configurations.

It is apparent from these findings that damage to the posterior part of the right cerebral hemisphere may cause very severe deficits in abilities although the nature of the deficit varies greatly from that seen in patients with left hemisphere lesions. Nevertheless, practical aspects of adjustment require one to deal with relationships in space and time as well as in the area of

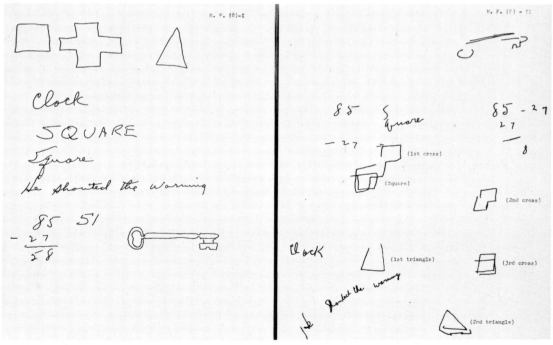

FIGURE 17–3 Simple performances in drawing and writing of a 52-year-old man before and after serious structural damage in the posterior part of the right cerebral hemisphere. Note the profound impairment of this patient's ability to copy simple figures such as a cross and triangle.

verbal communication, and lesions of the right cerebral hemisphere may have very profound significance in limiting the adequacy of adaptation to problems in everyday living.

Left Carotid Artery Stenosis

A wide range of vascular disorders affecting cerebral function can be identified in which psychological evaluation makes a significant contribution in the overall assessment of the patient. Repeated examination may be especially helpful because the initial testing can be used as a baseline for evaluating changes. Of particular importance would be the assessment of possible improvement, using objective testing procedures, following operative intervention or other treatment as in the case of the following patient.

This 60-year-old woman was admitted with a history of recent occasional episodes of dizziness. On the day of admission she had two episodes of vertigo, blurring of vision, and difficulty in verbal expression accompanied by severe occipital headaches. Physical neurological examination was essentially normal except that the patient had some difficulty in executing commands and showed some perseveration in her speech. Electroencephalographic tracings revealed delta waves, Grade II, in the left temporal area. Bilateral carotid arteriograms demonstrated a localized narrowing of the left internal carotid artery just distal to the bifurcation. A thromboendarterectomy of the left common carotid artery was performed, and a good retrograde flow as well as good pulsation above the lesion site was established following this procedure. From a clinical point of view the patient seemed to be improved.

The woman was examined psychologically both before and after the surgical procedure. She showed a number of deficits in the area of language functions and in the types of sensory-perceptual tests described earlier. While she had no highly specific symptoms of dysphasia, her abilities in dealing with symbolic and communicational aspects of language functions were somewhat impaired, suggesting some dysfunction of the left cerebral hemisphere. She also showed evidence of mild right-left confusion, a finding that is much more common in patients with left than right hemisphere lesions. Her strength of grip was scarcely greater in her right upper extremity than her left, although measures of lateral dominance indicated that she was strongly right-handed. She was reasonably intact in finger tapping speed, but this represented essentially her only adequate performance. Even in this instance, however, her tapping speed was scarcely faster with her right hand than with her left hand, a finding that suggested some impairment of function in the right (preferred) hand.

In testing the patient for perception of bilateral simultaneous sensory stimulation, she showed a marked tendency to fail to perceive an auditory stimulus to her right ear when it was given simultaneously with one to the left ear, although she made no mistakes with unilateral stimulation. She showed the same tendency with respect to visual stimulation, frequently failing to notice the stimulus toward her right side when it was given simultaneously with one on the left side. These findings implied that the left cerebral hemisphere was dysfunctional as compared with the right.

In terms of higher-level psychological functions, this patient was grossly impaired. She obtained a verbal IQ of 85 and a performance IQ of 91, although the detailed scores indicated that the IQ values were based largely on tests that are dependent upon accumulated and stored information. She was quite deficient in tasks that required immediate problem-solving ability. She was unable to make any satisfactory progress on either the Category Test or the Tactual Performance Test and was unable to sustain her attention to the task sufficiently to complete the Seashore Rhythm Test or the Speech-sounds Perception Test. Although she was able to complete Part A of the Trail Making Test, she worked for five minutes on Part B and was entirely bewildered by the requirement that she switch back and forth between the alphabetic and numerical sequences.

The second psychological examination was done 16 days following the endarterectomy. The patient obtained both verbal and performance IQ values of 96, indicating a modest increase in both instances. Inspection of the weighted scores for the individual subtests suggested that the patient was clearly more alert than she was at the time of the first examination although part of the "improvement" may have been due to positive practice-effect. The patient was able to complete nearly all the other tests in the battery even though she demonstrated serious impairment of adaptive abilities. This, in itself, represented a marked improvement in comparision with the initial test results.

The patient now demonstrated more marked disparities between the function of the right and left sides of the body than she had on the initial testing, in part because the general improvement she had shown permitted the disparities to become more clear. She continued to have very mild difficulty with language functions and a very mild tendency not to perceive auditory and visual stimuli on the right side when they were in competition with stimuli to the left side of the body.

In spite of her continued profound impairment in many areas of adaptive abilities, the test results provided objective verification of the clinical impression that this patient had shown improvement following the operation.

A Question of a Brain Tumor

This patient, a 14-year-and-5-month-old boy, had developed essentially within normal limits and without significant medical, psychological, or adjustment problems except that during the last one and one half years he had experienced four episodes of a tingling sensation in the right upper and lower extremities and right side of the face. He also had suffered rather frequent headaches during this time. Such an episode, followed by vomiting and headache, had led to his admission to the hospital. The night before admission he had experienced a nocturnal grand mal convulsive seizure.

This patient's history did not reveal any events that identified a likely cause although he had been unconscious briefly after running into a tree approximately two and one half years prior to his admission. He had sustained another head injury two years prior to admission when he had been hit on the left side of his head with a baseball and had been stunned. Physical neurological examination was entirely negative, but ophthalmological consultation revealed early bilateral papilledema. An electroencephalogram indicated the presence of a dysrhythmia, Grade I, generalized, and delta waves, Grade I, of the left temporoparietal area. This evidence raised very definite concern about the presence of an intracranial tumor.

Psychological examination was performed at this time, and the subject obtained a verbal IQ of 135 (well into the superior range), whereas his performance IQ was 112 (in the lower part of the high average range). The individual subtests of the Wechsler Scale showed some variability but did not provide any basis for inferring the presence of cerebral damage. The rest of the tests in the battery indicated that this child had good basic adaptive abilities. In terms of level of performance, the results did not indicate any serious brain lesion. The patient did extremely well on the Category Test; such an excellent performance, in its own right, would

almost certainly rule out an intrinsic cerebral tumor. In addition, the suggestive evidence from the electroencephalogram tended to implicate the left cerebral hemisphere, a finding that was inconsistent with the high verbal IQ and other excellent abilities shown by the subject in dealing with language symbols for communication. Further, he performed extremely well on Part B of the Trail Making Test, providing evidence of flexibility in thought processes and a degree of efficiency in his performances that rarely if ever is seen in persons with intrinsic cerebral neoplasms. Although our test results argued strongly against the presence of an intrinsic neoplasm of either cerebral hemisphere, certain of the findings did raise a question of the possible presence of much milder cerebral dysfunction. The patient was a little slow in finger tapping speed with the right hand as compared with his left hand, and he had just a little difficulty in tactile finger localization on his right hand but made no mistakes on his left hand. He had even more pronounced difficulty on the right hand in fingertip number writing perception. While the patient had no definite evidence of aphasia, he first identified a square as a rectangle and then spontaneously corrected himself, a type of error that may point to left cerebral dysfunction. These findings suggested that the patient had some mild disturbance of functioning in the left cerebral hemisphere as well as possible very mild right hemisphere dysfunction. This latter was suggested by the subject's tendency to fail to perceive a tactile stimulus to the left side of his face when it was given simultaneously with a stimulus to the right hand. The patient also had some very mild difficulty in tactile form recognition with his left hand as well as his right hand. Even though the overall findings suggested some mild cerebral dysfunction involving both hemispheres, they were hardly compatible with an acutely destructive or rapidly progressive focal lesion of either cerebral hemisphere. The interpretation of psychological findings indicated that the patient probably had some very minimal impairment of brain functions of a type that could be considered compatible with possible prior brain trauma or infectious disease involving the brain.

Because of the evidence of papilledema and the electroencephalographic findings, it was felt that contrast studies should be performed on this child. Angiograms were essentially normal and a decision was made to follow this patient closely rather than to undertake additional diagnostic procedures or possible operation. Repeated ophthalmological examination remained constant over the next two-month period. It was finally concluded that the peculiarities of the optic discs appeared to be within the range of normal variation and should be classified as pseudopapillitis rather than an indication of intracranial hypertension. Treated with anticonvulsive medication, the patient had no further difficulties of the type that had led to hospitalization. He was a freshman in high school at the time of the initial examination. This patient was available for repeated examinations and he was seen most recently just after graduation from college. His development neurologically and neuropsychologically has been essentially normal.

Although the eventual diagnosis would certainly have been reached even though neuropsychological examination had not been done, the results obtained were timely and helped in the eventual understanding of the patient. However, it is necessary to note that an interpretation of this type is dependent upon a good deal of prior experience and knowledge of psychological test results in patients with and without cerebral neoplasms, a type of experience that is not yet common to a great number of psychologists.

PSYCHOLOGICAL ASSESSMENT AS PART OF NEUROLOGICAL EVALUATION

The development of methods during the last generation for evaluating the psychological correlates of brain lesions now makes possible a fairly detailed and valid contribution from this area to total neurological evaluation. Neurological scientists have long recognized the importance of the brain as the organ of adaptive behavior. In the main, however, they have directed their attention toward diagnosis and treatment of the basic disease process or physical disorder rather than toward the aspects of brain functions concerned with intelligence and adaptive abilities. It would be fair to say, in terms of the behavioral aspects of neurological disorders, that disproportionate attention has been directed toward sensory and motor deficits as compared with the more important but more subtle aspects of higher brain functions. For example, there has been relatively little recognition by neurological scientists in a practical sense of the impact of impaired language functions and com-

municational abilities on problems of later adaptation to everyday living. While most neurological scientists would agree on the importance of loss of ability to organize diverse stimulus material and to analyze relationships in attempting to understand problems, relatively few have addressed their efforts toward this aspect of neurological disease and damage. Deficits in dealing with visuospatial and manipulatory aspects of the environment may also be critical in limiting the patient's adjustment to everyday living. Extensive information has become available regarding human brain-behavior relationships during the last three decades, but problems definitely exist in full utilization of this information.[1, 4, 10] Psychologists, in the main, have little background or training in the neurological sciences, and neurological scientists often have little detailed knowledge of the methods or procedures in psychology. Such circumstances raise the question whether our traditional disciplinary boundaries shall continue to fractionate the brain-behavior equation or whether the specialists in each aspect of the relationship, recognizing that both brain functions and behavior constitute integral elements of the functioning of every human being, will direct continued attention to exploring brain function and dysfunction within an appropriate and broad frame of reference.

Relatively little is known at present regarding the application of knowledge of the psychological effects of brain lesions in the area of rehabilitation. Rehabilitational efforts also continue to be directed toward the obvious deficits, the sensory and motor disorders, rather than losses that are more subtle, deficits in the ability to form reasonable concepts and to use good judgment. In terms of practical results, however, it may do little good to restore motor functions if higher-level psychological deficits (which, in practice, are not often even evaluated) doom the patient to failure. While formal programs have not been initiated to study the potential for the training of higher-level functions, it has been well documented that individual subjects, in selected instances, can make good progress in regaining intellectual and cognitive functions after structural damage to the cerebral hemispheres. The practical implications with respect to training and rehabilitation, of knowledge that has already been gained in the area of human brain-behavior relationships, need urgently to be studied.

Preparation of this paper and the research reported was supported in part by NIH research grants NB 01468, NB 05211, and NB 07178.

REFERENCES

1. Halstead, W. C.: Brain and Intelligence. Chicago, University of Chicago Press, 1947.
2. Heimburger, R. F., and Reitan, R. M.: Easily administered written test for lateralizing brain lesions. J. Neurosurg., *18*:301–312, 1961.
3. Matthews, C. G., Shaw, D. J., and Kløve, H.: Psychologic test performances in neurologic and "pseudoneurologic" subjects. Cortex, *2*: 244–253, 1966.
4. Mountcastle, V. B., ed.: Interhemispheric Relations and Cerebral Dominance. Baltimore, Johns Hopkins Press, 1962.
5. Reitan, R. M.: An investigation of the validity of Halstead's measures of biological intelligence. A.M.A. Arch. Neurol. Psychiat., *73*:28–35, 1955.
6. Reitan, R. M.: Psychological deficit. Ann. Rev. Psychol., *13*:415–444, 1962.
7. Reitan, R. M.: Problems and prospects in studying the psychological correlates of brain lesions. Cortex, *2*:127–154, 1966.
8. Reitan, R. M.: A research program on the psychological effects of brain lesions in human beings. *In,* International Review of Research in Mental Retardation. Vol. I. Ellis, N. R., ed.: New York, Academic Press, 1966, pp. 153–218.
9. Wheeler, L., and Reitan, R. M.: The presence and laterality of brain damage predicted from responses to a short aphasia screening test. Percept. Motor Skills, *15*:783–799, 1962.
10. Yates, A. J.: Psychological deficit. Ann. Rev. Psychol., *17*:111–144, 1966.

IV

Physiology and Homeostasis

The enlarged ventricles of hydrocephalus are accommodated primarily by expansion of the skull and only secondarily, if at all, by a reduction in total brain volume. Hypertonic solutions in infants cause not only dehydration of the brain but diminution in the size of the fontanelles and a reduction in total intracranial volume.

These and other observations on the Monro-Kellie doctrine can be summarized by stating that the craniospinal intradural space is *nearly* constant in volume and that its contents are *nearly* noncompressible. These qualifications, however, are very important and account for many of the clinically significant aspects of intracranial dynamics. Thus, the spinal dura is not in contact with the wall of the vertebral canal as it is in the intracranial space, permitting some changes in total volume at the expense of the blood volume in the spinal extradural veins. Since the dura can be stretched very little, these changes in volume are quite small. Furthermore, every substance can be either stretched or compressed if the applied force is large enough, and in physical terms these properties of the material are expressed in terms of elasticity.

A formula has been derived relating change in pressure in a hypothetical container the approximate size of a monkey skull to the volume of fluid injected.[156] The purpose was to examine the volume-pressure relationship in the intracranial space at a time when it behaved as a closed box, when reciprocal changes among compartments could no longer occur. The model consisted of a closed sphere with a capacity of 100 ml of water and a wall 3 mm in thickness. The elastic modulus of polymethylmethacrylate was substituted for bone, and the bulk modulus of elasticity of the contents was considered to be the same as water. In this closed system, volume can be added only by compressing the water or expanding the shell. Since Young's modulus of elasticity for the container is greater than the bulk modulus of water, the added volume is accommodated primarily by increasing the density of the contents. Applying the formula, it was found that adding 1 ml of water to the 100-ml filled container increased the pressure within the container to 2190 mm of mercury. Thus, within the

limitations of the model, when intracranial pressure in the monkey has been increased to about 200 mm of mercury, 0.1 ml of fluid has been added to the intracranial space. The fluid is accommodated by both distention of the skull and compression of its contents. It is apparent then that a mass is accommodated within the intracranial space by displacement of some of its normal contents, and if there is no change in pressure the volume of the displaced fluid is equal to the volume of the mass. By the same token, if the volume of the mass exceeds the volume of displaced fluid, intracranial pressure rises, but the difference in the two volumes required to produce a large change in pressure is very small indeed, only a fraction of a per cent of the total intracranial volume. Thus, the Monro-Kellie doctrine, with Burrows' modification, continues to be valid and useful.

Factors Responsible for Intracranial Pressure

A consideration of the factors responsible for normal intracranial pressure can begin with examination of a few simple models. Figure 18–1 *A* illustrates a model of a patient in the lateral decubitus position with a needle in the spinal subarachnoid space. The plane of the needle passes through the midsagittal plane of the skull. If the uppermost portion of the skull is open, forming a bowl, the pressure measured in the spinal canal is the distance between the midsagittal plane and the lateral wall of the skull. Thus, the pressure would be approximately 70 mm of water in this static open system. Water seeks its own level in a U-tube with both ends open to the atmosphere. When the model is tilted from the horizontal to the vertical position fluid rises in the manometer attached to the lumbar needle until it equals the fluid level in the skull (Fig. 18–1 *B*). On the other hand, if the skull were a completely closed, rigid container filled to capacity, no fluid would flow into the manometer when the model was tilted into the vertical position (Fig. 18–1 *C*). The reason is that the fluid in the needle in the spinal canal, but not the fluid in the head, is exposed to the atmosphere. If one places one end of a rubber

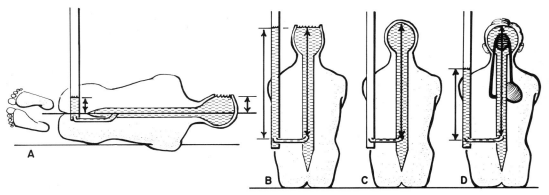

FIGURE 18-1 Models of craniospinal pressure. See text for explanation.

tube into an automobile gas tank and the other end into a pail, gasoline does not flow from the tank. But if the car is raised approximately 34 feet, the pressure in the gas tank exceeds normal atmospheric pressure, and gasoline flows into the pail. An easier way to achieve the same result is to reduce atmospheric pressure at the end of the tube by applying suction. Figure 18–1 *D* illustrates a normal patient in the sitting position. Spinal fluid in an open manometer attached to the lumbar puncture needle rises to about the level of the cervicothoracic junction. Thus, actual spinal fluid pressure in the sitting position is less than it would be if the intracranial space were an open system and greater than if it were a completely closed system.

Weed and his colleagues investigated these phenomena extensively in experimental animals and attributed the pressure changes that occur in tilting from the horizontal to the head-down and tail-down positions to the elasticity of the craniospinal contents.[284-286] Pollock and Boshes, in an excellent application of physical principles to biological research, concluded, on the contrary, that the skull is an imperfectly closed container, because a portion of atmospheric pressure is applied to the intracranial space through the blood vessels (Fig. 18–1 *D*).[216] Patients with large skull defects have higher than normal pressure in the sitting position, because the system is further exposed to the atmosphere.

Another matter having to do with the mechanics of pressure measurements is the relationship of "absolute" to "relative" intracranial or spinal fluid pressure. In order to measure pressure in an open manometer, fluid must be dislocated into the manometer, thereby reducing the volume of fluid in the craniospinal intradural space; also the higher the pressure, the more fluid is required to measure it. This is often termed the relative pressure and is less than absolute pressure. Absolute pressure can be measured if the method does not permit escape of fluid. Originally this was performed with a "bubble manometer." A bubble of air is introduced at the hub of the needle and rises in the manometer during measurement of relative pressure. The manometer is then elevated until the dislocated fluid flows back into the spinal canal, and the bubble again rests at the bottom of the manometer. The problem of distinguishing between relative and absolute pressures is of less concern today with the wide use of pressure transducers. A transducer is attached to the hub of the needle at the time of insertion so that no fluid is lost, except that which may leak around the shaft of the needle. The volume of fluid displaced then is only that contained within the needle plus the minute quantity required to displace the diaphragm of the transducer.

Many of the factors responsible for maintaining normal intracranial pressure in the horizontal position are unknown. The fact that the intracranial space is filled to capacity contributes, and the volume of continuously circulating blood is an important factor.

Methods of Measurement

The first spinal tap appears to have been performed by Corning for the purpose of anesthetizing the spinal cord.[119] The first treatise on lumbar puncture was published by Quincke who introduced the practice of measuring pressure with a fine glass pipet.[219] He described the normal pressure as 90 to 100 mm of water. In later years Jackson described spinal fluid pressure measurements with a mercury manometer in a variety of pathological conditions,[119] and the significance of examination of the spinal fluid in the diagnosis of intracranial tumors was thoroughly evaluated by Ayer.[4] However, the procedure was not used extensively until it began to be applied in the management of head injuries. Sharpe published a monograph on brain injuries in which he stated that his principal criterion for operation was increased spinal fluid pressure.[251] Numerous reports of spinal fluid pressure measurements in head injury patients followed, and there was much disagreement on the indications and danger of lumbar puncture and the reliability of the procedure in accurately measuring intracranial tension. Most authors did agree that a pressure in excess of 200 mm of water was definitely abnormal.

The two principal objections to lumbar puncture in the diagnosis of intracranial hypertension have been the danger of inducing acute brain stem compression, either at the tentorial incisura or the foramen magnum, and the contention that spinal fluid pressure is not an accurate reflection of intracranial pressure. The former concern has led to the admonition that a spinal tap should not be performed when there is clinical evidence of increased intracranial pressure, particularly in the presence of papilledema or signs of a tentorial pressure cone. Certainly the latter sign remains a contraindication to spinal tap under all except the most unusual circumstances. The value of analysis of the cerebrospinal fluid in patients with papilledema must be weighed against the dangers of the procedure. Lumbar puncture is not an innocuous procedure in patients with intracranial hypertension, but in experienced hands the danger appears to be minimal except in those patients who have a shift of the midline structure or those who already have signs of herniation or brain stem compression. The second reservation concerning lumbar puncture, that the spinal fluid pressure need not accurately reflect the intracranial pressure, is considered later.

Ventricular puncture for relief of increased intracranial pressure is one of the oldest practices in neurosurgery. Ventricular fluid pressure measurements during the procedure were described by a number of investigators, and occasionally ventricular and lumbar subarachnoid pressures were measured simultaneously. However, prolonged pressure measurements were performed infrequently, because water and mercury manometers were cumbersome for this purpose and because of the risk of intracranial infection. Lundberg reviewed the early history of direct intracranial pressure mensuration in his monograph, "Continuous recording and control of ventricular fluid pressure in neurosurgical practice," a major milestone in the story of intracranial hypertension.[172]

Lundberg uses a polyethylene cannula and stylet mounted on a stopcock. The cannula is inserted into the frontal horn of the right lateral ventricle through a burr hole. A rubber stopper through which the cannula is inserted is seated in the burr hole to prevent leakage of cerebrospinal fluid and to reduce the risk of infection. In 130 patients there were no hematomas that could be ascribed to the procedure. There were two cases each of extradural and intradural infections. Intracranial pressure can also be measured from a catheter in the subdural space, but the tip of the catheter tends to become obstructed at high levels of intracranial pressure and the method does not permit removal of cerebrospinal fluid for examination or rapid reduction of pressure.[152]

In recent years there has been much interest in solid-state transducers that are not dependent for their function on contact with intracranial fluid and do not require penetration of the brain. The ideal transducer must meet many demands, and the present goal is to develop transducers for different purposes rather than one all-purpose device. The requirements range from long-term measurement of intracranial pressure in hydrocephalic infants to a quick method of recording intracranial pressure in patients with severe head injuries. The pressure changes in hydrocephalus are subtle, and the intracranial pulse pressure may be as important as the mean pressure in determining the ventricular size. The device should be implantable within the intracranial space for periods of months or longer, should operate efficiently at low pressures, and should have minimal baseline drift. A transducer for measuring intracranial pressure in patients with severe head injuries or other major cerebral insults should be adaptable to use in the emergency ward or intensive care unit. It should be small enough to pass through a twist drill hole in the skull, thus avoiding open surgery in the operating room, and be rugged enough to withstand repeated use by personnel who have limited experience with the instrument.

A "passive pressure transensor" has been used to measure intracranial pressure in hydrocephalic patients.[2] It contains a parallel-tuned circuit consisting of a capacitance and an inductance. One plate of the capacitor is a flexible stainless steel diaphragm that is displaced by externally applied pressure. The transensor is implanted in a burr hole and connected to a catheter inserted into the lateral ventricle. Its frequency varies with the ventricular pressure, and the frequency variations are recorded with an inductor coil placed against the scalp over the transensor. The major advantage is the absence of external leads. It is, however, sensitive to changes in temperature and atmospheric pressure, and it records pulse pressure, not absolute pressure.

Experiences with other intracranial pressure transducers have been described in recent years.[31, 36, 122] One of these is a disc approximately 6 mm in diameter containing four arms of a Wheatstone bridge.[31, 122] Displacement of the sensing diaphragm by a change in intracranial pressure unbalances the bridge, and the voltage change is amplified and recorded. The device measures absolute pressure, but the baseline can be set to record only the intracranial pressure above standard atmos-

pheric pressure. It is sensitive to temperature changes, but they can be compensated for manually. The transducer appears to be stable over long periods. It is implanted into the intracranial space through a burr hole, and the leads are brought out through the scalp for connection to the recording apparatus.

Thus, several transducers are available for continuous monitoring of intracranial pressure, and others that employ different principles offer promise. Lack of stability, errors caused by changes in temperature and atmospheric pressure, and ease of insertion and removal are still problems with most of the devices.

PATHOPHYSIOLOGY

Intracranial Volume-Pressure Relationship

Reciprocal changes among compartments occur during physiological alterations in the intracranial contents. Hypercapnia increases intracranial blood volume to values at least twice the control volume and is accompanied by an increase in intracranial pressure.[291] The rise in intracranial pressure appears to be damped, however, by expression of cerebrospinal fluid as the vasodilatation and increase in cerebral blood volume occur. When the fluid has already been displaced by prior brain swelling or a mass lesion, hypercapnia produces a much greater rise in intracranial pressure.[155] Presumably the increase in cerebral blood volume is the same, but the increase in intracranial pressure is greater, because less cerebrospinal fluid is available to be displaced.

During gradual expansion of a mass lesion, the volume displaced may be cerebrospinal fluid, intravascular blood, or brain tissue water. Long-term compression of the brain can produce atrophy and perhaps some reduction in the mineral content of the brain, but changes in brain solids must be very small in terms of total volume. Rosomoff estimated the cerebrospinal fluid volume in the dog to be approximately 9 per cent of total intracranial volume.[230] If all of this fluid were displaceable, the intracranial space could accommodate a mass 9 per cent of the total intracranial volume without an increase in intracranial tension. Measurements of cerebral blood volume vary considerably according to the technique used, and the methodology has been reviewed recently by Sklar et al.[263] Most investigators have found an average cerebral blood volume of about 2 per cent in postmortem determinations in animals. The animals were sacrificed by quick freezing the head, or attempts were made to prevent drainage of blood from the head at sacrifice. In vivo measurements of cerebral blood volume in man have yielded values as high as 7 per cent.[202] If the latter value is correct, there is in fact considerable blood within the intracranial space that could be expressed during expansion of a mass lesion. Reduction in total brain water as a means of compensation for an expanding mass has not been adequately investigated. Since the subarachnoid space over the cerebral hemispheres is obliterated and the ventricles are narrowed by expansion of a mass or by brain swelling, it appears that cerebrospinal fluid is the principal spatial buffer, although reduction in blood volume may be an important factor under some circumstances.

Another important factor is the time required for spatial compensation to take place. If, for example, cerebrospinal fluid could not be rapidly displaced, rapid expansion of even the smallest mass would produce an increase in intracranial pressure incompatible with life; that is, the intracranial space would behave as a completely closed container. Ryder et al. injected fluid into the lumbar subarachnoid space and then immediately withdrew fluid in sufficient amount to return the pressure to the baseline.[242] Invariably the amount of fluid withdrawn was less than that injected, indicating that some of the fluid had rapidly escaped from the intradural space. Foldes and Arrowood infused the spinal subarachnoid space with saline and found that pressure remained constant at elevated levels during continuous infusion.[71] Equilibrium was reached with an infusion rate of 4 drops per minutes at 265 mm of cerebrospinal fluid, and with 16 drops per minute equilibrium pressure was 395 mm of cerebrospinal fluid. Their observations suggest that as much as 1 ml of cerebrospinal

fluid per minute can be expressed from the intradural space in the presence of elevated pressure. Thus, a large hematoma could be accommodated within a few hours without a dangerous rise in intracranial pressure. The complex anatomy of the cerebrospinal fluid spaces does not permit such a simple analogy, but the fact remains that the fluid can be driven rapidly out of the intracranial space, and were this not so, even the smallest extradural hematoma would cause rapid death from intracranial hypertension.

Figure 18–2 summarizes several of these observations in the monkey in the form of a volume-pressure graph. Water was added to a supratentorial extradural balloon by injecting 1 ml every hour or with a low-rate infusion pump. The graph is a composite of six experiments. Intracranial pressure did not increase significantly until the added volume approximated 5 ml, then rose progressively with additional increments. The horizontal portion of the curve is the period of spatial compensation, and the balloon is accommodated largely by expression of cerebrospinal fluid from the intracranial space. The essential features of the graph obtain with tumor, hematoma, hydrocephalus, and swelling of the brain parenchyma. The period of injection is as important as the volume in determining the

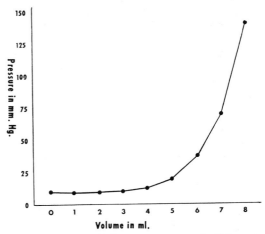

FIGURE 18–2 Volume pressure graph. Volume is given in milliliters (abscissa), and pressure in millimeters of mercury (ordinate) in this and all subsequent illustrations. (From Langfitt, T. W., Weinstein, J. D., and Kassell, N. F., *in* Caveness, W. F., and Walker, A. E., eds.: Head Injury: Conference Proceedings. Philadelphia, J. B. Lippincott Co., 1966.)

height of intracranial pressure. One milliliter injected in a few seconds can increase intracranial tension to the level of the blood pressure. By the same token, if the experiments had been carried out over a period of days rather than hours, it is likely that the balloon would have accommodated a somewhat larger volume before an increase in intracranial pressure occurred. Since the volume of displaceable fluid is finite, however, an increase in intracranial pressure must ultimately occur. Note in particular the marked change in pressure produced by a slight increase in the volume of the balloon on the vertical portion of the curve. The last 1-ml injection increased pressure an average of 70 mm of mercury. Thus, in the presence of a tumor that has slowly increased to such size that nearly all displaceable intracranial fluid has been eliminated, slight changes in brain tissue water or intravascular blood volume cause pressure alterations of great magnitude.

Transmission of Intracranial Pressure

The term intracranial pressure is meaningful only if one can assume that pressure is everywhere equal. The pressure in brain adjacent to an expanding mass might be elevated at a time when intraventricular pressure is normal. If so, one must speak of intracranial *pressures,* and in this case the important measurement in terms of function is in the compressed brain. Lumbar subarachnoid pressure is usually equated with intracranial pressure, but if for any reason there is failure of communication of pressure from the intracranial space to the spinal canal the spinal fluid pressure will be misleading.

Methods for recording intracranial and intraspinal pressures were developed in the latter part of the nineteenth century, and some investigators noted that increased pressure was not transmitted consistently from the intracranial to the intraspinal space. Hill maintained that rapid injections of fluid into the supratentorial subarachnoid space caused displacement of the cerebral hemispheres and the cerebellum with obstruction at both the tentorial incisura and foramen magnum.[108] Cushing stated that severe effects of compression could occur locally with little or no transmission to remote areas of the brain.[43] On the other hand, Eyster argued that displacement of the brain could not occur because of the incompressible fluid in the spinal canal, which he believed had no means of escape.[60] In the experiments of Kahn and Meyers an increase in pressure in the supratentorial space was not always fully communicated to the posterior fossa, but the difference in pressure was quite small.[136, 192]

There have been few reports of simultaneous measurements of intracranial and spinal fluid pressures in patients with pathological intracranial conditions. Hodgson reported some difference in the two pressures in the majority of patients with posterior fossa mass lesions, but failure of communication of pressure was rare with supratentorial lesions.[109] Smyth and Henderson found a lower lumbar pressure in 8 of 33 patients with intracranial space-occupying lesions, most of which were tumors, but the maximum difference in pressure was 100 mm of water.[265] These observations contrast with the high incidence of transtentorial herniation caused by supratentorial mass lesions. At autopsy, Finney and Walker found transtentorial herniation in 55.4 per cent of an unselected series of brain tumors, including an incidence of 88 per cent in glioblastomas of the cerebral hemispheres.[66] In 23 per cent of supratentorial tumors, herniations at both the tentorial incisura and foramen magnum were present. However, many herniations may not completely obstruct the basal cisterns. Recently Kaufmann and Clark found lumbar subarachnoid pressure to be significantly less than intraventricular pressure in the majority of a series of patients with severe head injury.[137]

Observations in animals have demonstrated that obstruction to communication of pressure at both the incisura and the foramen magnum occurs uniformly during the expansion of mass lesions, but the issue of pressure transmission within the supratentorial space has not been completely resolved.[159, 289] Pressure in an extradural mass may be manyfold the pressure recorded in the remainder of the intracranial space, because the dura is highly elastic* and is often firmly attached to the inner table of the skull. It would seem that the brain, particularly the cortical surface with its dense network of blood vessels, also has significant elastic properties that would resist displacement and deformation. If this is the case, it should be possible for pressure in the cortex beneath a subdural hematoma or meningioma to exceed the tension in the remainder of the brain. The elasticity of brain, in contrast to dura, is difficult to measure because of its heterogeneous architecture. There is some evidence, however, that the brain is more plastic than elastic; that it is easily deformed and displaced by a mass lesion, and persistent differences in pressure do not develop within its substance. Pressure has been measured in several small intracerebral balloons during the expansion of another balloon either in the subdural space or within the brain parenchyma.[289] When the pressure in the injection balloon was rapidly increased to 100 mm of mercury, the maximum difference in pressure measured across the brain was 35 mm of mercury. This contrasts with the large and persistent pressure gradient across the dura that is produced by injections of fluid into the extradural space. On the other hand, rapid expansion of an extracerebral mass produces ischemia confined to the brain beneath the mass.[289] Although intracerebral pressures were not measured in the latter experiments, the results suggest that whatever the difference in pressure across the supratentorial space, it is sufficient to account for collapse of blood vessels in brain subjacent to the balloon.

In the monkey, continued expansion of a supratentorial balloon invariably leads to obstruction at the tentorial incisura, and when obstruction is complete, elevating the intracranial pressure above the systolic blood pressure has no effect on the spinal fluid pressure.[159] In contrast, when the supratentorial pressure is raised to high levels by infusion of saline into the cerebrospinal fluid spaces, there is full communication of pressure throughout the craniospinal axis. These experiments demonstrate that the basal cisterns at the incisura must be blocked by brain tissue for a difference in pressure to occur and that this can be produced consistently by a mass lesion but not by infusion of the cerebrospinal fluid spaces. Injection of fluid into the spinal subarachnoid space or cisterna magna will reduce the block at the incisura created by a supratentorial mass, but the block redevelops immediately as long as the mass remains. Following evacuation of the mass, infusion of the cisterna magna with saline opens the tentorial cisterns, and free communication of pressure throughout the craniospinal axis is re-established.

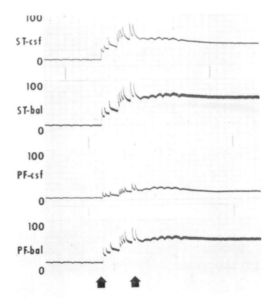

FIGURE 18–3 A supratentorial balloon had been expanded gradually until a difference in pressure was created between the supratentorial space and the posterior fossa. Pressures were recorded from a catheter in the supratentorial space (ST-csf), a supratentorial subdural balloon (ST-bal), a catheter in a posterior fossa cistern (PF-csf), and a posterior fossa balloon (PF-bal). This illustration demonstrates full communication of pressure from the supratentorial space to the posterior fossa balloon, with only minimal communication of pressure to the subarachnoid space surrounding the brain stem.

---

*An elastic substance is one that resists deformation in response to an applied stress and returns to its original shape and position when the stress is removed. Steel is highly elastic. Materials that are easily deformed and do not regain their original shape are termed plastic. The term "pressure" should be used only in a hydrostatic system. The generation and transmission of forces in elastic materials are expressed as stress-strain relationships. However, at the risk of oversimplification, pressure is used herein to describe forces within both the brain and the intracranial fluid compartments.

Herniation of brain through the tentorial incisura causes displacement and local compression of the brain stem and the familiar neurological signs of a tentorial pressure cone. If the pressure in the posterior fossa is normal, because of the obstruction at the incisura, the pons and medulla might be spared from the intracranial hypertension. In fact, increased supratentorial pressure is freely communicated through the brain stem to the medulla at a time when pressure in the cerebellopontine angle is normal by virtue of the incisural obstruction (Fig. 18–3).[289]

The gross anatomy of the intracranial space in man and monkey is sufficiently similar to make these observations applicable to human pathology. But the data cannot be extrapolated to man with the accuracy required to determine in what specific circumstances spinal fluid pressure is no longer an accurate index of intracranial pressure. Figure 18–4 does demonstrate that complete obstruction can occur clinically. Intracranial pressure equals the diastolic blood pressure, but lumbar subarachnoid pressure is normal. Thus, although the two pressures may be equal in many or even most patients with intracranial disease, one cannot assume this to be true in any given patient. Marked, spontaneous fluctuations in intracranial pressure have been demonstrated frequently in patients with a variety of intracranial lesions, and it is unlikely that these pressure waves are fully communicated to the spinal canal. The problem can be resolved only by simultaneous continuous measurement of both pressures under many circumstances.

Intracranial Pressure and Cerebral Blood Flow

The cerebral circulation is influenced by several anatomical and physiological features that are peculiar to the brain. It is the only major organ encased in a rigid container, and it is surrounded by the cerebrospinal fluid buffer that can expand and contract with changes in volume of the cerebrovascular bed. The organization of the vascular bed into arteries, capillaries, and veins is much the same as in other organs, but the collateral arterial and venous circulation is unusually rich. A unique feature is the final venous outflow track consisting of the thick-walled sinuses. Finally, the resistance vessels of the brain are exquisitely sensitive to metabolic changes, but influenced by the autonomic nervous system less than blood vessels in other organs.

The cerebrovascular mean pressure falls from approximately 90 mm of mercury in the carotid and vertebral arteries to 3 mm of mercury in the jugular and vertebral

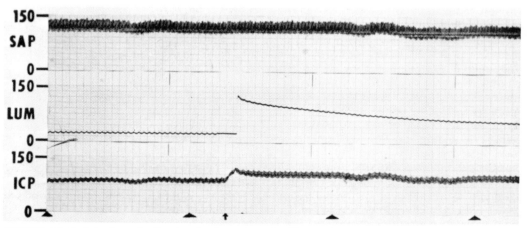

FIGURE 18–4 Injection of saline into lumbar subarachnoid space in a patient with complete obstruction to communication of pressure from the intracranial space to the spinal canal. Seven seconds after beginning of injection, intracranial pressure begins to rise (*arrow*), and at the completion of the injection, intracranial and lumbar pressures are equal. Spinal pressure then falls toward its previous level as intracranial tension remains at the level of the diastolic blood pressure. Time between triangles = one minute.

veins in normotensive subjects in the horizontal position. The largest fall in pressure per unit length of vessel is across the arterioles, but the loss of pressure across the arteries is also large. Small artery mean pressure in the dog averages 63 mm of mercury with a mean aortic pressure of 137 mm of mercury.[256] In other organs the peripheral resistance of the capillary bed is 20 to 30 per cent of total resistance, and presumably this holds true also for the brain.[150] The fall in pressure from the arterial to the venous end of the capillary is 15 to 20 mm of mercury, and mean cerebral capillary pressure is estimated to be 35 mm of mercury.[256]

The relationship of cerebral venous pressure to intracranial cerebrospinal fluid pressure has been controversial. It has been stated that the two pressures are always equal,[75, 108] that they are nearly always the same but that either pressure may exceed the other,[6] and that the sagittal sinus pressure is always greater than the cerebrospinal fluid pressure.[48] Cerebrospinal fluid pressure in man was found to always exceed jugular vein pressure.[200] It has been difficult to reconcile the observation that sagittal sinus or jugular vein pressure is higher than cerebrospinal fluid pressure with current concepts of bulk flow of the fluid into the sinuses through valves. The pressure gradient should always be from cerebrospinal fluid to blood. Recent detailed measurements by Shulman and Verdier in dogs indicate that sagittal sinus pressure is 60 per cent and torcular pressure 30 per cent of the cerebrospinal fluid pressure.[258] Pressures in cerebral veins and the sagittal sinus are about 14 mm and 7 mm of mercury respectively.[256, 258]

The arterioles are the most vasoactive portion of the vascular tree, but the arteries contribute significantly. This is evident in magnification angiography of cerebral vessels during procedures that alter vascular diameter. A venomotor system exists in some organs but not apparently in the brain, and the capillary bed is passive. The normal regulation of cerebral blood flow is considered elsewhere in this volume (Chapter 28). The following brief summary considers the physiology of cerebral blood flow as it is related to intravascular pressures, intracranial pressure, and brain volume. The cerebral resistance vessels have a high degree of resting vasoconstrictor tone. The origin of the tone is poorly understood and may be metabolic, myogenic, neurogenic, or some combination of the three mechanisms. An increase in the concentration of carbon dioxide, either in the blood or locally due to increased metabolism, dilates the resistance vessels and increases cerebral blood flow. The carbon dioxide may have a direct effect on the arteriolar wall, be mediated through a change in pH, or less likely, exert its effect through a chemoreceptor mechanism in the brain stem. Hypoxia also causes vascular dilatation, and hypocapnia and hyperoxygenation have the opposite effect.

A rise in systemic arterial pressure normally causes the resistance vessels to constrict. When the pressure falls, they dilate. This response, termed autoregulation, maintains blood flow constant through a wide range of perfusion pressures. The physiological basis of autoregulation has not been established, but a myogenic reflex seems to fit the facts best. The effective stimulus, according to this hypothesis, is a change in transmural pressure. A fall in cerebral arterial pressure lessens the difference between the intravascular and intracranial pressure, and the resistance vessels dilate. When the cerebral arterial pressure rises, the transmural pressure increases, and the vessels constrict.

The distribution of pressures across the cerebrovascular bed, from the large arteries to the jugular veins, is altered by changing the inflow pressure, the outflow pressure, the diameter of any segment of the system, or the external pressure (intracranial pressure). An increase in systemic arterial pressure is accompanied by constriction of the resistance vessels if autoregulation is intact. Cerebral venous pressure rises little if at all, indicating that the increased arterial pressure head is lost across the constricted vessels.[177] If autoregulation has failed, or during active dilatation of the resistance vessels as with carbon dioxide, a larger than normal portion of the arterial pressure head is communicated downstream to the capillary and venous beds, tending to dilate them. Cerebrovascular volume should then increase. Although capillaries appear not to dilate and constrict with changes in intraluminal tension, large portions of the capillary bed that are normally closed may open with increased inflow pressure.[303] Thus, capillary blood volume may be augmented by increased inflow pressure. There is evidence that the cerebral veins are nearly fully dilated at normal pressure, but congestion of surface veins has been described in many clinical and experimental circumstances.[258] Cerebral blood volume doubles with hypercapnia,[291] and carbon dioxide has a profound effect on intracranial pressure when the brain is swollen or a mass lesion is present.

Thus, dilatation of the resistance vessels is accompanied by an increase in pressure in capillaries and veins, and cerebral blood flow and blood volume increase. Obstruction of the venous outflow track also increases cerebral venous pressure and blood volume, but the pressure soon falls because of extensive venous collaterals. Occlusion of multiple cerebral veins, the sagittal sinus, or both lateral sinuses in the monkey fail to produce neurological deficits, demonstrating that cerebral blood flow is not critically reduced by these procedures.[205] However, sustained intracranial hypertension, presumably from cerebrovascular congestion and edema, occurs occasionally following bilateral radical neck dissections that include sacrifice of both internal jugular veins.[269]

These observations are helpful in understanding the effect of increased intracranial pressure on cerebral blood flow and the converse, the effect of changes in cerebral blood flow and blood volume on intracranial pressure. The equation for flow through rigid tubes only approximates the hemodynamics in organs and tissues, but is useful in attempting to define the effects of increased intracranial pressure on cerebral blood flow. The equation states:

$$\text{Flow} = \frac{(\text{inflow pressure} - \text{outflow pressure})\ \text{radius}^4}{\text{length} \times \text{viscosity}}$$

The total resistance to flow is the sum of the resistances in series from the carotid artery to the jugular vein. Thus, radius = r arteries + r arterioles + r capillaries + r veins + r dural sinuses. The length of the cerebrovascular tree changes very little.

Viscosity is an important factor, particularly in the capillary bed. It is ignored in the following discussion, however, because of lack of information on the effect of changes in intracranial pressure on cerebral blood viscosity. Then cerebral blood flow varies directly with changes in perfusion pressure and exponentially with the diameter of the cerebrovascular bed. If the arterioles (r arterioles) dilate and all the other factors in the equation remain the same, blood flow increases. If for any reason the diameter of another portion of the cerebrovascular bed is simultaneously diminished, this tends to counteract the arteriolar dilatation, because the total resistance to flow is the algebraic sum of all the resistances in series. Extravascular (intracranial) pressure does not appear in the equation. An increase in intracranial pressure can reduce flow either by decreasing the diameter of one or more portions of the cerebrovascular bed or by reducing the difference between the inflow and outflow pressures. The inflow pressure remains constant unless the intracranial hypertension induces a vasopressor response, and jugular vein pressure changes little during increased intracranial pressure.[155]

In early animal studies increased intracranial pressure was found to prolong cerebral circulation time, and by inference cerebral blood flow was believed to be decreased.[300] Cerebral blood flow was reduced slightly if at all in patients with increased intracranial pressure or supratentorial tumors in studies in which cerebral arteriovenous oxygen content differences were used.[37, 292] Kety et al. accurately measured cerebral blood flow in patients with the nitrous oxide technique and found subnormal values only when the intracranial pressure exceeded 450 mm of cerebrospinal fluid.[140] In recent animal experiments and clinical investigations, the relationship of intracranial pressure and cerebral blood flow has been found to be complex. Cerebral blood flow varied inversely with intracranial pressure in experiments in monkeys when electromagnetic flowmeters were used.[154] During rapid expansion of an extracerebral balloon, blood flow began to fall as soon as the intracranial pressure rose. These observations are at variance with those of Kety et al.[140] They were attributed to the rate of increase of intracranial pressure and the fact that the monkeys were under moderately deep barbiturate anesthesia. Huber et al. measured internal carotid and vertebral artery blood flow with electromagnetic flowmeters during expansion of an extradural balloon in different regions of the intracranial space.[114] The effect of increased pressure on blood flow varied with the location of the balloon, and this was attributed to differences in pressure across the intracranial space. Thus, blood flow was more reduced adjacent to the balloon, primarily because the difference between the arterial perfusion pressure and local tissue tension was less than in the opposite cerebral hemisphere. Zwetnow slowly infused artificial cerebrospinal fluid into the cisterna magna of dogs and demonstrated that cerebral blood flow, measured by the xenon-133 clearance method, did not fall until intracranial pressure reached a level within 40 to 50 mm of mercury of the mean arterial pressure.[304] Thus, the cerebral circulation is able to compensate, within limits, for rising intracranial pressure.

The complexity of the problem in human intracranial disease is emphasized by some early observations of Shenkin et al.[255] They found cerebral blood flow to be reduced in several patients with brain tumors and increased intracranial pressure, but blood flow was not significantly improved after the intracranial pressure had been reduced by ventricular drainage. Cronqvist and Lundberg found that spontaneous fluctuations in intraventricular pressure in brain tumor patients were accompanied by reciprocal changes in cerebral blood flow, but in several patients with prolonged sustained intracranial hypertension, reducing intracranial pressure with hypertonic mannitol had a paradoxical effect.[40] Fast flow (cerebral cortex) increased, but mean flow decreased with the fall in intracranial pressure. As intracranial pressure approaches the arterial pressure in patients with uncontrolled brain swelling, cerebral blood flow ceases. At this time the patient is comatose, and spontaneous respirations have ceased. Contrast material fails to enter the intracranial space.[153, 218, 279] A radioisotope injected into the carotid artery under high pressure does enter the intracranial space,

but fails to clear. This demonstrates total cerebral circulatory arrest and has been advocated as a test for brain death.[98]

What are the mechanisms responsible for maintenance of cerebral blood flow during rising intracranial pressure and for the decrease in blood flow that occurs when intracranial pressure exceeds certain limits? Wolff and Forbes observed the cortex through a cranial window during induced increases in intracranial pressure and noted consistent dilatation of the pial vessels.[301] When intracranial pressure was increased by injection of fluid into the spinal canal, diffuse cortical vascular dilatation was observed in monkeys in which the bone over a large portion of both cerebral hemispheres had been replaced by a transparent, watertight calvarium.[287] This vascular dilatation is the principal mechanism responsible for maintaining cerebral blood flow in the face or rising intracranial pressure and appears to represent a form of cerebral autoregulation dependent on the difference between the intravascular and extravascular pressures. If the pressure within small arteries and arterioles remains constant as intracranial pressure rises, the transmural pressure falls. This is equivalent to a decrease in arterial pressure, and the vessels dilate. In experiments in which the primary event is an induced rise in intracranial pressure, cerebral blood flow may be maintained, as noted, but it does not increase. According to the flow equation, therefore, the decrease in resistance manifested by arteriolar dilatation must be balanced by increased resistance elsewhere in the cerebrovascular tree.

Wright noted that bridging cerebral veins, observed through a cranial window, remained patent until rising intracranial pressure exceeded the blood pressure.[302] When collapse occurred, blood was forced proximally, indicating that the outflow resistance exceeded the resistance in the proximal vascular bed. He suggested that the intracranial hypertension caused constriction of the cerebral veins at their junction with the dural sinuses. This explanation has received support from more recent experiments by Hedges et al. and Greenfield and Tindall.[92, 107] Shulman and Verdier measured cerebral blood flow and cerebral venous pressure at various levels of intracranial pressure and derived values for resistances in the venous and prevenous beds.[258] During rising intracranial pressure the prevenous resistance decreased as the venous resistance rose. These observations further confirm the hypothesis that intracranial hypertension tends to collapse cortical veins and that the resultant increased resistance in the venous segment is counteracted by dilatation of the resistance vessels so as to maintain cerebral blood flow. Cerebral blood flow ultimately declines as intracranial tension continues to rise, because the region of maximum resistance shifts from the arterioles to the cerebral veins. Cerebral blood flow then becomes a function of intracranial pressure.

These observations apply to diffuse intracranial hypertension, in which it is assumed that pressure is distributed equally throughout the intracranial space and all vessels are subjected to the same physical forces. A space-occupying mass, however, produces vascular compression in the brain surounding the mass. Perhaps in the early stages these vessels are also able to dilate and maintain local cerebral blood flow, but ultimately the autoregulatory capacity of the vessels is overcome by the forces generated within the mass. Observations through the transparent calvarium demonstrate that the vascular collapse spreads circumferentially from a gradually expanding subdural balloon (Fig. 18–5).[287] At the same time cortical vessels remote from the balloon dilate as pressure rises throughout the intracranial space. If cerebral blood flow were measured at this time with the nitrous oxide technique, for example, total cerebral flow might be within the normal range. But regional cerebral blood flow measurements would demonstrate a marked reduction in flow in the vicinity of the mass. The local cerebral ischemia produces neurological signs appropriate to the region involved.

The collapse of vessels beneath the balloon is caused by the compressing force of the balloon. In cortex surrounding the balloon, the vessels are compressed by the overlying calvarium. The local increase in volume obliterates the subarachnoid space, and the surface of gyri adjacent to the balloon makes contact with the calvarium. Thus, the vascular collapse begins on the surface of gyri and involves arteries and

veins alike. It extends gradually from the vicinity of the balloon, in a circumferential manner, and at the same time the pallor spreads from the flattened gyri into the sulci. When most of the superficial vessels have been obliterated throughout much of the ipsilateral hemisphere, other vessels in deep sulci still contain blood. These observations were made in short-term experiments and simulate acute subdural and extradural hematomas, but they may not apply to chronic space-occupying lesions. Here there is more time for the cerebral vessels to compensate, and the amount of vascular compression may be less for a mass of the same size. Otherwise, it would be difficult to explain the absence of local neurological signs in so many patients with large chronic subdural hematomas and meningiomas.

Arteries resist compression more than veins because of higher intraluminal pressure and thicker walls. The dural sinuses have been considered to be essentially noncompressible because of their thick walls, internal trabeculations, and partial encasement in bone in the case of the transverse sinuses. Patterns of vascular collapse were studied in monkeys during marked changes in intracranial pressure produced by expansion and deflation of an extracerebral balloon.[160a] Sagittal sinus and intracranial pressures were measured continuously. The relationship of the two pressures was complex and seemed to be explained best by a combination of cerebral venous compression proximal to the sinus and compression of the sinus itself distal to the recording catheter.

Severe brain swelling developed in several animals.[250] When intracranial pressure had risen to the level of the diastolic pressure, after removal of the balloon, the animals were sacrificed by immersing their heads in liquid nitrogen. The frozen heads were sectioned in coronal planes with a band saw. Most of the cortical veins were obliterated by compression between the expanded brain and the inner table of the skull, and the lumen of the straight sinus was greatly narrowed. The sagittal sinus was narrow throughout much of its course. Obliteration of the lumen was found only in the region of the coronal suture (Fig. 18–6). This appears to occur because the

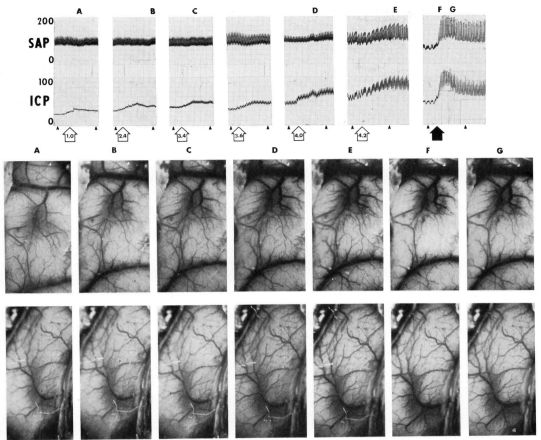

FIGURE 18–5 Gradual expansion of an intracranial balloon in a monkey with a watertight transparent calvarium. Balloon volume is indicated within the arrows. In *A* through *D*, intracranial pressure gradually rises, and cortical vessels dilate in both the right (*above*) and left (*below*) hemispheres. In *F*, prior to administration of norepinephrine, the animal is in shock, and intracranial pressure approaches the diastolic blood pressure. Vessels in sulci are still dilated at a time when vessels over the surface of gyri are collapsed. This is more marked on the side of the balloon (*above*). Following administration of norepinephrine (*black arrow*), systemic arterial pressure (SAP) and intracranial pressure (ICP) rise together, and some of the surface vessels are again filled with blood. Time between triangles in the polygraph tracings = two minutes.

sinus is partially encased in bone throughout much of its length, in the monkey, and is least so at the coronal suture. The transverse sinuses, which are surrounded by bone on three sides, were little affected. Arteries as well as veins were compressed, however, and in one animal the large single anterior cerebral artery characteristic of the rhesus monkey was nearly collapsed in its course over the corpus callosum. Sagittal sinus pressure is increased in hydrocephalic dogs and also has been attributed to partial collapse of the sinus.[259]

In summary, cerebral blood flow is maintained within normal limits, to rather high levels of intracranial pressure, by dilatation of the resistance vessels. This is probably a form of cerebral autoregulation that is induced by a decrease in the transmural pressure across the arteries and arterioles. At the same time as the arterioles dilate, the cerebral veins are compressed by the increase in intracranial pressure, and the decrease in resistance in the proximal vascular bed is matched by the increase in resistance in the veins. Net cerebrovascular resistance does not change, and cerebral blood flow remains constant. Pressure in the capillaries and veins increases because a larger portion of the arterial pressure head

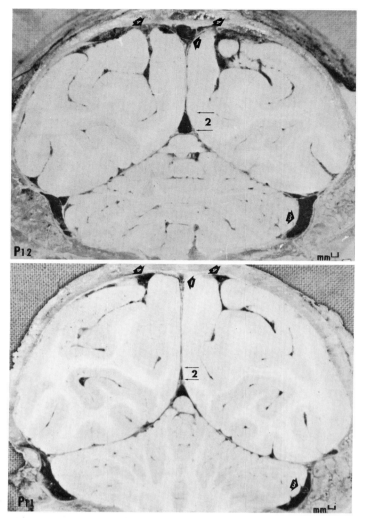

FIGURE 18–6 Coronal sections from a control (*top*) and a decompensated (*bottom*) animal at the level of the foramen magnum. In the latter, the sagittal sinus (1) and the straight sinus (2) are markedly constricted. Arrows indicate the vertical extent of the straight sinus. The sigmoid sinus (3) is patent. Two large sulci (4) persist in the decompensated animal and contain large fully patent veins that cannot be visualized at this magnification. The anteroposterior coordinate is indicated posterior (P) to the interaural line.

is released into the capacitance system by dilatation of the resistance vessels and because of the increased resistance in the venous outflow track. Cerebral blood volume increases, because blood is trapped between the arterioles and the sinuses, and the increased blood volume causes a further rise in intracranial pressure. Cerebral blood flow begins to fall because the increased resistance in the veins exceeds the vasodilatory capacity of the resistance vessels. As intracranial pressure approaches the blood pressure, the sinuses and arteries begin to collapse, and cerebral blood flow ceases when the two pressures are equal. This description undoubtedly is an oversimplification of the events and does not take into account regional differences in vasomotor reactivity and vascular compression. However, it does provide a model that can be used to evaluate a number of the clinical aspects of intracranial hypertension.

The final venous outflow pressure, in the jugular and vertebral veins, is affected little by the phenomena occurring within the intracranial space. Thus, the perfusion pressure to the brain varies only with the inflow pressure if the jugular vein pressure is accepted as a valid outflow pressure. But if one chooses the cerebral venous pressure as the outflow pressure, it rises in proportion to the rise in intracranial pressure. Applying the formula, cerebral blood flow ceases when the intracranial pressure equals the mean arterial pressure, because the perfusion pressure has been abolished. The alternative explanation, if the jugular vein pressure is used as the outflow pressure, is that one or more portions of the cerebrovascular bed have collapsed, and resistance is now infinite. This may be no more than an intellectual exercise, since the end-result is the same, but it does point up the importance of defining one's terms. It is often stated that the perfusion pressure to the brain is the difference between the arterial and intracranial pressure. This is true only if the pressure in the cerebral veins is accepted as the venous outflow pressure.

An increase in systemic venous pressure or obstruction of the great veins in the neck does increase cerebral venous outflow pressure and reduces perfusion pressure. In patients with venous obstruction produced by application of a tourniquet to the neck, however, cerebral blood flow did not fall with increases in jugular vein pressure of nearly 20 mm of mercury.[196] Similar observations have been made in dogs during transient occlusion of the superior vena cava.[121] This is probably another manifestation of autoregulation, but in this circumstance transmural pressure changes in the resistance vessels are difficult to predict. If the increased venous pressure is transmitted back along the cerebrovascular bed to the arterioles, increasing their intraluminal pressure, they should constrict, reducing cerebral blood flow. Intracranial pressure rises, however, because of the increased cerebral blood volume, and as noted, this should cause the arterioles to dilate.

Pressure Waves

It is customary to consider intracranial pressure as a rather steady phenomenon, but in clinical practice lumbar subarachnoid pressure is measured infrequently and for brief periods of time. Cerebrospinal fluid in a manometer pulsates synchronously with the heart rate, and superimposed respiratory oscillations are also present. When intracranial pressure is elevated both oscillations increase in amplitude. In addition, low amplitude 4 to 8 per second waves have been described by Lundberg in patients with intracranial hypertension.[172] They are synchronous with similar oscillations of blood pressure often referred to as Traube-Herring-Mayer waves. The latter were first described by several investigators in the nineteenth century in animals with experimental intracranial hypertension. They also occur in normal patients and seem to be of little clinical significance.

Over the years spontaneous fluctuations in cerebrospinal fluid pressure of greater magnitude have been described in occasional patients with intracranial lesions. Guillaume and Janny studied these pressure phenomena in some detail and commented particularly on large paroxysmal waves that developed for no apparent rea-

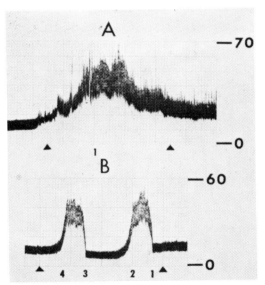

FIGURE 18-7 Continuous recording of intracranial pressure in a patient following removal of an acoustic neurinoma. *A.* Fall in intracranial pressure produced by respiratory assistance with 40 per cent oxygen (1). *B.* Rapid changes in intracranial pressure when the respirator was removed (1 and 3) and when respiratory assistance with 40 per cent oxygen was reinstituted (2 and 4). Time between triangles = 30 minutes.

son and were sometimes seen in association with flushing of the face.[97] They attributed them to disturbances in vasomotor control of the cerebral circulation. Lundberg recorded intraventricular pressure on a strip chart recorder for periods of days to weeks.[172] Three types of pressure waves (A, B, and C) were described in his patients. Only the A waves were found to be of clinical significance and were observed in 21 of 48 patients. The A waves were divided into two types: rhythmic fluctuations in pressure occurring in 15 to 30 minute intervals, and "plateau waves" that persisted for longer periods of time. The rhythmic 2 to 4 per hour waves began spontaneously from a base of mild to moderately elevated intracranial tension, rose to values of 60 to 100 mm of mercury, and then subsided. Plateau waves were often in excess of 100 mm of mercury. Evacuation of ventricular fluid was always accompanied by a prompt fall in pressure.

Pressure waves also have been observed in postoperative craniotomy patients. Frequently they develop without apparent cause and can almost always be induced by hypoxia and hypercapnia. Figure 18–7 illustrates the intracranial pressure record-

ing in a patient a few hours after excision of an acoustic neurinoma. Following the operation, intracranial pressure, recorded continuously with a catheter in the subdural space, gradually increased to approximately 50 mm of mercury, then fell promptly when respiratory assistance with 40 per cent oxygen and room air was instituted (*A*). In *B* intracranial pressure rose each time the respirator was removed, then fell to the control value when it was re-applied. Figure 18–8 illustrates intracranial and systemic arterial pressures, the latter recorded from a catheter in the radial artery, in a patient following removal of a recurrent pituitary adenoma. Respiration was assisted during the postoperative period. Intracranial pressure rose abruptly when the respirator was removed and fell immediately to the control value when it was reapplied. Subsequently a plateau wave developed, accompanied by an increase in blood pressure, and at this time the intracranial pressure was unresponsive to hyperventilation. Both pressures fell rapidly after administration of hypertonic mannitol.

The ease of inducing pressure waves by hypoxia and hypercapnia, their response to hyperventilation, and their enhancement by

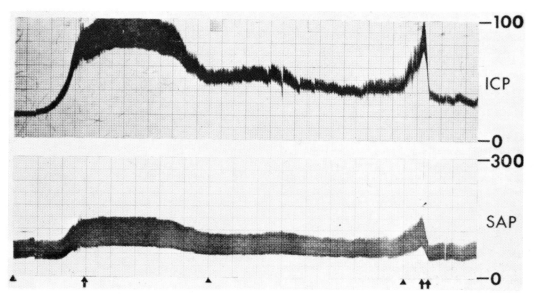

FIGURE 18–8 Continuous recording of intracranial pressure in a patient following removal of a recurrent pituitary adenoma. Response of intracranial pressure (ICP) and blood pressure (SAP) to withdrawal (*first arrow*), and reinstitution (*second arrow*) of respiratory assistance. Subsequently, a spontaneous increase in intracranial and blood pressures occurred. An infusion of mannitol was begun (*third arrow*), and both pressures fell rapidly. Time between triangles = two hours.

an arterial pressor response favor alterations in cerebral blood volume as the most likely cause. An increase in cerebral blood flow is accompanied by a rise in intracranial pressure, and the effect on intracranial pressure is greater if the initial pressure is elevated.[154, 241] Intracranial pressure rises during sleep, and in patients with space-occupying intracranial lesions, the pressure may increase to alarming levels.[36]

The intracranial hypertension is due to increased cerebral blood flow and blood volume either from respiratory depression and hypercapnia or from increased cerebral metabolism, as in rapid eye movement sleep. The increase in regional cerebral blood volume produced by increased metabolic activity has been demonstrated to be accompanied by augmentation of regional cerebral blood volume, and recently Risberg et al. have clearly demonstrated increased cerebral blood volume during plateau waves in one patient with intracranial hypertension of unknown origin and in a second patient with an unverified cerebral glioma.[225] Halothane anesthesia increases cerebral blood flow and produces a moderate rise in intracranial pressure.[183] In brain tumor patients, however, intracranial pressure may rise to dangerously high levels.[133] Thus, hypoxia and hypercapnia dilate cerebral vessels and in normal man and animals cause a small increase in intracranial pressure. However, on the vertical portion of the volume-pressure graph, when most of the displaceable cerebrospinal fluid has been eliminated from the intracranial space, a small increase in blood volume produces an enormous rise in pressure. Therefore, mild respiratory insufficiency that may have no effect on brain function in normal patients can cause severe intracranial hypertension and a critical reduction in cerebral blood flow in patients with brain swelling or a space-occupying mass.

The origin of the pressure waves that occur in adequately ventilated patients is unknown, but those who have studied the problem have attributed them to an instability of cerebral vasomotor tone. Cairns discussed the role of vascular factors in cerebral swelling and commented on the sudden increase in brain bulk that occurs occasionally during marked retraction over deep-seated tumors in the absence of airway obstruction.[25] The swollen brain was always congested in his experience, and he inferred that the retraction caused damage to a mechanism, perhaps in the brain stem, that influences the vasoconstrictor tone of cerebral vessels. Rapid generalized swelling of the brain was produced by LeBeau and Bonvallet with lesions in the midbrain of cats.[165] Obrador and Pi-Suñer caused the brain to swell acutely with mechanical lesions in the floor of the fourth ventricle.[203] Both groups of authors attributed the swelling to sudden vascular dilatation. Their observations are intriguing, because they suggest that cerebral vasomotor tone is in part regulated by a neurogenic mechanism in the brain stem. Recent attempts to reproduce their findings, however, have failed.[160a]

Cerebral Edema

The study of cerebral swelling has occupied investigators since the dawn of the neurological sciences. Because the brain is encased in bone and has little room for expansion, progressive brain swelling ultimately causes a rise in intracranial pressure, and in clinical practice and experimental studies, the signs and symptoms of cerebral edema are difficult to distinguish from those of intracranial hypertension. Thus, cerebral edema and increased intracranial pressure are inseparable problems.

In the past the terms cerebral swelling and cerebral edema have often been used interchangeably despite evidence that cerebrovascular congestion and multiple small hemorrhages contribute to the increase in brain bulk in many circumstances. The most important recent development has been demonstration of the interrelationship of changes in the cerebral circulation, brain volume, and intracranial pressure. Edema and intracranial hypertension, from whatever cause, damage the brain by interference with cerebral blood flow and metabolism, but of equal importance is the fact that primary injuries to the cerebral circulation can induce or aggravate edema so as to cause further embarrassment of cerebral blood flow.

Nearly all forms of insult to the brain

can upset cerebral water balance and lead to edema. The following clinical conditions have been chosen for discussion because they are common problems, and cerebral edema is or appears to be a significant part of the pathophysiology of each of them.

Head Injuries

The occurrence and clinical significance of cerebral edema following acute head injury has been a subject of debate for many decades. Analysis of the incidence of brain swelling has been based on pathological examination of the brain, clinical signs, including cerebrospinal fluid pressure measurements, and observations of the brain at the time of operation.

Some confusion has been generated in pathological studies by the failure to distinguish between focal cerebral edema in the vicinity of gross hemorrhages or contusions and diffuse cerebral edema with little or no evidence of structural brain damage. Edema was described in brain surrounding an intracerebral hemorrhage before the turn of the century.[108, 280] Courtney described the edema associated with cerebral contusions and emphasized the coalescence of perifocal edemas.[38] He stated that contusion and edema are constant features of severe head injury. Diffuse traumatic edema was described by Apfelbach, among others, but Greenfield stated that he had never seen diffuse cerebral edema following craniocerebral trauma.[1, 91]

Lumbar puncture has been performed frequently for measurement of intracranial pressure in patients with head injuries and is still employed routinely in many neurosurgical clinics. In the absence of a space-occupying hematoma, an increase in intracranial pressure has been considered indirect evidence of brain swelling or cerebral edema and has been one of the principal criteria used in the management of these patients. Moderate intracranial hypertension was described by many observers, but a marked increase in pressure was rare.[119, 181, 182] Browder and Meyers carefully studied several patients following acute head injury and measured the lumbar subarachnoid pressure on several occasions.[16, 17] Among four patients who died from their injuries, only one had elevated

pressure at the time of the last spinal tap prior to death. The authors concluded that increased intracranial pressure is not a significant cause of death following head injury. In contrast, at the operating table, Dandy found marked swelling of the brain to be the rule in severely injured patients and concluded that death in the acute stage following head injury is due almost entirely to brain swelling and increased intracranial pressure.[45a] Dandy and others stated that spinal fluid pressure is not an accurate index of intracranial pressure in the presence of marked elevation of the latter.[130, 204, 221, 260]

It seems safe to conclude that brain swelling is a frequent if not invariable sequela to severe craniocerebral trauma, and failure to recognize its presence by many investigators in the past probably is attributable to undue reliance on spinal fluid pressure measurements as a precise reflection of intracranial pressure and to disagreements on the pathological criteria of cerebral edema. The importance of continuous measurement of intracranial pressure in the evaluation of intracranial dynamics following head injury has been demonstrated clearly by Lundberg et al.[174] They observed marked intracranial hypertension, as high as 115 mm of mercury, during continuous recording of intraventricular pressure in patients with severe head injuries but without evidence of a space-occupying mass. Troupp found intracranial hypertension to be present in 15 of 18 patients with generalized brain injury, and similar observations were made by Kaufmann and Clark.[137, 278]

Ischemia and Anoxia

Cerebral edema occurs in a variety of clinical conditions that have as their common denominator cerebral hypoxia. Focal cerebral edema develops around a hemorrhagic or ischemic infarction, probably on the same pathological basis as the perifocal edema around contusions. Shaw et al. reviewed the time course and extent of edema following ischemic infarction in numerous previous clinical studies and presented a large series of their own patients.[253] Among those patients who died during the first week following onset of symptoms, there was almost always marked swelling of the brain with evidence of transtentorial herniation, and the authors concluded that nearly all these patients died as a direct result of brain swelling and increased intracranial pressure. In those who died more than two weeks after the onset of hemiplegia, evidence of brain swelling was minimal, and death was attributed to some other cause. Plum studied 106 patients who were diagnosed clinically to have relatively large cerebral infarctions.[213] Approximately 1 in 5 showed clinical signs of brain swelling manifested by a progressive rostrocaudal brain stem dysfunction starting in the upper diencephalon. Plum concluded that some cerebral edema probably develops in the vicinity of all acute cerebral infarcts, but most patients survive despite the edema. Since nearly all patients who die following cerebral infarction are comatose for a significant period of time prior to death, pulmonary insufficiency and diffuse cerebral hypoxia may contribute to the focal edema, and particularly to edema in brain tissue that might have been spared by the infarction. In Plum's series many patients had significant oxygen desaturation of the arterial blood, but he was unable to establish a consistent relationship between the blood gas values and the patient's clinical course. Severe abnormalities in acid-base balance and blood oxygenation also develop in the majority of comatose patients following craniocerebral trauma, and several investigations have established a good correlation between arterial oxygen saturation, level of consciousness, and survival.[35, 112, 201, 262] The contribution of cerebral edema to the mortality in these patients, however, has not been determined.

It has been generally accepted that many of the structural changes in the brain ordinarily associated with cerebral edema are indistinguishable from those produced by anoxia,[39] but the significance of cerebral edema, as opposed to primary neuronal damage, in the mortality from asphyxia has not been cleared established. Chronic pulmonary insufficiency can cause gradually progressive brain swelling and intracranial hypertension manifested by headache, drowsiness, and papilledema.[3, 33] In many of these patients all the neurological signs and symptoms appear to be attributable to the brain swelling. Therefore, this syndrome could represent clinical evidence of cerebral edema secondary to prolonged mild anoxia. However, these patients also have varying degrees of hypercapnia and increased venous pressure from cor pulmonale. On the basis of the present evidence the relative contributions of hypoxia, hypercapnia, and increased cerebral venous pressure to the syndrome cannot be stated.

Increased venous pressure has been implicated in the brain swelling observed in several clinical conditions. Evidence of increased intracranial pressure may follow extensive destruction of intracranial venous outflow in the neck, and bilateral jugular ligation alone may be sufficient to cause transient intracranial hypertension.[269] At one time thrombosis of the intracranial venous sinuses was considered the most common cause of pseudotumor cerebri, and there is still convincing evidence that thrombosis of the lateral sinus can cause this syndrome.[12, 274]

Tumors

Marked swelling of the brain surrounding intracranial mass lesions has been amply demonstrated. This form of perifocal edema has aroused particular interest, because it may occur in the absence of necrosis either within the tumor or the brain. This distinguishes it from the edema of contusion or ischemic necrosis, which might be considered simply as an outpouring of fluid from disrupted capillary walls into the surrounding brain. Metastatic carcinoma, in particular, causes such a profound reaction of the surrounding brain that a small metastasis may cause diffuse swelling of the entire hemisphere. A similar degree of swelling is also encountered with subdural hematomas, and the patient's signs and symptoms of increased intracranial pressure may be more the result of the swelling than of the hematoma.[18, 34, 184]

Arterial Hypertension

A form of cerebral swelling that continues to occupy considerable attention, mainly because of the difficulty in establishing its incidence and etiology, is that associated with arterial hypertension. Fishberg described a syndrome consisting of seizures and a variety of focal neurological signs and symptoms in patients with advanced hypertension, and subsequently described two major types of hypertensive encephalopathy.[67] The first of these probably is caused by intermittent cerebrovascular insufficiency and constitutes what are now called transient ischemic attacks. The second type, consisting of seizures, increased intracranial pressure, and a very high blood pressure was attributed by Fishberg to cerebral vasospasm. The vasospasm results in cerebral ischemia followed by edema. Byrom and Meyer and colleagues have provided experimental evidence to support this etiology.[23, 190, 191] Pharmacological agents such as caffeine and aminophylline that increase cerebrovascular resistance may be effective in the treatment of this form of hypertensive encephalopathy. Moyer and associates concluded that cerebral vasodilatation rather than vascular spasm was the underlying cause of brain swelling associated with hypertension.[197, 198] They postulated that decreased tone in the resistance vessels permitted transmission of pressure to the capillary and venous beds followed by passage of fluid into the brain parenchyma. If their hypothesis is correct, this is probably a form of cerebral vasomotor paralysis.[155]

Toxic and Metabolic Disorders

Cerebral edema has also been described in a wide variety of toxic and metabolic disorders. In most conditions the diagnosis has been made clinically by the presence of the usual signs of intracranial hypertension, but pathological examination of the brain has been carried out in a few patients who have died from the cerebral insult or from other effects of the toxic agent. Among the toxic encephalopathies, arsphenamine poisoning received the most attention at a time when this agent was used extensively in the treatment of syphilis. Scheinker described the pathological findings in the brains of five patients who died from arsphenamine poisoning.[245] The principal finding was severe damage to the small blood vessels of the brain, which Scheinker attributed to "central vasoparalysis." The brains were similar in appearance to those

of patients who died following severe craniocerebral trauma, and Scheinker postulated a common etiology of vascular stasis, capillary necrosis, and edema. Acute cerebral edema has also been described in association with severe allergic phenomena and has generally been attributed to cerebral vasodilatation and increased capillary permeability, perhaps secondary to histamine or a similar substance.[41] The form of toxic cerebral edema most commonly encountered today is in lead encephalopathy.

Pseudotumor Cerebri

The condition known as pseudotumor cerebri includes brain swelling produced by a variety of causes, many of which are not known or are incompletely understood. Continued study of this group of patients should help to elucidate the more obscure causes of cerebral edema. Numerous terms have been used to describe brain swelling or intracranial hypertension of uncertain cause, and several are of historical interest only. The condition was originally termed "serous meningitis" because of the belief that the increased intracranial pressure was due to excess cerebrospinal fluid.[219] The association of increased intracranial pressure with infections of the middle ear and mastoid led Symonds to suggest the term "otitic hydrocephalus," and he postulated that the principal pathological mechanism was thrombosis of the lateral sinus.[274] It was not until the report of Dandy, describing the radiographic appearance of the ventricles in these cases, that the location of the excess fluid was clearly understood.[46] The ventricles were normal, or somewhat reduced in size, and there was no evidence of an enlarged cerebral subarachnoid space. Thus, it was apparent that the cause of the intracranial hypertension was brain swelling. Since that time there have been numerous reports of large series of patients, and most authors have had as their primary objective a sorting out of the many possible etiological factors.

Initially an attempt was made to identify those cases secondary to middle ear infection. This appeared to be the cause of the pseudotumor in 61 per cent of the cases analyzed by Bradshaw, but in only 18 per cent of Foley's cases.[12, 72] A pseudotumor syndrome has been described following rather mild head injury, and in some patients there is a history of antecedent systemic infection.[72, 178] One of the striking features of this condition, noted by early observers and emphasized in nearly all recent studies, is the high incidence in obese females.[12, 46, 72, 244] Foley also remarked on the association of brain swelling with pregnancy and menstrual disturbances.[72] Interest is now centered on this group of patients and others who have pseudotumor in association with hormonal or metabolic abnormalities.

In 1899, Klippel described a patient with Addison's disease who died following a short illness consisting of delirium, convulsions, and coma.[143] At postmortem examination there was marked swelling of the brain. Numerous additional examples of brain swelling in association with adrenocortical insufficiency have been reported since that time.[85] Also, there have been many case reports of the development of a pseudotumor syndrome following reduction or discontinuation of prolonged corticosteroid therapy in children with asthma, eczema, nephrosis, rheumatoid arthritis, and other systemic disorders.[93, 282] Reduction in 17-ketosteroid excretion has been demonstrated during the period of increased intracranial pressure, and all those who have written on the subject agree that the cerebral edema is due to adrenocortical insufficiency rather than to a toxic effect of the steroid preparation. Rarely the syndrome has developed without a reduction in corticosteroid therapy, but this may be explained by an increased requirement for steroid, as during infection.[8] Greer presented several cases of pseudotumor developing at puberty and postulated that this also was on the basis of transient adrenal insufficiency; the increase in estrogen secretion inhibits the production of adrenocorticoids.[95] Pseudotumor has also been described in patients with dysmenorrhea and during pregnancy.[85, 94, 96]

Goldzieher et al. reported two patients with hyperthyroidism and central nervous system signs and symptoms suggesting pseudotumor cerebri.[88] This association, however, appears to be quite rare. Many neurological syndromes have been described in hypothyroidism, including psychiatric disorder, peripheral neuropathy, deafness, and vertigo. Somnolence, decrease in visual acuity, and increased spinal fluid pressure have also been considered, in several patients, as evidence of a pseudotumor syndrome. The finding that 17-ketosteroid excretion is diminished in myxedema suggests again a common cause of the pseudotumor produced by many hormonal disturbances. Glowacki et al. have proposed a combined hormonal-metabolic scheme of disorders to account for these edemas.[85]

In a recent review of 23 cases of pseudotumor in the pediatric age group, Rose and Matson found four children with otitis media, eight with infections other than otitis media, four with a recent history of craniocerebral trauma, and one in whom steroid therapy had been abruptly withdrawn.[229] The possible etiology was obscure in the remainder. A pseudotumor syndrome also has been described in patients with subacute sclerosing leukoencephalitis, as a complication of tetracycline therapy, and following bee sting.[65, 84, 86, 146]

It is common practice, in the absence of a space-occupying lesion, to attribute the signs and symptoms of increased intracranial pressure to cerebral edema. This raises the issue whether cerebral edema per se has a deleterious effect on brain function or whether it causes neurological signs and symptoms only by elevation of intracranial pressure or displacement of cerebral tissue. Few neuronal changes have been found in studies of both clinical and experimental cerebral edema. Windle et al. emphasized the morphological integrity of the neurons in edematous brain by comparing the histological appearance of animal brains swollen by water intoxication and those submitted to severe craniocerebral trauma.[295] Although most attention has been directed toward the glia in experimental brain edema, many investigators have commented that the neurons are normal in appearance or slightly shrunken. The shrinkage was attributed to fixation artifact.

Despite these observations, neuropathologists have generally accepted the concept that cerebral edema causes damage to the brain by producing capillary compression, reduced cerebral blood flow, neuronal damage, and more edema. The problem cannot be solved with the clinical information currently available, because any structural changes in the brain attributable to cerebral edema might just as well have been caused by ischemia induced by increased intracranial pressure. Furthermore, focal neurological signs attributable to cerebral edema surrounding a mass lesion may not be the result of the edema. If the expanding mass causes vascular collapse in the adjacent brain, the decrease in regional cerebral blood flow could account for both the edema and the neuronal damage. Both processes then are independent results of the ischemia. A similar problem is encountered in evaluating the origin of the signs and symptoms of cerebral edema produced by toxic agents. Assuming that the brain swelling is focal, or that diffuse edema is gradual in development and insufficient to cause significant intracranial hypertension, it is necessary to demonstrate that the toxic agent does not have a direct effect on neurons in order to attribute its deleterious effects to edema.

Despite the lack of convincing evidence that an increase in the water content of the brain disturbs neuronal function, there are several possible mechanisms whereby edema might cause brain damage. Microangiography of the brains of rats made edematous by triethyl tin poisoning has demonstrated severe changes in small cerebral vessels.[210] Marked tortuosity of small arteries was present in both gray and white matter, and segmental narrowing and dilatation of the vessels also were observed. However, these alterations were present only in the advanced stages of cerebral edema, at which time there was also evidence of increased intracranial pressure. Even though neurons may not become edematous, a change in their external environment incident to the edema could cause dysfunction. The resting and action potentials of the neuron depend on an unequal distribution of ions across its membrane. Thus, the inside of the neuron is approximately 70 mv negative to the outside by virtue of a high internal potassium concentration. The sodium content of the neuron is low in the resting state, but during depolarization of its membrane a rapid influx of sodium occurs. When the sodium or potassium concentration is changed in either the external or internal environment of the neuron, a corresponding alteration in neuronal excitation occurs. Investigations to date indicate that extracellular edema fluid contains these important cations in the same concentration as exists normally. Thus, the incomplete evidence available would suggest that neither the neurons nor the fluid in the extracellular space bathing them are significantly altered in composition. An exception is water intoxication, but the ratio of intracellular and extracellular ion concentrations in this condition is not known.

A strong argument could be made for interference in neuronal metabolism by cerebral edema if one assumes that the extracellular space in the brain is small to begin with and that the transport of nutrients to the nerve cells from the capillary must occur through glia. Swelling of the glia might well disrupt transport mechanisms sufficiently to deprive the neurons of oxygen and metabolites. The general acceptance now of a significant functional extracellular space in the brain decreases the possible significance of this mechanism. Even though the extracellular space serves as the pathway for exchange of materials between blood and the neurons, it could be argued that this space is obliterated by swelling of glial cells preventing adequate transport of metabolites to the neurons.

Finally, neurons may be displaced so far from a capillary that they are deprived of adequate nutrition. This theory is based on the Krogh model, which considers the diffusion of oxygen and metabolites from blood to neurons.[148] Since the maximum increase in cerebral volume that can be accommodated within the closed intracranial space is approximately 10 per cent, it is highly unlikely that a neuron would be significantly removed from its capillary by diffuse cerebral edema. Even with focal cerebral edema in which local volume may be increased by 50 per cent or more, this mechanism seems to be an unlikely explanation for neuronal dysfunction.

In neurosurgical experience, the gradual development, then subsidence, of focal neurological signs and symptoms following intracranial surgery for various disorders are strongly suggestive of cerebral edema. The time course is often similar to that described by Shaw et al. in patients with ischemic infarctions of the cerebral hemispheres.[253] If increased intracranial pressure can be ruled out in these patients, the clinical picture is most likely due to a direct effect of edema on neuronal function. However, diffuse cerebral edema, as in pseudotumor cerebri, may be severe enough to cause marked intracranial hypertension without evidence of cerebral dysfunction. This may be explained by the quantity of water that can accumulate within the closed intracranial space in diffuse and focal edema. Normally cerebrospinal fluid occupies no more than 10 per cent of the intracranial space. Thus, if expansion of the brain were sufficiently great to obliterate all these spaces including the ventricles, the increase in the volume of the brain would be 10 per cent. Assuming an average weight of the human brain of 1200 gm, 78 per cent or 936 gm is water. If the brain expands by 10 per cent of its original weight, it now weighs 1320 gm. If all of this increase in volume is water, the water content of the 1320-gm brain is 1056 gm. The water content is now 80 per cent compared to the 78 per cent in the control. Therefore, "maximum" diffuse cerebral edema is produced by a 2 per cent increase in water content. If the distribution of increased water were equal throughout gray and white matter, it should not interfere with brain function in the absence of raised pressure. On the other hand, if the edema is confined to a small region, a much greater accumulation of water can occur before the cerebrospinal fluid buffer space is exhausted. Using the same data, a 120-gm segment of brain could expand by 100 per cent of its original weight before all the cerebrospinal fluid had been expressed from the intracranial space. The water content under these circumstances would increase from 78 per cent to 91 per cent, and interference with metabolism would be more likely but by no means certain. In conclusion, there is no clear evidence that cerebral edema per se disturbs brain function, because it is difficult to evaluate the contributions of increased intracranial and local tissue pressures.

CLINICAL DIAGNOSIS

Signs and Symptoms of Increased Intracranial Pressure

Few of the signs and symptoms ordinarily attributed to intracranial hypertension are actually due to the increased pressure. Intracranial pressure may reach high levels in pseudotumor cerebri, yet the patient shows little evidence of it. Headache usually is not severe, certainly less so than in many patients with brain tumors and intracranial hypertension. Vomiting is uncommon, and the patient is alert and feels well. But papilledema may be severe enough to threaten the patient's vision. The benign course of pseudotumor is due to the fact that the brain swells diffusely, intracranial pressure is equal throughout the craniospinal axis, and the brain is displaced little if at all. Sixth nerve palsies occur and are attributed to stretching of the nerve by caudal displacement (axial distortion) of the brain stem, but sixth nerve palsy is uncommon.

The headache associated with changes in intracranial pressure was described in detail by Wolff.[299] The pain-sensitive structures within the intracranial space are the middle meningeal artery and its branches, the large arteries at the base of the brain, the sinuses and bridging veins, and the dura at the base of the cranial fossae. Headache was regularly induced in subjects in the erect position by withdrawal of cerebrospinal fluid. The headache was nearly always frontal or at the vertex. It developed at approximately the same reduction in pressure among all subjects and disappeared promptly when the pressure was returned to normal by injection of saline into the subarachnoid space.

Wolff elevated intracranial pressure to values as high as 850 mm of cerebrospinal fluid for one to two minutes by intrathecal injections of saline. Headache was never recorded. Similar observations were made by Ryder et al. in subjects whose intracranial pressure was elevated to values of 500 to 1000 mm of cerebrospinal fluid by inflation of a cuff around the neck or by the Valsalva maneuver.[236, 239] Nine per cent of patients with elevated pressure developed headache, but a skull defect was present in most of them, and the pain was localized to the region of the defect. Since intracranial pressure was elevated by artificial means in these patients for short periods of time, it could be argued that the procedures did not simulate clinical intracranial hypertension. The pressure waves described by Lundberg occurred spontaneously.[172] Pressure waves to 60 to 70 mm of mercury occurred in his patients without headache or other symptoms of increased intracranial pressure.

Thus, increased intracranial pressure even to very high levels is a rare cause of headache. This is explained by the postulated cause of headache with decreased intracranial pressure, or more properly with a decrease in cerebrospinal fluid volume. The brain rests on a cushion of fluid. When the volume of fluid is reduced, the brain sinks with the patient in the erect position or shifts to the dependent side when the patient is horizontal. At the same time cerebral vessels, particularly the veins, dilate to compensate for the reduction in cerebrospinal fluid volume. The combination of venous dilatation and traction on the bridging cerebral veins and stretching of the arteries at the base cause headache. When intracranial pressure is increased diffusely, displacement of and traction on blood vessels are minimal, insufficient to stimulate pain receptors, and headache does not occur. It follows that traction on blood vessels or compression and invasion of the pain-sensitive dura at the base of the cranium, not increased intracranial pressure, is the cause of headache in patients with space-occupying lesions.

The headache associated with increased intracranial pressure is often severe on awakening in the morning and is relieved by vomiting. Intracranial pressure increases during sleep and can reach dangerously high levels in patients with space-occupying lesions.[36] The most likely explanation is that there is brain swelling from vascular dilatation and perhaps edema that is secondary to carbon dioxide retention. Lundberg noted that pressure waves were terminated by vomiting when the vomiting was accompanied by hyperventilation.[172] Following on this argument, the headache is not due to the increased pressure but to increased traction or displacement of blood vessels produced by the brain swelling.

The cause of nausea and vomiting in patients with increased intracranial pressure is poorly understood. Vomiting that occurs without nausea suggests intracranial disease, particularly when it is precipitate. Since vomiting was not observed in the patients of Wolff and Ryder et al. with artificially induced increased intracranial pressure, it may also be more a function of displacement of intracranial structures than of pressure.

Papilledema is the only reliable clinical sign of increased intracranial pressure. The other neurological signs attributed to or associated with intracranial hypertension, such as sixth nerve palsy and the signs of tentorial or foramen magnum herniation, are due to displacement of brain tissue. The mechanisms of herniation are complex, and increased pressure albeit small may be necessary as the driving force behind the herniation. This raises again the issue of tissue pressure and intracranial pressure. If pressure or force in the medial temporal lobe adjacent to a tumor in the temporal fossa is increased, without elevated pressure in the rest of the intracranial cavity, herniation can occur without raised "intracranial pressure." In practice most patients with tentorial pressure cones do have a diffuse rise in intracranial tension.

Half of brain tumor patients have papilledema at the time the diagnosis is made. Some authors have attributed the absence of papilledema in the other half to anatomical variations of the optic nerve, sheath space, or papilla that preclude the development of papilledema. Local anomalies may account for the occasional finding of unilateral papilledema in a patient with a posterior fossa lesion, but most patients with brain tumor and no papilledema probably do not have increased intracranial pressure sufficient to cause it.

Changes in Vital Signs

Early clinical investigations of increased intracranial pressure suggested that changes in blood pressure, heart rate, and respiration might serve as an accurate index of the onset and degree of intracranial hypertension. Kocher defined four stages of cerebral compression and intracranial hypertension, based on changes in the vital signs and level of consciousness.[145] However his observations did not receive wide attention until the experiments of Cushing demonstrated that "an increase of intracranial tension occasions a rise of blood pressure which tends to find a level slightly above that of the pressure exerted above the medulla."[42–44] The increase in arterial pressure did not occur until the intracranial pressure approached or equalled the mean arterial pressure, and thereafter the two pressures rose together. Cushing also emphasized the importance of bradycardia and respiratory irregularities, but it is clear from his writings that he considered arterial hypertension the most diagnostic of the changes in vital signs. Cushing's observations were confirmed by many writers in the early part of the century, and Janeway stated that the highest blood pressures ever recorded were in patients with severe increased intracranial pressure.[123] The Cushing criteria were used particularly in the management of patients with head injuries, but several authors expressed the opinion that blood pressure was of little value in the management of head injuries.[119, 221, 252] Browder and Meyers recorded blood pressure and spinal fluid pressure intermittently in patients following head injury and found that blood pressure may be high without increased intracranial pressure, intracranial pressure may be elevated without a change in blood pressure, and blood pressure may increase as intracranial pressure is falling.[16] They concluded that changes in the arterial pressure were of no value in the diagnosis of cerebral compression and increased intracranial pressure. Evans and associates increased intracranial pressure to values in excess of 1000 mm of water by lumbar injections without necessarily altering the blood pressure.[59, 239]

Many of the clinical studies were limited by a failure to demonstrate that patients who did not have increased arterial pressure did in fact have increased intracranial pressure. Kjallquist et al. recorded intraventricular fluid pressure (VFP) and arterial pressure continuously in brain tumor patients preoperatively.[141] They related spontaneous fluctuations in intracranial pressure, previously described in detail by Lundberg, to the arterial pressure.[172] Blood pressure did not increase with VFP as high as 70 mm of mercury; but Lundberg, in a personal communication, has observed arterial hypertension at the peak of VFP "plateau waves" that often exceed 100 mm of mercury. In postcraniotomy patients an inconstant relationship was found between intracranial and blood pressures.[152] In some patients intracranial pressure rose to the level of the mean arterial pressure without provoking a pressor response, whereas in others marked sustained increases in blood pressure occurred with intracranial pressure waves of relatively low magnitude. One can conclude from these many clinical observations that arterial hypertension may be a direct result of rising intracranial pressure, a true "Cushing response," but that the vasopressor response is an inconstant phenomenon. Experimental data in animals suggest that the nature and location of the lesion are as important in determining the threshold and amplitude of the arterial pressor response as is the level of intracranial hypertension.[288]

Expansion of a supratentorial mass in experimental animals almost always causes an arterial pressor response. The response persists following removal of the cerebral hemispheres and progressive maceration of the brain stem to a level at the superior border of the inferior olive, but with further destruction of the medulla it disappears.[74] Therefore, the vasopressor response to cerebral compression appears to arise in the medulla. It is accompanied by marked peripheral vasoconstriction that appears to be neurogenic in origin, and it is abolished by sympathectomy.[19, 61, 76] Several mechanisms have been proposed to explain the vasopressor response. Cushing, following upon the earlier hypothesis of Kocher, believed that an increase in arterial pressure did not occur until the rise in intracranial pressure was sufficient to cause ischemia of the medullary vasomotor center. This was based primarily on the observation that arterial hypertension did not occur until intracranial pressure approached the level of the blood pressure, at which time it was assumed blood flow throughout the brain must be nearly abolished. Dickinson and McCubbin, however, found the vasopressor threshold in unanesthetized dogs to be far below the diastolic blood pressure.[47] There is experimental evidence that brain ischemia, produced by lowering the arterial pressure to the isolated dog head or by carotid and vertebral occlusion does cause a marked rise in arterial pressure, but this vasopressor response need not be elicited by the same mechanism operative in intracranial hypertension.[243, 273] Rodbard and Stone postulated a baroceptor mechanism responsible for the vasopressor response.[228] They described a three-fold cardiovascular response in the dog. Immediately after the onset of acute compression, blood pressure rises sharply, presumably owing to a direct neurogenic effect on peripheral arterioles. A secondary rise, coming on several seconds after the onset of compression, was attributed to the release of pressor substances into the blood. A final increase in blood pressure was attributed to an increase in circulating blood volume. They postulated the existence of an intracranial receptor that is sensitive to differences in pressure between the intravascular space and the cerebrospinal fluid. Thus, a rise in intracranial pressure would be interpreted by the receptor as a fall in intravascular pressure, and peripheral vasoconstriction would be elicited. Additional evidence in favor of the proposal by Rodbard and Stone is the demonstration by Weinstein et al. that during failure of the vasopressor mechanism a response still could be elicited by increasing intracranial pressure to several times the systolic arterial pressure, far beyond the level required for total cerebral ischemia.[288]

An important recent development has been demonstration of the relationship of the vasopressor threshold to brain stem displacement or compression. Meyers noted that an increase in arterial pressure could be elicited more readily by injecting fluid into the ventricles than into the lumbar subarachnoid space and that the rapid ventricular injections were accompanied by the establishment of a difference in pressure between the ventricle and the cisterna magna.[192] This is best explained by a downward displacement or kinking of the brain stem. Thompson and Malina introduced the term "dynamic axial brain stem distortion" to explain the cardiorespiratory changes pro-

duced by increased intracranial pressure.[277] They demonstrated that the arterial pressor response, bradycardia, and respiratory irregularities occurred at a lower threshold with expansion of a supratentorial balloon than did elevation of intracranial pressure with lumbar fluid injections. Weinstein et al. quantitated the vasopressor response in monkeys by alternating injections into a supratentorial extradural balloon and the lumbar subarachnoid space.[288] They found that a vasopressor response could be elicited by a balloon injection to an intracranial pressure 50 mm of mercury below the mean arterial pressure at a time when it was necessary to raise the intracranial pressure to within 5 mm of mercury of the mean arterial pressure by lumbar injection in order to obtain the same increase in blood pressure. Thus, patterns of brain stem distortion and displacement appear to be important in determining the nature and degree of the cardiorespiratory changes produced by an expanding mass. This mechanism cannot account for the vasopressor response produced by diffuse cerebral ischemia, however, nor for the fact that compression of the isolated spinal cord also causes a rise in arterial pressure.[288] The latter finding indicates that the medulla need not mediate the vasopressor response.

The changes in heart rate produced by intracranial hypertension have received less attention than the arterial pressor response, although it is well accepted that severe bradycardia may be the principal alteration in vital signs in acutely expanding lesions such as extradural hematoma. The bradycardia produced by intracranial hypertension in experimental animals is unaffected by denervation of the carotid sinuses, is abolished by section of the vagi, and is independent of the rise in blood pressure.[43, 55]

The occurrence of respiratory irregularities with increased intracranial pressure was recognized in the earliest clinical reports. Respiratory and vasomotor collapse were the principal criteria of the end-stage of cerebral decompensation in Kocher's schema. Periodic respiration of the Cheyne-Stokes type was recognized in the nineteenth century in patients with primary cerebral disease. Jackson postulated that

Cheyne-Stokes respiration is due to an interference in the neural connections between the respiratory center and higher levels.[120] Damage to the higher centers releases the respiratory mechanism in the medulla from a supranuclear control, and the periodic respiration is a manifestation of some inherent automatism within the medulla. A thorough study of levels of respiratory control was carried out by Hoff and Breckenridge who described respiratory disorders in dogs and cats decerebrated at various levels between the hypothalamus and the medulla.[110] Midpontine decerebration resulted in slow respirations that were succeeded by "ataxic" respirations when the level of section reached the pontomedullary level. Ataxic breathing is grossly irregular and inefficient, usually leading to early death of the animal. The concept that periodic respiration is a release phenomenon caused by damage to supramedullary mechanisms is also supported by clinical studies.

The most comprehensive clinical evaluation of respiratory disorders secondary to diencephalic and brain stem damage has been reported by Plum and associates.[186, 212, 214] They analyzed 52 cases with cerebral infarction, hemorrhage, trauma, or neoplasm. Level of consciousness, the status of the motor system, and numerous brain stem reflexes were analyzed in an attempt to establish the level of impairment within the brain stem or diencephalon. In the "diencephalic stage," a few patients respired normally, but the majority had Cheyne-Stokes respiration. As evidence of involvement of the midbrain and upper pons developed, periodic respiration was succeeded by sustained hyperventilation. When the level of dysfunction reached the upper medulla, respirations reverted to a nearly normal pattern, although somewhat more rapid and shallow, and in the final stage of medullary involvement breathing became ataxic. Clinical ataxic breathing consists of intermittent, irregularly spaced pauses, deep sighs or gasps, and prolonged periods of apnea.

Pulmonary edema may also occur with increased intracranial pressure. Ducker described 11 patients with intracranial hypertension who died from pulmonary edema.[49] None of them had had excess parenteral fluids, and all but two had normal central venous pressure. The only abnormality in the lungs at postmortem examination was diffuse noncellular edema. Based on studies of experimental increased intracranial pressure in animals, Ducker and colleagues concluded that the pulmonary vascular system shares in the systemic vascular responses to intracranial hypertension and that the edema is due primarily to increased pulmonary venous pressure.[50, 51]

Tentorial Pressure Cone

In early studies of brain swelling and increased intracranial pressure, emphasis was placed on direct involvement of the medulla as the principal cause of coma and alterations in the vital signs. This was attributed in large part to medullary compression from herniation of the cerebellar tonsils into the foramen magnum. In recent times emphasis has shifted to transtentorial herniation as the principal cause of brain stem dysfunction with supratentorial mass lesions and cerebral swelling. Since the earliest days of neurology, clinicians have been puzzled by a number of false localizing signs in patients with expanding supratentorial lesions. Collier found sixth and third nerve palsies to be the most common neurological signs that could not be attributed directly to the lesion.[32] Knapp described paresis of the ipsilateral oculomotor nerve as the most frequent sign of a temporal lobe tumor; occasionally both nerves or the contralateral one only were involved.[144]

Transtentorial herniation was first described by Meyer in autopsy specimens.[188] The significance of herniation in clinical terms was emphasized by the demonstration of grooving and an occasional partial transection of the contralateral cerebral peduncle by the edge of the tentorium.[139] Hasenjäger and Spatz brought attention to the marked displacement of both the diencephalon and midbrain that accompanies tentorial pressure cones, but lateral rather than caudal displacement was described.[102] Jefferson placed emphasis on transtentorial herniation as the cause of many signs and symptoms previously attributed to foramen magnum herniation, and his general discussion provided the first wide introduction of the problem to neurosurgeons.[132]

Many of the signs and symptoms often ascribed to transtentorial herniation and brain stem compression may be indistinguishable from those caused by the primary lesion. It is generally accepted that the most convincing evidence of herniation is a dilated pupil or other signs of third nerve dysfunction. Sunderland considered this the surest indicator of the onset and degree of herniation.[271] However, large tentorial pressure cones have been demonstrated in patients who did not exhibit evidence of oculomotor abnormalities.[66, 199] The third nerve palsy has been variously attributed to direct pressure by herniated tissue, midbrain ischemia, compression by the petroclinoid ligament, and compression or distortion of the nerve as it enters the cavernous sinus.[135, 163, 209, 224] The most frequently quoted explanation is that the nerve is kinked across a displaced posterior cerebral artery or trapped between the posterior cerebral and superior cerebellar arteries.[272]

Transient obscurations of vision, appearing as hemianopic defects or intermittent total blindness, also are caused by transtentorial herniation. Ethelberg and Jensen attributed the symptoms to intermittent obstruction of one or both posterior cerebral arteries,[58] and Lindenberg described the posterior cerebral artery as the most frequently compressed large vessel in patients with severe brain swelling.[168] Visual symptoms also have been attributed to displacement or compression of the optic tracts in association with herniation.[27]

Contralateral weakness is such a common accompaniment of supratentorial mass lesions that it is usually difficult to assess the contribution of transtentorial herniation to the patient's neurological signs. The observations of Kernohan and Woltman show clearly the pathological changes that can occur in the cerebral peduncles, but the "Kernohan notch" appears to be a rather rare finding.[139] Nevertheless, Cabieses and Jeri contended that 50 per cent of patients with transtentorial herniation have contralateral motor signs on the basis of ipsilateral involvement of the brain stem by the herniation.[24]

Transection of the upper midbrain is the classic means of producing decerebration in experimental animals, and severe midbrain ischemia produced by transtentorial herniation might be expected to produce a high incidence of preterminal decerebration in patients. In fact, it has been described infrequently or incompletely, and in the retrospective series of brain tumor patients reported by Finney and Walker decerebration was present in only 9 per cent.[66] General experience, however, suggests that the incidence is much higher. Ingvar and Lundberg have described intermittent decerebration in brain tumor patients at the peak of intracranial pressure waves.[117] Loss of consciousness and tonic extension of all four limbs occurred frequently, followed by complete recovery when intracranial pressure had returned to normal. Clonic convulsive movements were also observed in the presence of a remarkably normal electroencephalogram, and the authors identified the attacks with the "cerebellar fits" considered in detail by Penfield and Jasper.[208] Opisthotonus also was observed occasionally. The frequent occurrence of decerebrate phenomena in the material of Ingvar and Lundberg, both among patients and repeatedly in the same patient, emphasizes again the importance of brain stem dysfunction in the symptomatology of raised intracranial pressure.

The production of irreversible coma by brain stem injury has been clearly demonstrated in both experimental animals and man, and a decreasing level of consciousness would be expected to constitute one of the cardinal signs of brain stem dysfunction produced by transtentorial herniation. Munro and Sisson stated that nearly all patients with transtentorial herniations show progressive coma.[199]

Most authors who have written on the subject agree that the clinical diagnosis of transtentorial herniation is difficult in most cases, and the question arises whether the herniation is primarily responsible for the signs and symptoms of brain stem dysfunction.[66] In experimental animals, expansion of a supratentorial mass sufficient to cause transtentorial herniation always produced caudal displacement and distortion of the brain stem, and this direct effect on the brain stem might be sufficient to explain the clinical signs without need to invoke compression by herniated tissue.[277, 289] Scheinker emphasized downward displacement of the midbrain through the incisura, as opposed to herniation, and Howell demonstrated that longitudinal buckling of the brain stem may occur without temporal lobe herniation.[111, 246] Recently Hassler examined the vertebral-basilar circulation by postmortem angiography in patients who had died from supratentorial mass lesions.[103] In all patients there was severe caudal displacement and distortion of the brain stem and stretching of the paramedian branches of the basilar artery.

A third mechanism requiring consideration is the one originally proposed by Cushing to explain the effect of a mass lesion on remote regions of the brain.[44] He postulated, as had Kocher, that dysfunction in the brain surrounding the lesion is due to capillary stasis and ischemia that gradually spreads to involve adjacent brain. McNealy and Plum believed that this or a similar mechanism is the most likely explanation for the orderly spread of brain stem dysfunction from above downward in their patients.[186] Transtentorial herniation and caudal displacement of the brain stem were believed to play a minor role.

Thus, several different mechanisms might account for the clinical signs and symptoms ordinarily attributed to transtentorial herniation alone, and identification of the significance of each factor is difficult because they appear to develop concurrently. Animal experiments have been helpful, but most have been short-term studies in anesthetized animals, conditions far removed from the clinical problem.

TREATMENT

General Principles

The treatment of increased intracranial pressure is inseparable from the treatment of cerebral edema and, usually, from the problems associated with management of the comatose patient. Initial therapy must always be directed toward correction of those conditions most likely to kill the patient. The first steps are to insure adequate respiratory exchange and control external hemorrhage. Proper respiratory control and hyperventilation with high oxygen mixtures are often the most rapid means of reducing intracranial tension. Intravenously administered hypertonic solutions also reduce brain bulk rapidly. When time permits, hypothermia and corticosteroids may be effective, but these agents act too slowly to be of benefit in the moribund patient. None of these methods of treatment will be effective for any length of time if the patient has an expanding intracranial mass as the cause of his difficulty. In fact, hypertonic solutions can prove lethal in a patient with a rapidly expanding mass such as an extradural hematoma. The patient may improve temporarily with the treatment, but the reduction in brain bulk permits continued enlargement of the hematoma. When the osmotic gradient is reversed the brain expands into a space smaller than it previously occupied, and intracranial pressure rises acutely. Thus, a space-occupying mass must be ruled out as quickly as possible in all patients with suspected intracranial hypertension.

Nearly all treatment of severe head injuries and cerebrovascular accidents in the acute stage is with agents that have as their primary effect a reduction in the volume of the brain. But the contribution of brain swelling and increased intracranial pressure to the clinical course of patients with head injury and intracranial hemorrhage and thrombosis has not been established with certainty. A patient may be comatose with dilated fixed pupils because of a primary injury to the brain stem without brain swelling. It is doubtful that any form of therapy currently available alters the course of patients with brain stem hemorrhages or thrombosis. The coma may be secondary to brain stem compression caused by cerebral edema, increased intracranial pressure, and herniation. If the patient improves with an agent that is known to reduce intracranial pressure, one can assume that intracranial hypertension contributed to his neurological impairment. But failure to improve may be due to an underlying primary injury, failure of the agent to exert its usual effect, or brain damage from severe prolonged increased intracranial pressure that is no longer reversible when the pressure is reduced. The neurological examination does not permit a choice among these three alternatives.

Continuous measurement of intracranial

pressure, however, will supply many of the answers. If the initial intracranial pressure is normal, brain swelling and intracranial hypertension are not the cause of the patient's coma. Single or even multiple spinal fluid pressure measurements are not adequate to make this conclusion because of marked fluctuations in intracranial pressure, the pressure waves, that occur frequently in patients with brain injuries. Also, lumbar subarachnoid pressure may not accurately reflect intracranial pressure because of obstruction at either the tentorium or foramen magnum. If intracranial pressure is elevated initially and falls with treatment, but the patient does not improve, it is likely that the brain stem has been irreversibly damaged, either primarily or secondarily by compression. Finally, if the fall in intracranial pressure is accompanied by improvement in the patient's neurological status, and this obtains in a large number of patients with the same therapeutic agent, a cause and effect relationship is established. There is no substitute for continuous recording of intracranial pressure in the management of patients with brain swelling and intracranial hypertension.

Respiratory Control

Hypoxia and hypercapnia have a profound effect on intracranial pressure when a mass lesion is present or the brain is swollen and most of the cerebrospinal fluid buffer has been expressed from the intracranial space. The pathophysiology of brain swelling and intracranial hypertension secondary to respiratory insufficiency has not been adequately investigated in man, but data from experimental animals permit speculation on the sequence of events that might be expected. The comatose patient is unable to maintain an adequate respiratory toilet. Secretions accumulate within the trachea and large bronchi, producing an element of obstructive respiratory insufficiency, and in the bronchioles and alveoli, causing what is commonly termed secretory respiratory insufficiency. This leads to pulmonary venous shunts and oxygen hemoglobin desaturation of the arterial blood. The pulmonary problems are further complicated by decreased respiratory rate and depth or a rapid rate that is ineffectual because of de-

creased tidal volume. A cycle is now established in which reduced blood oxygen causes depression of the central nervous system, less respiratory effort, and a further reduction in oxygen exchange across the alveoli. Anoxia and hypercapnia cause cerebral vessels to dilate in order to provide more oxygen for the brain, but brain-blood volume also increases. Cerebrovascular congestion is accompanied by edema, and the brain continues to swell. When expansion of the brain is gradual, the rise in intracranial pressure is minimal because of expression of cerebrospinal fluid from the intracranial space. However, at this time a slight additional reduction in blood oxygen or increase in carbon dioxide causes the cerebral vessels to dilate further. In this "tight" situation within the intracranial space a minimal increase in blood volume now produces a marked increase in intracranial pressure, the pressure wave. Cerebral blood flow begins to slow, and the brain is subjected to ischemic as well as anoxic anoxia. Intracranial pressure is now a function of the oxygen and carbon dioxide content of the blood, and if adequate respiratory exchange is not restored the patient soon dies from uncontrolled intracranial hypertension and cerebral anoxia. The influence of respiratory insufficiency on intracranial pressure in patients with intracranial tumors and following intracranial surgery has been clearly demonstrated.[152, 172, 173]

Cyanosis is a certain sign of hypoxemia, but the reduction in blood oxygen must be severe. Advanced tracheal obstruction is manifested by forced stertorous breathing and retraction of the chest. Ataxic breathing is inefficient and obviously inadequate on clinical inspection. The need for tracheostomy and respiratory control is immediately apparent in these patients, but occult hypoxemia due to more subtle changes in respiratory pattern can be difficult to diagnose. Hyperventilation is often described in comatose patients. In fact, however, the patient is frequently tachypneic, not hyperventilating, and he is hypoxemic because air is exchanging within the tracheobronchial dead space; or he may actually be overbreathing, with a more than sufficient tidal volume, but secretory obstruction is creating large regions of atelectasis and pulmonary venous shunts.

Siris et al. measured arterial oxygen saturation in 10 patients with varying degrees of depression of consciousness following head injury and cerebrovascular accident.[262] Oxygen saturations ranged from 80.4 to 95.8 per cent. The highest value among the 5 stuporous patients was 87.1 per cent, and there was an excellent correlation between oxygen saturation and level of consciousness. In none of the patients was there convincing clinical evidence of respiratory insufficiency; even the patients with only 80 per cent oxygen saturation were not cyanotic. The most extensive investigations of the relationship of respiratory insufficiency to coma and death following head injury were carried out by Cook et al. and Huang et al.[35, 112] Sixty-eight patients with severe craniocerebral trauma were studied. Various parameters of respiratory function were measured, and arterial pH, PCO_2, and oxygen saturation were determined at frequent intervals. Arterial oxygen-hemoglobin desaturation was present in every patient, and among 36 cases studied within the first five days after injury, average oxygen saturation was 85 per cent. Tracheostomy alone had no effect on hypoxemia, but when the patients were mechanically ventilated with 100 per cent oxygen, the oxygen saturation of the arterial blood rose to normal within a few minutes. Acid-base balance in these patients was also studied, and the majority of patients had respiratory alkalosis due to hyperventilation, rather than respiratory acidosis from depression of respiration. All those patients with respiratory acidosis, without tracheostomy, died. Many patients with respiratory alkalosis survived. The overall mortality rate was 75 per cent. Tracheostomy greatly influenced the length of survival but not the survival rate. The reason is not entirely clear, but probably this was due to the failure of tracheostomy to relieve hypoxemia. The principal purposes of tracheostomy are removal of secretions and reduction in dead space, but the study of Huang et al. demonstrates that the critical problem in terms of brain function, hypoxemia, can be relieved only by respiratory assistance.

There has been a great increase in the number of tracheostomies performed in general hospitals during the past 15 years.

In the study by Head, covering several years, the number of tracheostomies for mechanical obstruction remained the same, probably because an inadequate airway is so clearly evident in these patients.[106] The greatest increase in the number of tracheostomies was in patients with secretional obstruction and central nervous system disease with secretions. This represents an increasing awareness of the incidence of occult hypoxemia. The benefits of tracheostomy in comatose patients following head injury have been repeatedly emphasized.[53, 54, 175, 176, 276] Dunsmore et al. described a mortality rate of 69 per cent in a series of patients with particularly severe head injury and postulated that the mortality might well have been close to 100 per cent without tracheostomy.[53] Maciver et al. obtained a decrease in mortality in severe head injury from 90 to 40 per cent over a period of several years and attributed the improvement to prompt tracheostomy.[175] Tracheostomies were performed on all patients who were deeply unconscious on admission and who did not show signs of regaining consciousness. Except in the study by Huang et al., blood gases were not determined nor were comparisons with comparable series of patients without tracheostomy described.[112] Walker and Black, in a retrospective study, found that tracheostomy did not significantly benefit neurosurgical patients with a wide variety of disorders.[281] Although more detailed studies are required, there are few neurosurgeons today who would deny the benefits of tracheostomy in comatose patients. Tracheostomy alone is only half the treatment, and mechanical ventilation including hyperventilation in appropriate cases may reduce the mortality rate even further.

Complications of tracheostomy include those directly attributable to the operation, such as wound bleeding and pneumothorax, and the more significant late complications, such as infection, occlusion of the cannula, tracheal bleeding, and tracheal stenosis. Fitz-Hugh and McLean had three deaths attributable to the tracheostomy among 300 procedures.[69] Two were caused by tracheal erosion and hemorrhage and one by bilateral tension pneumothorax. In the series of Head there were four deaths attributable to the procedure in 462 cases, and tracheostomy contributed to death in 22 additional cases.[106] It was more difficult to establish the salvage rate, but he believed that 175 patients, 38 per cent of the series, survived because of tracheostomy. The most common late complications were infection, ranging from minor wound sepsis to pneumonia, and occlusion of the cannula. Efforts to reduce the infection rate by adoption of rigid aseptic techniques for tracheal aspiration did not succeed, according to the statistics, but he attributed this to failure of the technique not the concept.

The choice between endotracheal intubation and tracheostomy depends on the urgency of the situation and the individual's competence with the procedures. The advantages of endotracheal intubation are avoidance of the operation and, in experienced hands, the rapidity of establishing an airway. However, aspiration through the endotracheal tube is more difficult, the lumen is more readily obstructed by concretions, and intracranial pressure may rise greatly during intubation.[267] The dead space is larger than in patients with tracheostomy, and if the tube is left in place too long, laryngeal edema and necrosis can occur.

Hyperventilation

Hyperventilation is the exchange of a larger volume of air in a given period of time by increased depth or rate of respiration. Positive-negative-pressure respiration, as used in anesthesia, consists of the application of negative pressure to each expiratory phase of the respiratory cycle. The advantages of hyperventilation are assurance of adequate blood oxygenation, increased venous return, and decreased jugular vein pressure.[113] Slocum et al. and Hayes and Slocum advocated hyperventilation to reduce brain bulk at the time of intracranial surgery.[105, 264] However, Rosomoff has produced evidence that reduction in brain bulk during craniotomy is more apparent than real.[233] In experiments in dogs he found that 30 minutes of hyperventilation to an arterial pH of 7.59 and a P_{CO_2} of 20 mm of mercury did not change the volume of brain water or solids.[232] Blood volume was decreased, and cerebro-

spinal fluid volume was proportionally increased, resulting in no net change in fluid volume within the intracranial space. The apparent decrease in the size of the brain at the operating table is due then to escape of a larger volume of cerebrospinal fluid than is present normally, particularly the hydraulic cushion of fluid on which the brain rests.

Although the effect of hyperventilation on brain volume and intracranial pressure under normal circumstances is small, it can be a lifesaving procedure in patients with severe intracranial hypertension, particularly at the peak of a pressure wave. Under these circumstances, even a slight reduction in brain volume will cause a profound fall in intracranial pressure, and hyperventilation is the most rapid means of reducing intracranial pressure at this time.[152]

Hyperbaric Oxygen

Several studies in recent years have demonstrated a beneficial effect of hyperbaric oxygen in animals with head injury, brain swelling, and cerebral compression.[30, 52, 270] In the experiments of Sukoff et al. cerebral edema was produced in dogs by implantation of psyllium seeds, and in a second group of animals cerebral compression was produced by expansion of an extradural balloon.[270] Mortality rate was greatly reduced in animals treated with hyperbaric oxygen at 3 atm compared to the control groups. The authors suggested that the beneficial effects of hyperbaric oxygen were probably due to a combination of increased oxygen availability and decreased cerebral blood flow. Further studies are required.

Fluid Therapy

In the past, there has been some fear of using isotonic saline in the fluid therapy of patients with increased intracranial pressure and following craniotomy because of the belief that saline promotes cerebral edema. Experimental studies in both animal and man do not support this assumption. Intravenous administration of a solution of 5 per cent glucose in water increases intracranial pressure in dogs.[283, 294] Fishman compared the effects of isotonic saline, 5 per cent dextrose in water, and 5 per cent dextrose in isotonic saline on cisterna magna pressure in dogs.[68] The rise in pressure following glucose water administration was half again as great as that produced by infusion of saline. There was no difference between isotonic saline and 5 per cent glucose in saline. Bakay et al. made similar observations in patients with malignant brain tumors, hematomas, and subarachnoid hemorrhage.[5] Infusions of 5 per cent glucose in distilled water and 5 per cent glucose in isotonic saline were compared. The volume of the infusion varied from 1000 to 1500 ml. Resting intracranial pressures in both groups were comparable. Glucose in saline caused a maximum increase in spinal fluid pressure of 200 mm of water, whereas the increase in pressure with glucose and water varied from 270 to 800 mm of water. The difference was attributed to the rapid metabolism of the glucose. Although 5 per cent glucose in water is an isotonic solution, the elimination of the glucose caused plasma hypoosmolality and an increase in brain water.

Administration of salt-free solutions following routine intracranial surgery can cause water intoxication. McLaurin et al. administered 2000 to 4000 ml of glucose and water solution for a period of several days to 10 unselected postcraniotomy patients.[185] Four patients showed unmistakable evidence of water intoxication consisting of drowsiness and seizures, and the signs were reduced by administration of sodium chloride. Three other patients had mild signs of intoxication. Numerous measurements of water and electrolyte balance were made, and the most consistent relationship was between intoxication and the per cent of lowering of serum osmolality. There was no relationship between the type of pathologic condition and the occurrence of intoxication. They recommended mild restriction of fluids and the administration of at least 500 ml of isotonic saline daily during the first few days after intracranial surgery or brain injury. The evidence is convincing enough to warrant treatment of patients with increased intracranial pressure with isotonic saline or Ringer's solution rather than glucose and water alone.

Hypertonic Solutions

In the course of investigations of the effect of various solutions on intracranial pressure, Weed and McKibben described a marked fall in pressure in cats following the administration of hypertonic solutions of sodium chloride, sodium bicarbonate, sodium sulfate, and glucose.[285] A decrease in brain volume was also observed in animals with the skull open. The high concentrations of sodium salts caused respiratory and cardiac disturbances, but hypertonic glucose appeared to be without untoward effect. There followed many reports describing the effect of hypertonic glucose and other solutions on intracranial pressure and the clinical course of patients with many neurological disorders. Most of the studies were in patients with severe head injury. The fall in intracranial pressure following 50 per cent glucose administration was often of brief duration, and rebound in pressure above the control value was described.[15, 90] Although the secondary increase in intracranial pressure usually was not very great, Browder and Meyers described one patient in whom the resting intracranial pressure was approximately 475 mm of water, and following administration of hypertonic glucose the pressure rebounded to nearly 900 mm of water.[17] Browder and Meyers also maintained that most patients with severe head injury did not have increased intracranial pressure; therefore, the rationale for the use of dehydrating agents was questionable. Jefferson also pleaded for an intelligent use of hypertonic solutions based on careful evaluation of the patient's intracranial disease.[131] Masserman described a variety of untoward signs and symptoms in patients who had received large quantities of hypertonic glucose, including headache, backache, peripheral nerve pains, and transient fever.[180] Fay recommended magnesium sulfate together with restricted fluid intake for lowering intracranial pressure and maintained that a secondary rise in pressure did not occur.[62, 63] However, severe vomiting occurred frequently with this treatment, and occasional patients developed peripheral shock. Sodium arabinate solutions were also used, but were considered too difficult and expensive to prepare.[115]

Several investigators postulated that the rebound of intracranial pressure with hypertonic glucose was due to the rapid passage of the glucose into the brain and cerebrospinal fluid. As the plasma concentration of glucose fell, the osmotic gradient was reversed, and water entered the brain and cerebrospinal fluid in larger quantities than were present prior to treatment. Bullock et al. introduced sucrose as a material that does not diffuse into the brain or cerebrospinal fluid to a significant degree.[21] The effects of hypertonic glucose, sodium chloride, and sucrose on spinal fluid pressure were compared in dogs. Sucrose caused the greatest reductions in pressure for the longest period of time, and a secondary increase in pressure did not occur. Despite these encouraging results in animals Patterson failed to find a consistent reduction in spinal fluid pressure with sucrose in both normal patients and those with increased intracranial pressure.[207] Bragdon concluded that no dehydrating agent available at that time produced a consistent reduction in intracranial pressure, nor was any without some side effects.[13] Albumin was also suggested as a brain dehydrating material, because it does not cross the blood-brain barrier, but 25 per cent human serum albumin causes a marked increase in plasma volume and no reduction in intracranial pressure.[64, 171]

In recent years urea and mannitol have been used more frequently than any other hypertonic agents in the management of increased intracranial pressure. Fremont-Smith and Forbes first demonstrated, in 1927, that intraperitoneal injections of 50 per cent urea caused marked reductions in cerebrospinal fluid pressure in cats.[77] Little further work was done with urea until the demonstration by Smythe et al. that it caused a more pronounced and more prolonged fall in intracranial pressure in monkeys than did 50 per cent sucrose or dextrose.[266] Urea was introduced clinically by Javid, and his extensive investigations of the agent in animals and man led to its adoption as the hypertonic agent of choice in most neurology and neurosurgery clinics around the world.[124–126, 128, 129] In 1961 he reported results in 700 patients and described a marked sustained fall in intracranial pressure in nearly all cases.[126] Many

vehicles were investigated, and 30 per cent urea in 10 per cent invert sugar at a dose of 1 gm per kilogram body weight appeared to give optimum results. Several complications have been described. Infiltration of the subcutaneous tissue during intravenous therapy can cause sloughing of the skin, at times so severe as to require a skin graft. Dehydration has been described with repeated doses of urea, but is readily combated by adequate fluid therapy. Hemoglobinuria has been described frequently and was attributed by Javid and Anderson to the combination of urea and the solution that contained it rather than the urea alone.[127] They studied 30 per cent urea in 10 different vehicles in monkeys and found that only a combination of urea and 10 per cent invert sugar did not produce this complication. Mason and Raaf studied the effect of urea on clotting time, clot retraction, and prothrombin time in patients and found that only the prothrombin time was significantly abnormal.[179] It was reduced in 65 per cent of patients who received a single infusion of 30 per cent urea. A major objection to other hypertonic solutions, such as glucose and sucrose, was a rebound in intracranial pressure above the control level. Javid did not observe rebound, but it has been clearly described in both clinical and animal studies.[151, 187] The rebound is greater when the initial intracranial pressure is elevated.

The effects of hypertonic urea on the electroencephalogram and cerebral blood flow have also been studied. A slow wave focus can be diminished or abolished in brain tumor patients,[261] and in patients with a clinical diagnosis of cerebral edema from many different causes, an abnormal EEG often returns to normal with hypertonic urea.[274] This improvement was attributed to a reduction in cerebral edema, either diffuse or peritumoral edema, but as described later, this explanation may be incorrect. Harper and Bell found no change in cortical blood flow or oxygen consumption in normal animals, whereas Goluboff et al. found a significant increase in cerebral blood flow with hypertonic urea in glioma patients.[89, 106] The difference in results may be explained by the fact that control cerebral blood flow in the glioma patients was reduced, probably because of increased intracranial pressure that was relieved by the urea.

A single intravenous infusion of 30 per cent urea has little effect on serum electrolytes.[7, 82, 83, 179] Gilboe and Javid recorded serum electrolytes and urinary electrolyte excretion in patients undergoing surgery and compared a group that received a single infusion of urea with a group of untreated patients.[82] Water excretion was twice as great in the urea-treated patients, as expected, but sodium and potassium excretion were about the same in the two groups. There was no significant difference in serum electrolytes. Repeated doses of urea can, however, cause prolonged diuresis, negative water balance, and severe serum hyperosmolarity.[179]

The mode of action of urea in dehydrating the brain has been studied extensively in recent years. Javid and Anderson demonstrated that the reduction in intracranial pressure is not dependent on diuresis.[128] In fact, reduced pressure was better maintained in monkeys with bilateral nephrectomy than in controls. Urea is a nonpolar, un-ionized, water-soluble material that readily penetrates most cell membranes. It is generally assumed that in the steady state cellular and extracellular concentrations of urea are the same. Thus, it has often been used to measure total body water. If urea penetrated brain as freely as other organs and tissues, however, dehydration of nervous tissue would not occur, and the effect of hypertonic urea on intracranial pressure could not be explained by a difference in osmotic pressure between blood and brain. The steady state concentration of urea in brain and cerebrospinal fluid is different from that in other tissues. Kleeman et al., using ^{14}C-labeled urea, found that the steady state concentration in the water of white matter was about equal to the concentration in plasma water, but gray matter contained a higher (ratio 1.18) and cerebrospinal fluid a lower (ratio 0.78) concentration of urea.[142] They suggested that some of the urea might be adsorbed on intracellular proteins in neurons but not in glial cells. The decreased concentration of urea, from gray matter to white matter to cerebrospinal fluid, could then be explained by the number of neurons in each compartment, from a large number in the gray matter to none, of course, in the fluid. This explanation also permits the assumption that there is equilibration between free brain urea and cerebrospinal fluid, a necessary condition if the absence of a barrier between brain and cerebrospinal fluid is accepted. It also follows that the concentration of urea in cerebrospinal fluid and free urea in the brain are less than plasma, indicating a blood-brain barrier to urea.

A barrier to diffusion of urea from brain to blood, in fact, has been amply confirmed. Carbon-14-labeled urea penetrates the brain far more slowly than muscle and enters white matter more slowly than gray matter.[83, 142, 247] Equilibration in gray matter takes place in less than 6 hours but not until 12 hours in white matter. The difference may be explained by the greater vascularity of gray matter, but it is likely that other factors contribute.[11] Reed and Woodbury studied the penetration of hypertonic urea (2 gm per kilogram) into the brain of rats and recorded brain urea concentration, brain water volume, and cerebrospinal fluid pressure at various times following administration of the agent.[222] The kinetics of urea uptake by the brain indicated a two-compartment system with half-times of 23 minutes and 2.5 hours. Figure 18–9 shows that cerebrospinal fluid pressure and brain water volume fell rapidly following injection of the urea. However, both pressure and water volume began to return toward normal at a time when a large urea osmotic gradient from brain to blood still existed. They postulated that both the fast and slow compartments of the brain were rapidly dehydrated by the initial high concentration of urea in the plasma. After equilibrium had been reached in the fast compartment, urea continued to enter the slow compartment carrying water with it and accounting for the parallel rise of brain water and urea concentration over the next several hours. The rapid return of cerebrospinal fluid pressure toward normal was explained by some vasodilatation and particularly by either increased production or decreased absorption of cerebrospinal fluid, as first demonstrated by Rosomoff.[231] In a subsequent paper, Reed and Woodbury confirmed this hypothesis by demonstrating that the return of cerebrospinal fluid pressure to normal following hypertonic urea

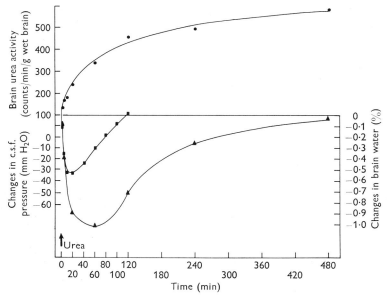

FIGURE 18–9 The upper curve represents the ^{14}C-labeled urea radioactivity of brain tissue. The lower curve shows the change in the percentage water content of the brain cortex. Urea was administered at time zero. Each point on either curve represents the mean of four determinations; vertical bars showed 95 per cent fiducial limits. (From Reed, D. J., and Woodbury, D. M.: J. Physiol., *164*:252–264, 1962.)

was delayed by reducing the fluid formation with acetazolamide.[223] Probably, this is also the explanation for the rebound in intracranial pressure above control levels. As the water content of the brain returns to normal, the brain expands into a space made smaller by the accumulation of cerebrospinal fluid and by dilatation of cerebral vessels. Also, a slightly reversed osmotic gradient for urea, from blood to brain, most likely is contributory.

Goldstein et al. compared the water and electrolyte content of dog brains dehydrated by urea with control values and found that the fluid removed contained sodium, potassium, and chloride in normal cerebral concentrations when the vehicle was invert sugar.[87] Urea dissolved in saline, however, removed fluid that was rich in sodium and poor in chloride. In contrast, Pappius and Dayes found that the fluid removed by urea in invert sugar was sodium free.[206]

The effect of hypertonic urea on experimental cerebral edema also has been studied. In rabbit brains made edematous by triethyltin intoxication, hypertonic urea reduced the water content of edematous white matter.[167] During the initial period of dehydration the sodium content of the

edematous tissue did not change, but three hours after administration of the urea a secondary sharp reduction in both sodium and water content of edematous white matter occurred. The authors had no explanation for this late mobilization of sodium. Their observations that urea dehydrates edematous brain contrast with those of Pappius and Dayes.[206]

In the clinical literature hypertonic solutions are described as effective in the management of cerebral edema and increased intracranial pressure. This implies that they reduce the water content of edematous tissue, perhaps even selectively compared to normal brain. There is experimental evidence that this is not the case.[29, 206] In the experiments of Pappius and Dayes cerebral edema was produced by a freezing lesion of the cortex in cats.[206] Large amounts of water were removed from normal brain by hypertonic urea, but the water content of edematous brain was unchanged. Thus, hypertonic urea dehydrates normal but not edematous brain, at least in this experimental situation. The authors attributed the results to a breakdown of the blood-brain barrier in edematous brain so that urea entered all compartments rapidly. However, the blood-brain barrier in white matter made edematous by necrotic lesions of the cortex remains impermeable to albumin. Either the barrier is partially disrupted so as to prevent passage of urea, a smaller molecule than albumin, or some other mechanism must be sought.

In recent years mannitol has replaced urea as the cerebral dehydrating agent of choice in many institutions. It is the alcohol of the 6-carbon sugar mannose. Its molecular configuration is similar to that of glucose, but it is not metabolized to any extent, and unlike urea, it appears to remain entirely in the extracellular compartment. Thus, mannitol is an excellent diuretic and has been used in research in renal physiology since 1945.[249] It was introduced into neurosurgery by Wise and Chater.[297] They demonstrated in dogs that in comparison with urea, mannitol decreased cerebrospinal fluid as effectively, for longer periods of time, with no rebound in pressure. McQueen and Jeanes compared urea and mannitol in normal dogs and those with intracranial hypertension produced by subarachnoid injections of blood.[187] The decrease in pressure was about the same with equivalent amounts of the two agents, but the effect of mannitol lasted longer. Some rebound in pressure occurred with mannitol in the animals with intracranial hypertension, but it was minimal compared to the large rebound observed with urea. In contrast, Beks and terWeeme found that increased intracranial pressure produced by cold lesions in cats was reduced more rapidly and more profoundly by urea than by mannitol and the duration of action was about equal with the two agents.[6a]

Mannitol has been used extensively in the management of clinical intracranial hypertension.[254, 298] In contrast to urea, it causes increased urinary excretion of sodium for the first 24 hours following intracranial surgery, but serum sodium concentration changes very little because it opposes the sodium retention that normally follows a major operation.[296] Recently a solution containing both fructose and mannitol has been said to be a better agent than mannitol alone.[193] Hypertonic sorbitol has about the same effect as mannitol in reducing intracranial pressure, but the rebound in pressure is greater with sorbitol.[211]

Glycerol was introduced by Italian investigators to reduce intracranial pressure.[26] It has the advantage that it can be administered orally for long periods of time without apparent toxicity or a rebound in pressure.[20]

Hypothermia

Hypothermia has been used principally in the treatment of patients with severe craniocerebral trauma or anoxia, and in intracranial and cardiovascular surgery. Despite encouraging reports of the effectiveness of hypothermia in reducing the morbidity and mortality of head injury and in intracranial surgery, particularly for aneurysms, it has fallen into disfavor among many neurosurgeons during the past decade. The principal reason appears to be a lack of convincing evidence that hypothermia is in fact an effective treatment of brain injury, cerebral swelling, and increased intracranial pressure. Sedzimir treated 30 consecutive patients with severe head injury with hypothermia.[248] He found it difficult to interpret the contributions of hypothermia, but believed that it was probably beneficial. He emphasized, however, that tracheostomy was also performed in these patients and could well have accounted for the lower mortality rate, compared to another series of patients who received neither hypothermia nor tracheostomy. Lazorthes and Campan were more enthusiastic about the beneficial effects of hypothermia in patients with severe head injuries and stated that the results in their series probably would have been even better if the patients had come to treatment earlier following the injury.[162] Lundberg et al. observed a dramatic reduction in intracranial pressure, including cessation of pressure waves, with hypothermia in one patient with a head injury.[174] Pressure was normal about two hours after cooling was begun. Gaavel et al. and Williams and Spencer reported improvement in patients with cardiac arrest treated with hypothermia.[79, 293]

Experimental studies of hypothermia are more impressive than clinical results reported to date. During a fall in body temperature from normal to 25° C, systemic arterial and venous pressures fall, cerebral blood flow declines, and the cerebral metabolic rate for oxygen also decreases.[9, 189, 235, 268] Cerebral glucose metabolism decreases in proportion to oxygen consumption.[9] Polarographic measurements of oxygen availability in the cortex show no change, again demonstrating the parallel response of cerebral blood flow and metabolism to the hypothermia.[189] Thus, neuronal metabolism is significantly reduced, and Meyer and Hunter presented evidence that the neurons are affected in a descending manner, the cortex first and the medullary centers and spinal cord only at deep levels of hypothermia.[189]

Under hypothermia, the brain idles and should be able to function for longer periods of time with a reduction in available oxygen and metabolites. This is the basis for the use of hypothermia in intracranial and cardiovascular surgery in which periods of systemic or local cerebral circulatory arrest may be necessary. The protective effect of hypothermia in this regard has been clearly demonstrated in experimental animals. Ganshirt et al. demonstrated that survival time after total cerebral ischemia was a function of the depth of hypothermia and was particularly significant below 30° C.[81] Recovery time was also measured in their experiments and was found to increase rapidly below 30° C. They concluded, therefore, that optimum protection of the brain, in terms of both survival and revival, was produced by temperatures between 27° and 30° C. Hypothermia also reduces brain bulk and intracranial pressure.[234] Lowering of the temperature in dogs to 25° C resulted in a reduction in brain volume of 4.1 per cent. Lemmen and Davis, however, measured lumbar cerebrospinal fluid pressure in patients during hypothermia induced in preparation for craniotomy.[166] It fell in patients with little or no initial pressure elevation, but when intracranial hypertension was present, the pattern varied considerably, and in some patients there was no significant fall in pressure. In comparison with animal studies, however, the period of hypothermia was brief.

Shulman and Rosomoff demonstrated that hypothermia at 25° C significantly reduces mortality in dogs with brain swelling produced by a cold lesion of the cerebral cortex.[257] These results were confirmed by Laskowski et al.[161] The amount of edema was less in the protected animals, blood-brain barrier permeability was less affected, and the enlargement and PAS-positive staining of glial cells was less pronounced than in the control animals. Recently Rosomoff et al. emphasized the reduction in inflammatory response of the hypothermic animals, compared to controls, with cold lesions of the cortex.[236] Hypothermia also protects the blood-brain barrier against Diodrast.[134]

The discrepancy between the experimental studies of hypothermia, that clearly show reduced cerebral metabolism and protection against mechanical and anoxic injury, and the clinical results is probably due to the timing of the treatment and the nature of the lesions being treated. Hypothermia is most effective in experimental animals if it precedes the injury. This is not possible in clinical head injuries, for example and the effects of multiple contusions may be largely irreversible before treatment can be effected. Where intracranial hypertension is the problem, hypothermia can reduce intracranial pressure, but several hours are required, and more rapid means of reducing intracranial tension are available.[174] Since most investigations of hypothermia and head injury were reported several years ago, a re-evaluation of the treatment would appear to be in order, particularly in light of a more complete understanding of intracranial and cerebral circulatory dynamics. In particular a combination of hypothermia and adequate respiratory control might be more effective than either method of treatment alone.

Steroids

Although corticosteroids are now used routinely in most institutions in the management of cerebral edema, and there has been strong clinical evidence to support their use, there is still some reluctance to accept the evidence that steroids do in fact prevent or reduce cerebral edema and lower intracranial pressure. Most clinical studies have relied upon improvement in the patient's neurological status or failure to develop signs and symptoms of cerebral edema as the criteria for effective therapy. This lack of objective measurement of the effect of the agents appears to be the main reason for the unwillingness to accept the results completely. The first reports of the clinical effectiveness of steroids were in stroke patients.[226, 238] Kofman et al. described a marked improvement in the neurological status of patients with cerebral metastases from carcinoma of the breast.[147] The reports of Galicich et al. and Rasmussen and Gulati were principally responsible for the introduction of steroid therapy into neurosurgery.[80, 220] In the former study 14 patients with brain tumors and increased intracranial pressure were treated with dexamethasone. Thirteen of them showed definite clinical improvement, and in two cases angiography during treatment showed a decrease in the size of the total mass. Rasmussen and Gulati compared steroid treated patients who underwent temporal lobectomy for epilepsy with a series of untreated patients. The incidence of hemiparesis, early seizures, and other signs ordinarily attributed to edema during the postoperative period was reduced in the treated patients. In 1964 French and Galicich reviewed their experience with 300 neurosurgical patients treated with dexamethasone.[78] They concluded that the treatment was effective in the medical and postoperative management of a variety of intracranial disorders that frequently cause cerebral edema. The usual dose was 16 mg of dexamethasone a day in divided doses. There were a few complications. Several patients on long-term treatment developed water retention, but arterial hypertension was not observed, and serum electrolyte abnormalities were rare. Wound healing was delayed in a few patients, but factors other than the catabolic and antifibroblastic action of the glucocorticoid appeared to be the explanation. The incidence of wound infection was not increased. Gastrointestinal hemorrhage was seen in only four patients and was apparent in only one of them prior to death. In this author's experience, the incidence of gastrointestinal hemorrhage is much larger and constitutes the major risk with steroid therapy in neurosurgical patients.

A few clinical studies have attempted to provide more objective criteria for the effect of steroids on cerebral edema and increased intracranial pressure. Long et al. compared brain biopsy specimens from patients with brain tumors who were treated with dexamethasone with those from untreated patients.[170] The study was difficult to control because evidence that the patients had peritumoral edema before treatment was based entirely on the clinical signs. There was little evidence of edema in brain adjacent to the tumors in treated patients, in contrast to the high incidence of peritumoral edema in another series of patients studied by the same group. Kullberg and West administered dexamethasone preoperatively to brain tumor patients during continuous recording of ventricular fluid pressure.[149] Intracranial pressure fell during treatment. In particular, the large dangerous plateau waves described by Lundberg were attenuated by the treatment.

The effects of steroids on experimental brain injury and cerebral edema have been studied in numerous models. They appear to be quite effective in preventing or reducing cerebral edema in some models but not others, perhaps based on the pathophysiology of the edema. The first study of this type was carried out by Prados et al. in 1945.[217] They demonstrated that an extract of the anterior pituitary lobe reduced the swelling and the increased permeability to trypan blue of brain exposed to the atmosphere. Grenell and McCawley confirmed the prevention of exposure edema by using adrenal cortical extract.[96a] Steroids have also been found effective in preventing the edema associated with experimental brain wounds, injection of cottonseed oil into the carotid artery, castor oil emboli in the carotid artery, sodium diatrizoate injury, and triethyltin intoxication.[10, 73, 99, 104] There was little or no effect of steroids on the brain swelling associated with experimental infarction and implantation of a foreign body into the cerebral hemisphere.[169, 215] As noted, these results may be due to the nature of the lesion and perhaps even more importantly to the criteria used for cerebral edema.

The effect of steroids on blood-brain barrier permeability was reported recently in two studies in which accurate methods for assessing barrier permeability were used effectively. Harris produced a severe, rapidly reversible lesion of the barrier using intracarotid sodium acetrizoate.[101] The extent and time course of the injury were measured with trypan blue and autoradiographs of the brains of animals injected with ^{125}I serum albumin. The time course of penetration and the distribution of these indicators was not affected by pretreatment of the animals with methylprednisolone. Rovit and Hagan used autoradiographs to evaluate the migration of ^{131}I-labeled serum albumin from lesions produced by electrocoagulation of the brain.[237] Animals treated with dexamethasone were compared to controls. During the first four days after production of the lesion the extravascular radioactivity in the steroid treated animals was reduced by as much as 50 per cent compared to controls, and the radioactivity was more restricted to the brain immediately adjacent to the lesion.

The mechanism of steroid action is poorly understood but appears to be a direct effect on the brain rather than on systemic factors. It has been known for a long time that erythrocytes swell when adrenocortical hormones are deficient, and the swelling is reversed by replacement therapy.[227] A large influx of sodium and water into the toad bladder occurs when it is poisoned by various means, and the transport functions of the bladder can be reconstituted by large quantities of glucosteroids.[164] In vitro brain slices from adrenalectomized animals swell more than those from normal animals, and the swelling is reduced by adding cortisone to the bathing medium.[57] In the brain, adrenalectomy causes an increase in intracellular sodium, a decrease in extracellular sodium, and increased brain excitability. Thus, steroids have a marked effect on cell membranes, and this could account for a redistribution of water and electrolytes in those types of cerebral edema in which cell membrane permeability is altered. As noted by Rovit and Hagan,[237] it is unlikely that steroids influence the basic pathological process in necrotic edema, namely the extravasation of fluid, electrolytes, and protein from ruptured blood vessels into the surrounding brain. However, the migration of these elements through the brain, particularly the white matter, may be transcellular as well as extracellular, and the former mechanism may be influenced by steroid treatment. Necrotic lesions also excite an inflammatory response that could be influenced by the treatment, but one would expect that if a response does occur it should be impairment of the healing process. A specific effect on the blood-brain barrier within the capillary wall must also be considered. Recently Eisenberg et al. studied the effect of dexamethasone on barrier permeability in cats with prolonged seizure activity.[56] In the untreated animals permeability to ^{131}I albumin was greatly increased; it was reduced by 60 per cent in animals treated with dexamethasone. Finally, a recent study by Weiss and Nulsen demonstrated that cerebrospinal fluid production is significantly reduced by glucocorticoids.[290]

Surgical Decompression

Internal and external cranial decompressions have been used to combat brain swelling and increased intracranial pressure. Internal decompression, resection of brain tissue, is employed most frequently at craniotomy for brain tumors and for better access to lesions at the base of the brain. The surgeon may elect to do an anterior temporal lobectomy, for example, in a patient with a large deep glioma in the temporocentral region of the brain that cannot be removed completely, particularly when the brain is swollen. Experience has taught that the survival rate in patients with marked brain swelling at the time of closure of the craniotomy is poorer than in patients with a slack brain, despite the various treatments to combat cerebral edema that have just been described.

Acute brain swelling occurs occasionally during craniotomy. The most common causes are airway obstruction and bleeding within the intracranial space that is not immediately visible. Occasionally neither of these etiologies can be proved, and the brain continues to swell despite hyperventilation and rapid administration of a hypertonic solution. Anterior frontal or temporal lobectomy can be a lifesaving procedure at this time.

External cranial decompression is used routinely in neurosurgical practice. Some neurosurgeons prefer to leave the dura open and do not wire down the bone flap in most of their craniotomy cases. Others, probably the majority, are guided by the circumstances in each patient. They do a reconstructive closure if the brain is slack, and leave a large opening for decompression if it is swollen. If swelling is severe, the craniotomy can be enlarged. From time to time external decompression has been advocated for uncontrollable brain swelling, particularly in patients with severe craniocerebral trauma. Recently the method was tested experimentally in dogs by Moody et al.[195] Marked increased intracranial pressure was produced by inflating an extracerebral balloon. The entire cranial vault except for a strip of bone over the sagittal sinus was removed in half the animals. The survival rate among these animals was significantly higher than among the controls, but the quality of survival was poor. All animals remained comatose, and fungus cerebri developed routinely within 10 days following surgery. Clark et al. reported a similar discouraging experience in two patients with severe head injuries who had "circumferential craniotomy."[28] In one patient there was marked upward displacement of the brain stem.

Surgical decompression of the brain can be a life-saving procedure, but always causes or at least runs the risk of brain damage. Removal of "silent" regions of the brain is not without complications, and protrusion of brain tissue through even the largest external opening usually results in damage to the herniated tissue. One can hope that in the future chemical means for combating brain swelling will become so effective that surgical decompression of the brain is no longer required.

CONCLUSION

It seems safe to conclude that uncontrolled intracranial hypertension is one of the most common causes of death in patients with a wide variety of disorders of the central nervous system. Undiagnosed or incompletely treated space-occupying lesions continue to be significant in the mortality of increased intracranial pressure, but less so in recent years owing to improved diagnostic techniques and greater general awareness of the signs and symptoms of an intracranial mass. The major problem is brain swelling, which includes not only cerebral edema but the increase in brain bulk caused by cerebrovascular congestion or multiple contusions and petechial hemorrhages.

Increased intracranial pressure disturbs brain function by reducing cerebral blood flow and thereby, cerebral metabolism. The neurons "run down" for lack of metabolites, and anaerobic glycolysis leads to tissue acidosis. The glial cells swell, perhaps because of failure of ionic pumps or the acidosis, and intracellular edema is superimposed on the underlying process. The homeostatic mechanisms that control the cerebral circulation (autoregulation, vasomotor tone) are disrupted by the anoxia, and ordinarily the result is more brain edema. The edema causes a further rise in intracranial pressure and reduction in cerebral blood flow. Respiratory exchange becomes inadequate as the patient loses consciousness, and anoxic anoxia, superimposed on ischemic anoxia, causes another round of the cycle.

Increased intracranial pressure does not cause a critical reduction in cerebral blood flow until the pressure reaches very high levels, near the diastolic blood pressure, as long as the pressure is equally distributed throughout the craniospinal space. The intracranial hypertension causes dilatation of the resistance vessels of the brain, probably a form of autoregulation, that maintains cerebral blood flow.

A space-occupying mass produces cerebral dysfunction that is independent of the level of intracranial pressure, at least pressure recorded from a lateral ventricle. The changes that occur in the brain underlying the mass, and their cause, are poorly understood. There is evidence that the mass produces local vascular compression from which one infers that the pressure or force in that portion of the brain is greater than in the remainder of the cerebral hemispheres. Focal cerebral edema is common and may also disrupt metabolism by still unknown mechanisms. As the mass continues to expand the brain is distorted and displaced, along the path of least resistance, toward the tentorial incisura. The upper brain stem is pushed downward into the posterior fossa and compressed from side to side by herniating tissue.

The amount of brain stem displacement and compression is primarily a function of the size of the mass and the volume of displaceable fluid within the supratentorial space, not the intracranial pressure. The brain can be greatly distorted without disturbing its function if it has the time and space to accommodate to the mass. It is common to see an elderly patient with a large chronic subdural hematoma and marked transtentorial herniation, manifested by caudal displacement of a posterior cerebral artery; yet the patient has no brain stem signs and does have normal intracranial pressure. The reason is that the hematoma develops slowly, and because the patient has cerebral atrophy, a large amount of cerebrospinal fluid is available to be displaced by the expanding hematoma. This picture contrasts with an acute extradural hematoma in a young patient. The hematoma is relatively small, but it develops rapidly, and the amount of displaceable cerebrospinal fluid is limited. The volume of herniated tissue is also less than in the former patient, but brain stem signs are present because the brain stem does not have sufficient time to accommodate to the effect of the mass.

Intracranial pressure is a variable phenomenon. Pressure waves of large magnitude are common and often arise from a base of normal pressure. Increased intracranial pressure may not be fully communicated to the spinal canal because of obstruction at either the tentorial incisura or foramen magnum. Thus, in order to properly diagnose and treat intracranial hypertension, pressure should be recorded directly and continuously from one of the intracranial compartments.

The cause of increased intracranial pressure is brain swelling, in the absence of a space-occupying mass. No single method of treatment or combination of methods currently available is adequate to treat brain swelling. The approach is empirical, often "shotgun," because we do not fully understand either the pathophysiology of the cerebral edemas or the mechanism of action of the many forms of therapy. Angiography and air study can suggest the diagnosis of cerebral edema, but it is impractical to perform frequent studies at short intervals to chart the course of cerebral edema during treatment. At present one must rely on intracranial pressure as the index of brain volume; thus, in clinical practice the treatment of cerebral edema and increased intracranial pressure are inseparable.

Supported by the John A. Hartford Foundation, Incorporated.

REFERENCES

1. Apfelbach, C. W.: Studies in traumatic fractures of the cranial bones. I. Edema of the brain; II. Bruises of the brain. Arch. Surg., 4:434–450, 1922.
2. Atkinson, J. R., Shurtleff, D. B., and Foltz, E. L.: Radio telemetry for the measurement of intracranial pressure. J. Neurosurg., 27:428–432, 1967.
3. Austen, F. K., Carmichael, M. W., and Adams, R. D.: Neurologic manifestations of chronic pulmonary insufficiency. New Eng. J. Med., 257:579–590, 1957.
4. Ayer, J. B.: Analysis of the lumbar cerebrospinal fluid in sixty-seven cases of tumors and cysts of the brain. Ass. Res. Nerv. Ment. Dis., 8:189–199, 1927.
5. Bakay, L., Crawford, J. D., and White, J. C.: The effects of intravenous fluids on cerebrospinal fluid pressure. Surg. Gynec. Obstet., 99:48–52, 1954.
6. Becht, F. C.: Studies on the cerebrospinal fluid. Amer. J. Physiol., 52:1–125, 1920.
6a. Beks, J. W. F., and terWeeme, C. A.: The influence of urea and mannitol on increased intraventricular pressure in cold-induced cerebral oedema. Acta Neurochir., 16:97–107, 1967.
7. Beks, J. W. F., Groen, A., Huizinga, T., Noordhoek, K. H. N., Smit, J. M., and Walter, W. G.: Effects of intravenously administered hypertonic urea solution. Acta Neurochir., 13:1–10, 1965.
8. Benson, P. F., and MacKeith, R. C.: Pseudotumor cerebri. Lancet, 2:55–56, 1961.
9. Bering, E. A., Jr., Taren, J. A., McMurrey, J. D., and Bernhard, W. F.: Studies on hypothermia in monkeys. II. The effect of hypothermia on the general physiology and cerebral metabolism of monkeys in the hypothermic state. Surg. Gynec. Obstet., 102:134–138, 1956.
10. Blinderman, E. E., Graf, C. J., and Fitzpatrick, T.: Basic studies in cerebral edema. Its control by a corticosteroid (Solu-Medrol). J. Neurosurg., 19:319–324, 1962.
11. Bradbury, M. W. B., and Coxon, R. V.: The penetration of urea into the central nervous system at high blood levels. J. Physiol., 163:423–435, 1962.
12. Bradshaw, P.: Benign intracranial hypertension. J. Neurol. Neurosurg. Psychiat., 19:28–41, 1956.

13. Bragdon, F. H.: Alterations observed in cranio-cerebral injuries following the use of dehydrating agents. Ass. Res. Nerv. Ment. Dis., *24*:545–561, 1943.
14. Brock, M., Fieschi, C., Ingvar, D. H., Lassen, N. A., and Schurmann, K.: Cerebral Blood Flow. New York, Springer-Verlag, 1969.
15. Browder, J.: Dangers in the use of hypertonic solutions in the treatment of brain injuries. Amer. J. Surg., *8*:1213–1217, 1930.
16. Browder, J., and Meyers, R.: Observations on behavior of the systemic blood pressure, pulse and spinal fluid pressure following craniocerebral injury. Amer. J. Surg., *31*:403–426, 1936.
17. Browder, J., and Meyers, R.: A revaluation of the treatment of head injuries. Ann. Surg., *110*:357–375, 1939.
18. Browder, J., and Rabiner, A. M.: Regional swelling of the brain in subdural hematoma. Ann. Surg., *134*:369–375, 1951.
19. Brown, F. K.: Cardiovascular effects of acutely raised intracranial pressure. Amer. J. Physiol., *185*:510–514, 1956.
20. Buckell, M., and Walsh, L.: Effect of glycerol by mouth on raised intracranial pressure in man. Lancet, *2*:1151–1152, 1964.
21. Bullock, L. T., Gregersen, M. I., and Kinney, R.: The use of hypertonic sucrose solution intravenously to reduce cerebrospinal fluid pressure without a secondary rise. Amer. J. Physiol., *112*:82–96, 1935.
22. Burrows, G.: Disorders of the Cerebral Circulation. London, 1846.
23. Byrom, F. B.: The pathogenesis of hypertensive encephalopathy and its relation to the malignant phase of hypertension: Experimental evidence from hypertensive rat. Lancet, *2*:201–211, 1954.
24. Cabieses, F., and Jeri, R.: Transtentorial temporal lobe herniation. Acta Neurol. Lat. Amer., *1*:167–179, 1955.
25. Cairns, H.: Raised intracranial pressure: Hydrocephalic and vascular factors. Brit. J. Surg., *27*:275–294, 1939.
26. Cantore, G., Guidetti, B., and Virno, M.: Oral glycerol for the reduction of intracranial pressure. J. Neurosurg., *21*:278–283, 1964.
27. Carrillo, R.: Hernias cisternales. Arch. Neurocir., *7*:498–590, 1950.
28. Clark, K., Nash, T. M., and Hutchison, G. C.: The failure of circumferential craniotomy in acute traumatic cerebral swelling. J. Neurosurg., *29*:367–371, 1968.
29. Clasen, R. A., Prouty, R. R., Bingham, W. G., Martin, F. A., and Hass, G. M.: Treatment of experimental cerebral edema with intravenous hypertonic glucose, albumin, and dextran. Surg. Gynec. Obstet., *104*:591–606, 1957.
30. Coe, J. E., and Hayes, T. M.: Treatment of experimental brain injury by hyperbaric oxygenation. Preliminary report. Amer. Surg., *32*:493–495, 1966.
31. Coe, J. E., Nelson, W. J., Rudenberg, F. H., and Garza, R.: Technique for continuous intracranial pressure recording. Technical note. J. Neurosurg., *27*:370–375, 1967.
32. Collier, J.: The false localizing signs of intracranial tumors. Brain, *27*:490–508, 1904.
33. Conn, H. O., Dunn, J. P., Newman, H. A., and Belkin, G. A.: Pulmonary emphysema simulating brain tumor. Amer. J. Med., *22*:524–533, 1957.
34. Cook, A. W., Browder, E. J., and Carter, W. B.: Cerebral swelling and ventricular alterations following evacuation of intracranial extracerebral hematoma. J. Neurosurg., *19*:419–423, 1962.
35. Cook, A. W., Browder, E. J., and Lyons, H. A.: Alterations in acid-base equilibrium in craniocerebral trauma. A determinant in survival. J. Neurosurg., *18*:366–370, 1961.
36. Cooper, R., and Hulme, A.: Intracranial pressure and related phenomena during sleep. J. Neurol. Neurosurg. Psychiat., *29*:564–570, 1966.
37. Courtice, F. C.: The effect of raised intracranial pressure on the cerebral blood flow. J. Neurol. Psychiat., *3*:293–305, 1940.
38. Courtney, J. W.: Traumatic cerebral edema: Its pathology and surgical treatment—a critical study. Boston Med. Surg. J., *140*:345–347, 1899.
39. Courville, C. B.: Structural changes in the brain consequent to traumatic disturbances of intracranial fluid balance. Bull. Los Angeles Neurol. Soc., *7*:55–76, 1942.
40. Cronqvist, S., and Lundberg, N.: Regional cerebral blood flow with intracranial tumours with special regard to cases with intracranial hypertension. Scand. J. Clin. Lab. Invest., *22*:Suppl. 102, 1968.
41. Crowe, W. R.: Cerebral allergic edema. J. Allerg., *13*:173–176, 1941–1942.
42. Cushing, H.: Concerning a definite regulatory mechanism of the vasomotor centre which controls blood pressure during cerebral compression. Bull. Johns Hopk. Hosp., *12*:290–292, 1901.
43. Cushing, H.: Some experimental and clinical observations concerning states of increased intracranial tension. Amer. J. Med. Sci., *124*:375–400, 1902.
44. Cushing, H.: The blood-pressure reaction of acute cerebral compression, illustrated by cases of intracranial hemorrhage. Amer. J. Med. Sci., *125*:1017–1045, 1903.
45. Cushing, H.: Studies in Intracranial Physiology and Surgery. London, Oxford University Press, 1925.
45a. Dandy, W. E.: Diagnosis and treatment of injuries of the head. J.A.M.A., *101*:772–775, 1933.
46. Dandy, W. E.: Intracranial pressure without brain tumor. Diagnosis and treatment. Ann. Surg., *106*:492–513, 1937.
47. Dickinson, C. J., and McCubbin, J. W.: Pressor effect of increased cerebrospinal fluid pressure and vertebral artery occlusion with and without anesthesia. Circ. Res., *12*:190–202, 1963.
48. Dixon, W. E., and Halliburton, W. D.: The cerebro-spinal fluid. II. Cerebro-spinal pressure. J. Physiol., *48*:128–153, 1914.
49. Ducker, T. B.: Increased intracranial pressure

and pulmonary edema. Part I: Clinical study of 11 patients. J. Neurosurg., *28*:112–117, 1968.

50. Ducker, T. B., and Simmons, R. L.: Increased intracranial pressure and pulmonary edema. Part 2: The hemodynamic response of dogs and monkeys to increased intracranial pressure. J. Neurosurg., *28*:118–123, 1968.

51. Ducker, T. B., Simmons, R. L., and Anderson, R. W.: Increased intracranial pressure and pulmonary edema. Part 3: The effect of increased intracranial pressure on the cardiovascular hemodynamics of chimpanzees. J. Neurosurg., *29*:475–483, 1968.

52. Dunn, J. E., Jr., and Connolly, J. M.: Effects of hypobaric and hyperbaric oxygen on experimental brain injury. Proceedings of Third International Conference on Hyperbaric Medicine, Duke University Medical Center, 1965, p. 447.

53. Dunsmore, R. H., Scoville, W. B., Reilly, F., and Whitcomb, B. B.: Tracheotomy in neurosurgery. J. Neurosurg., *10*:228–232, 1953.

54. Echols, D. H., Llewellyn, R., Kirgis, H. D., Rehfeldt, F. C., and Garcia-Bengochea, F.: Tracheotomy in the management of severe head injuries. Surgery, *28*:801–811, 1950.

55. Edholm, O. G.: The relation of heart rate to intracranial pressure. J. Physiol., *98*:442–445, 1940.

56. Eisenberg, H. M., Barlow, C. F., Lorenzo, A.: Effects of dexamethasone (Decadron) on altered brain vascular permeability. Meeting of Amer. Ass. Neurol. Surg. and Amer. Soc. Neuroradiologists, Cleveland, Ohio, April, 1969, p. 62.

57. Elliott, K. A. C., and Yrarrazaval, S.: An effect of adrenalectomy and cortisone on tissue permeability in vitro. Nature, *169*:416–417, 1952.

58. Ethelberg, S., and Jensen, V. A.: Obscurations and further time-related paroxysmal disorders in intracranial tumors. Syndrome of initial herniation of parts of the brain through the tentorial incisure. Arch. Neurol. Psychiat., *68*:130–149, 1952.

59. Evans, J. P., Espey, F. F., Kristoff, F. V., Kimbell, F. D., and Ryder, H. W.: Experimental and clinical observations on rising intracranial pressure. Arch. Surg., *63*:107–114, 1951.

60. Eyster, J. A. E.: Clinical and experimental observations upon Cheyne-Stokes respiration. J. Exp. Med., *8*:565–613, 1906.

61. Eyster, J. A. E., Burrows, M. T., and Essick, C. R.: Studies on intracranial pressure. J. Exp. Med., *11*:489–514, 1909.

62. Fay, T.: Comparative values of magnesium sulphate and sodium chloride for relief of intracranial tension. J.A.M.A., *82*:766–769, 1924.

63. Fay, T.: The control of intracranial pressure. J.A.M.A., *84*:1261, 1925.

64. Fender, F. A., and MacKenzie, A. S.: Effect of albumin solution on cerebrospinal fluid pressure. Arch. Neurol. Psychiat., *59*:529–531, 1948.

65. Fields, J. E.: Bulging fontanel: A complication of tetracycline therapy in infants. J. Pediat., *58*:74–76, 1961.

66. Finney, L. A., and Walker, A. E.: Transtentorial Herniation. Springfield, Ill., Charles C Thomas, 1962.

67. Fishberg, A. M.: Hypertension and Nephritis. Ed. 5., Philadelphia, Lea & Febiger, 1954.

68. Fishman, R. A.: Effects of isotonic intravenous solutions on normal and increased intracranial pressure. Arch. Neurol. Psychiat., *70*:350–360, 1953.

69. Fitz-Hugh, G. S., and McLean, W. C.: Tracheostomy: Indications and comments. J. Mich. Med. Soc., *56*:1400–1404, 1957.

70. Flexner, L. B., Clark, J. H., and Weed, L. H.: The elasticity of the dural sac and its contents. Amer. J. Physiol., *101*:292–303, 1932.

71. Foldes, F. F., and Arrowood, J. G.: Changes in cerebrospinal fluid pressure under the influence of continuous subarachnoidal infusion of normal saline. J. Clin. Invest., *27*:346–351, 1948.

72. Foley, J.: Benign forms of intracranial hypertension—"toxic" and "otitic" hydrocephalus. Brain, *78*:1–41, 1955.

73. Foley, J. M., Chambers, R. A., and Adams, R. D.: The effects of cortisone on the early repair of brain wounds in guinea pigs. J. Neuropath. Exp. Neurol., *12*:101–102, 1953.

74. Forster, F. M.: The role of the brain stem in arterial hypertension subsequent to intracranial hypertension. Amer. J. Physiol., *139*:347–350, 1943.

75. Frazier, C. H., and Peet, M. M.: The action of glandular extracts on the secretion of cerebrospinal fluid. Amer. J. Physiol., *36*:464–487, 1915.

76. Freeman, N. E., and Jeffers, W. A.: Effects of progressive sympathectomy on hypertension produced by increased intracranial pressure. Amer. J. Physiol., *128*:662–671, 1939–1940.

77. Fremont-Smith, F., and Forbes, H. S.: Intraocular and intracranial pressure. An experimental study. Arch. Neurol. Psychiat., *18*:550–564, 1927.

78. French, L. A., and Galicich, J. H.: The use of steroids for control of cerebral edema. Clin. Neurosurg., *10*:212–223, 1964.

79. Gaavel, J. A., Dechêne, J. P., and Beaulieu, N.: L'hypothermie dans la prévention des lesions cérébrales consécutives à l'arrêt cardiaque. Laval Med., *29*:48–60, 1960.

80. Galicich, J. H., French, L. A., and Melby, J. C.: Use of dexamethasone in treatment of cerebral edema associated with brain tumors. Lancet, *81*:46–53, 1961.

81. Ganshirt, H., Hirsch, H., Krenkel, W., Schneider, M., and Zylka, W.: Über den Einfluss der Temperatursenkung auf die Erholungsfähigkeit des Warmblütergehirns. Arch. Exp. Path. Pharmark., *222*:431–449, 1954.

82. Gilboe, D., and Javid, M.: Electrolyte studies following a single administration of hypertonic urea. Surg. Gynec. Obstet., *116*:693–700, 1963.

83. Gilboe, D., Javid, M., and Frechette, P.: The fate and distribution of hypertonic urea solutions: A preliminary report. Surg. Forum, *11*:390–391, 1960.

84. Glowacki, J., Guazzi, G. C., and Van Bogaert, L.:

Pseudo-tumoural presentation of certain cases of subacute sclerosing leucoencephalitis. J. Neurol. Sci., *4*:199–215, 1967.

85. Glowacki, J., Guazzi, G. C., Alvisi, C., Gambetti, P., Jonckheer, M., and Tassinari, C. A.: L'oedème cérébral pseudotumoral endocrinien et/ou metabolique. Acta Neurol. Belg., *65*:873–910, 1965.

86. Goldstein, N. P., Rucker, C. W., and Klass, D. W.: Encephalopathy and papilledema after bee sting. J.A.M.A., *188*:1083, 1964.

87. Goldstein, S. I., Himwich, W. A., Knapp, F. M., and Rovine, B. W.: Effects of urea and other dehydrating agents upon dog brain. J. Neurosurg., *21*:672–677, 1964.

88. Goldzieher, M. A., McGavack, T., Paterson, C. A., Goldzieher, J. W., and Miller, H. R.: Retrobulbar neuritis associated with hyperthyroidism. Arch. Neurol. Psychiat., *65*:189–196, 1951.

89. Goluboff, B., Shenkin, H. A., and Haft, H.: The effects of mannitol and urea on cerebral hemodynamics and cerebrospinal fluid pressure. Neurology, *14*:891–898, 1964.

90. Grant, F. C.: Value of hypertonic solutions in reducing intracranial pressures. Res. Publ. Ass. Res. Nerv. Ment. Dis., *8*:437, 1927.

91. Greenfield, J. G.: The problem of cerebral oedema in neuro-surgery. Proc. Roy. Soc. Med., *40*:695–697, 1947.

92. Greenfield, J. C., and Tindall, G. T.: Effect of acute increase in intracranial pressure on blood flow in the internal carotid artery of man. J. Clin. Invest., *44*:1343–1351, 1965.

93. Greer, M.: Benign intracranial hypertension. II. Following corticosteroid therapy. Neurology, *13*:439–441, 1963.

94. Greer, M.: Benign intracranial hypertension. III. Pregnancy. Neurology, *13*:670–672, 1963.

95. Greer, M.: Benign intracranial hypertension. IV. Menarche. Neurology, *14*:569–573, 1964.

96. Greer, M.: Benign intracranial hypertension. V. Menstrual dysfunction. Neurology, *14*:668–673, 1964.

96a. Grenell, R. G., and McCawley, E. L.: Central nervous system resistance. III. The effect of adrenal cortical substances on the central nervous system. J. Neurosurg., *4*:508–518, 1947.

97. Guillaume, J., and Janny, P.: Manométrie intracranienne continue. Intérêt physiopathologique et clinique de la méthode. Press Méd., *59*:953–955, 1951.

98. Hadjidimos, A. A., Brock, M., Baum, P., and Schürmann, K.: Cessation of cerebral blood flow in total irreversible loss of brain function. *In* International Symposium on Clinical Application of Isotope Clearance Measurement of Cerebral Blood Flow, Mainz, 1969. Cerebral Blood Flow: Clinical and Experimental Results. Berlin, Springer-Verlag, 1969.

99. Hammargren, L. L., Geise, A. W., and French, L. A.: Protection against cerebral damage from intracarotid injection of Hypaque in animals. J. Neurosurg., *23*:418–424, 1965.

100. Harper, A. M., and Bell, R. A.: The failure of intravenous urea to alter the blood flow

through the cerebral cortex. J. Neurol. Neurosurg. Psychiat., *26*:69–70, 1963.

101. Harris, A. B.: Steroids and blood brain barrier alterations in sodium acetrizoate injury. Arch. Neurol., *17*:282–297, 1967.

102. Hasenjäger, T., and Spatz, H.: Über örtliche Veränderungen der Konfiguration des Gehirns beim Hirndruck. Arch. Psychiat., *107*:193–222, 1937.

103. Hassler, O.: Arterial pattern of human brainstem. Normal appearance and deformation in expanding supratentorial conditions. Neurology, *17*:368–375, 1967.

104. Hatanaka, H.: Steroids and cerebral edema. Brain Nerve, *15*:624–633, 1963.

105. Hayes, G. J., and Slocum, H. C.: The achievement of optimal brain relaxation by hyperventilation technics of anesthesia. J. Neurosurg., *19*:65–70, 1962.

106. Head, J. M.: Tracheostomy in the management of respiratory problems. New Eng. J. Med., *264*:587–591, 1961.

107. Hedges, T. R., Weinstein, J. D., Kassell, N. F., and Stein, S.: Cerebrovascular responses to increased intracranial pressure. J. Neurosurg., *21*:292–297, 1964.

108. Hill, L.: The Physiology and Pathology of the Cerebral Circulation: An Experimental Research. London, J. and A. Churchill Ltd., 1896.

109. Hodgson, J. S.: The relation between increased intracranial pressure and increased intraspinal pressure. Changes in the cerebrospinal fluid in increased intracranial pressure. Res. Publ. Ass. Res. Nerv. Ment. Dis., *8*:182–188, 1927.

110. Hoff, H. E., and Breckenridge, C. G.: Intrinsic mechanisms in periodic breathing. Arch. Neurol. Psychiat., *72*:11–42, 1954.

111. Howell, D. A.: Longitudinal brain stem compression with buckling. Arch. Neurol. Psychiat., *4*:116–123, 1961.

112. Huang, C. T., Cook, A. W., and Lyons, H. A.: Severe craniocerebral trauma and respiratory abnormalities. I. Physiological studies with specific reference to effect of tracheostomy on survival. Arch. Neurol., *9*:113–122, 1963.

113. Hubay, C. A., Waltz, R. C., Brecher, G. A., Praglin, J., and Hingson, R. A.: Circulatory dynamics of venous return during positive-negative pressure respiration. Anesthesiology, *15*:445–461, 1954.

114. Huber, P., Meyer, J. S., Handa, J., and Ishikawa, S.: Electromagnetic flowmeter study of carotid and vertebral blood flow during intracranial hypertension. Acta Neurochir., *13*:37–63, 1965.

115. Hughes, J., and LaPlace, L.: Effect of hypertonic solutions of sodium arabinate on cerebrospinal fluid pressure. J. Pharmacol. Exp. Ther., *38*:363–383, 1930.

116. Hulme, A., and Cooper, R.: A technique for the investigation of intracranial pressure in man. J. Neurol. Neurosurg. Psychiat., *29*:154–156, 1966.

117. Ingvar, D. H., and Lundberg, N.: Paroxysmal symptoms in intracranial hypertension,

studied with ventricular fluid pressure recording and electroencephalography. Brain, *84*: 446–459, 1961.

118. Ingvar, D. H., Lassen, N. A., Siesjo, B. K., and Skinhoj, E.: Cerebral blood flow and cerebrospinal fluid. Scand. J. Clin. Lab. Invest., Suppl. 102, 1968.

119. Jackson, H.: The management of acute cranial injuries by the early exact determination of intracranial pressure, and its relief by lumbar drainage. Surg. Gynec. Obstet., *34*:494–508, 1922.

120. Jackson, J. H.: Neurological fragment. XV. Superior and subordinate centres of the lowest level. Lancet, *1*:476–478, 1895.

121. Jacobson, I., Harper, A. M., and McDowall, D. G.: Relationship between venous pressure and cortical blood flow. Nature, *200*:173–175, 1963.

122. Jacobson, S. A., and Rothballer, A. B.: Prolonged measurement of experimental intracranial pressure using a subminiature absolute pressure transducer. J. Neurosurg., *26*:603–608, 1967.

123. Janeway, T. C.: The Clinical Study of Blood Pressure. New York, Appleton, 1904.

124. Javid, M.: Urea—new use of an old agent. Reduction of intracranial and intraocular pressure. Surg. Clin. N. Amer., *38*:907–928, 1958.

125. Javid, M.: A valuable new method for the reduction of intracranial and intraocular pressure by the use of urea. Trans. Amer. Neurol. Ass., pp. 113–116, 1958.

126. Javid, M.: Urea in intracranial surgery. A new method. J. Neurosurg., *18*:51–57, 1961.

127. Javid, M., and Anderson, J.: Observations on the use of urea in rhesus monkeys. Surg. Forum, *9*:686–690, 1958.

128. Javid, M., and Anderson, J.: The effect of urea on cerebrospinal fluid pressure in monkeys before and after bilateral nephrectomy. J. Lab. Clin. Med., *53*:484–489, 1959.

129. Javid, M., and Settlage, P.: Effect of urea on cerebrospinal fluid pressure in human subjects. Preliminary report. J.A.M.A., *160*:943–949, 1956.

130. Jefferson, G.: Discussion on diagnosis and treatment of acute head injuries. Proc. Roy. Soc. Med., *25*:735–762, 1932.

131. Jefferson, G.: The treatment of acute head injuries. Brit. Med. J., pp. 807–812, 1933.

132. Jefferson, G.: Tentorial pressure cone. Arch. Neurol. Psychiat., *40*:857–876, 1938.

133. Jennett, W. B., McDowall, D. G., and Barker, J.: The effect of halothane on intracranial pressure in cerebral tumors. Report of two cases. J. Neurosurg., *26*:270–274, 1967.

134. Jeppsson, P. G., and Nielsen, K.: The effect of hypothermia on lesions of the blood-brain barrier produced by Umbradil. Excerpta Med., sec. *8*:848–849, 1955.

135. Johnson, R. T., and Yates, P. O.: Tentorial herniation and midbrain deformity. A clinicopathological study. Proceedings of the Second International Congress of Neuropathology, London, 1955, pp. 329–332.

136. Kahn, A. J.: Effects of variations in intracranial pressure. Arch. Neurol. Psychiat., *51*:508–527, 1944.

137. Kaufmann, G. E., and Clark, W. K.: Transmission of increased intracranial pressure across the tentorium in man. Surg. Forum, *20*:437, 1969.

138. Kellie, G.: An account of the appearances observed in the dissection of two of three individuals presumed to have perished in the storm of the 3D, and whose bodies were discovered in the vicinity of Leith on the morning of the 4th, November 1821 with some reflections on the pathology of the brain. Trans. Med. Chir. Soc. Edinb., *1*:84–169, 1824.

139. Kernohan, J. W., and Woltman, H. E.: Incisura of the crus due to contralateral brain tumor. Arch. Neurol. Psychiat., *21*:274–287, 1929.

140. Kety, S. S., Shenkin, H. A., and Schmidt, C. F.: The effects of increased intracranial pressure on cerebral circulatory functions in man. J. Clin. Invest., *27*:493–499, 1948.

141. Kjallquist, A., Lundberg, N., and Ponten, U.: Respiratory and cardiovascular changes during rapid spontaneous variations of ventricular fluid pressure in patients with intracranial hypertension. Acta Neurol. Scand., *40*:291–317, 1964.

142. Kleeman, C. R., Davson, H., and Levin, E.: Urea transport in the central nervous system. Amer. J. Physiol., *203*:739–747, 1962.

143. Klippel, M.: Encephalopathie addisonienne. Rev. Neurol., *7*:898–899, 1899.

144. Knapp, A.: Die Tumoren des Schläffenlappens. Z. Ges. Neurol. Psychiat., *42*:226–289, 1918.

145. Kocher, T.: Hirnerschütterung, Hirndruck and chirurgische Eingriffe bei Hirnerkrankungen Nothnagel's specielle Pathologie und Therapie. Bid. ix, 3 Teil, 2 Abteilung, s 81, 1901.

146. Koch-Weser, J., and Gilmore, E. B.: Benign intracranial hypertension in an adult after tetracycline therapy. J.A.M.A., *200*:345–347, 1967.

147. Kofman, S., Garvin, J. S., Nagamani, D., and Taylor, S. G., III: Treatment of cerebral metastases from breast carcinoma with prednisolone. J.A.M.A., *163*:1473–1476, 1957.

148. Krogh, A.: The active and passive exchanges of inorganic ions through the surfaces of living cells and through living membranes generally. Proc. Roy. Soc., *133*:140–200, 1946.

149. Kullberg, G., and West, K. A.: Influence of corticosteroids on the ventricular fluid pressure. Acta Neurol. Scand., *41*:445–452, 1965.

150. Landis, E. M.: Capillary pressure and capillary permeability. Physiol. Rev., *14*:404–481, 1934.

151. Langfitt, T. W.: Possible mechanisms of action of hypertonic urea in reducing intracranial pressure. Neurology, *11*:196–209, 1961.

152. Langfitt, T. W., and Kassell, N. F.: Acute brain swelling in neurosurgical patients. J. Neurosurg., *24*:975–983, 1966.

153. Langfitt, T. W., and Kassell, N. F.: Non-filling of cerebral vessels during angiography: Correlation with intracranial pressure. Acta Neurochir., *14*:96–104, 1966.

154. Langfitt, T. W., Kassell, N. F., and Weinstein, J. D.: Cerebral blood flow with intracranial hypertension. Neurology, 15:761–773, 1965.

155. Langfitt, T. W., Weinstein, J. D., and Kassell, N. F.: Cerebral vasomotor paralysis produced by intracranial hypertension. Neurology, 15:622–641, 1965.

156. Langfitt, T. W., Weinstein, J. D., and Kassell, N. F.: Vascular factors in head injury: Contribution to brain swelling and intracranial hypertension. In Caveness, W. F., and Walker, A. E., eds.: Head Injury: Conference Proceedings. Philadelphia, J. B. Lippincott Co., 1966. pp. 172–194.

157. Langfitt, T. W., Weinstein, J. D., Kassell, N. F., and Gagliardi, L. J.: Transmission of increased intracranial pressure. II. Within the supratentorial space. J. Neurosurg., 21:998–1005, 1964.

158. Langfitt, T. W., Weinstein, J. D., Kassell, N. F., and Jackson, J. L. F.: Contributions of trauma, anoxia, and arterial hypertension to experimental acute brain swelling. Trans. Amer. Neurol. Ass., pp. 257–259, 1967.

159. Langfitt, T. W., Weinstein, J. D., Kassell, N. F., and Simeone, F. A.: Transmission of increased intracranial pressure. I. Within the craniospinal axis. J. Neurosurg., 21:989–997, 1964.

160. Langfitt, T. W., Shawaluk, P. D., Mahoney, R. P., Stein, S. C., and Hedges, T. R.: Experimental intracranial hypertension and papilledema in the monkey. J. Neurosurg., 21:469–478, 1964.

160a. Langfitt, T. W., Weinstein, J. D., Kassell, N. F., Gagliardi, L. J., and Shapiro, H. M.: Compression of cerebral vessels by intracranial hypertension. I. Dural sinus pressures. Acta Neurochir., 15:212–222, 1966.

161. Laskowski, E. J., Klatzo, I., and Baldwin, M.: Experimental study of the effects of hypothermia on local brain injury. Neurology, 10:499–505, 1960.

162. Lazorthes, G., and Campan, L.: Hypothermia in the treatment of craniocerebral traumatism. J. Neurosurg., 15:162–167, 1958.

163. Lazorthes, G., and Gaubert, J.: Les rapports du III de la clinoide posterieure à sa penetration dans le sinus caverneux. Bull. Ass. Anat., 40:161–164, 1953.

164. Leaf, A., Anderson, J., and Page, L. B.: Active sodium transport by the isolated toad bladder. J. Gen. Physiol., 41:657–668, 1958.

165. LeBeau, J., and Bonvallet, M.: Oedeme aigu du cerveau par lesion due tronc cérébral. C. R. Soc. Biol., (Paris), 127:126–130, 1938.

166. Lemmen, L. J., and Davis, J. S.: Studies of cerebrospinal fluid pressure during hypothermia in intracranial surgery. Surg. Gynec. Obstet., 106:555–558, 1958.

167. Levy, W. A., Taylor, J. M., Herzog, I., and Scheinberg, L. C.: The effect of hypertonic urea on cerebral edema in the rabbit induced by triethyl tin sulfate. Arch. Neurol., 13:58–64, 1965.

168. Lindenberg, R.: Compression of brain arteries as pathogenetic factor for tissue necroses and their areas of predilection. J. Neuropath. Exp. Neurol., 14:223–243, 1955.

169. Lippert, R. G., Svien, H. J., Grindlay, J. H., Goldstein, N. P., and Gastineau, C. F.: The effect of cortisone on experimental cerebral edema. J. Neurosurg., 17:583–589, 1960.

170. Long, D. M., Hartmann, J. F., and French, L. A.: The response of human cerebral edema to glucosteroid administration. An electron microscopic study. Neurology, 16:521–528, 1966.

171. Lowell, A., Cournand, A., and Richards, D. W., Jr.: Changes in plasma volume and mean arterial pressure after the intravenous injection of concentrated human serum albumin in thirty-eight patients with oligemia and hypotension. Surgery, 22:442–452, 1947.

172. Lundberg, N.: Continuous recording and control of ventricular fluid pressure in neurosurgical practice. Acta Psychiat. Scand., suppl. 149, 36:1–193, 1960.

173. Lundberg, N., Kjallquist, A., and Bien, C.: Reduction of increased intracranial pressure by hyperventilation. Acta Psychiat. Scand., 34:4–64, 1959.

174. Lundberg, N., Troupp, H., and Lorin, H.: Continuous recording of the ventricular-fluid pressure in patients with severe acute traumatic brain injury. A preliminary report. J. Neurosurg., 22:581–590, 1965.

175. Maciver, I. N., Frew, I. J. C., and Matheson, J. G.: The role of respiratory insufficiency in the mortality of severe head injuries. Lancet, 1:390–393, 1958.

176. Mack, E. W., Smith, N. B., and Rosenauer, A.: Tracheotomy in severe head injuries. Rocky Mountain Med. J., 56:69–72, 1959.

177. Marshall, W. J. S., Jackson, J. L. F., and Langfitt, T. W.: Brain swelling caused by trauma and arterial hypertension. Arch. Neurol., 21:545–553, 1969.

178. Martin, J. P.: Signs of obstruction of the superior longitudinal sinus following closed head injuries (traumatic hydrocephalus). Brit. Med. J., 2:467–470, 1955.

179. Mason, M. S., and Raaf, J.: Physiological alterations and clinical effects of urea-induced diuresis. J. Neurosurg., 18:645–653, 1961.

180. Masserman, J. H.: Effects of intravenous administration of hypertonic solutions of dextrose. With special reference to the cerebrospinal fluid pressure. J.A.M.A., 102:2084–2086, 1934.

181. McClure, R. D., and Crawford, A. S.: The management of craniocerebral injuries. Arch. Surg., 16:451–468, 1928.

182. McCreery, J. A., and Berry, F. B.: A study of 520 cases of fractures of the skull. Ann. Surg., 88:890–901, 1928.

183. McDowall, D. G., Barker, J., and Jennett, W. B.: Cerebro-spinal fluid measurements during anaesthesia. Anaesthesia, 21:189–201, 1966.

184. McLaurin, R. L.: Contributions of angiography to the pathophysiology of subdural hematomas. Neurology, 15:866–873, 1965.

185. McLaurin, R. L., King, L. R., Knowles, H. Jr., and Elam, E. B.: Water intoxication following intracranial surgery. Neurology, 11:630–638, 1961.

186. McNealy, D. E., and Plum, F.: Brain stem dys-

function with supratentorial mass lesions. Arch. Neurol. Psychiat., 7:10–32, 1962.

187. McQueen, J. D., and Jeanes, L. D.: Dehydration and rehydration of the brain with hypertonic urea and mannitol. J. Neurosurg., 21: 118–128, 1964.

188. Meyer, A.: Herniation of the brain. Arch. Neurol. Psychiat., 4:387–400, 1920.

189. Meyer, J. S., and Hunter, J.: Effects of hypothermia on local blood flow and metabolism during cerebral ischemia and hypoxia. J. Neurosurg., 14:210–227, 1957.

190. Meyer, J. S., Waltz, A. G., and Gotoh, F.: Pathogenesis of cerebral vasospasm in hypertensive encephalopathy: I. Effects of acute increases in intraluminal blood pressure on pial blood flow. Neurology, 10:735–744, 1960.

191. Meyer, J. S., Waltz, A. G., and Gotoh, F.: Pathogenesis of cerebral vasospasm in hypertensive encephalopathy: II. Nature of increased irritability of smooth muscle of pial arterioles in renal hypertension. Neurology, 10:859–867, 1960.

192. Meyers, R.: Systemic vascular and respiratory effects of experimentally induced alterations in intraventricular pressure. J. Neuropath. Exp. Neurol., 1:241–264, 1942.

193. Miyazaki, Y., and Matsumoto, N.: Reduction of intracranial pressure with fructose-mannitol solution. J. Neurosurg., 26:306–312, 1967.

194. Monro, A.: Observations on the Structure and Function of the Nervous System. Edinburgh, Creech and Johnson, 1783.

195. Moody, R. A., Ruamsuke, S., and Mullan, S. F.: An evaluation of decompression in experimental head injury. J. Neurosurg., 29:586–590, 1968.

196. Moyer, J. H., Miller, S. I., and Snyder, H.: Effect of increased jugular pressure on cerebral hemodynamics. J. Appl. Physiol., 7:245–247, 1954.

197. Moyer, J. H., Miller, S. I., Teshnek, A. B., Snyder, D., and Bowman, R. O.: Malignant hypertension and hypertensive encephalopathy: Cerebral hemodynamic studies and therapeutic response to continuous infusion of intravenous Veriloid. Amer. J. Med., 14: 175–183, 1953.

198. Moyer, J. H., Teshnek, A. B., Miller, S. I., Snyder, H., and Bowman, R. O.: Effect of theophylline with ethylenediamine and caffeine on cerebral hemodynamics and cerebrospinal fluid pressure in patients with hypertensive headaches. Amer. J. Med. Sci., 224:377–385, 1952.

199. Munro, D., and Sisson, W. R., Jr.: Hernia through the incisura of the tentorium cerebelli in connection with craniocerebral trauma. New Eng. J. Med., 247:699–708, 1952.

200. Myerson, A., and Loman, J.: Internal jugular venous pressure and its relationship to cerebral spinal fluid pressure. J. Nerv. Ment. Dis., 74:192–194, 1931.

201. Naeraa, N.: Blood-gas analysis in unconscious neurosurgical patients on admission to hospital. Acta Anaesth. Scand., 7:191–199, 1963.

202. Nylin, G., Hedlund, S., and Regnström, O.: Studies of the cerebral circulation with labeled erythrocytes in healthy man. Circ. Res., 9: 664–674, 1961.

203. Obrador, S., and Pi-Suñer, J.: Experimental swelling of the brain. Arch. Neurol. Psychiat., 49:826–830, 1943.

204. Ody, F.: Atlanto-occipital evacuation trepanation in contusions of the brain. Arch. Neurol. Psychiat., 28:112–119, 1932.

205. Owens, G., Stahlman, G., Capps, J., and Meirowsky, A. M.: Experimental occlusion of dural sinuses. J. Neurosurg., 14:640–647, 1957.

206. Pappius, H. M., and Dayes, L. A.: Hypertonic urea. Arch. Neurol., 13:395–402, 1965.

207. Patterson, J. H.: An investigation into the effect of intravenous injection of sucrose on the cerebrospinal fluid pressure as measured by the lumbar puncture. Proc. Roy. Soc. Med., 35:530, 1942.

208. Penfield, W., and Jasper, H.: Epilepsy and the Functional Anatomy of the Human Brain. Boston, Little, Brown and Co., 1954.

209. Penfield, W., and MacEachern, D.: Intracranial Tumors. Oxford Medicine, Chap. VI, pp. 137–216, 1938.

210. Perez, C. A., Hodges, F. J., and Margulis, A. R.: Microangiography in experimental cerebral edema in rats. Radiology, 82:529–535, 1964.

211. Perkins, R. K., Chater, N. L., and Wise, B. L.: The effect of hypertonic sorbitol solution on cerebrospinal fluid pressure in the dog. J. Neurol. Sci., 3:511–514, 1966.

212. Plum, F.: Neural mechanisms of abnormal respiration in humans. Arch. Neurol., 3:484–487, 1960.

213. Plum, F.: Brain swelling and edema in cerebral vascular disease. Ass. Res. Nerv. Ment. Dis., 41:318–348, 1961.

214. Plum, F., and Swanson, A. G.: Central neurogenic hyperventilation in man. Arch. Neurol. Psychiat., 81:535–549, 1959.

215. Plum, F., Alvord, E. C., and Posner, J. B.: The effect of steroids on experimental cerebral infarction. Arch. Neurol., 9:571–573, 1963.

216. Pollock, L. J., and Boshes, B.: Cerebrospinal fluid pressure. Arch. Neurol. Psychiat., 36: 931–974, 1936.

217. Prados, M., Strowger, B., and Feindel, W.: Studies on cerebral edema. II. Reaction of the brain to exposure to air; physiologic changes. Arch. Neurol. Psychiat., 54:290–300, 1945.

218. Pribram, H. F. W.: Angiographic appearances in acute intracranial hypertension. Neurology, 11:10–21, 1961.

219. Quincke, H.: Ueber Meningitis serosa und verwandte Zustande. Deutsch. Z. Nervenheilk., 9:149, 1897.

220. Rasmussen, T., and Gulati, D.: Cortisone in the treatment of postoperative cerebral edema. J. Neurosurg., 19:535–544, 1962.

221. Rawling, L. B.: Cerebral oedema (excess cerebrospinal fluid). Its causation and surgical treatment. Brit. Med. J., 1:499–502, 1918.

222. Reed, D. J., and Woodbury, D. M.: Effect of

hypertonic urea on cerebrospinal fluid pressure and brain volume. J. Physiol. (London), *164*:252–264, 1962.

223. Reed, D. J., and Woodbury, D. M.: Effect of urea and acetazolamide on brain volume and cerebrospinal fluid pressure. J. Physiol. (London), *164*:265–273, 1962.

224. Reid, W. L.: Cerebral herniation through the incisura tentorii. Surgery, *8*:756–770, 1940.

225. Risberg, J., Lundberg, N., and Ingvar, D. H.: Regional cerebral blood volume during acute transient rises of the intracranial pressure (plateau waves). J. Neurosurg., *31*:303–310, 1969.

226. Roberts, H. J.: Supportive adrenocortical steroid therapy in acute and subacute cerebrovascular accidents, with particular reference to brain-stem involvement. J. Amer. Geriat. Soc., *6*:686–702, 1958.

227. Robinson, J. R., and McCanoe, R. A.: Water metabolism. Ann. Rev. Physiol., *14*:115, 1932.

228. Rodbard, S., and Stone, W.: Pressor mechanisms induced by intracranial compression. Circulation, *12*:883–889, 1955.

229. Rose, A., and Matson, D. D.: Benign intracranial hypertension in children. Pediatrics, *39*:227–237, 1967.

230. Rosomoff, H. L.: Method for simultaneous quantitative estimation of intracranial contents. J. Appl. Physiol., *16*:395–396, 1961.

231. Rosomoff, H. L.: Effect of hypothermia and hypertonic urea on distribution of intracranial contents. J. Neurosurg., *18*:753–759, 1961.

232. Rosomoff, H. L.: Distribution of intracranial contents with controlled hyperventilation: Implications for neuroanesthesia. Anesthesiology, *24*:640–645, 1963.

233. Rosomoff, H. L.: Adjuncts to neurosurgical anaesthesia. Brit. J. Anaesth., *37*:246–261, 1965.

234. Rosomoff, H. L., and Gilbert, R.: Brain volume and cerebrospinal fluid pressure during hypothermia. Amer. J. Physiol., *183*:19–22, 1955.

235. Rosomoff, H. L., and Holaday, D. A.: Cerebral blood flow and cerebral oxygen consumption during hypothermia. Amer. J. Physiol., *179*:85–88, 1954.

236. Rosomoff, H. L., Clasen, R. A., Hartstock, R., and Bebin, J.: Brain reaction to experimental injury after hypothermia. Arch. Neurol., *13*:337–345, 1965.

237. Rovit, R. L., and Hagan, R.: Steroids and cerebral edema: The effects of glucocorticoids on abnormal capillary permeability following cerebral injury in cats. J. Neuropath. Exp. Neurol., *27*:277–299, 1968.

238. Russek, H. I., Zohman, B. L., and Russek, A. S.: Cortisone in the immediate therapy of apoplectic stroke. J. Amer. Geriat. Soc., *2*:216–228, 1954.

239. Ryder, H. W., Rosenauer, A., Penka, E. J., Espey, F. F., and Evans, J. P.: Failure of abnormal cerebrospinal fluid pressure to influence cerebral function. Arch. Neurol. Psychiat., *70*:563–586, 1953.

240. Ryder, H. W., Espey, F. F., Kimbell, F. D.,

Penka, E. J., Rosenauer, A., Podolsky, B., and Evans, J. P.: Effect of changes in systemic venous pressure on cerebrospinal fluid pressure. Arch. Neurol. Psychiat., *68*:175–179, 1952.

241. Ryder, H. W., Espey, F. F., Kimbell, F. D., Penka, E. J., Rosenauer, A., Podolsky, B., and Evans, J. P.: Influence of changes in cerebral blood flow on the cerebrospinal fluid pressure. Arch. Neurol. Psychiat., *68*:165–169, 1952.

242. Ryder, H. W., Espey, F. F., Kimbell, F. D., Penka, E. J., Rosenauer, A., Podolsky, B., and Evans, J. P.: The mechanism of the change in cerebrospinal fluid pressure following an induced change in the volume of the fluid space. J. Lab. Clin. Med., *41*:428–435, 1953.

243. Sagawa, K., Ross, J. M., and Guyton, A. C.: Quantitation of cerebral ischemic pressor response in dogs. Amer. J. Physiol., *200*:1164–1168, 1961.

244. Sahs, A. L., and Joynt, R. J.: Brain swelling of unknown cause. Neurology, *6*:791–803, 1956.

245. Scheinker, I. M.: Genesis of encephalopathy due to arsphenamine (central vasoparalysis due to arsphenamine). Arch. Path., *37*:91–98, 1944.

246. Scheinker, I. M.: Transtentorial herniation of the brain stem. Characteristic clinico-pathological syndrome. Pathogenesis of hemorrhages in brain stem. Arch. Neurol. Psychiat., *53*:289–303, 1945.

247. Schoolar, J. C., Barlow, C. F., and Roth, L. J.: The penetration of carbon-14 urea into cerebrospinal fluid and various areas of the cat brain. J. Neuropath. Exp. Neurol., *19*:216–227, 1960.

248. Sedzimir, C. R.: Therapeutic hypothermia in cases of head injury. J. Neurosurg., *16*:407–414, 1959.

249. Selkurt, E. E.: The changes in renal clearance following complete ischemia of the kidney. Amer. J. Physiol., *144*:395–403, 1945.

250. Shapiro, H. M., Langfitt, T. W., and Weinstein, J. D.: Compression of cerebral vessels by intracranial hypertension. II. Morphological evidence for collapse of vessels. Acta Neurochir., *12*:223–233, 1966.

251. Sharpe, W.: The Diagnosis and Treatment of Brain Injuries. Philadelphia, J. B. Lippincott Co., 1920, pp. 108–137.

252. Sharpe, W.: Repeated lumbar punctures and spinal drainage; Diagnostic and therapeutic value in traumatic and allied lesions of the central nervous system. J.A.M.A., *104*:959–965, 1935.

253. Shaw, C., Alvord, E. C., Jr., and Berry, R. G.: Swelling of the brain following ischemic infarction with arterial occlusion. Arch. Neurol., *1*:53–69, 1959.

254. Shenkin, H. A., Goluboff, B., and Haft, H.: The use of mannitol for the reduction of intracranial pressure in intracranial surgery. J. Neurosurg., *19*:897–901, 1962.

255. Shenkin, H. A., Novack, P., and Goluboff, B.: Relation of cerebral circulation to cerebrospinal fluid pressure: Clinical considerations. Arch. Neurol. Psychiat., *68*:408, 1952.

256. Shulman, K.: Small artery and vein pressures in the subarachnoid space of the dog. J. Surg. Res., 5:56–61, 1965.

257. Shulman, K., and Rosomoff, H. L.: Effect of hypothermia on mortality in experimental injury to the brain. Amer. J. Surg., 98:704–705, 1959.

258. Shulman, K., and Verdier, G. R.: Cerebral vascular resistance changes in response to cerebrospinal fluid pressure. Amer. J. Physiol., 213:1084–1088, 1967.

259. Shulman, K., Yarnell, P., and Ransohoff, J.: Dural sinus pressure. In normal and hydrocephalic dogs. Arch. Neurol., 10:575–580, 1964.

260. Sieber, P. R.: Pulse rate and blood-pressure observations as an aid in the treatment of head traumas. Ann. Surg., 67:51–62, 1918.

261. Silverman, D., Parandian, S., Shenkin, H., and Mellies, M.: Effect of intravenous urea on the EEG of brain tumor patients. Electroenceph. Clin. Neurophysiol., 13:587–590, 1961.

262. Siris, J. H., Henry, E. I., and Cukier, D. S.: Occult hypoxemia complicating acute and subacute intracranial lesions. New York J. Med., 62:1440–1443, 1962.

263. Sklar, F. H., Burke, E. F., Jr., and Langfitt, T. W.: Cerebral blood volume: Values obtained with ^{51}Cr-labeled red blood cells and RISA. J. Appl. Physiol., 24:79–82, 1968.

264. Slocum, H. C., Hayes, G. J., and Laezman, B. L.: Ventilator techniques of anesthesia for neurosurgery. Anesthesiology, 22:143–145, 1961.

265. Smyth, G. E., and Henderson, W. R.: Observations on the cerebrospinal fluid pressure on simultaneous ventricular and lumbar punctures. J. Neurol. Psychiat., 1:226–237, 1938.

266. Smythe, L., Smythe, G., and Settlage, P.: The effect of intravenous urea on cerebrospinal fluid pressure in monkeys. J. Neuropath. Exp. Neurol., 9:438–442, 1950.

267. Stephen, C. R., Woodhall, B., Golden, J. B., Martin, R., and Nowill, W. K.: The influence of anesthetic drugs and techniques on intracranial tension. Anesthesiology, 15:365–377, 1954.

268. Stern, W. E., and Good, R. G.: Studies of the effects of hypothermia upon cerebrospinal fluid oxygen tension and carotid blood flow. Surgery, 48:13–30, 1960.

269. Sugarbaker, E. D., and Wiley, H. M.: Intracranial-pressure studies incident to resection of internal jugular veins. Cancer, 4:242–250, 1951.

270. Sukoff, M. H., Hollin, S. A., and Jacobson, J. H., Jr.: The protective effect of hyperbaric oxygenation in experimentally produced cerebral edema and compression. Surgery, 62:40–46, 1967.

271. Sunderland, S.: The tentorial notch and complications produced by herniations of the brain through that aperture. Brit. J. Surg., 45:422–438, 1958.

272. Sunderland, S., and Hughes, E. S. R.: The pupilloconstrictor pathway and the nerves to the ocular muscles in man. Brain, 69:301–309, 1946.

273. Symon, L., Ischikawa, S., and Meyer, J. S.: Cerebral arterial pressure changes and development of leptomeningeal collateral circulation. Neurology, 13:237–250, 1963.

274. Symonds, C. P.: Otitic hydrocephalus. Brain, 54:55–71, 1931.

275. Szabo, L., and Mathe, A.: The effect of urea-mannitol on the electrical activity of the brain in cerebral oedema. Electroenceph. Clin. Neurophysiol., 15:538–539, 1963.

276. Taylor, G. W., and Austin, G. M.: Treatment of pulmonary complications in neurosurgical patients by tracheostomy. Arch. Otolaryng., 53:386–392, 1951.

277. Thompson, R. K., and Malina, S.: Dynamic axial brain-stem distortion as a mechanism explaining the cardiorespiratory changes in increased intracranial pressure. J. Neurosurg., 16:664–675, 1959.

278. Troupp, H.: Intraventricular pressure in patients with severe brain injuries. II. J. Trauma, 7:875–883, 1967.

279. Troupp, H., and Heiskanen, O.: Cerebral angiography in cases of extremely high intracranial pressure. Acta Neurol. Scand., 39:213–223, 1963.

280. Von Bergmann, E.: Allgemeine traumatisch bedingte Störungen des endocraniellen Nervensystems. In Billroth, T., and Luecke, G. A.: Deutsche Chirurgie. Stuttgart, F. Enke, 1880, No. 30, p. 226.

281. Walker, A. E., and Black, P.: The heroic treatment of acute head injuries: A critical analysis of the results. Amer. Surg., 26:184–188, 1960.

282. Walker, A. E., and Adamkiewicz, J. J.: Pseudotumor cerebri associated with prolonged corticosteroid therapy. J.A.M.A., 188:779–784, 1964.

283. Webster, J. E., and Freeman, N. E.: Studies on the cerebrospinal fluid pressure in unanesthetized dogs. Ann. Surg., 113:556–571, 1941.

284. Weed, L. H.: Some limitations of the Monro-Kellie hypothesis. Arch. Surg., 18:1049–1068, 1929.

285. Weed, L. H., and McKibben, P. S.: Pressure changes in cerebrospinal fluid following intravenous injection of solutions of various concentrations. Amer. J. Physiol., 48:512–530, 1919.

286. Weed, L. H., Flexner, L. B., and Clark, J. H.: The effect of dislocation of cerebrospinal fluid upon its pressure. Amer. J. Physiol., 100:246–261, 1932.

287. Weinstein, J. D., and Langfitt, T. W.: Responses of cortical vessels to brain compression: Observations through a transparent calvarium. Surg. Forum, 18:430–432, 1967.

288. Weinstein, J. D., Langfitt, T. W., and Kassell, N. F.: Vasopressor response to increased intracranial pressure. Neurology, 14:1118–1131, 1964.

289. Weinstein, J. D., Langfitt, T. W., Bruno, L., Zaren, H. A., and Jackson, J. L. F.: Experimental study of patterns of brain distortion and ischemia produced by an intracranial mass. J. Neurosurg., 28:513–521, 1968.

290. Weiss, M. H., and Nulsen, F. E.: Effect of glucocorticoids on CSF flow. Presented at the

meeting of the American Association of Neurological Surgeons, Cleveland, April, 1969.

291. White, J. C., Verlot, M., Selverstone, B., and Beecher, H. K.: Changes in brain volume during anesthesia: The effects of anoxia and hypercapnia. Arch. Surg., *44*:1–21, 1942.

292. Williams, D., and Lennox, W. G.: The cerebral blood-flow in arterial hypertension, arteriosclerosis and high intracranial pressure. Quart. J. Med., *8*:185–194, 1939.

293. Williams, G. R., and Spencer, F. C.: The clinical use of hypothermia following cardiac arrest. Amer. J. Surg., *148*:462–465, 1958.

294. Wilson, B. J., Jones, R. F., Coleman, S. T., and Moyer, C. A.: Effects of various hypertonic sodium salt solutions on cisternal pressure. Surgery, *30*:361–366, 1951.

295. Windle, W. F., Rambach, W. A., de Ramirez de Arellano, R. M. I., Groat, R. A., and Becker, R. F.: Water content of the brain after concussion and its noncontributory relation to the histopathology of concussion. J. Neurosurg., *3*:157–164, 1946.

296. Wise, B. L.: Effects of infusion of hypertonic mannitol on electrolyte balance and on osmolarity of serum and cerebrospinal fluid. J. Neurosurg., *20*:961–967, 1963.

297. Wise, B. L., and Chater, N.: Effect of mannitol on cerebrospinal fluid pressure. Arch. Neurol., *4*:96–98, 1961.

298. Wise, B. L., and Chater, N.: The value of hypertonic mannitol solution in decreasing brain mass and lowering cerebrospinal-fluid pressure. J. Neurosurg., *19*:1038–1043, 1962.

299. Wolff, H. G.: Headache and Other Head Pain. New York, Oxford University Press, 1963.

300. Wolff, H. G., and Blumgart, H. L.: The cerebral circulation. VI. The effect of normal and of increased intracranial cerebrospinal fluid pressure on the velocity of intracranial blood flow. Arch. Neurol. Psychiat., *21*:795–804, 1929.

301. Wolff, H. G., and Forbes, H. S.: Cerebral circulation. V. Observations of the pial circulation during changes in intracranial pressure. Arch. Neurol. Psychiat., *20*:1035–1047, 1928.

302. Wright, R. D.: Experimental observations on increased intracranial pressure. Aust. New Zeal. J. Surg., *7–8*:215–235, 1938.

303. Zweifach, B. W.: Microcirculatory aspects of tissue injury. Ann. N. Y. Acad. Sci., *116*: 831–838, 1964.

304. Zwetnow, N.: CBF autoregulation to blood pressure and intracranial pressure variations. CSF and CBF. Scand. J. Clin. Lab. Invest., Suppl. 102, 1968.

19

NUTRITION AND PARENTERAL THERAPY

The importance of maintaining body fluid homeostasis following trauma or operation has been emphasized for more than three decades. Kerpel-Fronius, in 1935, distinguished between the two "pure" types of dehydration, the first being due to water depletion alone, and the second resulting from the depletion of electrolytes.[15] Nadal, Pedersen, and Maddock and Marriott aided in the clinical differentiation of these two types of dehydration by defining the characteristic symptoms and physical findings in each.[19, 24] The work of Moore and Ball in 1952 further elucidated the metabolic reactions occurring in response to trauma.[23] Even though physicians are now increasingly aware of the occurrence of metabolic, fluid, and electrolyte disturbances in the post-traumatic or post-operative period, occasions still arise when the clinical patterns or laboratory findings prove to be confusing, and this often times results in failure to give the patient proper replacement therapy.

During the past 30 years a large body of evidence has been reported that indicates the metabolic response to head injury, cerebral disease, or cerebral operation to be similar to that occurring after general body trauma, usually differing only in the degree of response. Recent investigations have indicated without question that cerebral areas are involved in body fluid and metabolic homeostasis.[42]

HISTORICAL BACKGROUND

Lewy and Gassman were among the earliest investigators to establish a rela-

tionship between central nervous system lesions and electrolyte and metabolic regulation.[17] They found that unilateral stimulation and subsequent destruction of the paroptic ganglion of cats was followed by an increase of blood chlorides with a decrease in urinary chloride. There was no effect upon the blood sugar. They also noted that unilateral stimulation and subsequent destruction of the periventricular nucleus was associated with an increase of the blood sugar with no effect upon the blood chloride. Since that time numerous reports have been made noting the association of electrolyte and metabolic abnormalities occurring in patients with cerebral lesions.

Allott was the first to associate cerebral lesions with hypernatremia and hyperchloremia in the absence of renal disease.[1] He reported five cases in which hypernatremia, hyperchloremia, and azotemia occurred with decreased urinary excretion of sodium and chloride. Three of his patients had ruptured aneurysms of the anterior cerebral artery, one a recent cerebral infarct, and the other a tumor of the choroid plexus.

Sweet et al. found gastrointestinal hemorrhages, hyperglycemia, azotemia, hyperchloremia, and hypernatremia following lesions of the frontal lobe in humans.[35] They presented data on four patients and suggested that these changes occurred with lesions confined to the anterior portion of the frontal lobes. Wolfman and Schoch reported the case of a patient with closed head trauma and midbrain injury who developed hypernatremia, hyperchloremia, azotemia, and hypochloruria.[40] They felt this most likely resulted from water deple-

E. F. WOLFMAN, JR.

tion in a comatose patient. MacCarty and Cooper also found hypernatremia, hyperchloremia, hypochloruria, uremia, and moderate hypopotassemia in a patient in whom both anterior cerebral arteries were ligated proximal to the site of the anterior communicating artery during the removal of a pituitary adenoma.[18] These authors reported upon two additional cases that same year and suggested that cerebral dysfunction concerned with the control of water balance might be responsible for their findings.[7]

Cooper and Crevier, in 1952, reviewed 14 cases of marked hypernatremia or hyperchloremia or both associated with cerebral lesions and added four additional cases.[6] Although they did not elucidate upon the mechanisms involved, they suggested they were neurogenic in origin and perhaps caused by damage to cerebral osmoreceptor mechanisms. They further noted that the cerebral lesions associated with these disturbances usually involved the frontal lobes or hypothalamus.

Simultaneous with the aforementioned documentation of hypertonicity of the extracellular fluid, other reports of "cerebral salt-wasting" were being presented. Peters et al., in 1950, described three cases of excessive sodium excretion in the presence of hyponatremia.[28] The cerebral lesions associated with these disturbances were encephalitis, stroke, and bulbar poliomyelitis. Cort, in 1954, described similar findings in a patient with a glioma of the thalamus.[8]

In addition to the marked derangement of the extracellular electrolytes that occurred in association with cerebral lesions, similar disturbances were found in protein and carbohydrate metabolism. The work of Lewy and Gassman established experimentally a relationship between the brain and glucose metabolism.[17] Sweet et al. found a severe hyperglycemia without acetonuria occurring in a patient 15 days following bilateral frontal lobotomy.[35] Wolfman and Schoch further noted urinary nitrogen excretions ranging between 27 and 34 gm per 24 hours in their patient with a midbrain injury.[40]

These basic reports served to call attention to a relationship between the central nervous system and body fluid, electrolyte, and metabolic homeostasis and to alert the clinician to severe derangements that may occur in association with operation, trauma, or disease of the brain.

METABOLIC RESPONSE TO CRANIOCEREBRAL TRAUMA

McLaurin et al. and Wise, as well as others, have well documented the metabolic changes occurring in patients with craniocerebral injury and have found that in general these changes are similar to those occurring in patients responding to general body trauma or operation.[21, 22, 39] The metabolic response to trauma or operation includes the following:

1. Increased protein catabolism and urine nitrogen excretion.
2. Increased urinary excretion of potassium.
3. Increase in blood sugar.
4. Decreased urinary excretion and decreased serum concentration of sodium and chloride.
5. Decreased body weight.
6. Decreased renal excretion of water.

It has long been assumed that the increased output of adrenal steroids (17-hydroxycorticosteroids and aldosterone) occurring in response to the stress of operation or trauma is responsible for these electrolyte, carbohydrate, and protein metabolic changes. Antidiuresis has been attributed to pain, emotion, and anesthesia producing central stimulation leading to an increased output of antidiuretic hormone.

Sodium

Sodium retention usually begins on the day of operation or injury and lasts between two and four days. The degree of sodium retention may range from minimal to maximal and is related to a number of factors: the status of the functional or circulating extracellular fluid volume before injury or operation, increased output of adrenal cortical steroid hormones, and the area of the brain injured.

Although decreased renal excretion of sodium is a well-known feature of the postoperative and post-traumatic state, the mechanisms responsible for this retention have not yet been clearly defined. There is evidence that the changes in sodium excretion observed under these circumstances can occur *independently* of variation in the supply of adrenal cortical hormones. In normal individuals the renal excretion of sodium is directly related to the functional or circulating extracellular fluid volume.[32,33] Sodium retention that occurs postoperatively also relates directly to a diminution of the effective extracellular fluid volume.[31] Randall and Papper have offered further evidence that the postoperative and post-traumatic retention of sodium is due to a contraction of the circulating extracellular fluid volume, rather than to an augmented output of adrenal cortical steroids.[29] These workers studying healthy young males before and after major orthopedic procedures found that the usual postoperative sodium and chloride retention could be prevented if extracellular fluid losses were restored.

There is now experimental evidence that sodium retention can be due to a cerebral lesion per se. Because of the earlier findings of hypernatremia occurring in patients with lesions of the frontal lobes or hypothalamus, Wolfman et al. have studied the correlation of retention of sodium and chloride, edema of the contralateral leg, and a negative nitrogen balance with a destructive lesion in the precommissural septum.[42] When the precommissural septum was spared, no metabolic derangements were detected.

On the basis of balance studies of humans and experimental animals subjected to craniocerebral injury or operation, the following conclusions may be reached:

1. Sodium retention does occur in most patients for two to three days followed by diuresis and then equilibrium.

2. During this phase of sodium retention the serum sodium tends, paradoxically, to fall, probably owing to water retention.

3. The magnitude of retention is related both to the degree of trauma and the area of the brain injured, i.e., the precommissural septum or its connections.[20,42]

Potassium

Immediately following cerebral operations or trauma, negative potassium balances are common for one or two days, but seldom of enough magnitude to assume clinical significance. It is, therefore, seldom necessary to administer potassium under these circumstances unless extra-renal losses, i.e., diarrhea or vomiting, are occurring. A serum potassium level of less than 3.5 mEq. per liter indicates an extracellular potassium deficit. It should be remembered that serum potassium levels can be misleading and a deficit of total body potassium can be present despite normal serum concentrations of this ion. This can occur when acidosis is present and a shift of potassium occurs from the cells into the circulating extracellular fluid. Under these circumstances the serum potassium concentration may be found to be normal or high, associated with decreased total body potassium. Alkalosis, on the other hand, is associated with a movement of potassium from the extracellular compartment into the cells, resulting in a hypokalemia without loss of potassium from the body. The electrocardiogram is more accurate in detecting serum potassium abnormalities than are serum levels. Low flat T waves, prolonged Q-T intervals, and a depressed RS-T segment are characteristic of hypokalemia. In contrast, hyperkalemia is indicated by tall peaked T waves, absence of P waves, aberrant QRS complexes, and an idioventricular rhythm. Potassium intoxication is most often seen with the cerebral salt-losing syndrome, diabetic coma, or acute renal insufficiency.

Nitrogen

Nitrogen losses are a common accompaniment of craniocerebral trauma, operation, or disease. The usual losses are similar to those following major general surgical procedures, i.e., approximately 10 gm per day, and this catabolic condition lasts from 7 to 10 days. Patients, after cerebral injury or cerebral operations, however, are apt to excrete massive amounts of urinary nitrogen in a manner closely paralleling that of burn patients. The excretion of up to 34 gm of nitrogen per day has been reported and this amounts to an endogenous body protein breakdown of over 200 gm per day.[40] The situations under which this degree of catabolism occurs do not relate directly to the degree of trauma sustained, but are related more to the specific areas of the brain involved. This is confirmed by experiments of Wolfman et al. in which monkeys were subjected first to unilateral and then bilateral destruction of the precommissural septum without hemispherectomy.[43] Sodium and chloride retention and negative nitrogen balances again occurred even though this operation was traumatically a much less extensive operation than hemispherectomy.

Although there is no evidence that the usual period and degree of negative nitrogen balance jeopardizes the patient's postoperative convalescence, it would seem wise to attempt to minimize the effects of massive body protein breakdown, i.e., in excess of 100 gm of body protein per day. The catabolism of large quantities of body protein delivers to the kidneys excessive amounts of urea for excretion. The resultant osmotic diuresis, forced diuresis caused by the osmotic attraction for water of the large quantities of urea being excreted, may produce marked losses of body water. Administration of a high protein diet (1.5 to 2.0 gm protein per kilogram body weight per day) combined with enough calories to meet metabolic demands (2000 to 2500 calories per day) will reduce the negativity of the nitrogen balance sustained and may even produce a positive nitrogen balance.[30]

In summary, negative nitrogen balance is seldom prolonged or excessive, and usually no attempts are necessary to minimize or reverse these losses in the usual neurosurgical patient. One must always be alert for massive losses or situations characterized by chronic negative nitrogen balance (paraplegia). In these latter instances a high protein, high caloric diet, and anabolic steroids may be required to avoid complications.

Water

The response of the neurosurgical patient subjected to craniotomy or craniocerebral trauma is not unlike that of other surgical patients in regard to postoperative water retention. The usual response is that of retaining water for 12 to 36 hours following craniotomy and perhaps somewhat longer following cranial trauma.[20, 45] The response in each instance is presumably caused by the release of antidiuretic hormone from the posterior lobe of the pituitary gland after activation of the supraopticohypophyseal tract. McLaurin found that water retention does occur and that it closely coincides with the period of sodium retention, but different mechanisms are responsible for each.[20] He noted a lack of dependency of water retention on salt metabolism because water balance statistically correlated with sodium balance only on the third postoperative day. Oliguria does not occur if diabetes insipidus is produced by a lesion of the pituitary, the infundibulum, or the supraoptic nucleus of the hypothalamus.

Hormones

The hormonal response of patients to brain injury or operation is also similar to that in other surgical patients. Following injury or operation, the pituitary secretes increased amounts of adrenocorticotropic hormone, which acts upon the adrenal glands to increase their output of the adrenal steroid hormones. Of these, the 11-oxy-17-hydroxycorticosterone known also as cortisol, compound F, or hydrocortisone, is produced in greatest amounts. This hormone is largely responsible for the increased nitrogen excretion, decreased glucose tolerance, and alteration in the formed elements of the blood (decreased lymphocytes, decreased eosinophiles) and involution of lymphoid tissue. It has only a moderate effect on the postoperative retention of sodium and excretion of potassium. Aldosterone, the most potent of the adrenal mineral corticoids, is produced in smaller quantities and is probably primarily responsible for the postoperative electrolyte changes previously mentioned. There is some evidence to suggest that aldosterone cannot account for *all* these changes. For example, postoperative sodium retention has been reported in patients with Addison's disease who have undergone subsequent operations while receiving constant dosages of steroids.[29] There is little question that aldosterone is intimately involved in the regulation of the extracellular fluid volume. Barrter has demonstrated that aldosterone secretion decreased if the

TABLE 19-1 *DIFFERENTIAL DIAGNOSIS OF HYPERTONIC EXTRACELLULAR FLUID*

	COMA PER SE		DIABETES INSIPIDUS WITH THIRST LOSS OR COMA		"OSMOREGULATORY" DEFECT	
	Early	*Late*	*Early*	*Late*	*Early*	*Late*
24-hour urine volume	Oliguric	Increased	Increased	Increased	Normal	Oliguric to increased
Urine specific gravity	Increased	Increased	Decreased	Decreased	Decreased to normal	May be increased
Urine osmolality	Increased	Increased	Decreased	Decreased	Decreased to normal	May be increased
Urinary NaCl	Normal to increased	Decreased to absent	Normal	Normal	Decreased to normal	Normal to increased
Dry mouth and membranes	Present	Severe	Present	Severe	Absent	Minimal
Blood pressure	Normal	Hypotension	Normal to mild hyper-tension	Shock	Normal	Normal
Proper treatment	Water	Water	Water and Pitressin	Water and Pitressin	Water	Water

extracellular fluid volume was increased, regardless of the associated intracellular volume changes, and increased with a contraction of the extracellular fluid volume.[2] Some evidence exists that suggests aldosterone secretion is under the control of volume receptors in the afferent renal arterioles, which respond to changes in the renal arterial pressure and blood flow.[9] A decreased renal arterial blood pressure or flow has been found to increase the release of renin from the juxtaglomerular cells causing the formation of angiotensin II and this substance stimulates the secretion of aldosterone by the adrenal glands. Similarly, an increase in pressure results in a decreased secretion of aldosterone. Probably none of the metabolic responses to operation are regulated entirely by hormones, but rather these substances serve as catalysts to the metabolic and other phenomena occurring.

FLUID AND ELECTROLYTE DERANGEMENTS IN THE NEUROSURGICAL PATIENT

The metabolic responses to cerebral injury and operation are usually unnoticed and most often are of little clinical significance. There are, however, instances in which marked derangements occur and must be recognized and treated if severe sequelae are to be avoided. Often these metabolic abnormalities are of a temporary nature, and if fluid and electrolyte homeostasis can be maintained during the acute phase, the patient will subsequently recover. The electrolyte aberrations encountered can be classified simply as hypertonicity or hypotonicity of the extracellular fluid (Table 19-1).

Hypertonicity of the Extracellular Fluid

Severe hypertonicity of the extracellular fluid has often been observed in patients with cerebral lesions.* Although the etiological mechanisms are largely unknown, enough information is available to permit treatment of these patients in a rational manner. The degree of hypertonicity of the extracellular fluid reported in patients with cerebral lesions has seldom been noted in those without cerebral disease. Most of the reported cases of hypernatremia and hyperchloremia, with or without azotemia, hyperglycemia, and hypokalemia, have had lesions either in the frontal lobes or in the hypothalamus or both.[1, 6, 7, 13, 18, 26, 35, 40, 44] There is no available data to indicate the frequency of hypertonicity occurring in association with cerebral disease, but it has most usually been encountered under the following circumstances: (1) after closed head injury with midbrain involvement; (2) after removal of a craniopharyngioma or a chromophobic adenoma of the pituitary gland; and (3) after rupture of an aneurysm of the anterior cerebral artery.[41]

*See references 1, 5-7, 11-13, 18, 25, 26, 35, 36, 40, 41, 44.

Since awareness of the potential for this complication to develop is essential to early diagnosis in all the foregoing clinical situations, serum electrolytes should be determined routinely after trauma or an operation. Measurement of the 24-hour fluid intake and urine output is also mandatory. In this manner the onset of the metabolic abnormality can be detected and corrective measures instituted early. The hyperosmolal or hypertonic condition has been observed most often in the following three groups of patients: the comatose patient per se; the patient with diabetes insipidus and coma or the patient with diabetes insipidus and the concomitant loss of the sensation of thirst; and in the patient with "osmoregulatory" defects.

The Comatose Patient Per Se

Coma may result from trauma or operation. It is usually necessary to maintain these patients on parenteral fluids for prolonged periods, and many clinicians prefer to limit the quantity of fluids administered to minimize the possibility of producing cerebral edema. In normal subjects, complete fluid restriction does not result in hypertonicity of the extracellular fluid. Nadal et al. withheld all fluids from a normal subject for four days without producing significant extracellular fluid hypertonicity.[24] Thirst, however, became marked and this necessitated the administration of oral fluids.

There are several reasons why the comatose patient is more likely to develop a hyperosmolal extracellular fluid than normal persons. First, since he is unable to express the thirst of which he would complain if conscious, water deficits can progress to more advanced stages without recognition than in patients with an intact thirst mechanism. The thirst mechanism is presumably actuated by losses of intracellular and extracellular fluid and not by the degree of hypertonicity of the extracellular fluid itself.[34] The regulation of the tonicity of the extracellular fluid, in the early stages of water depletion, is dependent upon two physiological processes: renal excretion of sodium and chloride ions equivalent to the deficit of body water, and maximal water reabsorption. As water deprivation continues, the kidneys, presumably under the influence of antidiuretic hormone, continue to reabsorb water. In addition, sodium and chloride ions are reabsorbed, and the urine is concentrated maximally in a compensatory attempt to prevent further depletion of the volume of extracellular fluid. Since obligatory water losses continue in the absence of an adequate intake of water, and since reabsorption of sodium and chloride ions is maximal under these circumstances, the extracellular fluid becomes hypertonic. The comatose patient, unable to express thirst, may progress to the late stages of dehydration before the disproportion between fluid intake and output is recognized. Second, patients with cerebral damage may excrete massive amounts of urinary nitrogen. Such quantities of urinary nitrogen, excreted largely as urea, produce an osmolal diuresis increasing obligatory urinary water losses. Third, some patients, i.e., those with midbrain damage, lose control of the mechanisms regulating body temperature. Consequently, marked elevations in body temperature result in large losses of body water. Finally, with midbrain damage, hyperpnea, with or without polypnea, is commonly seen and serves to greatly increase the quantity of water vaporized from the lungs. Therefore, since water requirements may be increased in comatose patients, dehydration and associated hyperosmolality of the extracellular fluid may develop rapidly if adequate quantities of water are not given.

Many comatose patients excrete large urinary volumes, frequently as high as 3000 ml daily.[40] However, regardless of the volume of urine excreted, if the extracellular fluid is hypertonic, the urine specific gravity or osmolality will be high unless diabetes insipidus or chronic renal disease is present. Excretion of a large volume of highly concentrated urine does not indicate adequate body hydration, but merely represents the least urinary volume in which the contained solute load can be excreted—obligatory losses.

Since the hypernatremia occurring under these circumstances is due to a primary water depletion, the early physical examination of the patient reveals little in the way of positive findings. The greatest absolute water losses are sustained from the intracellular compartment (70 per cent) and only about 7 per cent of the total losses are derived from the plasma volume. Consequently, the physical findings are minimal early and the diagnosis is best confirmed by detecting serum hypertonicity and the high urinary specific gravity or osmolality. As the body water deficit increases, dryness of the mouth, tongue, and mucous membranes will be present. In more advanced stages, hypotension may result from the reduction in total circulatory blood volume (Table 19-1).

Proper therapy will correct the dehydration, and the quantities of fluid necessary to achieve this are determined by correlating the urinary specific gravity or osmolal concentration with the amount of fluid administered. When water balance is re-established, concentrations of the serum electrolytes will decrease and the urine will become more dilute. Patients who are extremely dehydrated, with associated hyperpyrexia or large obligatory urinary losses, frequently require 4000 to 6000 ml of water daily. Water may be administered intravenously as 5 per cent dextrose in water, but cerebral edema is less likely to occur if it is given slowly into the gastrointestinal tract via a small caliber nasogastric tube.

The ideal fluid for replacement not only supplies adequate quantities of water, but also contains enough calories to minimize endogenous protein catabolism, thus reducing the associated osmolal diuresis. For this reason, intravenous solutions of 10 per cent glucose given slowly serve well. If replacement therapy is to be given by way of the intestinal tract, many commercial formulas are available. Many of the commercial formulas cause diarrhea; Youmans has suggested one that seldom does.[46] It is a blended mixture of the regular hospital diet of the day. The low incidence of diarrhea and other complications probably is due to the fact that the gastrointestinal tract is accustomed to this diet. In preparing the blended diet, only the bones and decorations are removed. The remainder is pulverized in a blender. Enough water is added to increase breakfast to 400 ml, lunch to 1000 ml, and dinner to 1000 ml. The tube feeding is begun in small amounts, 10 to 30 ml each two hours as the intravenous fluids are decreased. Ten milli-liters of water is injected in one quick bolus after each feeding. This method is used to clear the feeding tube. Gradually the feeding is increased until 200 ml is given each two hours throughout the day and night. It is important to give the feeding in 200 ml boluses rather than larger doses that may distend the stomach and increase the probability of regurgitation and aspiration of the gastric contents. Experience has shown that if the patient develops diarrhea on this diet, one of the more likely causes is an unauthorized change in the diet by the personnel in the kitchen. In order to decrease the work of blending the diet, such items as milk, raw eggs, or emulsified fat have been substituted for the regular hospital diet. A check with the kitchen personnel can identify and remedy the problem.

A patient on nasogastric tube feeding requires the addition of sodium chloride in the same amount as a normal patient. The diet kitchen personnel must be kept informed of this need. Periodic checks of the serum electrolytes are necessary to insure that adequate sodium and potassium are included in the diet. Additional discussion of nasogastric and gastrotomy feedings is given in Chapter 40.

As the accumulated water deficit is being corrected, replacement of electrolytes may also be required since, in the early stages of water depletion, electrolytes have been excreted by the kidneys in a compensatory attempt to maintain isotonicity of the extracellular fluid.[27] Later, even though the extracellular fluid is hypertonic, the total body quantities of sodium and chloride are reduced. The quantity of electrolytes that must be replaced can be estimated by determining the serum electrolyte concentrations and correlating these values with the urinary excretion of the same ions; a persistently positive sodium or chloride balance occurring while the serum levels of these electrolytes are decreasing indicates the need for larger quantities to be administered.

Interestingly, the clinical condition of patients who have been presumed to have hopeless cerebral damage frequently improves with correction of the dehydration and return of the concentrations of the extracellular electrolytes to normal.

Diabetes Insipidus Associated with Loss of Thirst Sensation or Coma

Patients with diabetes insipidus excrete large urinary volumes of low specific gravity or osmolality. These individuals usually do not become dehydrated because the thirst mechanism, actuated by intracellular and extracellular fluid losses, serves as a compensatory device.[34] However, if because of cerebral injury, the sensation of thirst is not present or the patient is comatose and unable to express thirst, dehydration may occur within 24 to 48 hours unless an adequate amount of exogenous water is supplied. If the necessary supplies of water are lacking, the extracellular fluid becomes concentrated; severe hypertonicity develops more rapidly in this type of patient than in the comatose patient per se who is still able to concentrate urine.

In patients with diabetes insipidus, the osmolality of the urine is usually less than that of the serum. Examination of the mouth shows dryness of the mucous membranes. If the patient is conscious, dysphagia may be present. A 2- to 5-pound loss of body weight may occur in a 24-hour period of time. Occasionally, increasing lethargy or coma in a previously conscious patient results from hypertonicity of the extracellular fluid. Later, sudden circulatory collapse and profound shock may follow a gradual but marked decrease in the total circulating blood volume. Unless appropriate therapeutic measures are immediately undertaken, most of these patients die in "irreversible shock."

Appropriate management of these cases is contingent upon early recognition of this abnormality and correction of the fluid deficits. Since there is insufficient antidiuretic hormonal activity, administration of vasopressin (Pitressin) will prevent the large losses of body fluid that might otherwise occur. Vasopressin may be given either intramuscularly or intravenously. The most commonly used preparation is Pitressin tannate in oil, which is administered intramuscularly. The amount of this drug required and the frequency with which it is administered varies with each patient. It must be given cautiously, and the patient's response carefully evaluated. The average duration of action of Pitressin tannate in oil is 48 hours. If the patient is highly sensitive to Pitressin, or if it is given too frequently or in excessive amounts, water intoxication may occur. Fluids must be given cautiously after Pitressin therapy has been instituted, and the specific gravity, or osmolality, and volume of the urine should be determined daily. If the urinary specific gravity rises and then returns to low levels, more Pitressin must be given. Contrariwise, if oliguria occurs, fluid administration should be limited so that excessive retention of fluid and subsequent water intoxication do not occur.

In the later stages of dehydration, if shock occurs, fluids must be given rapidly to restore the circulating blood volume. If the administered fluids are to be retained, then Pitressin must also be given. Under these circumstances intravenous aqueous Pitressin is preferred, since its action is immediate and of short duration, and cumulation of the drug will not occur. If Pitressin tannate in oil is administered to a hypotensive patient, absorption occurs slowly and usually only after large quantities of fluid have been given. Consequently, significant water retention may occur 24 to 48 hours later and cause water intoxication. Once hypotension has been corrected and the extracellular fluid volume restored, periodic intramuscular Pitressin tannate in oil serves well for maintenance.

The type and quantity of solutions to be replaced are similar to those recommended for the comatose patient per se. If the patient is conscious, oral administration is preferred. If the patient is comatose, replacement may be given enterally via a nasogastric tube of small caliber. If more than 4000 or 5000 ml of fluid must be administered daily, the intravenous route should also be used to prevent troublesome diarrhea. By titrating the dosage of Pitressin with the volume of fluid given, it is possible to correct the deficits of body fluid. With proper titration of pitressin and intravenous and oral fluid, the patient should excrete a 24-hour urinary volume of 1000 to 1500 ml; this urine should have a specific gravity of approximately 1.010 to 1.015.

Patients with "Osmoregulatory" Defects

Although there is no conclusive evidence to indicate the presence of osmoreceptors in the human diencephalon, Verney has presented indirect evidence that favors the presence of osmoreceptors in that portion of the dog brain supplied by the internal carotid arteries.[37] If osmoreceptors do exist in human beings, they should respond to small deviations in the concentration of the extracellular electrolytes. Presumably, increases in the tonicity of the extracellular fluid may normally be prevented by an osmoregulatory response to small increases in the concentration of the extracellular electrolytes. This response may be manifested by either an increased renal excretion of sodium and chloride ions or an inhibition of urine flow or both. If a defect in osmoregulatory function exists, then relatively small deficits of body water could cause hypertonicity of the extracellular fluid, since compensatory urinary losses of sodium and chloride would not occur or because antidiuresis does not result. It is possible then that the severe hypertonicity of the extracellular fluid that is observed in certain patients with cerebral damage is related to a disturbance of some osmoregulatory system that is operative in individuals without cerebral disorders. Such a thesis would explain those cases of extreme extracellular fluid hypertonicity occurring in the absence of clinical signs of dehydration.[6]

The development of hyperosmolality of the extracellular fluid in association with an inadequate supply of water may occur even more rapidly in individuals with postulated osmoregulatory defects than in persons in the other two groups. Since minor deficits of water remain uncompensated, hypernatremia or hyperchloremia or both may develop within 48 hours after injury or operation.

Osmoregulatory defects should be suspected in patients who fail to regain consciousness after head injury or cerebral operation, even though other more common causes exist. The diagnosis can be made by determining the serum electrolyte values and correlating them with urinary concentration. A low urinary osmolality or specific gravity associated with hypertonicity of the extracellular fluid is highly suggestive. For reasons yet unexplained, hyperchloremia usually precedes the hypernatremia. In the early stages of development of this pattern urinary volumes appear adequate, usually ranging from 1000 to 5000 ml daily; urinary specific gravity is low. Later, after the serum becomes more hypertonic, the urine becomes more concentrated; it is not uncommon to find the specific gravity to be 1.020 to 1.035 or the osmolality to exceed 1200 mOsm per liter. In some instances it appears that osmoregulatory response to *moderate changes* in serum osmolality is impaired; when osmolal changes in the serum become great enough, some compensatory response occurs.

Treatment is aimed at correcting the fluid deficits and establishing a positive water balance. The amount of fluid required varies, but approximately 3000 ml daily is sufficient if adequate calories are given to lessen endogenous catabolism of nitrogen and subsequent osmolar diuresis. The fluids may be given either orally as a liquid formula or intravenously in the form of 10 per cent glucose or invert sugar. Again, serum electrolyte levels and urinary concentration serve as a guide to the quantity of fluid required. Once water balance has been established, a progressive fall in the serum electrolyte and urinary concentrations will be noted. To avoid cerebral edema one should attempt to lower the serum electrolyte concentrations gradually over an interval of several days rather than attempting to correct the entire water deficit in a 24-hour period. Concomitant with a return of the serum electrolytes to normal values, improvement in the patient's clinical condition usually occurs.

Hypotonicity of the Extracellular Fluid

Hyponatremia, hypochloremia, hyperchloruria, and hypernatruria may also be seen in association with cerebral disease, injury, or operation, but less commonly than the hypertonic state. Hyponatremia may result from: excessive loss of sodium from the body; an excessive or abnormal retention of body water; the over-administration of electrolyte-free solutions; and any combination of these factors.

Excessive Loss of Body Sodium

Any patient who has been on prolonged diuretic therapy or sodium restriction may have serious depletion of the total body sodium and would be especially susceptible to postoperative hypotonicity of the extracellular fluid. Patients with liver disease or adrenal insufficiency may likewise become hypotonic.

Excessive Retention of Body Water

Peters et al. observed a number of patients with cerebral hyponatremia.[28] They identified this entity as cerebral salt-wasting and postulated that the brain lesion decreased the renal tubular reabsorption of sodium either indirectly by depressing adrenocortical function or directly by way of the renal nerves. Welt et al., in 1952, reported two additional cases and, since these patients excreted large amounts of potassium when given desoxycorticosterone acetate, concluded the salt wastage was due to the impaired proximal renal tubular reabsorption of sodium.[38] In 1954 Cort described a patient with a glioma of the thalamus with hyponatremia.[8] Carter et al. performed balance studies on two patients with cerebral hyponatremia.[4] One of these had a metastatic brain carcinoma and the other a basilar skull fracture. They found that in each instance the hyponatremia resulted from water retention rather than from significant salt wastage. Their studies suggested that the water retention resulted from a persistently high secretion of antidiuretic hormone, but the manner in which the cerebral injury produced this result was not determined. Initially in both patients the secretion of antidiuretic hormone appeared to be autonomous of both osmotic and volume control. In one of their patients the secretion of antidiuretic hormone in the later stages appeared to be under the control of extracellular volume, but remained independent of plasma osmolality. It has been postulated also that the expanded extracellular fluid volume causes increased sodium excretion by inhibiting aldosterone secretion and increasing the glomerular filtration rate.

Overadministration of Electrolyte-Free Solutions

Probably the most common cause of hyponatremia in the neurosurgical patient is the injudicious administration of glucose solutions in the immediate postoperative or post-traumatic period. Water intoxication results when the hyponatremia is marked enough to produce clinical symptoms. Postoperative hyponatremia is a well-known sequela following other major surgical procedures. It is particularly important to recognize hyponatremia in neurosurgical patients because the signs and symptoms closely mimic those of postoperative intracranial hemorrhage or other complications. Furthermore, hyponatremia postoperatively produces cerebral edema and increased intracranial pressure. Since water diffuses freely across the capillary and cell membranes, most of any excess water administered becomes intracellular and, consequently, water intoxication is due to intracellular water rather than to any measurable changes in the extracellular electrolytes.

The signs and symptoms of hypotonicity of the extracellular fluid vary depending upon its cause, the rate with which it develops, and whether or not there is associated intracerebral disease or injury. If total body sodium depletion is contributory to the hyponatremia, there will be a more marked associated decrease in the circulating blood volume. Under these circumstances symptoms of hypovolemia such as tachycardia, weakness, decreased peripheral venous filling, peripheral vasoconstriction, oliguria, and hypotension will be present. The severity of the symptoms relates directly to the extent of the hypovolemia produced by the salt deficit. The most common type of hyponatremia occurring in the neurosurgical patient is dilutional with only minor electrolyte deficits and, depending upon its severity, produces the symptom complex referred to as water intoxication. The more rapidly the serum electrolyte concentration is lowered, the more severe the symptoms. The brain is most sensitive to osmolal changes while the blood-brain barrier is slowly permeable to sodium. Consequently, with rapid decreases in the extracellular fluid tonicity due to overhydration, the brain imbibes water, because it contains a relative excess of sodium, and this produces cerebral swelling. The cerebral swelling is responsible for the neurological symptoms produced.

These vary from subtle manifestations of apprehension, restlessness, depression, and irritability to confusion, disorientation, delirium, seizures, lethargy, coma, and death. Objective findings include serum hypotonicity, elevated cerebrospinal fluid pressure, and decreased voltage and frequency of electroencephalographic activity. Symptoms seldom appear until the serum sodium concentration is less than 128 to 130 mEq per liter. Since the symptomatology produced by hyponatremia is not distinguishable from that due to intracranial hematoma, serum sodium concentration and serum osmolality should be determined before re-exploration of suspected postoperative intracranial hemorrhage.

Treatment of hypotonicity depends upon its cause. Since the symptoms may confuse the surgeon with postoperative or posttraumatic complications, all measures should be employed to prevent the development of hypotonicity. This may be done in most circumstances by the intravenous administration of only sufficient 5 per cent glucose, after injury or operation, to provide for an adequate urinary volume. In general, 1500 ml of 5 per cent glucose will suffice to cover insensible losses and water of vaporization and to provide enough urine to clear metabolic wastes from the body. The urine specific gravity should be monitored simultaneously and, in a glucose-free, protein-free, 24-hour urine sample, should be kept in the 1.015 to 1.020 range. If water intoxication does occur, one can raise the tonicity of the extracellular fluid by either the addition of electrolytes or the restriction and removal of water. All hyponatremic states do not require aggressive treatment, and the use of hypertonic salt solutions should be reserved for those situations in which central nervous system signs are present. A patient in whom a hyponatremia is found by examination of the serum sodium should be treated by water restriction and isotonic electrolyte administration if electrolyte replacement is important (i.e., if total body sodium is reduced).

When central nervous system signs are present, immediate treatment is indicated with hypertonic salt solutions. The type of solution employed depends upon the acid-base balance of the patient. Disturbances in acid-base balance are best diagnosed by determining the serum bicarbonate level along with the serum pH. If neither acidosis or alkalosis is present, therapy can be initiated by the intravenous administration of 500 ml of a solution containing 250 ml of $\frac{1}{3}$ molar sodium lactate and 250 ml of 3 per cent sodium chloride. If acidosis is present, 500 ml of $\frac{1}{3}$ molar sodium lactate should be given. Conversely, if the patient is alkalotic, then 500 ml of 3 per cent sodium chloride is administered. Infusion time should be one and one half hours. Hypertonic solutions are effective because they remove water from the cells, thus reducing intracellular edema as well as expanding the extracellular fluid volume. Certain precautions should be observed during their administration. A central hyperpyrexia may result from the too-rapid withdrawal of fluid from the brain. Therefore, the body temperature should be monitored and, if it exceeds 102° to 103° F, administration should be slowed or discontinued. In elderly patients or those with borderline cardiac status, monitoring of the central venous pressure is advisable so as not to expand the extracellular fluid volume too rapidly.

PARENTERAL NUTRITION

Some patients may be unable to ingest an oral diet in the post-traumatic or postoperative period, and parenteral therapy must be employed. During this interval the metabolic derangements previously mentioned may occur, and careful attention must be given to the metabolic state of the patient. Simple screening techniques such as recording the 24-hour fluid intake and urinary output, and determination of the urine specific gravity and body weight provide helpful guides to clinical management. Ideally, biochemical evaluation of the serum and urine should be obtained preoperatively or in the immediate post-traumatic period and be repeated periodically until the well-being of the patient is evident.

The aim of parenteral therapy is to maintain metabolic homeostasis and to correct any deviations that may occur. In the past it has been impossible to maintain adequate body nutrition by the parenteral route alone over long periods. In recent years, however, much progress has been made in this field until at the present time numerous reports have indicated that appropriate parenteral fluid therapy can achieve and maintain metabolic homeostasis even for a prolonged time.[3, 10, 14, 16]

Dudrick et al. have recently reported upon the administration of a hypertonic nutrient solution into the superior vena cava of over 300 patients for periods of time varying between 7 and 210 days.[10] With this solution, containing large amounts of nitrogen, calories, and vitamins along with the required amounts of electrolytes, they were able to achieve weight gain, positive nitrogen balance, and growth and development. In these patients, neither anabolic steroids nor fat emulsions were required to obtain these results. Despite these advances, parenteral feeding should be used only to maintain the nutritional and metabolic balance of the patient until oral alimentation can be resumed.

REFERENCES

1. Allott, E. N.: Sodium and chloride retention without renal disease. Lancet, *1*:1035–1037, 1939.
2. Barrter, F. C.: The role of aldosterone in normal homeostasis and in certain disease states. Metabolism, *5*:369–383, 1956.
3. Beal, J. M., Payne, M. A., Gilder, H., Johnson, G., Jr., and Carver, W. L.: Experience with administration of an intravenous fat emulsion to surgical patients. Metabolism, 6:673–681, 1957.
4. Carter, N. W., Rector, F. C., Jr., and Seldin, D. W.: Hyponatremia in cerebral disease resulting from the inappropriate secretion of antidiuretic hormone. New Eng. J. Med., *264*: 67–72, 1961.
5. Cooper, I. S.: Disorders of electrolyte and water metabolism following brain surgery. J. Neurosurg., *10*:389–396, 1953.
6. Cooper, I. S., and Crevier, P. H.: Neurogenic hypernatremia and hyperchloremia. J. Clin. Endocr., *12*:821–830, 1952.
7. Cooper, I. S., and MacCarty, C. S.: Unusual electrolyte abnormalities associated with cerebral lesions. Proc. Mayo Clin., 26:354–358, 1951.
8. Cort, J. H.: Cerebral salt wasting. Lancet, *1*: 752–754, 1954.
9. Davis, J. O.: Aldosterone and angiotensin. Interrelationships in normal and diseased states. J.A.M.A., *188*:1062–1068, 1964.
10. Dudrick, S. J., Wilmore, D. W., Vars, H. M., and Rhoads, J. E.: Can intravenous feeding as the sole means of nutrition support growth in the child and restore weight loss in an adult. Ann. Surg., *169*:974–984, 1969.
11. Engstrom, W. W., and Liebman, A.: Chronic hyperosmolarity of the body fluids with a cerebral lesion causing diabetes insipidus and anterior pituitary insufficiency. Amer. J. Med., *15*:180–186, 1953.
12. Gordon, G. L., and Goldner, F.: Hypernatremia, azotemia and acidosis after cerebral injury. Amer. J. Med., *23*:543–553, 1957.
13. Higgins, G., Lewin, W., O'Brien, J. R. P., and Taylor, W. H.: Metabolic disorders in head injury. Hyperchloremia and hypochloremia. Lancet, *1*:1295–1300, 1951.
14. Holden, W. D., Krieger, H., Levey, S., Abbott, W. E.: The effect of nutrition on nitrogen metabolism in the surgical patient. Ann. Surg., *146*: 563–579, 1957.
15. Kerpel-Fronius, E. Ö.: Über die Beziehungen Zwischen Salz- und Wasserhaushalt bei experimentellen Wasserverlusten. Z. Kinderheilk., *57*:489–504, 1935.
16. Larsen, V., and Brockner, J.: The effect of pre- and postoperative parenteral nutrition on the nitrogen balance following major surgery. Acta Chir. Scand., Suppl., *357*:247–251, 1966.
17. Lewy, F. H., and Gassman, F. K.: Experiments on the hypothalamic nuclei in the regulation of chloride and sugar metabolism. Amer. J. Physiol., *112*:504–510, 1935.
18. MacCarty, C. S., and Cooper, I. S.: Neurologic and metabolic effects of bilateral ligation of the anterior cerebral arteries in man. Proc. Mayo Clin., *26*:185–190, 1951.
19. Marriott, H. L.: Water and Salt Depletion. Springfield, Ill., Charles C Thomas, 1950.
20. McLaurin, R. L.: *In* Coveness, W. E., and Walker, A. E., eds.: Head Injury. Conference Proceedings. Philadelphia, J. B. Lippincott Co., 1966, Chapter 11.
21. McLaurin, R. L., King, L., Elam, E. B., and Budde, R. B.: Metabolic response to craniocerebral trauma. Surg. Gynec. Obstet., *110*: 282–288, 1960.
22. McLaurin, R. L., King, L., Tutor, F. T., and Knowles, H., Jr.: Metabolic response to intracranial surgery. Surg. Forum, *10*:770–773, 1960.
23. Moore, F. D., and Ball, M. R.: The Metabolic Response to Surgery. Springfield, Ill., Charles C Thomas, 1952.
24. Nadal, J. W., Pedersen, S., and Maddock, W. G.: Comparison between dehydration from salt loss and from water deprivation. J. Clin. Invest., *20*:691–703, 1941.
25. Natelson, S., and Alexander, M. O.: Marked hypernatremia and hyperchloremia with damage to the central nervous system. A.M.A. Arch. Int. Med., *96*:172–175, 1955.
26. Peters, J. P.: The role of sodium in the production of edema. New Eng. J. Med., *239*:353–362, 1948.
27. Peters, J. P.: Water balance in health and disease. *In* Duncan, G. C.: Diseases of Metabolism. 2nd Ed. Philadelphia, W. B. Saunders Co., 1947, pp. 271–346.
28. Peters, J. P., Welt, L. G., Sims, E. A. H., Orloff,

J., and Needham, J. A.: Salt-wasting syndrome associated with cerebral disease. Trans. Ass. Amer. Physicians, *63*:57–64, 1950.

29. Randall, R. E., and Papper, S.: Mechanism of postoperative limitation in sodium excretion: The role of extracellular fluid volume and of adrenal cortical activity. J. Clin. Invest., *37*: 1628–1641, 1958.

30. Rhoads, J. E.: Protein nutrition in surgical patients. Fed. Proc., *11*:659–665, 1952.

31. Shires, T., Williams, J., and Brown, F.: Acute changes in extracellular fluid associated with major surgical procedures. Ann. Surg., *154*: 803–810, 1961.

32. Smith, H. W.: Salt and water volume receptors. Amer. J. Med., *23*:623–652, 1957.

33. Strauss, M. B.: Body Water in Man: The Acquisition and Maintenance of the Body Fluids. Boston, Little, Brown & Co., 1957.

34. Strauss, M. B.: Body Water in Man. Boston, Little, Brown and Co., 1957, pp. 29–49.

35. Sweet, W. H., Cotzias, G. C., Seed, V., and Yakovlev, P. I.: Gastrointestinal hemorrhages, hyperglycemia, azotemia, hyperchloremia, and hypernatremia following lesions of the frontal lobe in man. (1947). Ass. Res. Nerve. Dis. Proc., *27*:795–831, 1948.

36. Ullmann, T. D.: Hyperosmolarity of the extracellular fluid in encephalitis. Amer. J. Med., *15*:885–890, 1953.

37. Verney, E. B.: Croonian Lecture: Antidiuretic hormone and factors which determine its re-lease. Proc. Roy. Soc. London, s.B. *135*:25–105, 1947.

38. Welt, L. G., Seldin, D. W., Nelson, W. P., German, W. J., and Peters, J. P.: Role of the central nervous system in metabolism of electrolytes and water. Arch. Int. Med., *90*:355–378, 1952.

39. Wise, B. L.: Fluids and Electrolytes in Neurological Surgery. Springfield, Ill., Charles C Thomas, 1965.

40. Wolfman, E. F., Jr., and Shoch, H. K.: Water depletion in the comatose patient. Univ. Mich. Med. Bull., *17*:73–82, 1951.

41. Wolfman, E. F., Jr., Coon, W. W., and Kahn, E. A.: The recognition and management of severe hypertonicity of the extracellular fluid associated with cerebral lesions. Surgery, *47*:410–416, 1960.

42. Wolfman, E. F., Jr., Coon, W. W., and Schwartz, S.: Sodium retention following experimental lesions of the precommissural septum in the monkey. J. Surg. Res., *6*:2–18, 1966.

43. Wolfman, E. F., Jr., Coon, W. W., and Sloan, C.: Unpublished data.

44. Wolfman, E. F., Jr., Coon, W. W., Reifel, E., Iob, V., and McMath, M.: Severe hypertonicity of the extracellular fluid associated with cerebral lesions. Surgery, *47*:929–939, 1960.

45. Wynn, V., and Rob, C. G.: Water intoxication: Differential diagnosis of the hypotonic syndromes. Lancet, *1*:587–594, 1954.

46. Youmans, J. R.: Personal communication.

V

Anesthesia and Operative Technique

20

ANESTHESIA

The anesthetic management of the neurosurgical patient should concern the neurosurgeon as well as the anesthesiologist. Probably in no other field can the skills of the anesthesiologist so profoundly affect the work of the surgeon. This is particularly true for intracranial surgery because all anesthetic agents and techniques may significantly alter normal cerebral physiology and, secondarily, intracranial dynamics. Intelligent management of the patient requires that the anesthesiologist fully understand the procedure planned by the surgeon and know the patient's preoperative neurological status. When he has this information, consultation with the neurosurgeon will permit selection of the proper anesthetic agents and techniques, and determination of possible need for special techniques and monitoring devices. The neurosurgeon should be aware of the major effects of anesthesia on cerebral physiology and should be familiar with both the cerebral and systemic effects of the various special techniques available to him.

GENERAL PRINCIPLES

Airway

Providing an adequate airway is vitally important in all phases of the care of patients with intracranial disease. This is so not only because of the undesirable effects of hypoxia and carbon dioxide accumulation but also because of the direct relationship of intracranial pressure to intrathoracic

J. D. MICHENFELDER
G. A. GRONERT
K. REHDER

and intra-abdominal pressure. Any degree of airway obstruction may trigger the vicious circle of increased intracranial pressure, cerebral hypoxia, and irreversible edema. Managing the airway in the comatose patient requires careful evaluation of the depth of coma and the prognosis. In light coma the presence of adequate muscle tone, active protective reflexes, and adequate tidal volume and respiratory rate permits a "wait and watch" approach. Deeper coma associated with deterioration of any of these factors or the presence of excessive tracheobronchial secretions requires endotracheal intubation. In general, any patient who requires an oropharyngeal or nasopharyngeal airway should be intubated unless immediate improvement is anticipated. If the prognosis indicates a long-term problem (more than 48 hours), elective tracheostomy should be done after intubation. If the patient is expected to improve within 48 hours, or is dying, an endotracheal tube is sufficient.

The use of armored endotracheal tubes has solved most of the problems related to unusual operative positions or inaccessibility of the airway. Specific airway problems may be encountered in patients with fixed cervical spine, fracture of the cervical spine, limited mandibular motion, or head and neck trauma; these patients must have careful preoperative evaluation to determine the feasibility of intubation. If loss of the airway is likely when general anesthesia is induced, the patient should be intubated while awake. Rarely, intubation is mechanically impossible or carries sufficient potential hazard to warrant an elective preoperative tracheostomy.

Postoperative airway problems may result from dysfunction of the ninth, tenth, or twelfth cranial nerve, usually caused by operative trauma during the removal of a tumor of the fourth ventricle.[3] Damage to the vagus nerve is most important to assess since it may result in loss of protective airway reflexes and interfere with swallowing. The potential hazard of aspiration in these patients makes tracheostomy mandatory. Bilateral damage to the twelfth cranial nerve may also make tracheostomy necessary because of the resulting loss of motor function and inability to maintain an airway.

Premedication

As in all surgical procedures, the purpose of premedication in neurosurgery is to ensure that the patient is in a suitable state for smooth induction of anesthesia, is protected from harmful reflexes, and is free of anxiety. In the patient with intracranial disease, there is often a narrow margin between inadequate medication, resulting in struggling or straining, and excessive medication, resulting in airway obstruction, hypoventilation, or circulatory depression. In general, excessive medication should be avoided by using narcotics or hypnotics minimally if at all in infants, in patients with increased intracranial pressure, and in comatose patients. Atropine is a useful drug in most patients; it reduces tracheobronchial secretions and, in sufficient dosage, will minimize vagal effects on the heart secondary to anesthetic drugs or surgical manipulation. Such vagal reflexes may be expected during pneumoencephalography, carotid angiography, carotid surgery, orbital exploration or decompression, trigeminal nerve surgery, and posterior fossa exploration. Antiemetics may be a useful addition to the premedications to prevent nausea and retching, which are particularly likely to occur during pneumoencephalography and ventriculography under regional anesthesia.

Local Anesthesia

Before World War II, regional anesthesia was often the anesthetic method of choice for intracranial surgery, in part because of the deficiencies in techniques and personnel available for administering general anesthesia. In some respects local anesthesia is particularly well suited for brain surgery: the brain itself is insensitive to pain, and with adequate infiltration of the extracranial tissues, surgical pain is minimal; the patient's response to manipulation and retraction of the brain can be assessed accurately; and central nervous system depression by anesthetic agents is minimized. The disadvantages of local anesthesia are equally apparent: uncooperative patients may require sedation to the point of uncontrolled depression of the central nervous system; cooperative patients become increasingly uncomfortable from prolonged maintenance of a rigid position; any patient may experience nausea with retching, straining, and coughing; control of the airway is not always possible; and the maintenance of adequate ventilation is not assured. With the introduction of new agents and techniques and the increasing availability of trained personnel for the administration of general anesthesia, the desirability of regional anesthesia in most institutions has decreased to the point at which it now is reserved for only a few neurosurgical procedures. These generally include procedures that require continuous evaluation of the patient's neurological status, such as carotid ligation, percutaneous cordotomy, stereotaxic operations, and electrocorticography; or brief uncomplicated procedures such as pneumoencephalography, cerebral angiography, myelography, and drilling of burr holes for extracerebral hematomas, ventricular drainage, or ventriculography.

The *use of regional anesthesia in no way reduces the need for continuous monitoring and care of the patient.* Premedication for patients scheduled for operation under regional anesthesia should not be excessive; it is preferable to provide sedation intravenously as required during surgery. Selection of the proper local anesthetic for infiltration should be based primarily on the anticipated length of the procedure. For a craniotomy of several hours' duration, intermittent fortification of the initial anesthetic by infiltration is necessary. The addition of epinephrine to the local anesthetic is optional, but its use prolongs the anesthesia and significantly reduces loss of blood from the highly vascular tissues of the scalp.

It is a common misconception that "sick"

or comatose patients will not tolerate general anesthesia and must, therefore, be operated upon under regional anesthesia. This may have been true in past years; however, current techniques of general anesthesia permit a significantly greater degree of control of the patient's vital functions than is possible with any regional technique. If regional anesthesia is selected for a comatose patient, an adequate airway must be provided, either by preoperative tracheal intubation or by tracheostomy.

Neuroleptanalgesia

In recent years, a new group of drugs has been introduced which is capable of producing a sedated but rousable patient with emotional detachment or psychic indifference.[30] Such a state is produced by the combination of a so-called neuroleptic drug such as droperidol or haloperidol and a narcotic, specifically phenoperidine or fentanyl. The latter drugs are in themselves emetics; the addition of a neuroleptic drug counteracts this effect and, in addition, provides a cataleptic state, diminishes sensitivity to epinephrine and norepinephrine, and may produce undesirable extrapyramidal effects. Operations not requiring muscular relaxation may be performed using these agents alone. Circulation is said to be stable, but drug antagonists may be needed on emergence. Properly administered, neuroleptanalgesia does not interfere with the patient's ability to cooperate; hence, it has been recommended for electrocorticography and for diagnostic neurosurgical procedures. Because these drugs may either induce or remove tremor, their use during thalamotomy is questionable. Supplemental nitrous oxide, relaxants, and controlled respiration produce satisfactory anesthesia for both adult and pediatric neurosurgical procedures. Neuroleptanalgesia has become accepted increasingly in many areas; its rational use implies that the agents be administered separately for specific patient needs.

General Anesthesia

The ideal agent for general anesthesia in neurosurgery should be potent, nonirritating, nonexplosive, stable, and nontoxic; should permit rapid, smooth induction and awakening (without coughing, retching, or vomiting); should abolish laryngeal and pharyngeal reflexes at light levels of anesthesia; and should be compatible with epinephrine. It should not increase intracranial pressure or unduly depress the cardiovascular or other organ systems of the body. No agent meets all these criteria; accordingly, individual preferences generally include the combination of two or more agents in an attempt to approach the ideal. Basic to most combinations is nitrous oxide. Variation exists primarily in the selection of supplementary agents. Recommended agents include halothane, ethyl ether, trichloroethylene, methoxyflurane, and various intravenously administered drugs such as hydroxydione, narcotics, thiopental, muscle relaxants, and neuroleptanalgesics.

Nitrous oxide is generally administered in a 60 to 70 per cent concentration; the resultant limitation on the inspired oxygen concentration is the primary disadvantage to its use. Relative contraindications to nitrous oxide arise during and after air encephalography and in procedures in which air embolism is a possible complication.[34] In severely depressed semicomatose patients, supplementation with other agents may not be required, particularly if ventilation is controlled. Similarly, in alert patients, nitrous oxide may be used along with large doses of muscle relaxants and controlled ventilation; this combination provides adequate analgesia and amnesia for most neurosurgical procedures, although some recommend supplementation with an opiate. The combination of nitrous oxide and a relaxant also may be used for electrocorticography because it rarely interferes with the observation of significant electrical patterns.[5]

Of the volatile anesthetics, halothane is probably selected most frequently, because it approaches several of the ideal requirements. It is potent and nonexplosive; it reduces pharyngeal reflexes at light levels of anesthesia; and it is characterized by a smooth, rapid induction and emergence. Objections to its use include the possibility that it produces an increase in cerebrospinal fluid pressure, an increased incidence of hypotension, and possible hepatic necrosis.

The effect on the cerebrospinal fluid pressure presumably is secondary to a mild degree of cerebral vasodilatation and is therefore probably countered by moderate hyperventilation.[48] Hepatic necrosis may be a remote risk (possibly only after repeated administration).[25]

Methoxyflurane has been recommended as a satisfactory substitute for halothane, primarily because of a reportedly lower incidence of hypotension at similar anesthetic levels. The outstanding disadvantage to its use is the prolonged emergence from the depressive effects on the central nervous system. This is a crucial consideration after intracranial surgery because the anesthetic effects cannot be differentiated from the effects of cerebral edema, infarction, or hemorrhage. Delayed recognition of such complications will postpone corrective measures, possibly beyond reversibility. Instances of renal failure after methoxyflurane anesthesia have been reported, but their relation to this agent is unknown. Ethyl ether is objectionable because of the prolonged emergence associated with its use and the hazard of explosion. Trichloroethylene was at one time frequently selected for neurosurgery. Its incompatibility with soda lime and the occurrence of tachypnea and ventricular arrhythmias associated with its use caused most anesthesiologists to abandon it after halothane was introduced.

Regardless of the primary agent selected, there are certain requirements of every general anesthetic administered for intracranial surgery. Induction should be as rapid and smooth as is possible; in adults this is best accomplished with intravenously administered barbiturates such as thiopental or methohexital. Endotracheal intubation should be attempted only when laryngeal reflexes are completely abolished or when total paralysis of the skeletal muscles has been produced. Intubation should be preceded by topical application of a local anesthetic, such as 4 per cent lidocaine, to the trachea and larynx. Considerations regarding techniques of ventilation are discussed elsewhere in this chapter.

The pediatric neurosurgical patient may be anesthetized with the same agents, with some modifications, as the adult. An induction technique using rectally administered thiopental, thioamylal, or methohexital, although generally smooth, is not well suited because of possible depression of vital centers and prolongation of postoperative recovery. Routine considerations include the monitoring and maintenance of body temperature and careful attention to blood loss and replacement. Special techniques such as deliberate hypotension and hypothermia are rarely, if ever, required in children, and control of intracranial pressure (assuming the existence of adequate ventilation) is seldom a problem.

Some neurosurgeons advocate the injection of epinephrine into and around the incision to produce local hemostasis. Epinephrine is compatible with most anesthetic agents under certain conditions, notably control of dosage and adequate ventilation. It is not generally recommended for use with halothane, as instances of ventricular fibrillation have been reported. Nonetheless, epinephrine has been used by some in combination with both halothane and methoxyflurane.

SPECIAL CONSIDERATIONS

Electrocorticography and Stereotaxis

Anesthesia for electrocorticography and stereotaxic procedures may present special problems that require significant alterations in the usual anesthetic techniques. These alterations are necessitated by the potential need for an "awake" electroencephalographic pattern or a rational response from the patient during the procedure. This has been accomplished by a variety of techniques, none entirely satisfactory. The objections to local anesthesia have been discussed. These can be partly remedied by inducing general endotracheal anesthesia after completing that part of the procedure that requires an awake patient; this can be technically difficult and hazardous because of the limitations imposed by the draped open head. The opposite approach has also been used: beginning with general endotracheal anesthesia and then, when needed, arousing the patient; then completing the operation using local infiltration or reinducing general anesthesia. This is an unpredict-

changes in pleural pressure from changes in endotracheal pressure without knowledge of pulmonary resistance (airway plus pulmonary tissue resistance), pulmonary compliance, and respiratory effort.

Potential harmful effects of hyperventilation are cerebral vasoconstriction with possible cerebral hypoxia, tetany, shift of the hemoglobin dissociation curve to the left (Bohr effect), decrease in cardiac output, increase in fixed acids, and decrease in arterial oxygen tension. Some of these effects warrant further comment.

An abrupt decrease in Pa_{CO_2} results in an exponential decrease in PCO_2 of tissue and cerebrospinal fluid and a concomitant decrease in hydrogen ion in the cerebrospinal fluid. After a few hours of hyperventilation, a "normal" pH results from a decrease in bicarbonate ion of the cerebrospinal fluid that is proportional to the lowered PCO_2. If hyperventilation ceases, the Pa_{CO_2} will rise initially; this is followed a few minutes later by the PCO_2 of the cerebrospinal fluid. However, the bicarbonate ion in the cerebrospinal fluid remains low. This produces an acidotic cerebrospinal fluid and stimulation of the central chemoreceptors; thus, a transient period of active hyperventilation may be observed despite normal chemical composition of the blood. It was recently suggested that the obligatory hypoventilation eventually necessary, after hyperventilation, to restore depleted supplies of body carbon dioxide, can last as long as an hour and may result in arterial hypoxia.[38]

Reported biochemical changes in the blood associated with hyperventilation vary and include a decrease in standard bicarbonate, a progressive decrease of buffer base and an increase of lactic acid, a decrease of bicarbonate with unchanged buffer base and only slightly elevated lactic acid levels, and a bicarbonate deficit with a rise in lactic and pyruvic acids. Recently, striking increases in brain and cerebrospinal fluid lactate, independent of blood levels, were found in anesthetized dogs hyperventilated for six hours.[28]

The reported effects of hyperventilation on cerebral function are inconsistent. Clutton-Brock found, in conscious volunteers, increased pain thresholds with active hyperventilation; he suggested that cerebral hypoxia may be produced by hyperventilation.[7] Robinson and Gray found similar responses in passively hyperventilated, conscious subjects, although increases of pH above 7.55 did not further raise the pain threshold.[31] Retinoscopy showed constricted retinal vessels. Contrary to the findings of Clutton-Brock, these authors did not find any change in pain response when they hyperventilated their patients with oxygen; they did not believe that the cerebral effects of passive hyperventilation were due to hypoxia. Barach and associates concluded that all degrees of hyperventilation at normal atmospheric pressure were detrimental to cerebral function.[4] Allen and Morris found a depression of the critical flicker-fusion test in 17 of 21 hyperventilated patients and concluded that hyperventilation in a patient under anesthesia can cause demonstrable cerebral malfunction, which is, however, minor in degree and duration.[2] Whitwam and associates, however, were unable to demonstrate any deterioration in cerebral function after passive hyperventilation in five volunteers, as measured by the critical flicker-fusion test.[47] Alteration of the blood-brain barrier after hyperventilation was recently described in cats, when Pa_{CO_2} was maintained below 20 mm of mercury for five hours. Cohen and associates were unable to demonstrate biochemical evidence for cerebral hypoxia during halothane anesthesia at a Pa_{CO_2} of 25 mm of mercury.[8] Alexander and co-workers observed, during nitrous oxide anesthesia with Pa_{CO_2} levels below 20 mm of mercury, an insignificant decrease in aerobic utilization of glucose accompanied by mild, readily reversible electroencephalographic changes consistent with mild hypoxia.[1] These authors concluded that only minimal hyperventilation should be used in patients with arterial hypotension or central-nervous-system disease, in the patient of advanced age, or in the febrile patient whose cerebral metabolic rate is increased. Sugioka and Davis found decreased cerebral oxygen tension in dogs during hyperventilation with room air, and an increase in cerebral oxygen tension when 5 per cent carbon dioxide was added to the inspired gas mixture.[37] These authors believed that cerebral hypoxia was produced by cerebral vasoconstriction caused by hypocapnia. The validity of their methods has been questioned.

Apparently, no generalizations regarding the consequences of passive hyperventilation can be made. Variability in the observed effects relates to the degree of hypocapnia, the duration of hyperventilation, the presence or absence of muscle relaxants, the presence or absence of a negative expiratory phase, the position of the patient, his condition, the nature of the operative procedure, and the interrelationship of respiratory rate, tidal volume, and airway pressure. However, based on the extensive clinical experience involving the use of passive hyperventilation, it is reasonable to conclude that this technique is hazardous only when used at the extremes of the previously mentioned variables. Its use in neurosurgery has virtually abolished the previously common complications related to inadequate ventilation and hypercapnia. It is likely that continuing investigations ultimately will resolve most of the existing controversies.

Deliberate Hypotension

The indications for induced hypotension in neurosurgery are not clearly defined. Those who make use of the technique generally recommend it for the removal of highly vascular tumors (meningiomas and hemangioendotheliomas) and the repair of vascular lesions (aneurysms and arteriovenous anomalies). Its application for the sole purpose of reducing brain bulk has been condemned; such an effect has never been substantiated and if it does occur, probably results from a reduction in cerebral blood flow only. The primary objections to hypotension in neurosurgery result from the uncertainties regarding the adequacy of cerebral blood flow, and the possible complications of "retractor anemia" or reactionary hemorrhage.

The effect of hypotension on cerebral blood flow is an important consideration. In normotensive supine persons a reduction in the mean arterial pressure to 60 mm of mercury is well tolerated. At pressures below this level, the variation in opinion, experience, and results suggests that, in at

least some patients, ischemic damage may occur. The work reported by Eckenhoff and associates is an outstanding exception to this generalization.[10] In this study, use of a 24-degree head-up tilt and ganglionic blockade lowered the systolic pressure to 70 mm of mercury in 23 patients and to 50 mm of mercury in 6 patients; these pressures were maintained for average periods of 42 and 39 minutes, respectively. Oxygen tension of jugular blood was used as an index of cerebral blood flow, and in no patient did the P_{O_2} decrease below a level of 27 mm of mercury, well above the presumed critical level of 15 to 20 mm of mercury. Rosomoff has cautioned against a direct application of this work to neurosurgery, since these patients were not studied during craniotomy.[33] Furthermore, the demonstration of an "adequate" jugular blood oxygen tension does not guarantee that regional cerebral blood flow is adequate. The potential untoward effects of hypotension on the heart, kidneys, and liver are well known and need not be reviewed here.[18]

Techniques recommended for the induction and maintenance of hypotension for neurosurgery vary; familiarity with the method selected is probably the most important consideration. Most anesthesiologists prefer either ganglion-blocking agents or deep anesthesia with halothane, supplemented by positive-pressure ventilation and varying degrees of head-up tilt. Although both these techniques are associated with a decrease in cardiac output, there is some evidence that ganglionic blockade produces a less significant decrease and may, therefore, be preferred to deep anesthesia with halothane as the primary method. Of the several ganglion-blocking agents available, the most commonly used are hexamethonium (100 to 300 mg), pentolinium (3 to 20 mg), or trimethaphan given as 0.1 to 0.2 per cent solution by intravenous drip. Trimethaphan offers a distinct advantage because the rapid onset and brief duration of action permit momentary control in accordance with surgical requirements. Disadvantages associated with its use include the common occurrence of tachyphylaxis and an unpredictable degree of sensitivity to vasopressors. If vasopressors are administered, subsequent induction of hypotension with trimethaphan is often difficult or impossible. The theoretic disadvantage of histamine release with this drug has not been demonstrated to provide a significant contraindication to its use in man.

Supplementation of drug-induced hypotension by increasing the mean airway pressure has been recommended by Enderby as a method of maintaining a stable level of hypotension.[13] The resultant increase in central venous pressure with this technique may be undesirable in neurosurgery, depending primarily on the degree of head-up tilt. The latter not only is an important consideration in providing an adequate venous drainage but also is an obvious means of reducing intracranial arterial blood pressure. The proper degree of head-up tilt can be determined only in relation to the arterial pressure as measured in the arm since, for every inch of elevation of the head above the heart (assuming the arm cuff to be level with the heart), a decrease of 2 mm of mercury in intracranial arterial pressure occurs. Thus, the arbitrary placement of limits on the "safe" degree of head-up tilt has little significance; rather, this limit varies directly with the arterial pressure. It is equally apparent that for intracranial surgery the judicious use of head-up tilt is an important supplement to induced hypotension, regardless of the primary method selected.

For most neurosurgical procedures, the duration of hypotension required is brief; hence, the selection of long-acting agents or methods that do not permit rapid reversal should be avoided. For the same reason, the combination of hypothermia with hypotension is rarely desirable. This method has been recommended as a theoretical means of reducing the possibility of ischemic damage to vital organs secondary to hypotension; this has not been proved clinically. The combination converts a brief, relatively simple procedure into a prolonged complicated one and probably introduces as many hazards as it is intended to overcome. Exceptions are the techniques described by Brown and Horton and Small and Stephenson, in which hypotension is produced intermittently by rapid intracardiac pacing of the heart, resulting in virtual arrest of the circulation; in these procedures, hypothermia is essential to provide sufficient time for surgical correction of an aneurysm.[6, 35]

There can be no absolute contraindications to induced hypotension in neurosurgery, since at any time it may provide the only chance for a successful surgical outcome. As an elective procedure, it should be restricted to patients without significant systemic disease. Its use in patients with increased intracranial pressure should be avoided until the dura has been incised and the brain decompressed. After the definitive surgical procedure, the pressure must be returned to normal before the dura is closed and the surgical field is lost to view. If ganglion-blocking agents are used, the possibility of postoperative cycloplegia should be anticipated and not misinterpreted as evidence of an intracranial disaster.

Hypothermia

Hypothermia has been a controversial technique since first introduced in 1940 by Smith and Fay.[36] In neurosurgery the method enjoyed periods of great enthusiasm: in 1955, after the initial use of moderate hypothermia in the surgical repair of aneurysms;[20] in 1957, after experimental evidence indicated its efficacy in the treatment of cerebral infarction and injury; and in 1960, after profound levels of hypothermia and circulatory arrest were utilized in the repair of aneurysms. In each instance, initial interest has been followed by disenchantment because of disappointing results and unexpected complications. The current status of hypothermia is difficult to evaluate, but a continuing interest in techniques that permit selective profound cooling of the brain or safe periods of circulatory arrest during moderate hypothermia suggests that a new wave of enthusiasm may be gathering.

Despite this continuing controversy, the therapeutic basis of hypothermia is well established. A reduction in body temperature is accompanied by a significant, predictable reduction in oxygen requirements of the whole body including the brain. Thus, if the brain can safely withstand 4 minutes without perfusion at 38° C, this period will be approximately doubled at 30° C, quadrupled at 22° C, and at 16° C more than 30 minutes of continuous circulatory arrest is tolerated. The promise of a bloodless surgical field for the intricate repair of intracranial vascular lesions assures a continuing interest in hypothermic techniques.

Studies concerned with the systemic effects of induced hypothermia have not uncovered any significant deleterious effects within well-defined limits. Above 28° C, and in the absence of shivering, cardiac output is maintained in relation to oxygen requirements, and cardiac arrhythmias, although frequent, are rarely serious problems. Below 28° C, progressive impairment of myocardial function and increasing myocardial irritability necessitate support of the circulation by extracorporeal techniques. This significant alteration in technical requirements provides a convenient point for the separation of moderate and profound hypothermic techniques.

Acid-base alterations relate primarily to the temperature achieved rather than the technique used. Confusion on this subject results from an inability to define normal values at an abnormal temperature. A decrease in temperature is accompanied by an increase in solubility of carbon dioxide, an increase in carbon dioxide combining power, a decrease in buffer capacity, and an increase in pK. Correction factors are available for these changes, but interpretation of the resulting values is controversial. Significant alterations in the metabolic component of the acid-base profile have not been found in the immediate posthypothermia period so long as shivering, inadequate tissue perfusion, or prolonged periods of circulatory arrest were avoided. Progressive respiratory alkalosis will accompany cooling if normothermic levels of ventilation are maintained. The combined effect of decreasing temperature and increasing pH on the binding of oxygen by hemoglobin (leftward shift of the dissociation curve) has been considered a possible cause of tissue hypoxia. This is, in part, counteracted by the increased solubility of oxygen; nonetheless, some investigators have recommended either the addition of carbon dioxide to the inspired gases or the intravenous infusion of dilute solutions of hydrochloric acid during hypothermia.

Function of the kidneys, liver, and endocrine system is depressed during hypothermia but returns to normal within 24 hours after rewarming.[45] Disturbances of blood coagulation have been encountered after profound hypothermia.[44] This appears to be a multifaceted problem that may result from inadequate doses of heparin during cooling, inadequate reversal of heparin after cooling, release of fibrinolysins, or the destruction of platelets and other clotting factors secondary to either mechanical trauma or extreme temperatures.

Shivering, easily recognized on the electrocardiogram by the characteristic disturbance of the baseline, is common during cooling and rewarming. It must be corrected, either by increasing the depth of anesthesia or by administering muscle relaxants. The potential deleterious effects of shivering result from an increase of 50 to 200 per cent in oxygen requirements that may not be accompanied by an appropriate increase in cardiac output. In this situation, a vicious circle of increasing anaerobic metabolism, progressive metabolic acidosis, and further cardiac depression may result. If shivering occurs during cooling, the decrease in temperature may be halted or reversed. The practice of permitting a patient to rewarm by allowing him to shiver is potentially hazardous and may account for the syndrome of "rewarming shock."

The anesthetic requirements for hypothermia in neurosurgery are not importantly different from those already discussed for intracranial procedures. Premedication with the so-called lytic cocktail, consisting of large doses of promethazine, chlorpromazine, and meperidine, is not necessary and probably should be avoided because of the risk of severe respiratory and cardiovascular depression. Light premedication, induction with a short-acting barbiturate, and maintenance with inhalation agents will minimize the potential problem of delayed destruction and excretion of depressant drugs secondary to cooling of the liver and kidneys. Since cold itself is an anesthetic, the maintenance concentration of the selected agent can be diminished when the patient's temperature is below 30° to 32° C; below 18° to 22° C, probably no anesthetic is required. Monitoring of the patient ideally should include the use of the electrocardiogram and multiple temperature probes, and measurement of direct arterial pressure and central venous pressure. The temperatures monitored should, at a minimum, include the nasopharyngeal temperature (as an index of brain temperature) and the esophageal temperature (as an index of heart temperature).

Techniques for cooling differ. Moderate levels of hypothermia (28° to 30° C) are almost always accomplished by surface cooling methods, generally with blankets that permit the circulation of a cooling liquid, or by direct immersion in an ice bath. The latter, although more rapid, is less controllable and is associated with a significant downward drift in temperature because of the large surface-to-core gradients created. The production of profound whole-body levels of hypothermia requires an extracorporeal circuit and the open-chest technique of Drew and Anderson or, as is more common, the closed-chest technique, as described by Patterson and Ray and by Michenfelder and associates.[9, 23, 26] Using these methods, large temperature gradients opposite to those encountered with surface cooling are commonly observed. For this reason, after induction of profound hypothermia an upward drift of core temperature is to be expected during the period of circulatory arrest. Selective cooling of the brain to profound levels of hypothermia is also possible and requires an extracorporeal system similar to that described by Kristiansen and co-workers.[17]

The primary indication for hypothermia in neurosurgery is for those procedures in which temporary cessation or significant reduction in part or all of the cerebral blood flow is contemplated. The level of hypothermia produced should be determined by the anticipated duration of reduced or absent blood flow required by the surgeon for repair of the lesion. This is, admittedly, a restricted indication and applies primarily, if not exclusively, to intracranial vascular lesions. Its use as a means of protecting the brain during the removal of large cerebral tumors, craniopharyngiomas, and tumors close to the vital centers is of questionable validity. Although a reduction in brain bulk occurs with hypothermia, hypothermia should not be used for this purpose alone since simpler and safer techniques are available. Even its use in the repair of aneurysms has been questioned because of a failure to demonstrate an associated decrease in morbidity and mortality.

Monitoring

The success or failure of a number of the techniques and procedures previously discussed depends, in part, upon adequate monitoring of the patient. Standard monitoring techniques are not always satisfactory: Indirect measurement of blood pressure may be misleading, particularly during induced hypotension or hypothermia; palpation of the radial pulse or auscultation of the heart sounds will not always reveal cardiac arrhythmias or permit accurate diagnosis; and respiratory rate and rhythm provide only modest information about the adequacy of alveolar ventilation. These deficiencies have particular significance in neurosurgery because of the frequent application of special techniques, the common occurrence of alterations in cardiac rate and rhythm, and the continuous necessity to provide adequate alveolar ventilation.

Intelligent use of the electrocardiogram permits immediate recognition and diagnosis of significant cardiac arrhythmias. Intracranial surgical manipulation may at any time produce sudden changes in cardiac rhythm or rate; however, they occur most commonly and with greatest significance in posterior fossa surgery, because of pressure, distortion, or traction on the brain stem and cranial nerves. Other procedures or complications frequently associated with cardiac arrhythmias include orbital decompression, carotid ligation, sudden intracranial decompression, trigeminal nerve surgery, tonsillar herniation, and air embolism. Stimulation of the trigeminal nerve is a common cause of ventricular arrhythmias and is always associated with hypertension, perhaps a response to painful stimulation under light anesthesia rather than true reflex arrhythmia. Additional indications for monitoring with the electrocardiogram in neurosurgery are induced hypothermia (for the recognition of both arrhythmias and shivering), induced hypotension, procedures associated with massive transfusion, and procedures for the localization of right atrial catheters or ventriculoatrial shunts.

The importance of adequate and proper ventilation in neurosurgery has been emphasized. The use of a mechanical ventilator provides an indirect but useful means of monitoring certain aspects of ventilation, including pressures, volume, and rate. A simple accurate means for continuous monitoring of Pa_{CO_2} would provide the ideal monitor. Detection of end-expired carbon dioxide with an infrared analyzer is cumbersome and does not necessarily reflect Pa_{CO_2}. Direct measurement of Pa_{CO_2} is not practical and in many institutions not possible. There is not yet a satisfactory solution to this problem; clinical impression continues to be the primary "monitoring device."

Direct, continuous monitoring of arterial pressure is indicated primarily in procedures requiring induced hypothermia or hypotension. This need not require elaborate equipment, and, as experience is gained, the indications may be expanded to include posterior fossa surgery and procedures associated with significant loss of blood. As in other surgical procedures, knowledge of central venous pressure is of value in determining proper fluid and blood replacement. For this purpose, right atrial catheterization offers the additional option of monitoring central venous oxygen levels and, in the event of air embolism, will permit the aspiration of intracardiac air. Additional useful monitoring devices include the esophageal stethoscope and esophageal or rectal thermistors; the monitoring of temperature is particularly valuable in children and, of course, during induced hypothermia. Interest in the electroencephalogram as a clinical monitoring device has waned, but Wyke has argued strongly in its favor.[49]

Interest has been expressed recently in monitoring the oxygen levels of jugular bulb blood as an index of cerebral blood flow, particularly during operations on the carotid artery. The validity of the method is based upon a number of assumptions, the most important of which are that the cerebral metabolic rate is steady, that there is no significant contamination by extra-

cerebral blood, and that the sample is representative of "mixed" cerebral venous blood. The last of these is known to be false and may cause erroneous interpretations. Normally, two thirds of the blood collected by an internal jugular vein is from the ipsilateral hemisphere, hence complete mixing does not occur, and a single jugular sample may fail to reflect significant changes in flow occurring in the contralateral hemisphere. Of greater concern is the failure of oxygen levels of the jugular blood to reflect absence or diminution of flow to a part of the brain; in this event, if total flow remains unchanged, venous oxygen levels may actually increase because of a reduction in the amount of brain tissue that consumes oxygen. These sources of misinterpretation have been emphasized by Larson and co-workers; in their patients undergoing carotid endarterectomy, the measurement of oxygen levels of the jugular bulb was of little or no value.[19] Similarly, the detection of localized changes in cerebral blood flow during intracranial surgery could not be accomplished by the monitoring of oxygen levels of jugular blood.

POSITION

Patients undergoing neurosurgical operations frequently must be placed in positions that may interfere with circulation and respiration. Respiratory mechanics may be altered by changes in the pulmonary blood volume, by interference with the movements of the thoracic wall and diaphragm, or by changes in lung volume. The distribution of pulmonary blood and of inspired gases may change with the posture of the anesthetized and ventilated patient; however, most of these changes can probably be adequately compensated for by judicious use of artificial ventilation. Usually, the normal anesthetized patient can compensate for the effects on the systemic circulation. Individuals with low cardiac reserve or inadequate nervous control of the peripheral circulation frequently cannot make appropriate adjustments. Immediate and sometimes dramatic effects, such as severe arterial hypotension, can result if the compensatory mechanisms fail, particularly during the positioning of the anesthetized patient. Adequate blood volume, occasional administration of vasopressors, and gradual rather than abrupt changes of body position allow the use, in most instances, of the position optimal for the operative procedure.

Improper positioning may result in injury to peripheral nerves (brachial plexus, common peroneal nerve, saphenous nerve, and so forth). Ocular complications such as retinal artery thrombosis may result from pressure over the eyeballs, particularly in conjunction with arterial hypotension. Closure of the eyelids after application of eye ointment usually will prevent corneal abrasions. Patients with systemic arteriosclerosis must be positioned with particular care to avoid arterial occlusion from pressure on diseased vessels.

For craniotomies done with the patient supine, a 10- to 15-degree elevation of the head will facilitate cerebral venous drainage. Venous pooling in the lower extremities can be minimized by correct wrapping of the legs with elastic bandages, applied while the patient is in the supine or slightly head-down position, before induction of anesthesia. No untoward alterations in circulatory or pulmonary function have been associated with the supine position.

The lateral position is likewise fairly benign as regards cardiopulmonary function. Hemodynamic studies in anesthetized (halothane) man in the right lateral position have shown a decrease in mean arterial pressure and systemic resistance, but an unchanged cardiac index.[11] Support of the pelvis and shoulder is necessary with this position and can be accomplished by means of sandbags and pillows. Excessive flexion of the head should be avoided so that cerebral venous drainage is not obstructed. The patient's head should be slightly elevated.

The prone position may compromise normal cardiopulmonary function. The flat prone position interferes with respiratory mechanics and possibly predisposes to atelectasis. It is particularly dangerous for the spontaneously breathing emphysematous patient who is primarily a diaphragmatic breather. Posner and co-workers found a decrease in total compliance of the chest in patients who were anesthetized, paralyzed, ventilated with a constant volume, and then turned from the supine to the prone position.[29] Abdominal compression may occur and result in obstruction of the inferior vena cava, which can cause arterial hypotension and excessive epidural bleeding. Various pads and devices have been described for support of the iliac crest and chest. Proper support of the iliac crest and the chest lessens the embarrassment to circulatory and respiratory function. Only the occasional obese patient presents an added risk.

The sitting position is preferred by many neurosurgeons for operations in the posterior fossa, middle fossa, and cervical spine because of improved venous drainage and better exposure. A variety of methods are available to hold the anesthetized patient in the sitting position. The legs should be wrapped with elastic bandages and placed at the level of the heart to facilitate venous return from the lower extremities. The patient should be put into the sitting position slowly, and the blood pressure measured frequently. With this precaution, arterial hypotension is rarely a problem. However, with the sitting position, even short periods of hypotension may result in cerebral hypoxia. The effect of the sitting position on internal carotid artery flow and pressure was recently determined in nine anesthetized and hyperventilated (Pa_{CO_2}, 22.5 mm of mercury) subjects.[42] Anesthesia (nitrous oxide and halothane) and hyperventilation alone resulted in an average decrease of 34 per cent in the internal carotid blood flow. The sitting position resulted in an additional reduction of 18 per cent. In healthy, unmedicated subjects, the change from the supine to the sitting position resulted in a decrease of 21 per cent in stroke volume and 10 per cent in cardiac index. An increase of 18 per cent in heart rate partially compensated for the decreased stroke volume.

Perhaps the greatest hazard associated with the sitting position is the potential for venous air embolism. This occurs most frequently in posterior fossa surgery because of the increased likelihood of opening into a noncollapsible venous channel (diploic veins and dural sinuses), which, in the presence of a negative venous pressure, may aspirate air. In a series of 751 such procedures, the incidence of air embolism was

4.1 per cent, whereas in over 1200 cervical laminectomies and middle fossa explorations, only one episode of air embolism was recognized.[24]

Morbidity and mortality due to venous air embolism can be minimized by appropriate prophylactic measures, early diagnosis, and vigorous treatment. Useful prophylactic measures include proper positioning of the patient, wrapping of the legs with elastic bandages or the application of a "G" suit, maintenance of adequate blood volume, positive pressure ventilation, intermittent compression of the internal jugular veins, frequent flushing of the surgical wound with saline, and liberal application of bone wax. When, despite these measures, air embolism occurs, the presence of a right atrial catheter is useful both for early confirmation of the diagnosis and for treatment. The diagnosis should be suspected when any sudden changes occur in the heart tones; small volumes of air impart a tympanitic quality to the heart sounds, and with increasing volumes a coarse systolic murmur becomes evident. The classic "mill-wheel" murmur is not a consistent diagnostic sign and, when present, usually indicates a large volume of intracardiac air. Less consistent diagnostic signs associated with air embolism include arrhythmias (usually ventricular), hypotension, increased central venous pressure, cyanosis, and tachypnea. With a right atrial catheter, immediate and certain confirmation of a suspected diagnosis of venous air embolism can be achieved by aspirating air from the right atrium.

Treatment of air embolism should be directed at preventing further entry of air and dispersing or removing the intracardiac air. Prevention may be accomplished by a variety of measures designed to increase the venous pressure in the surgical wound, thus permitting identification and occlusion of the open venous channel. These measures include compression of the internal jugular veins, continuous positive-pressure ventilation, and lowering the patient's head. If a right atrial catheter is present, continuous aspiration will remove a portion of the intracardiac air; the remainder must ultimately be ejected into the pulmonary circulation. The administration of a vasopressor that has a positive inotropic action will aid the heart in ejecting the air as well as improve the perfusion pressure. If these measures are effectively implemented, the catastrophic events usually associated with air embolism can be avoided.

ANESTHETICS, CEREBRAL METABOLISM, AND BLOOD FLOW

There is no invariable response of either cerebral blood flow or metabolism to anesthesia; rather, a different response is associated with each agent and, in the frequent clinical circumstance of multiple anesthetic agents, the end-result may be unknown. Cerebral metabolism may be unchanged, depressed, or stimulated by anesthetic drugs. The most common response is metabolic depression and the most potent depressant drugs known are the barbiturates. Thiopental, in man, may reduce cerebral oxygen consumption as much as 55 per cent; however, the degree of metabolic (as well as functional) depression may be significantly reduced by the method of drug administration, because of the phenomenon of acute tolerance.[27] The volatile anesthetic agents such as halothane and ether have generally been reported to reduce cerebral oxygen consumption 10 to 20 per cent. When concentrations of these agents increase, further metabolic depression is slight and, in the case of ether and cyclopropane, a return to normal oxygen consumption has been observed at high concentrations. Nitrous oxide is an exceptional agent and has been found to increase cerebral oxygen consumption.[41] Other researchers have found either no change or minimal depression. With the possible exception of barbiturates, anesthetic agents cannot provide significant protection of the brain against hypoxic stress.

The effect of anesthetic agents on cerebral circulation has not been as well documented as the metabolic effects, owing to the concomitant effects on cerebral vascular resistance produced by changes in perfusion pressure, arterial blood carbon dioxide tension, and metabolic rate. The barbiturates tend to reduce cerebral blood flow in relation to the reduced cerebral metabolic rate. The volatile anesthetic agents produce either no change or a moderate decrease in cerebral vascular resistance. Halothane has been consistently observed to produce moderate cerebral vasodilatation and has accordingly been condemned by some for use in intracranial surgery. This objection is probably only valid in the presence of spontaneous ventilation and a normal or elevated Pa_{CO_2}. Since anesthesia does not significantly alter the normal cerebral vascular response to carbon dioxide, the effects of halothane (and other agents) are presumably countered by a moderate degree of hyperventilation.

Portions of this chapter are reproduced with permission from Anesthesiology, 30:65–100, 1969.

REFERENCES

1. Alexander, S. C., Cohen, P. J., Wollman, H., Smith, T. C., Reivich, M., and Vander Molen, R. A.: Cerebral carbohydrate metabolism during hypocarbia in man: Studies during nitrous oxide anesthesia. Anesthesiology, 26:624–632, 1965.
2. Allen, G. D., and Morris, L. E.: Central nervous system effects of hyperventilation during anaesthesia. Brit. J. Anaesth., 34:296–304, 1962.
3. Baker, G. S.: Physiologic abnormalities encountered after removal of brain tumors from the floor of the fourth ventricle. J. Neurosurg., 23:338–343, 1965.
4. Barach, A. L., Fenn, W. O., Ferris, E. B., and Schmidt, C. F.: The physiology of pressure breathing: A brief review of its present status. J. Aviat. Med., 18:73–87, 1947.
5. Bozza Marrubini, M.: General anaesthesia for intracranial surgery. Brit. J. Anaesth., 37:268–287, 1965.
6. Brown, A. S., and Horton, J. M.: Elective hypotension with intracardiac pacemaking in the operative management of ruptured intracranial aneurysms. Acta Anaesth. Scand., suppl. 23, pp. 665–670, 1966.
7. Clutton-Brock, J.: The cerebral effects of overventilation (preliminary communication). Brit. J. Anaesth., 29:111–113, 1957.
8. Cohen, P. J., Wollman, H., Alexander, S. C., Chase, P. E., and Behar, M. G.: Cerebral carbohydrate metabolism in man during halothane anesthesia: Effects of Pa_{CO_2} on some aspects of carbohydrate utilization. Anesthesiology, 25:185–191, 1964.
9. Drew, C. E., and Anderson, I. M.: Profound hypothermia in cardiac surgery: Report of three cases. Lancet, 1:748–750, 1959.
10. Eckenhoff, J. E., Enderby, G. E. H., Larson, A., Davies, R., and Judevine, D. E.: Human cerebral circulation during deliberate hypotension and head-up tilt. J. Appl. Physiol., 18:1130–1138, 1963.
11. Eggers, G. W. N., Jr., deGroot, W. J., Tanner, C. R., and Leonard, J. J.: Hemodynamic changes associated with various surgical positions. J.A.M.A., 185:1–5, 1963.
12. Elwyn, R. A.: Personal communication to the authors.
13. Enderby, G. E. H.: Safety in hypotensive anaesthesia. In Proceedings World Congress of Anaesthesiologists, 1955. Minneapolis, Minn., Burgess Pub. Co., 1956, pp. 227–230.
14. Galloon, S.: Controlled respiration in neurosurgical anaesthesia. Anaesthesia, 14:223–230, 1959.
15. Gilbert, R. G. B., Brindle, G. F., and Galindo, A.: Anesthesia for Neurosurgery. Boston, Little, Brown and Co., 1966.
16. Hayes, G. J., and Slocum, H. C.: The achievement of optimal brain relaxation by hyperventilation technics of anesthesia. J. Neurosurg., 19:65–69, 1962.
17. Kristiansen, K., Krog, J., and Lund, I.: Experiences with selective cooling of the brain. Acta Chir. Scand., Suppl. 253, pp. 151–161, 1960.
18. Larson, A. G.: Deliberate hypotension. Anesthesiology, 25:682–706, 1964.
19. Larson, C. P., Jr., Ehrenfeld, W. K., Wade, J. G., and Wylie, E. J.: Jugular venous oxygen saturation as an index of adequacy of cerebral oxygenation. Surgery, 62:31–38, 1967.
20. Lougheed, W. M., Sweet, W. H., White, J. C., and Brewster, W. R.: The use of hypothermia in surgical treatment of cerebral vascular lesions: A preliminary report. J. Neurosurg., 12:240–255, 1955.
21. Lundberg, N., Kjällquist, Å., and Bien, C.: Reduction of increased intracranial pressure by hyperventilation: A therapeutic aid in neurological surgery. Acta Psychiat. Scand., 34: suppl. 139:1–64, 1959.
22. Michenfelder, J. D., Gronert, G. A., and Rehder, K.: Neuroanesthesia. Anesthesiology, 30:65–100, 1969.
23. Michenfelder, J. D., Kirklin, J. W., Uihlein, A., Svien, H. J., and MacCarty, C. S.: Clinical experience with a closed-chest method of producing profound hypothermia and total circulatory arrest in neurosurgery. Ann. Surg., 159:125–131, 1964.
24. Michenfelder, J. D., Martin, J. T., Altenburg, B. M., and Rehder, K.: Air embolism during neurosurgery: An evaluation of right-atrial catheters for diagnosis and treatment. J.A.M.A., 208:1353–1358, 1969.
25. National Research Council: Summary of the National Halothane Study: Possible association between halothane anesthesia and postoperative hepatic necrosis. J.A.M.A., 197:775–788, 1966.
26. Patterson, R. H., Jr., and Ray, B. S.: Profound hypothermia for intracranial surgery: Laboratory and clinical experiences with extracorporeal circulation by peripheral cannulation. Ann. Surg., 156:377–391, 1962.
27. Pierce, E. C., Jr., Lambertsen, C. J., Deutsch, S., Chase, P. E., Linde, H. W., Dripps, R. D., and Price, H. L.: Cerebral circulation and metabolism during thiopental anesthesia and hyper-

ventilation in man. J. Clin. Invest., *41*:1664–1671, 1962.

28. Plum, F., and Posner, J. B.: Blood and cerebrospinal fluid lactate during hyperventilation. Amer. J. Physiol., *212*:864–870, 1967.

29. Posner, A., Brody, D., and Ravin, M.: Effect of prone position with constant volume ventilation on paO_2 in man. Anesth. Analg. (Cleveland), *44*:435–439, 1965.

30. Ritsema van Eck, C. R.: Neuroleptanalgesia. Int. Anesth. Clin., *3*:659–673, 1965.

31. Robinson, J. S., and Gray, T. C.: Observations on the cerebral effects of passive hyperventilation. Brit. J. Anaesth., *33*:62–68, 1961.

32. Rosomoff, H. L.: Distribution of intracranial contents with controlled hyperventilation: Implications for neuroanesthesia. Anesthesiology, *24*:640–645, 1963.

33. Rosomoff, H. L.: Adjuncts to neurosurgical anaesthesia. Brit. J. Anaesth., *37*:246–261, 1965.

34. Saidman, L. J., and Eger, E. I., II.: Change in cerebrospinal fluid pressure during pneumoencephalography under nitrous oxide anesthesia. Anesthesiology, *26*:67–72, 1965.

35. Small, J. M., and Stephenson, S. C. F.: Circulatory arrest in neurosurgery. Lancet, *1*:569–570, 1966.

36. Smith, L. W., and Fay, T.: Observations on human beings with cancer, maintained at reduced temperatures of 75°–90° Fahrenheit. Amer. J. Clin. Path., *10*:1–11, 1940.

37. Sugioka, K., and Davis, D. A.: Hyperventilation with oxygen: A possible cause of cerebral hypoxia. Anesthesiology, *21*:135–143, 1960.

38. Sullivan, S. F., Patterson, R. W., and Papper, E. M.: Posthyperventilation hypoxia. J. Appl. Physiol., *22*:431–435, 1967.

39. Symbas, P. N., Abbott, O. A., and Leonard, J.: The effects of artificial ventilation on cerebrospinal fluid pressure. J. Thorac. Cardiov. Surg., *54*:126–131, 1967.

40. Terry, H. R., Jr., Daw, E. F., Michenfelder, J. D., Baker, H. L., Jr., and Holman, C. B.: The evolution of anesthesia for neuroradiologic procedures. Surg. Clin. N. Amer., *45*:907–918, 1965.

41. Theye, R. A., and Michenfelder, J. D.: The effect of nitrous oxide on canine cerebral metabolism. Anesthesiology, *29*:1119–1124, 1968.

42. Tindall, G. T., Craddock, A., and Greenfield, J. C., Jr.: Effects of the sitting position on blood flow in the internal carotid artery of man during general anesthesia. J. Neurosurg., *26*:383–389, 1967.

43. Ueyama, H., and Loehning, R. W.: Effect of hyperventilation on cerebrospinal fluid pressure and brain volume. Anesth. Analg. (Cleveland), *42*:581–587, 1963.

44. Uihlein, A., Owen, C. A., Jr., Cooper, T., and Thompson, J. H., Jr.: Bleeding tendencies associated with profound-hypothermia technics in neurologic surgery. Ann. N.Y. Acad. Sci., *115*:337–340, 1964.

45. Vandam, L. D., and Burnap, T. K.: Hypothermia. New Eng. J. Med., *261*:546–553, 595–603, 1959.

46. Werkö, L.: The influence of positive pressure breathing on the circulation in man. Acta Med. Scand., suppl. 193, pp. 1–125, 1947.

47. Whitwam, J. G., Boettner, R. B., Gilger, A. P., and Littell, A. S.: Hyperventilation, brain damage and flicker. Brit. J. Anaesth., *38*:846–852, 1966.

48. Wollman, H., Alexander, S. C., Cohen, P. J., Chase, P. E., Melman, E., and Behar, M. G.: Cerebral circulation of man during halothane anesthesia: Effects of hypocarbia and of d-tubocurarine. Anesthesiology, *25*:180–184, 1964.

49. Wyke, B.: Neurological principles in anaesthesia. *In* Evans, F. T., and Gray, T. C., eds.: General Anaesthesia. 2nd Ed. Washington, D.C., Butterworth & Co., Ltd., 1965, vol. 1, pp. 157–299.

21

GENERAL OPERATIVE TECHNIQUE

A wide variety of neurosurgical operations has been performed during the centuries since prehistoric man first began trephination.[1-7] As a result of this broad experience, many safe and reliable techniques have been developed. The following is a discussion of basic neurosurgical procedures as practiced today.

CRANIAL OPERATIONS

Preoperative Preparation, Positioning, and Draping

After an appropriate diagnostic work-up, the neurosurgical patient is prepared for his operation. As with any other type of surgery, the patient must give informed consent, but if he is unconscious or mentally incompetent, it must be obtained from the relative or institution that is legally responsible for him. His blood is typed and cross-matched, and, if possible, his oral intake is stopped at least eight hours before the operation. The pertinent x-ray films and brain scans are taken to the operating room.

In addition to the usual premedications for local or general anesthesia, it may be necessary to give special medications before certain operations. For example, cortisone acetate is usually given to patients scheduled for pituitary surgery (e.g., for an adult, 100 to 200 mg IM, 48, 24, and 2 hours before operation), and a steroid preparation may be given to patients with cerebral edema one or two days before surgery (e.g., for an adult, dexamethasone sodium phosphate, up to 4 mg IM, every six hours, or methylprednisolone sodium succinate, up to 40 mg intramuscularly every six hours). Patients scheduled for retrogasserian neurotomy for tic douloureux under local anesthesia are usually given additional analgesic and sedative medications preoperatively. Such a patient might be given 100 mg of sodium secobarbital intramuscularly, two hours and one hour before the operation, and 50 mg of meperidine hydrochloride one and one half hours and one half hour before the operation.

Immediately prior to operation, the appropriate areas, which have previously been clipped and washed, are carefully shaved. It may be desirable in some cases to clip and shave only one area of the scalp. For example, if only the posterior half is shaved, a woman undergoing suboccipital craniectomy can comb her remaining hair back after her bandage has been removed, with a better initial cosmetic result than if all her hair had been removed. Any hair that is cut off should be saved in an adequately labeled bag and taped to the patient's chart. The eyebrows should not be shaved, even when a supraorbital incision is to be made, because of the poor cosmetic result.

The lower extremities are wrapped with elastic bandages to prevent the pooling of blood in these limbs. Two sites for intravenous fluid administration should be prepared if unusual blood loss is anticipated. After anesthesia has been induced, the eyes should be protected from accidental injury by a bland ophthalmic ointment and a cover over the closed eyelids. An indwelling catheter is placed in the urinary bladder

R. H. WILKINS

G. L. ODOM

if hypertonic solutions might be given intravenously during the operation.

In many cerebral operations, the drainage of cerebrospinal fluid will greatly facilitate exposure and prevent cerebral herniation through the surgical opening in the dura mater. In these cases, a lumbar puncture needle is introduced preoperatively and is connected by sterile plastic tubing to a stopcock so that lumbar drainage can be started and stopped at will during the operation. If the patient is to be on his side, folded sheets are used to protect the lumbar needle from the weight of the drapes. If he is to be supine, a split mattress may be used. As an alternative, a malleable spinal needle or a plastic spinal catheter can be employed instead of a regular spinal needle.

Correct positioning of the patient is essential to achieve maximum surgical exposure and to avoid confusing distortions of normal anatomical relationships. If the patient is placed in the supine or lateral position, his head may be stabilized to some extent by placing it on a head ring. A pillow is placed between the patient's lower extremities if he is in the lateral position, and the area where the common peroneal nerve crosses the neck of the fibula is protected from the pressure of restraining straps. In the prone position, the patient's head may be supported by a cerebellar frame, allowing the anesthetist access to the patient's face. Undue pressure on the patient's eyes by the cerebellar frame should be avoided. His shoulders, thorax, and iliac crests should be supported laterally, allowing the center of the thorax and abdomen room for respiratory excursions. Forward flexion of the head on the neck and caudal traction of the shoulders with wide adhesive tape increase the exposure in suboccipital and cervical operations, but pressure on the jugular veins should be avoided since this will increase intracranial venous pressure. In this position a footboard is usually advantageous to prevent the patient from sliding toward the foot of the operating table, especially if the head of the table is elevated during the operation.

The sitting position offers the advantage of decreased cranial venous pressure, with decreased operative blood loss. But it also has the distinct disadvantages of decreased cerebral arterial blood flow and possible venous air embolism or rapid ventricular decompression with subdural hematoma formation. For this position, the Craig frame or Gardner chair may be used to stabilize the patient's body and head. As in the prone position, flexion of the head on the neck will increase the suboccipital and cervical operative exposure. It is important to avoid rotation or lateral flexion of the head, especially in preparation for the subtemporal approach to retrogasserian neurotomy, because the resulting anatomical distortion can confuse the surgeon.

The surgeon should look at the patient and examine his chart, x-ray films, and brain scans carefully just prior to operation to verify the side and location of the lesion. He should also remember two pertinent facts about craniocerebral topography

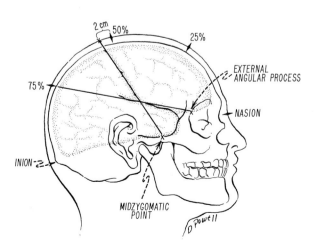

FIGURE 21–1 Craniocerebral topography showing approximate locations of the sylvian and rolandic fissures (see text for explanation).

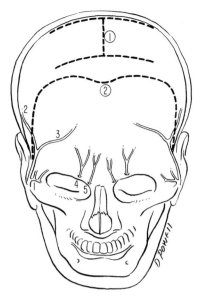

FIGURE 21-2 Basic incisions: (1) biparietal and (2) coronal. Arteries: 1, Superficial temporal; 2, parietal branch; 3, frontal branch; 4, supraorbital; 5, frontal.

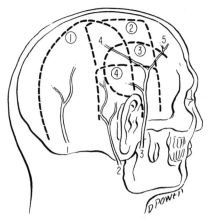

FIGURE 21-4 Basic incisions: (1) occipital, (2) parietal, (3) and (4) temporal. Arteries: 1, occipital; 2, posterior auricular; 3, superficial temporal; 4, parietal branch; 5, frontal branch.

(Fig. 21–1).[3] The fissure of Sylvius lies roughly along a line between the external angular process of the frontal bone and a point along the sagittal midline 75 per cent of the total nasoinionic distance posterior to the nasion. The fissure of Rolando lies along the superior portion of a line beginning along the sagittal midline about 2 cm posterior to the midpoint of the nasoinionic line, and extending laterally to cross the middle of the zygomatic arch. With these facts in mind, the surgeon should be able to plan a flap that will satisfactorily expose the pathological lesion without unnecessary exposure of the adjacent brain (Figs. 21–2 to 21–5).

If the patient with an intracranial mass has undergone ventriculography or pneumoencephalography shortly prior to opera-

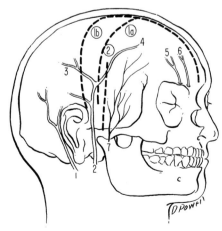

FIGURE 21-3 Basic incisions: (1a) standard frontal, (1b) large frontal, (2) temporal. Arteries: 1, posterior auricular; 2, superficial temporal, 3, parietal branch; 4, frontal branch; 5, supraorbital; 6, frontal. Nerves: 7, temporal branches of facial nerve.

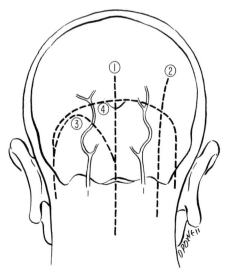

FIGURE 21-5 Basic incisions: (1) midline linear, (2) unilateral linear, (3) unilateral flap, and (4) bilateral flap. Arteries: 1, occipital.

tion, it is usually best to let him breathe spontaneously during surgery. Respiratory irregularities may be a sign of rapidly changing intracranial dynamics and may indicate that the patient should have an immediate ventricular puncture.

The skin in the primary operative and appropriate donor areas (e.g., lateral thigh if a fascia lata graft to the dura is anticipated) is cleansed several times with antiseptic solutions, care being taken to keep these solutions out of the eyes. Tincture of iodine may cause blistering of the skin and should be avoided in infants. Since iodine and thimerosol are incompatible, one should not be used to cleanse the skin if the other has been used on the same area a short time previously (e.g., for ventriculography before a craniotomy). A colorless antiseptic solution may be used on the face to avoid staining it (e.g., benzalkonium chloride in aqueous solution).

The proposed incision and appropriate landmarks, such as the sagittal midline, should be marked with a sterile dye. Cross marks should be made along the incision line every few centimeters to insure correct approximation of the edges of the scalp at the end of the operation. A sterile adhesive plastic film may be used to cover the cleansed areas after they have dried.

Appropriate sterile towels and drapes are then applied to isolate the operative field. These drapes are held up by an ether screen, poles, or angled bars to create a tent under which the anesthetist can reach the patient without entering the sterile operative field. The lowest edges of the drapes below the patient's head should be placed into a bucket or similar container on the floor to catch the irrigation fluid and blood that overflows the operative field. The sterile portions of the suction and cautery lines are attached to their unsterile counterparts away from the operative field. Two suction lines should be set up if brisk hemorrhage might be encountered during operation, as from a ruptured intracranial aneurysm.

Illumination of the operative field is initially achieved by overhead lights, but as the operation proceeds, other methods, such as a head light or illuminated retractors, may be required. Magnification may also be necessary for certain portions of a neurosurgical operation. Spectacles of various types are available for low-power magnification, and the operative microscope can be used to supply greater magnification as well as illumination of the operative field.[22]

The bactericidal effects of irradiation from ultraviolet lights in the operating room can be used during surgery, but the eyes and skin of all persons in the operating room must be protected against accidental burns.[24]

Exposure and Resection of the Brain

Each layer between the scalp and the brain presents a barrier against infection, and if an infection is localized to one plane, the underlying barrier should not be breached unless there is good evidence that infection is also present beneath it. For example, the arachnoid should be kept intact during the evacuation of a subdural empyema. If no such precautions are necessary, however, the brain can be exposed by the systematic opening of all the overlying tissue layers.

Whether or not general anesthesia is used, a local anesthetic agent, with or without epinephrine, may be injected along the proposed scalp incision for hemostasis as well as anesthesia. Such an injection will, however, limit the use of scalp clips because of the resulting local increase in the thickness of the scalp, so this technique is not used often.

In general, scalp incisions are either straight or are curved to outline a scalp flap that is based on a broad vascular pedicle (Figs. 21-2 to 21-5). Two incisions that meet or cross each other, such as Cushing's original crossbow incision, are now usually avoided because of poor healing at the angular tips of the scalp flaps. Excision of abnormal areas of the scalp (e.g., devitalized from trauma or distorted by an underlying neoplasm or encephalocele) should be as limited as feasible because of the difficulty encountered in closing even small scalp defects over the convex calvarium. In these situations, extensive undermining of the scalp, a relaxing incision elsewhere in the scalp, or a large scalp flap may be required for adequate closure. If it

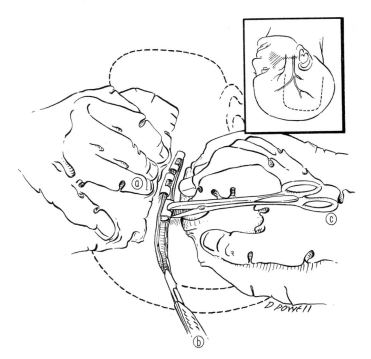

FIGURE 21-6 Standard craniotomy: (a) digital compression, (b) scalp incision, (c) application of scalp clips.

is possible, scalp incisions should be made so they will be hidden by the patient's hair when it grows back postoperatively.

As the scalp is incised, digital compression through sterile gauze pads or towels is maintained by assistants to control bleeding until the galea aponeurotica can be undermined a short distance on each side and hemostats or scalp clips can be applied (Fig. 21-6). These scalp clips should be used with care since they can lead to ischemic necrosis of the scalp edge if they are too tight. Exposed areas of the scalp should be covered with sterile skin towels. Large arteries supplying the scalp, such as the superficial temporal artery, should not be cut as the scalp is incised, if it is possible to avoid them. When they do cross the path of the incision they should be securely ligated or cauterized before they are divided.

The temporal and nuchal muscles should be incised in such a way that adequate muscular and fascial cuffs are retained for closure of the wound. This applies in particular to incisions adjacent to the inferior temporal line and the superior nuchal line. The scalp, musculature, and periosteum can be reflected together, allowing the bone to be removed piecemeal or as a free bone flap. More commonly, the scalp is reflected

first, and then the bone flap is hinged on the temporalis musculature and periosteum in order to preserve some of its blood supply and maintain its viability (Fig. 21-7). In this situation, the exposed surfaces of the

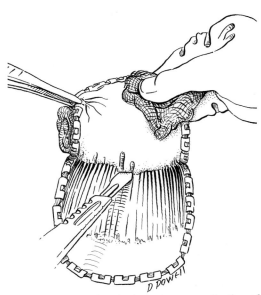

FIGURE 21-7 Standard craniotomy: reflection of the scalp flap (over a rolled gauze to prevent ischemia due to angulation of the base of the flap).

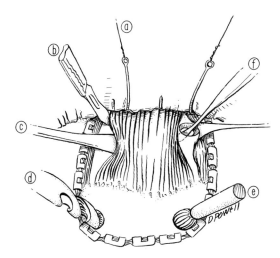

FIGURE 21–8 Standard craniotomy: (a) retraction of the scalp flap, which is wrapped in moist gauze and covered with a towel, by barbless fish hooks on rubber bands; (b) incision of the temporalis muscle; (c) separation of some of the muscle fibers from the bone with a periosteal elevator; (d) and (e) trephination with perforator and burr; (f) separation of the dura mater from the skull.

galea aponeurotica, the periosteum, and the temporalis fascia will ooze blood and serum, and careful hemostasis with cautery and the temporary application of strips of oxidized cellulose is necessary to prevent blood loss at operation as well as the postoperative accumulation of fluid under the scalp flap. Occasionally the bone flap is elevated and reflected together with all the overlying

soft tissues. As just noted, whenever the bone flap is hinged on the adjacent periosteum and musculature, it retains its vascularity and should be waxed to prevent continuous oozing of blood from its exposed surfaces.

Trephine openings are frequently made with the perforator and burr (Fig. 21–8). Newer electrical and air drills are also used, but more attention is required to avoid dural laceration with these powerful instruments. After an adequate number of trephine openings have been made, the dura mater is carefully separated from the inner table of the skull along the lines of the proposed bony opening, using a No. 3 Penfield dissector. This maneuver, done to prevent accidental dural laceration when the overlying bone is sawed, is especially important at cranial suture lines, over the dural venous sinuses, and in areas where the dura is unusually thin (e.g., frontal and subfrontal areas in elderly individuals).

The bone is removed with rongeurs, or a bone flap is formed with a Gigli saw or an air-driven craniotome (Fig. 21–9). Saw cuts are made between the outermost edges of the burr holes to permit as large an exposure as possible. If only a small cranial opening is required, a crown trephine may be used to remove a circular button of bone, which may be replaced at the end of the operation.

If the edge is beveled as a bone flap is

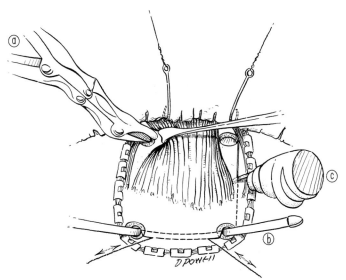

FIGURE 21–9 Standard craniotomy: (a) linear subtemporal craniectomy with rongeurs, (b) and (c) beveled division of bone with a Gigli saw or a craniotome.

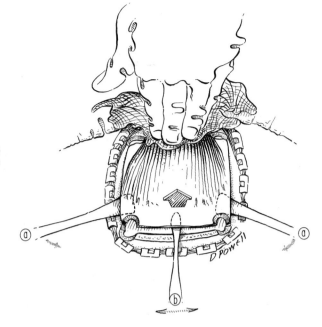

FIGURE 21–10 Standard craniotomy: (a) elevation of the bone flap, (b) separation of the dura mater from the flap.

sawed, the flap will sit more securely when it is replaced. In general, areas of the skull over the dural venous sinuses or middle meningeal arteries are sawed last, so that, if profuse bleeding occurs, the bone flap can be quickly removed and hemostasis achieved. When a bone flap is to be hinged laterally on the temporalis muscle, it can be divided along the other three sides and

then broken across the thin squamous portion of the temporal bone by prying up its medial edge with periosteal elevators as the dura is gently stripped from the inner table of the bone flap with a No. 1 or No. 2 Penfield dissector (Fig. 21–10).

After the bone flap has been elevated, the margins of the bony openings are waxed to prevent diploic bleeding (Figs. 21–11 and

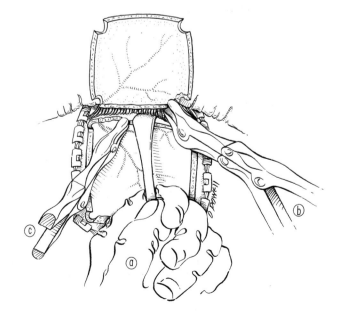

FIGURE 21–11 Standard craniotomy: (a) further separation of temporalis muscle from bone, (b) and (c) subtemporal craniectomy for postoperative decompression.

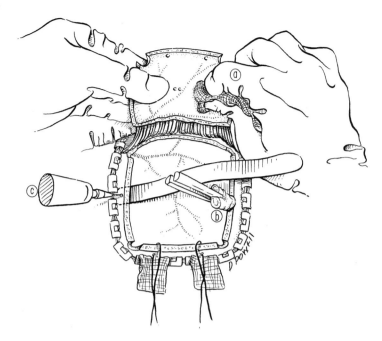

FIGURE 21-12 Standard craniotomy: (a) and (b) waxing of the bone, (c) drilling of wire holes.

21–12). If the surgeon applies the wax with his finger, he should put a gauze sponge between his glove and the wax to prevent sharp bone spicules from tearing the glove. He may also apply the wax with a short segment of dental roll or a cotton pledget held with forceps.

If the bone flap is to be replaced at the end of the operation, a few small drill holes are made in the skull around the periphery of the opening, avoiding contaminated areas such as the frontal sinus and mastoid air cells. The dura mater and brain are protected from injury as each hole is drilled, by the temporary insertion of a metal ribbon or similar instrument immediately beneath the bone in the area being drilled. A steel wire placed through each of these holes is bent double and is held out of the way with a hemostat. A small gauze pad beneath each wire protects it from contact with the potentially contaminated skin edge. Matching holes are drilled in the bone flap, and additional holes are made centrally so the dura mater can be sutured to the center of the bone flap when it is replaced at the end of the operation. A hinged bone flap is then wrapped in moist gauze and a surgical towel, and is retracted away from the operative field with barbless fishhooks on heavy rubber bands. A free bone flap is

similarly wrapped and is placed on the instrument table.

In cases of cranial trauma, the opening of the skull may require a few additional maneuvers. Linear skull fractures may overlie dural lacerations, especially if the edges of the bone are separated by more than 1 or 2 mm. The surgeon should be careful in these areas not to insert a rongeur, Gigli saw, or craniotome through the dura as he is opening the bone. In the case of comminuted or depressed fractures, the trephine openings should be made and connected in normal bone adjacent to the traumatized area before removal of the fractured bone is begun. This will permit the surgeon to recognize the anatomical planes more easily and will give him adequate room to control bleeding or cerebral herniation if either occurs when the fractured bone fragments are removed. Irregular extensions of the craniectomy may also be required in order to follow underlying dural lacerations to their limits.

Bone involved by tumor or infection should be discarded after specimens have been taken for pathological or bacteriological examination. If possible, the line of bony resection should pass through normal bone adjacent to the involved area. A saw or craniotome should be used rather than rongeurs, which might squeeze the tumor cells or bacteria into the adjacent healthy bone during the removal of the diseased bone.

If an intravenous hyperosmotic agent is to be used to combat increased intracranial pressure during the operation, it is given slowly as the scalp and bone flaps are being turned so that its maximum effect is exerted as the cerebral cortex is exposed. For this purpose, 40 gm of urea can be given as a 30 per cent solution in a solvent containing 10 per cent dextrose or invert sugar. However, it must drip through an adequate intravenous line. Infiltration into the perivenous tissues may result in extensive sloughing.

Lumbar drainage is not begun until the surgeon is ready to open the dura mater, and it is done slowly in order to avoid possible uncal or tonsillar herniation. This drainage should be performed cautiously for other reasons as well. Rapid shrinkage of the brain may precipitate annoying extradural or subdural venous bleeding, and, in cases of intracranial aneurysm, may cause a perianeurysmal clot to be pulled away from

the ruptured dome of the aneurysm, resulting in renewed arterial hemorrhage.

The dura mater is then picked up with a sharp hook and incised with a scalpel, using a No. 15 blade (Fig. 21–13). In most supratentorial craniotomies, the dura is cut with scissors 1 to 2 cm within the entire circumference of the bony defect, except for a small pedicle on which it is reflected away from the exposed brain. Vessels in the dural margins are occluded directly with tantalum clips. Large vessels are easily seen, but bleeding from small dural vessels may be identified more clearly as the dural edge is gently irrigated with clear fluid. Bleeding points on the dural surface should not be cauterized unless the underlying cerebral cortex can be protected from simultaneous thermal injury. In simple trephinations and suboccipital craniectomies, the dura mater may be opened in cruciate fashion instead of as a flap.

Veins bridging from the brain to the dural venous sinuses should be left intact, if possible. The dural opening may therefore have to be contoured around these areas and around pacchionian granulations. If the

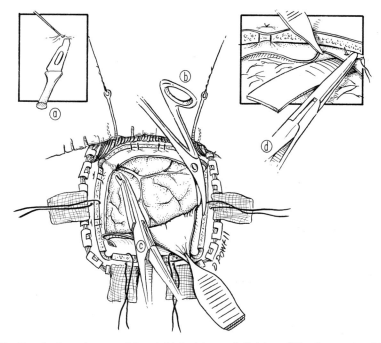

FIGURE 21–13 Standard craniotomy: (a) and (b) incision and division of the dura mater, (c) clip ligation of dural vessels, (d) suturing of the dura mater to the pericranium.

bridging veins must be divided, they should be clipped or coagulated and cut a few millimeters from the venous sinus to avoid a rent in the sinus wall.

Bleeding from the pacchionian granulations or the dural sinuses usually can be controlled by strips of absorbable gelatin sponge and gentle compression. In addition, the head of the operating table may be elevated to reduce intracranial venous pressure, though this maneuver increases the risk of air embolization. When simpler methods fail, a tear in a dural sinus may be closed with sutures, with or without an interposed stamp of autogenous muscle. As a last resort, it may even be necessary to ligate the sinus. The superior sagittal sinus usually may be ligated without complication in its anterior third, but acute ligation at any point more posterior may lead to a severe neurological deficit due to venous stasis in both cerebral hemispheres.

After the dura mater has been opened, it is tacked up to the pericranium around the circumference of the bony opening with interrupted silk sutures to minimize operative and postoperative extradural bleeding. The dural flap is reflected away from the brain, and is covered with moist cotton strips to minimize shrinkage. In addition, the peripheral dural edges may be held back with temporary sutures if further expo-

sure is necessary. Moist cotton strips may then be placed over the full thickness of the cutaneous, muscular, and bony edges of the cranial defect down to the brain, both to isolate the operative field and to prevent blood, pus, and other fluids from entering the subdural space or contaminating adjacent tissues.

The exposed brain should be constantly moistened by irrigation or by the application of moist cotton strips to prevent cortical injury due to drying. The irrigation fluid should be at a temperature of 105° to 115° F to be effective as a hemostatic agent, but fluid warmer than 120° F should not be used since this will damage neurons in the most superficial cortical layers.[28] With practice, the surgeon can judge the approximate temperature of the irrigation fluid by squirting a small amount on his gloved hand.

Frequently, extradural lesions can be exposed by simple retraction of the brain without cerebral resection. Strips of moist cotton should be placed between each retractor and the brain to prevent accidental cerebral laceration by the retractor. Lumbar drainage of cerebrospinal fluid and the intravenous administration of urea or mannitol markedly facilitate this cerebral retraction. If these techniques do not provide adequate exposure of the lesion, addi-

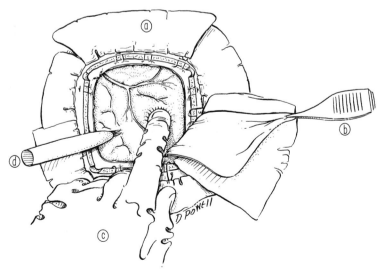

FIGURE 21–14 Standard craniotomy: (a) moist cotton strips, (b) reflection of the dural flap, (c) and (d) palpation and electrical stimulation of the brain.

tional cerebrospinal fluid may be released by puncturing the adjacent subarachnoid cisterns or a cerebral ventricle.

Before any cortical incision is made, the exposed cerebral gyri should be identified anatomically for the surgeon's orientation, using landmarks such as the fissure of Sylvius, vein of Trolard, and vein of Labbé (Fig. 21–14). Electrical stimulation may also be used to identify the motor cortex.

The neurosurgeon's next task is to find the patient's lesion, which often does not present on the cortical surface. However, widening or discoloration of the gyri in one area usually indicates that a mass lies beneath them. If the cortical surface appears normal, palpation with the moistened gloved finger or the use of ultrasonic encephalography may disclose the underlying lesion. In patients undergoing cerebral ablations for the control of epileptic seizures, electrocorticography is a very sensitive guide to the abnormal areas. If no other method is sufficient, a blunt ventricular needle may be passed into the brain in several different directions. When it encounters the lesion, the cerebral dissection may be made along its course. A subcortical mass should be approached by the most

direct route except when this is through a vital region such as a motor or speech area. In these cases, the cortical incision should be made in a less important area and the dissection performed obliquely down to the lesion.

The cortex adjacent to the proposed cerebral incision or resection should be protected with moist cotton strips (Fig. 21–15). Then the cortical surface along the line of the proposed incision may be cauterized superficially to coagulate the small pial vessels. In general, as many of the larger cortical vessels as possible should be saved; the line of the incision should pass along the plateau of the gyri, avoiding the vessels hidden in the sulci. The larger blood vessels usually cannot be coagulated by simple surface cauterization. The pia mater must be opened and a small amount of adjacent gray matter removed by suction so that each of these vessels may be grasped with forceps and coagulated. Even this technique may not be sufficient for major arteries and veins, which must be clipped before they are cauterized and divided. In the case of vascular lesions or large cerebral resections, the major arteries should be divided before the veins to avoid vascular engorgement of the portion being

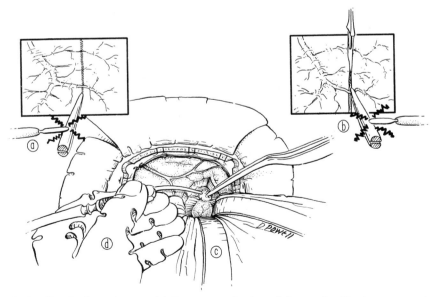

FIGURE 21–15 Standard craniotomy: (a) linear cauterization of the arachnoid, pia mater, and cortex; (b) cortical incision and cauterization of cortical vessels; (c) retraction of the brain; (d) suction in the depths of the wound.

removed. The pia mater and gray matter are usually incised with a scalpel or with the cutting electrocautery current. Normally the white matter is relatively avascular and soft, and it can be easily divided by any firm instrument such as a Penfield dissector or a metal suction tip. As the white matter along the line of resection is removed by suction, the deep vessels tend to remain as a fragile network. It saves unnecessary and annoying bleeding if these vessels can be drawn against the sucker, cauterized, and divided before they are accidentally torn.

Moist cotton balls and patties are employed routinely during cerebral resections. They usually are used in combination with irrigation and suction to keep the field clear of blood and tissue debris. They are also used to tamponade individual bleeding vessels, or are placed into one area of a resection to restrict capillary oozing while another area is being dissected. If bleeding is pronounced, several cotton balls may be placed into the area to tamponade the vessels, and then as these are removed one by one, hemostasis is achieved in each small sector uncovered. In obscure areas deep in the operative defect, it may be wise to use cotton balls and patties with attached sutures, which are brought out through the cranial opening as a reminder to remove them before closure.

Irrigation may also be quite helpful during cerebral resections. This fluid can be used to rinse the operative field, and it can be pooled in a resected area so that residual bleeding from individual vessels can be identified as the blood streams out into the clear fluid. In addition, irrigation fluid at a temperature of 105° to 115° F has intrinsic hemostatic properties since it induces vascular constriction and hastens blood coagulation.[28]

Retractors are customarily used to separate the incised cerebral surfaces so that deeper areas may be seen. This should be done gently, using cotton strips beneath the retractors to protect the brain from accidental laceration. The greatest degree of traction should be directed toward the lesion in order to spare relatively normal cerebral areas from undue compression. In particular, traction against the motor cortex should be avoided since this may produce postoperative hemiparesis ("traction palsy"). During the resection of a brain tumor, the center of the neoplasm may be gutted or a neoplastic cyst aspirated to provide more room for dissection and reduce the amount of retraction required.

If a ventricle is entered, an attempt should be made to prevent blood and tissue debris from entering it by temporarily occluding the opening with a large cotton ball or some similar material. This maneuver will reduce the severity of the resulting postoperative sterile ventriculitis.

In cases complicated by incisural herniation of the uncus and hippocampal gyrus, these swollen structures must be disimpacted under direct vision to prevent progressive mesencephalic compression and death. Simple removal of the overlying lesion (e.g., epidural hematoma) is usually not adequate for this purpose.

When the cerebral resection has been completed, all residual bleeding should be controlled. Irrigation fluid placed into the surgical defect must remain clear before efforts at hemostasis are ended. Also, any blood that has entered the subdural space during the operation should be washed out. A final check should be made to be certain that all cotton balls and strips have been removed.

Radiopaque markers may then be inserted for postoperative evaluation. Sterile tantalum dust can be placed along the surfaces of resection after the total or subtotal removal of brain tumors and held in place by overlying strips of oxidized cellulose. Postoperative recurrence of these tumors can then be identified by changes in the radiographic location of the tantalum. Similarly, tantalum dust may be placed on the surface of the cortex at the site of a craniectomy or craniotomy for evacuation of a subdural hematoma.[36] The distance between the layer of tantalum dust and the tantalum clips on the edges of the overlying dura mater can be measured postoperatively as an index of absorption or further accumlation of the subdural fluid.

Closure of the Operative Defect

Frequently the flap of dura mater that was turned at the beginning of the operation is inadequate to fill the dural defect at

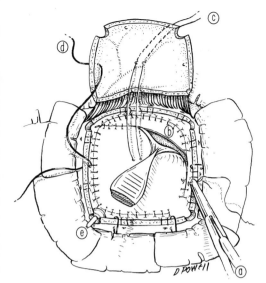

FIGURE 21–16 Standard craniotomy: (a) suturing of the dura mater, (b) dural graft, (c) central tack-up suture, (d) bone wires, (e) bottom of silicone rubber button.

using temporalis fascia, periosteum, fascia lata, or an artificial dural substitute. The dural flap and graft are usually sewn into position so the suture line is fairly water-tight. In supratentorial operations, this dural closure prevents outward cerebral herniation and minimizes the formation of a cortical cicatrix. These considerations are not as important in the suboccipital area. The dura mater is commonly left open after surgery in the posterior fossa, and if an adequate closure of the nuchal muscles is achieved, no adverse effects can be detected. The dura mater is also usually left open following a craniectomy for a subdural hematoma and beneath simple trephine openings.

The bone flap is wired back into place, and the dural flap is simultaneously sutured up to its central drill holes (Figs. 21–16 and 21–17). Silicone rubber or tantalum buttons, methylmethacrylate, or autogenous bone chips can be used to fill in the trephine openings and other bony defects for a better cosmetic result. Frequently, a portion of the bone under the temporalis muscle will be removed at some stage of the operation before the bone flap is closed, to provide a subtemporal decompression. This type of decompression has limited value, however, unless it is combined with dural grafting. In general, it is best to replace at

the end (Fig. 21–16). The tack-up sutures cause retraction of the dural margins, and some shrinkage of the dural flap occurs despite its coverage with moist cotton strips during the operation. In this situation and when dural decompression is necessary, a dural graft can be inserted,

FIGURE 21–17 Standard craniotomy: (a) twisting the bone wires, (b) central tack-up suture, (c) and (d) application of button tops, (e) suturing of the temporalis muscle and fascia.

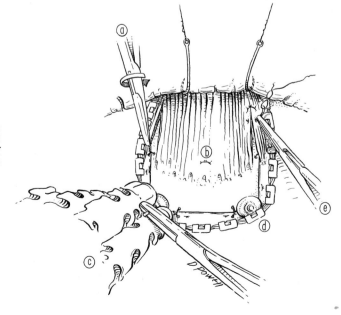

least part of the bone flap after operations for malignant brain tumors in order to prevent a long terminal period with a large bulging scalp flap.

If there is marked cerebral swelling, the bone flap should be removed. It can be wrapped in sterile towels and a sterile plastic bag, stored in a freezer, and replaced at a later time.[30] As an alternative, this bone flap can be used as a model for the postoperative construction of a methylmethacrylate cranioplasty plate.[32]

Silk is usually used for dural tack-up sutures and for closure of the dura, musculature, and scalp. In contaminated or infected cases, a less reactive type of suture material should be used, such as nylon or stainless steel wire. Interrupted inverted galeal sutures are an important part of the scalp closure in clean cases, but these buried sutures should not be used in the presence of gross contamination or infection since they may form a nidus for subcutaneous or subgaleal abscesses.

If there has been gross bacterial contamination or infection, devitalized bone should not be replaced unless it is important for cosmetic reasons (e.g., portions of the supraorbital ridge). Similarly, plastics and other foreign materials should be avoided. Copious irrigation of the operative field with sterile Ringer's solution or isotonic saline at the various anatomical levels of the operation is advisable, and irrigation with a relatively nonepileptogenic antibiotic (e.g., bacitracin, 50,000 units in about 10 ml of sterile Ringer's solution or isotonic saline) may also be helpful. Iodoform gauze packing may be placed in the epidural space before the scalp is closed, with one end brought out through a dependent limb of the incision or a separate stab wound. It may then be withdrawn gradually over several days and perhaps replaced with fresh iodoform gauze. Cranioplasty should be delayed for at least 6 to 12 months in these cases to avoid the risk of a second infection around the cranioplasty plate.

As the scalp is closed, the skin clips or hemostats should be removed systematically in small groups to avoid continuous bleeding from the rest of the incision while one area is being sutured (Fig. 21–18). Extensive cauterization of the bleeding scalp vessels is not advisable since it may delay

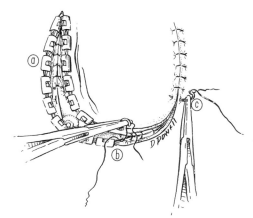

FIGURE 21–18 Standard craniotomy: (a) sutures in the temporalis fascia, (b) suturing of the galea aponeurotica, (c) suturing of the skin.

healing and result in sloughing along the scalp edges.

After the scalp has been sutured, sterile gauze pads, a loosely knit gauze wrap, and strips of adhesive tape are then applied. For the patient's comfort, his ears should be padded with cotton as the dressing is put on. An extra layer of fine-mesh gauze may also be wrapped over the dressing to hold it more firmly in place. This turban should come below the ears to keep the dressing from sliding off, but it should not be so tight that it is uncomfortable for the patient. As an aid to scalp hemostasis, if the bone flap has been replaced, an elastic bandage can be applied over the head dressing for one to two hours postoperatively. Small scalp incisions can be covered by simple collodion dressings. Intraoral incisions are usually closed with catgut sutures and require no dressing.

Ordinarily the gauze dressings are not taken off until it is time to remove the skin sutures. This is usually on the fifth day after operation for silk sutures in uncomplicated cases, or at a later time for nylon or wire sutures, especially if delayed wound healing is expected. The suture line should be painted with an antiseptic solution and the sutures removed using sterile technique. Even a small stitch abscess, which would be only a nuisance elsewhere in the body, may lead to osteomyelitis of the bone flap and necessitate its removal.

When drains are used, they may be brought out through a dependent portion of the scalp incision or through a separate stab wound in a dependent area of the scalp. Drains in clean cases (e.g., from the subdural space after evacuation of a subdural hematoma) should be removed within 24 to 36 hours because of the danger of retrograde infection along the drain. Loose scalp sutures that are placed in each drain incision at the time of operation should be tied as soon as the drain is removed to seal the incision. While the drains are in, a bulky head dressing should be employed, and this should be changed whenever the drainage stains through to the outer layers of gauze.

General Remarks about Specific Operative Approaches

Frontal Approach

A curved scalp incision is frequently used for a unilateral frontal approach (Fig. 21-3).[29] It arches posteriorly and then inferolaterally from a point on the forehead to end just anterior and superior to the ipsilateral ear. The vertical limb in the exposed portion of the forehead is least conspicuous if it is in the midline, and it will not result in denervation of any part of the frontalis muscle as will a more lateral incision. A coronal scalp incision, running from one anterior temporal area to the other at about the level of the coronal suture line, may be used for either unilateral or bilateral frontal operations (Fig. 21-2). This incision is entirely hidden behind the normal hair line, but is curved forward at the sagittal midline to allow easier anterior reflection of the frontal scalp.

With either type of incision, accidental injury to the anterior temporal branches of the facial nerve should be avoided by keeping the incision superior to the zygomatic process and no further than about 1.5 cm anterior to the ear. If these branches are damaged, noticeable postoperative paralysis of the ipsilateral frontalis muscle will result.

A supraorbital saw cut through the frontal bone should not enter the frontal sinus unless low exposure is necessary in a patient with large frontal sinuses (e.g., frontal craniotomy in an acromegalic patient). If the frontal sinus is entered, this contaminated area should be isolated from the sterile intracranial contents. The mucosa of the exposed portion of the sinus can be simply stripped away from the bone and collapsed if it has not been opened. However, if it has been opened, the mucosa in the sinus and any mucosal strips still adhering to the bone flap should be exenterated. In either case, the sinus can then be packed with autogenous muscle or gelatin sponge, or, if the mucosa has been opened, the sinus may be drained through the frontonasal duct into the nose, using a small catheter. In sealing off a surgical opening into the sinus, a flap of frontal periosteum or temporalis fascia may be placed across the defect and sutured to the periosteum superiorly and the dura mater inferiorly.

If bifrontal bone flaps are made, the medial bony incision is made 1 to 2 cm lateral to the sagittal midline. This cut should be beveled so the two flaps can be wired tightly together at the end of the operation. The smaller bone flap is turned first, and then the superior sagittal sinus and dura mater are carefully separated from the sagittal sulcus and frontal crest of the remaining bone flap before it is similarly reflected laterally on its attached temporalis muscle fibers.

Parietal and Occipital Approaches

An inverted U–shaped parietal scalp incision is usually used (Fig. 21-4).[29] The base should not be narrower than the apex to insure against ischemia of the edges of the scalp flap. Since there is no parietal musculature on which to hinge a bone flap, a free flap of parietal bone is generally employed. Parasagittal lesions may be approached through a biparietal H-shaped flap or a unilateral flap which has been extended across the midline (Fig. 21-2).

The usual occipital scalp incision begins just above and lateral to the inion, and extends parallel to the midline into the posterior parietal region where it curves temporally (Fig. 21-4). The bone flap is reflected laterally on the attached posterior fibers of the temporalis muscle.

In parietal and occipital operations, the superior sagittal and transverse sinuses should be carefully spared from injury because of the grave consequences of obstruction of these venous channels.

Temporal Approach

Depending on the nature of the operation and the extent of exposure necessary, the temporal scalp incision can be linear, U-shaped, or in the configuration of a question mark (Figs. 21–3 and 21–4).[29] All three begin anterior to the superior portion of the pinna, and care must be taken to avoid injury to the temporal branches of the facial nerve. The linear incision extends directly toward the sagittal midline; the U-shaped incision arches superomedially, posteriorly, and then inferolaterally to end behind the ear; and the question mark incision curves posteriorly just above the ear and then turns superiorly, medially, and anteriorly to end in the anterolateral frontal area.

Since the squamous portion of the temporal bone is thin and the heavy temporalis muscle will provide postoperative protection of the underlying brain, craniectomy is frequently used in the temporal area rather than craniotomy. When subtemporal craniectomy is performed for retrogasserian neurotomy, bone should be removed down to the floor of the middle fossa to provide adequate exposure.

No matter which method of bony opening is used, the contaminated mastoid air cells should not be intentionally entered, and injury to the transverse sinus should be avoided. If the mastoid air cells are opened, they should be sealed off with bone wax.

Suboccipital Approach

In many suboccipital operations, supratentorial ventricular drainage is required to reduce increased intracranial pressure, especially if a ventriculogram has been performed preoperatively. Usually at the beginning of the operation an indwelling ventricular needle or catheter is inserted into the right lateral ventricle through a right occipital trephine opening so that supratentorial ventricular pressure can be reduced at any time.

Several different types of incisions are used for suboccipital operations (Fig. 21-5).[18] Bilateral exposure is possible through a relatively avascular midline linear incision, or a U-shaped incision arched across the inion and based inferolaterally at the mastoid tips. Unilateral exposure can be achieved through a unilateral linear or hockey-stick incision, or a narrow U-shaped flap that has its lateral limb in the mastoid region and its medial limb along the nuchal midline.

By any approach, the emissary veins in the mastoid, suboccipital, and condylar areas may be encountered. These must be controlled with cautery and bone wax to prevent significant venous bleeding. A cuff of nuchal musculature (the trapezius and semispinalis capitis medially; the sternocleidomastoid and splenius capitis laterally) should be left as the muscle is incised to insure adequate closure of the wound.

The bone in the suboccipital area is removed piecemeal with rongeurs after multiple trephine openings have been made. Usually the posterior arch of the atlas is also removed to provide adequate exposure and decompression. Injury to the vertebral artery must be avoided when this arch is uncovered and removed. Any mastoid air cells exposed during a suboccipital craniectomy should be plugged with bone wax. Besides creating a route of entry into the posterior cranial fossa for bacteria and air, an opening into these air cells can provide an avenue for the persistent leakage of cerebrospinal fluid into the middle ear, eustachian tube, and pharynx.

The dura mater is opened in cruciate fashion over one or both cerebellar hemispheres and tonsils. The dural leaves are turned back and sutured to the adjacent periosteum, fascia, or muscles. As the dural incision is carried inferiorly, the circular dural venous channels at the level of the foramen magnum should be clipped. Likewise, the occipital sinus should be ligated and divided if bilateral exposure is required. Transfixion sutures are useful for occluding the occipital sinus since they are less likely to slip off than is a tantalum clip. The posterior arachnoidal wall of the cisterna magna is opened to provide additional decompression and exposure of the posterior fossa.

The patient's respiration should not be controlled by the anesthetist during operations in the vicinity of the medulla. Abnormal changes in spontaneous respiratory rate and rhythm are important signs of medullary injury and will serve as a warning to the surgeon to alter his operation accordingly.

The dura mater is usually left open at the completion of the suboccipital operation. If it is closed partially there is an increased tendency for cerebrospinal fluid to become trapped under the musculocutaneous flap. It is important that the nuchal muscles and scalp be closed well to prevent a cerebrospinal fluid fistula. If a ventriculocisternal shunt has been performed in association with the posterior fossa surgery, the nuchal muscles must be closed snugly about the shunt tube to keep cerebrospinal fluid from dissecting superiorly along its course. If the cuff of fibromuscular tissue is inadequate for a firm closure, a row of drill holes may be made along the superior and lateral bony margins of the craniectomy defect so the nuchal muscles can be sutured to these margins instead.

After the cranial dressing has been applied, a "checkrein" of adhesive tape can be attached to this dressing and to the posterior cervical skin to prevent undue tension on a transverse suboccipital incision.

A few combined supratentorial-infratentorial approaches have been devised for exposure of lesions extending through the tentorial incisura, but these are seldom necessary. They are somewhat difficult technically and may be associated with injury to the transverse sinus. Also, if an incision is made to outline two adjacent scalp flaps (one supratentorial and one infratentorial), wound healing may not be optimal.

Basal Approach

Several types of operation may be performed through the base of the skull anterior to the foramen magnum.[34, 35] The reader is referred to the references at the end of this chapter and to the other chapters in this book for the details of these procedures.

Postoperative Considerations

The very important subject of postoperative management is discussed elsewhere in this book. However, it does seem appropriate to mention a few points about the postoperative care of the surgical flap or incision.[21, 26, 37]

If fluid collects in the subgaleal space beneath the patient's scalp flap, it should not be aspirated unless the incision is in danger of separation. This fluid will be gradually reabsorbed spontaneously, and the insertion of a needle through the potentially contaminated scalp is rarely justified because of the possible introduction of infection.

The postoperative leakage of cerebrospinal fluid through the scalp incision frequently indicates an inadequate closure of the dura mater, and perhaps of other layers of the wound as well. This complication usually can be controlled by placing additional sutures along the scalp incision. Occasionally the entire wound must be reopened for careful closure of each of its layers. Since persistently elevated cerebrospinal fluid pressure may also be a contributing factor, periodic lumbar punctures may be useful to reduce cerebrospinal fluid pressure and decrease its force against the healing wound. Antibiotics should be given until satisfactory healing has occurred.

If the leakage of cerebrospinal fluid is due to a wound infection, a more serious situation exists. The wound must be reopened, culture specimens must be taken, and the wound must then be thoroughly cleansed. A tight dural closure must be achieved, using relatively nonreactive suture material. The more superficial sutures and other foreign material should be removed. The scalp may then be closed with a single layer of interrupted wire sutures, with or without drains or packs. Antibiotic therapy should also be used under these circumstances.

Postoperative radiotherapy for intracranial tumors should be delayed until the operative incision is well healed in order to prevent wound dehiscence.

Reoperation may become necessary in the immediate postoperative period because of intracranial hemorrhage or edema of the brain, or later because of postoperative persistence or recurrence of the patient's original lesion or the development of complications such as infection or hydrocephalus. In general, portions of the patient's original operative incision are reopened, and it is a definite advantage to the surgeon if he has a detailed report of the original operation to review before the second procedure. If the bone flap has been removed previously, accidental dural laceration should be avoided as the scalp is reflected. In reoperations performed several months or years after the initial procedure, the dura mater may be quite adherent to the underlying cerebral cortex or neoplasm, necessitating careful dissection to separate the two. This dissection should be as limited as possible to prevent unnecessary cortical damage.

In closing a second operation done for acute postoperative hemorrhage or edema, it may be desirable to graft the dura mater and leave out part or all of the bone flap. When infection is present, all devitalized and foreign material should be removed except for the necessary dural and scalp sutures, which should be of a relatively nonreactive material. The infected wound should be treated as outlined previously. After any secondary procedure, the scalp incision may be slower to heal, and the removal of scalp sutures should be delayed accordingly.

SPINAL OPERATIONS

Preoperative Preparation, Positioning, and Draping

As for cranial operations, informed consent for a spinal operation is required. The patient's blood should be typed and cross-matched, his stomach should be empty, he should be given appropriate premedications, and his pertinent x-ray films should be taken to the operating room. Unless his lesion is close to the upper or lower end of the spinal column, where the surgeon can recognize the vertebral level exactly by counting up from the sacrum or down from the occiput, the patient's skin should be marked preoperatively at the level of the lesion, using radiographic identification. Just before operation, the surgeon should consult the patient, his chart, and his x-rays to verify the side and level of his lesion.

General anesthesia is usually induced with the patient supine, and spinal anesthesia is achieved with the patient in the prone jackknifed or the lateral position. Patients with cervical fracture-dislocations

are commonly intubated with a nasotracheal tube while they are still awake; topical anesthesia is used. By this maneuver, the use of direct laryngoscopy with dangerous extension of the neck is avoided, and accidental aspiration of vomitus by the patient is minimized. As an alternative in this type of patient, a tracheostomy may be performed. A patient with a meningomyelocele may be intubated in the semilateral position to prevent unnecessary pressure on the spinal sac.

The patient's lower extremities are wrapped with elastic bandages to prevent pooling of blood in these limbs. As for other operations, the eyes of the anesthetized patient should be protected from accidental injury.

Patients with spinal fractures or dislocations must be moved into position for surgery with great care to avoid further injury to the spinal cord. Several strong persons, working simultaneously, should move the patient without unnecessary flexion, extension, or rotation of the spinal column. Cervical traction should also be maintained as the patient with cervical injuries is moved onto the operating table.

Spinal operations are generally performed with the patient in a prone or sitting position, but anterior spinal discectomy and stereotaxic cervical cordotomy are done with the patient supine, and posterior spinal operations are accomplished by some surgeons using the lateral position.

If the prone position is used, the patient's trunk should be supported laterally on pads or folded sheets, allowing space between them for free thoracic and abdominal respiratory excursions and avoiding compression of the inferior vena cava with its resulting distention of the intraspinal venous plexus. A footboard can be used to prevent the patient from sliding down the operating table if the head of the table is raised. Such elevation of the head can be used advantageously to reduce venous distention in the cervical area and to fill out the entire spinal subarachnoid space with cerebrospinal fluid to tamponade the extradural veins.

For most thoracic and lumbar operations done with the patient prone, the patient's head can be turned to the side and his arms extended to rest beside his head. Care must be taken to prevent overextension of the shoulder with pressure on or stretching of the vascular and nervous elements of the axilla. To avoid spinal rotation and distortion, upper thoracic and cervical operations should be performed with the patient's head flexed forward on the cerebellar frame and his arms by his sides. By the appropriate use of folded sheets and pads, an infant can be placed in a similar position on the operating table without the cerebellar frame. If the cerebellar frame is used, pressure on the patient's eyes should be avoided. Compression of the jugular veins by the mattress or pads should likewise be prevented in order to eliminate unnecessary cervical venous distention that might cause increased bleeding during the operation. Moderate caudal traction of the shoulders with wide adhesive tape can be used to increase the operative exposure in the cervical area, but the tape should not restrict respiratory movements of the posterior thorax and should not cover the iliac crests if an iliac bone graft is anticipated.

If cranial tongs were inserted prior to operation for skeletal traction, this traction can be maintained during the procedure by suspending the weight over a pulley attached to an extension beyond the cerebellar frame. The amount and direction of cervical traction can be altered during the operation to suit the surgeon.

During practically any spinal operation with the patient prone, the table may be flexed or extended, and the cerebellar frame or traction pulley can be lowered or elevated to separate or approximate the laminal arches. The surgeon can use these changes in position to gain a mechanical advantage. With the spine flexed and the laminal arches separated, the intervertebral disc is more easily exposed and dislocated facets can be more easily reduced. With the spine moderately extended, reduced facets can be locked in position and the laminal arches can be more easily wired or fused together.

The lateral position for spinal surgery avoids a number of the problems encountered in the prone position. There is less jugular and caval venous obstruction, better control over the patient's airway, and natural drainage of blood and cerebrospinal fluid out of the wound. Subarachnoid-peritoneal shunts are performed in this position since it permits simultaneous exposure of the back and the abdomen. However, adequate bilateral exposure of the spine and spinal cord is usually more difficult by this approach.

The sitting position can also be used for cervical spinal operations. As opposed to the prone position, there is less venous bleeding and little pooling of blood and cerebrospinal fluid in the wound. Yet there is a greater danger of cerebral ischemia, venous air embolism, and rapid loss of cerebrospinal fluid leading to an intracranial subdural hematoma.

After the patient has been positioned for operation, the primary and donor (e.g., iliac crests if a bone graft is anticipated) operative areas should be shaved and cleansed with antiseptic solutions. The anal area must be carefully excluded from the operative field with skin towels. Next, the important anatomical landmarks and the proposed incision should be marked with a sterile dye. Because of the incompatibility between thimerosol and iodine, if one or the other has been used to cleanse the skin for a lumbar puncture shortly before lumbar spinal surgery, the same solution should again be used for the operative skin preparation. After the operative area is draped, the suction and cautery lines are attached, and the field is illuminated. As with cranial operations, ultraviolet lights may be used during spinal surgery for their bactericidal effects.

General Remarks About Specific Operative Approaches

Posterior Approach

The skin and subcutaneous tissues are usually divided in the longitudinal midline, although this incision may be deviated in an elliptical fashion around each side of a midline dermal sinus. One exception to this approach is the incision generally used for a meningomyelocele. A generous transverse incision is made for this, and its ends may be curved in opposite directions to create skin flaps adequate to cover the central defect left after the sac has been resected.

Superficial subcutaneous bleeding is controlled with hemostatic clamps. These are then laid back over sterile towels that are brought up to the edges of the wound on each side to cover all the previously exposed skin. The edges of the incision are retracted, and bleeding vessels in the deeper layers of the subcutaneous tissue are cauterized.

The next layer encountered is the fascial layer overlying the paravertebral muscles (lumbodorsal or nuchal fascia). This is divided in the midline in preparation for a bilateral laminectomy. However, if a hemilaminectomy is planned, the fascia is divided a few millimeters lateral to the midline, leaving a cuff to aid in suturing this fascia during closure of the wound. In the cervical area, dissection is then carried through the relatively avascular ligamentum nuchae down to the spinous processes.

The paravertebral muscles are stripped away from the spines and laminae by subperiosteal dissection. This step is usually performed using a periosteal elevator and gauze packs to bluntly dissect away the muscle fibers, and a scalpel or scissors to divide their tendinous insertions. However, if the posterior arches are open, as with a spina bifida, or are unstable, as with a spinal fracture, only sharp dissection under direct vision should be used. The paravertebral muscles should be stripped from the spinous processes in the acute angle between their insertions and the bone. If the scalpel or periosteal elevator is used in the opposite direction, it will tend to follow the direction of the fibers away from the vertebral spines out into the vascular muscle mass. Bleeding from the detached muscles is controlled by cautery and by temporarily packing the paravertebral gutters with gauze pads. These muscles are then retracted laterally and the laminae are cleaned of overlying connective tissue and fat out to and including the intervertebral facets. The transverse processes must also be exposed when a fusion of these elements is to be performed.

The exact vertebral level may be established by counting up or down from a recognizable landmark such as the occiput, the spine of C2, the spine of C7, or the sacrum. The level of a cervical operation may also be verified by examining preoperative anteroposterior and lateral roentgenograms to identify individual characteristics of the various cervical spines (i.e., long or short, single or bifid). In the thoracic area, the exact level is more difficult to establish. Reference can be made to marks placed on the skin preoperatively, or roentgenograms may be made in the operating room using a metal object to mark one of the spines or laminae.

If a wide opening between or through the spinal arches does not already exist, portions of them must be removed with rongeurs or drills to create an entrance into the spinal canal. As a general rule, as little bone as possible is removed to provide adequate exposure, especially if an ensuing posterior spinal fusion is planned. To uncover a posterolateral herniation of an intervertebral disc, it is generally necessary to excise only the edges of one or two laminae and perhaps a portion of the adjacent intervertebral facet. For unilateral cordotomy or rhizotomy, adequate exposure can be achieved by removing one or more laminae on just one side, but any larger procedure usually requires removal of the laminae, spines, and the attached ligaments of several vertebrae bilaterally.

The excision of the spinous processes is facilitated by the preliminary division of the supraspinous and interspinous ligaments. Similarly, removal of the laminal arches is made easier if a plane is first established between one of the laminae and its underlying ligamentum flavum. Since the ligamenta flava attach like shingles to the anterior surfaces of the superior laminae and the posterior surfaces of the inferior laminae, the inferior laminal edges are the more easily separated from these ligaments by the posterior approach. Thus, the removal of each lamina should begin along its caudal edge. Care must be taken to avoid compression of the spinal cord or nerve roots as the spines and laminae are removed. Typically, there is an emissary vein that perforates each lamina laterally. Bleeding from these veins and from the edges of the divided bones can be controlled with bone wax.

After the bony opening has been created, portions of one or more of the ligamenta flava should be removed. If two adjacent ligaments are exposed, a gap between them can usually be found, and, starting at that point, they can be peeled away from the underlying epidural veins. This is especially true in the cervical region where the ligamenta flava are not as well developed as in other areas of the spine. If only a single ligamentum flavum has been exposed, it should be elevated with a sharp hook or forceps and incised carefully to avoid accidental laceration of the underlying dura mater. This ligament should be cut in a plane perpendicular to its surface; if not, it may fray into laminations and prolong the time required for its removal.

No matter how the ligamenta flava are excised, care should be taken not to lacerate the underlying epidural veins. Bleeding from these vessels will obscure the operative field and will increase the risk of paraplegia or quadriplegia due to the formation of a postoperative epidural hematoma.

If such a vein is accidentally opened, the bleeding usually can be controlled by compression. Direct pressure may be applied with a cotton patty; simultaneous compression of the spinal cord or its nerve roots must be avoided. As an alternative, the dura mater may be sutured laterally against the neighboring wall of the spinal canal after the dura has been opened. Pieces of gelatin sponge or oxidized cellulose may also be placed over the bleeding vein immediately before either of these maneuvers is performed. Frequently, individual epidural veins can be isolated and identified easily enough to permit clip ligation or cauterization of these structures. However, before being cauterized, they should be held away from the adjacent dura mater to prevent thermal injury to the underlying nervous tissue. After the venous bleeding has been controlled, cotton strips are placed over the epidural space and intervertebral facets along each side of the exposed dura.

When the dura mater is to be opened, it may be picked up with a sharp hook, incised with a scalpel with a No. 15 blade, and divided with scissors or a blunt hook. It is frequently advantageous to leave the arachnoid membrane intact while the dura is being opened. By this maneuver, the hydrostatic pressure compressing the epidural veins is maintained and blood is kept out of the subarachnoid space. The cut edges of the dura mater are elevated and held apart with traction sutures. This provides exposure of the spinal cord and forms a small barrier to prevent the blood that collects in the depths of the incision from flowing over the surface of the cord. Usually, the dura is then tacked up to the adjacent periosteum and paravertebral muscles in several places along each side of the bony opening in order to minimize epidural venous bleeding.

If possible, the arachnoid should not be incised immediately beneath the dural opening. This will allow an intact strip of arachnoid to seal off the inner surface of the dural incision after the dura has been sutured shut. When the patient is in the sitting position, only a small arachnoidal opening should be made at first, to prevent the sudden loss of cerebrospinal fluid and the possible development of an intracranial subdural hematoma. If a spinal tumor is present, the initial arachnoidal opening should be made cephalad to it, to avoid the occasional increase in neurological deficit associated with the release of cerebrospinal fluid below a spinal block.

The same techniques are applied in operating upon the spinal cord as upon the brain, but on a much smaller and more exact scale. The spinal cord is extremely sensitive to compression and other forms of injury, and the destruction of only a small amount of white or gray matter in the spinal cord may result in a significant neurological deficit. For this reason, great care must be taken to avoid injury to the normal nervous elements as pathological tissue is manipulated or removed from the spinal canal. Even minor retraction of the spinal cord may interfere with its function.

Adequate illumination is essential for this type of surgery and magnification can be of great value in avoiding unnecessary injury to normal structures. The cord should be kept moist with warm irrigation solution during operation to minimize desiccation. Suction should be performed through a cotton patty to prevent accidental aspiration of normal nervous tissue. Cauterization should be as limited as possible, using bipolar current ("cold cautery") and forceps with fine points. In order to avoid unnecessary hemorrhage, myelotomy should be performed in relatively avascular areas, and catheters should not be randomly passed into the epidural, subdural, or subarachnoid spaces away from the exposed areas of the spinal canal. Usually nerve roots are clipped before they are divided, to control bleeding from the radicular arteries that accompany them.

The dura mater may be left open at the end of the operation, but usually it is sutured shut to prevent blood and fibrous tissue from entering the subarachnoid space and cerebrospinal fluid from leaving it. If it appears that compression of the spinal cord might occur if the dura is sutured primarily, a graft of paravertebral fascia or an artificial dural substitute may be sutured into the dural defect. Whether or not a graft is used, a few of these dural sutures can also be tacked up to the overlying muscles as they are closed to aid in preventing postoperative epidural hemorrhage. Tantalum clips may be attached to the dura mater or paravertebral tissues to serve as postoperative radiographic markers.

If a posterior spinal fusion is planned, it can be done at this point. Next, the wound is carefully checked to make certain that all cotton strips and gauze sponges have been removed. The muscles, fascia, subcutaneous tissue, and skin are then sutured in anatomical layers. If a gap exists, as in the case of a meningomyelocele, additional maneuvers may be necessary to close it. Flaps of lumbodorsal or nuchal fascia can be elevated and sutured across such a defect. Also, the skin can be extensively undermined and cutaneous flaps can be created to obtain adequate coverage. Wire or another strong inert suture material should be used to close the laminectomy wound in debilitated patients and in those who will be given postoperative radiotherapy.

It is not advisable to place devitalized bone or foreign material into contaminated or infected laminectomy incisions. In these cases, the wound should be thoroughly irrigated with sterile Ringer's solution or isotonic saline before closure. An antibiotic solution, such as 50,000 units of bacitracin in 10 ml of fluid, may also be instilled into the wound. Because of the length of time required for a deep posterior spinal incision to fill with granulation tissue, an effort should be made to achieve some type of primary closure in minimally contaminated

cases, using a relatively nonreactive suture material such as wire. If the wound is left open, it may be packed with iodoform gauze to reduce the numbers of bacteria present and to stimulate the formation of granulation tissue.

In clean cases, the sterile gauze dressing placed on the skin incision is not disturbed until it is time for the skin sutures to be removed. For silk sutures in uncomplicated cases, this is usually on the sixth day after operation.

The postoperative management of patients with posterior spinal operations varies depending on the nature of the pathological process and the location and extent of the operation. As soon as the effects of anesthesia have abated, the patient's neurological status should be tested. Frequent examinations should then be performed periodically over the ensuing hours and days to spot any neurological deterioration that may be a sign of a postoperative extradural hematoma.

Narcotics are usually necessary for postoperative analgesia, but because of possible respiratory depression from these drugs, they should not be given following a cervical laminectomy until the patient is awake and it is obvious that he is having no difficulty breathing. As after other types of surgery, various measures should be taken to prevent postoperative pulmonary atelectasis and thrombophlebitis in the lower extremities. The paraplegic or quadriplegic patient will also require additional care, as discussed elsewhere in this book.

If the dura mater has not been opened, and the bony resection has been minor, the patient can stand and walk with assistance within a day after the operation. Following extensive laminectomies, however, the patient is usually kept at bed rest for several days to allow the paravertebral muscles time to begin healing together before being subjected to their normal stresses and strains. A back or neck brace may also be of considerable value for mechanical support after some types of spinal surgery.

The postoperative leakage of cerebrospinal fluid through a laminectomy incision should be managed in the same way as when it occurs following a cranial operation.

If reoperation in the same area and by the same approach becomes necessary, the patient's previous incision may be reopened. As with cranial reoperations, a detailed report of the original operation is of value to the surgeon planning a second procedure. Dense fibrous connective tissue may be encountered against the dura mater where the laminae and ligamenta flava have been removed; such tissue may distort normal anatomical relationships. Therefore it is wise to begin a second exploration in relatively normal tissue adjacent to the scarred area and to extend the dissection gradually from normal anatomical planes into the scar. This maneuver will usually prevent accidental laceration of the dura mater and its contents. The skin incision may take longer to heal after a second operation, and the removal of the skin sutures should be delayed accordingly.

Anterior Approach

The anterior approaches to the lower lumbar and lower cervical spine are considered in detail elsewhere in this book. Additional information may be found in the pertinent references at the end of this chapter.[20, 23, 31]

An anterior approach to the first two cervical vertebrae may be made through the oropharynx. This has been used primarily for the drainage of tuberculous and other types of abscesses, though a few surgeons have used this approach to resect tumors or to perform anterior spinal fusions. The procedure is not exceptionally difficult, but it is rarely necessary. Also, this approach is made through a contaminated area, with an appreciable chance of an operative infection.

Lateral Approach

The *direct lateral* approach to the spinal cord is made in some types of percutaneous stereotaxic cervical cordotomy. This, of course, does not involve an open surgical exposure.

However, for some conditions, such as spinal tuberculosis or ruptured thoracic intervertebral disc, a *posterolateral* exposure of the spinal canal may be optimal. The details of these operations may be found in the appropriate references at the end of this chapter.[19, 25, 27]

More *extensive posterolateral and anterolateral* approaches have also been devised for the treatment of spinal tuberculosis and other spinal deformities, but these operations are primarily of interest to the orthopedic surgeon and are not discussed here.

SUMMARY

This chapter briefly outlines some of the techniques used in cranial and spinal operations. Specific operations are dealt with in subsequent chapters. Discussion of current techniques has been in general terms. These methods are under constant refinement and revision by practicing neurosurgeons and must be individualized according to the nature and location of the disease process, the physiological and psychological status of the patient, the skill and experience of the surgical team, and the availability of various neurosurgical instruments and equipment.

It must also be stressed that skillful preoperative and postoperative management are necessary to achieve the best results from any type of neurosurgical operation no matter how well the operative techniques have been performed.

The illustrations used in this chapter have been patterned primarily after those of Gurdjian and Webster,[12, 13] Cushing,[3] and Asenjo.[9]

REFERENCES

Historical

1. Bennett, G.: History. *In* Howorth, M. B., and Petrie, J. G., eds.: Injuries of the Spine. Baltimore, Williams & Wilkins Co., 1964, pp. 1–59.
2. Bick, E. M.: Source Book of Orthopaedics. 2nd Ed. Baltimore, Williams & Wilkins Co., 1948.
3. Cushing, H.: Surgery of the head. *In* Keen, W. W., ed.: Surgery, Its Principles and Practice. Philadelphia, W. B. Saunders Co., 1908, 3:17–276.
4. Dandy, W. E.: Surgery of the brain. *In* Lewis' Practice of Surgery. Hagerstown, Md., W. F. Prior Co., Inc., 1932, 12:1–682.
5. Elsberg, C. A.: Diagnosis and Treatment of Surgical Diseases of the Spinal Cord and Its Membranes. Philadelphia, W. B. Saunders Co., 1916.
6. Walker, A. E.: A History of Neurological Surgery. Baltimore, Williams & Wilkins Co., 1951.
7. Wilkins, R. H.: Neurosurgical Classics. New York, Johnson Reprint Corp., 1965.

Review

8. Alexander, E., Jr.: Neurosurgical techniques. J. Neurosurg., *24*:818–819, 1966.
9. Asenjo, A.: Neurosurgical Techniques. Springfield, Ill., Charles C Thomas, 1963.
10. Bancroft, F. W., and Pilcher, C.: Surgical Treatment of the Nervous System. Philadelphia, J. B. Lippincott Co., 1946.
11. Crenshaw, A. H.: Campbell's Operative Orthopaedics. 4th Ed. St. Louis, C. V. Mosby Co., 1963.
12. Gurdjian, E. S., and Thomas, L. M.: Operative Neurosurgery. 3rd Ed. Baltimore, Md., Williams & Wilkins Co., 1970.
13. Gurdjian, E. S., and Webster, J. E.: Operative Neurosurgery, with Emphasis on Procedures in Trauma. Baltimore, Md., Williams & Wilkins Co., 1952.
14. Irsigler, F. J.: Allgemeine Operationslehre. *In* Olivecrona, H., and Tönnis, W., eds.: Handbuch der Neurochirurgie. Berlin, Springer-Verlag, 1960, Vol. IV, Part I, pp. 1–121.
15. Kempe, L. G.: Operative Neurosurgery. New York, Springer-Verlag, 1968–1970.
16. Poppen, J. L.: An Atlas of Neurosurgical Techniques. Philadelphia, W. B. Saunders Co., 1960.
17. Rowbotham, G. F., and Hammersley, D. P.: Pictorial Introduction to Neurological Surgery. Edinburgh, E. & S. Livingstone, Ltd., 1953.

General

18. Bucy, P. C.: Exposure of the posterior or cerebellar fossa. J. Neurosurg., *24*:820–832, 1966.
19. Capener, N.: The evolution of lateral rachotomy. J. Bone Joint Surg., *36-B*:173–179, 1954.
20. Cloward, R. B.: The anterior approach for removal of ruptured cervical disks. J. Neurosurg., *15*:602–614, 1958.
21. Davidoff, L. M.: The brain and spinal cord. *In* Rothenberg, R. E., ed.: Reoperative Surgery. New York, Blakiston, 1964, pp. 40–70.
22. Donaghy, R. M. P., and Yasargil, M. G.: Microvascular Surgery. Report of first conference, October 1–7, 1966. Mary Fletcher Hospital, Burlington, Vermont. St. Louis, C. V. Mosby Co., 1967.
23. Goldner, J. L., McCollum, D. E., and Urbaniak, J. R.: Anterior intervertebral discectomy and arthrodesis for treatment of low back pain with or without radiculopathy. Clin. Neurosurg., *15*: 352–381, 1968.
24. Hart, D., and Nicks, J.: Ultraviolet radiation in the operating room. Intensities used and bactericidal effects. Arch. Surg., *82*:449–465, 1961.
25. Hodgson, A. R., Stock, F. E., Fang, H. S. Y., and Ong, G. B.: Anterior spinal fusion. The operative approach and pathological findings in 412 patients with Pott's disease of the spine. Brit. J. Surg., *48*:172–178, 1960.
26. Horwitz, N. H., and Rizzoli, H. V.: Postoperative Complications in Neurosurgical Practice. Recognition, Prevention and Management. Baltimore, Williams & Wilkins Co., 1967.
27. Hulme, A.: The surgical approach to thoracic intervertebral disc protrusions. J. Neurol. Neurosurg. Psychiat., *23*:133–137, 1960.
28. Light, R. U.: Hemostasis in neurosurgery. J. Neurosurg., *2*:414–434, 1945.
29. Odom, G. L., and Woodhall, B.: Supratentorial skull flaps. J. Neurosurg., *25*:492–501, 1966.
30. Odom, G. L., Woodhall, B., and Wrenn, F. R., Jr.: The use of refrigerated autogenous bone flaps for cranioplasty. J. Neurosurg., *9*:606–610, 1952.
31. Robinson, R. A., and Southwick, W. O.: Surgical approaches to the cervical spine. Instr. Course Lect., *17*:299–330, 1960.
32. Schupper, N.: Cranioplasty prostheses for replacement of cranial bone. J. Prosth. Dent., *19*:594–597, 1968.
33. Spiegel, E. A.: Development of stereoencephalotomy for extrapyramidal diseases. J. Neurosurg., *24*:suppl., 433–439, 1966.
34. Stevenson, G. C., Stoney, R. J., Perkins, R. K., and Adams, J. E.: A transcervical transclival approach to the ventral surface of the brain stem for removal of a clivus chordoma. J. Neurosurg., *24*:544–551, 1966.
35. Van Buren, J. M., Ommaya, A. K., and Ketcham, A. S.: Ten years' experience with radical combined craniofacial resection of malignant tumors of the paranasal sinuses. J. Neurosurg., *28*:341–350, 1968.
36. Vieth, R. G., Tindall, G. T., and Odom, G. L.: The use of tantalum dust as an adjunct in the postoperative management of subdural hematomas. J. Neurosurg., *24*:514–519, 1966.
37. Wright, R. L.: Postoperative craniotomy infections. Springfield, Ill., Charles C Thomas, 1966.

22

MICRO-OPERATIVE TECHNIQUE

It is a well-established aphorism of surgery that adequate exposure of the operative site is essential. The success of an operation depends largely on the surgeon's ability to gain the proper exposure and to relate his knowledge of functional anatomy to the exposed tissues. In gaining the exposure, the neurological surgeon has more and different problems than other surgical specialists. The brain fills the cranial cavity and its tissue is easily injured by excessive retraction—at great biological cost.

SELECTION OF MICROSCOPE AND ACCESSORIES

The use of microtechniques in neurological surgery is rapidly expanding the neurosurgical frontier. To keep pace, the neurosurgeon must become master of the operating microscope in the neurosurgical setting. Quite often, in the beginning, he borrows the microscope from an ophthalmological or otological surgeon. In this event two considerations should be kept in mind:

1. Application of the surgical microscope to eye and ear operations is simple compared to its use on the brain and spinal cord. Since demands for range and patterns of mobility are small in these specialities, the delivery system (stand and carrying arms) of the standard microscope is often inadequate for neurosurgical use. If this fact is not appreciated, the neurosurgeon may be surprised and discouraged in his first attempts to use this equipment.

T. KURZE

2. If the instrument has been in use for some time, operating instructions may be unavailable, and the neurosurgeon must learn to operate the complex apparatus by trial and error. This should *never* be done during a regular neurosurgical procedure. It will be frustrating for the neurosurgeon and may be hazardous to the patient. The neurosurgeon should seek expert advice from his colleagues in otolaryngology or ophthamology or from an experienced neurosurgeon, obtain operating instructions, and become familiar with the instrument in his leisure time rather than during a microsurgical operation. A careful reading of pages 12 to 31 in M. G. Yasargil's text *Microsurgery* is highly recommended.[4]

When the neurosurgeon purchases his own instrument, he should never rely on the advice of an instrument salesman or an institutional purchasing agent. He should visit the operating room of a neurosurgeon who is an expert in this field. The neophyte should discuss his needs with and obtain the help of the more experienced colleague in selecting an instrument with appropriate accessories. If this is not possible, lists giving catalogue numbers and prices of recommended instruments and accessories are available from most teachers of microneurosurgery.

The need for specific recommendations is recognized.[1,2,4] The reader can appreciate, however, that they become dated in a short time and are not appropriate in this type of reference. Instead, several general comments on type and style of instrument may be useful and of more enduring value.

In selecting an instrument consider the following: (1) magnification (range), (2) light (intensity, coaxial or extra-axial

551

source, homogeneity, and heat), (3) objective, (4) eyepiece (straight or angled), (5) mounting (floor or ceiling), (6) carrying arms, (7) maneuverability, (8) mobility, (9) auxiliary scopes, (10) photographic and television accessories, and (11) manufacturer.

Enlargement of the image is always acquired at the expense of depth and breadth of field. Some systems of magnification are not worth the expense, limited mobility, mechanical complexity, and limitations of the light source. Undoubtedly, engineering improvements will nullify most of these objections in the future; however, at this time they are valid.

Experience increases one's ability to work well at the higher ranges of magnification. It should be remembered that the magnification control knob settings of 6, 10, 16, 25, 40 do not indicate true magnification values. These values are dependent on focal length of the objective, tube, eyepiece, and magnification.[4]

The coaxial light source is an asset of the operating microscope that is equal to the advantages of the magnification it provides. Intensity is determined by the surgeon's needs. A regular 30-watt light source in the instrument is adequate for operating in shallow fields and at low magnification without photography. However, for neurosurgery, a 50-watt bulb with adequate power boosters for photography is more desirable. In selecting an instrument one should carefully ascertain that the field of light within focal range of the objective to be used is homogeneous and without scotomata or dark spots.

If the surgeon prefers to work with a draped scope, he should devise or purchase a cooling device for the bulb.

Selection of the objective is a very important decision since it influences magnification, working distance between front of scope and operative field, and width and intensity of illumination. The author's preference is 250 mm and 300 mm. The 300-mm objective is particularly desirable in transtentorial approaches to the pineal area. A 200-mm objective does not provide an adequate working distance between the field and the front of the scope.

Angled and straight eyepiece tubes are available. The straight tube is preferable. Its image is oriented to the direct axis of the surgeon's vision, thus bringing the manual maneuvers into planes congruous with the surgeon's image. Adaptation to the angled image is easy for the experienced surgeon;

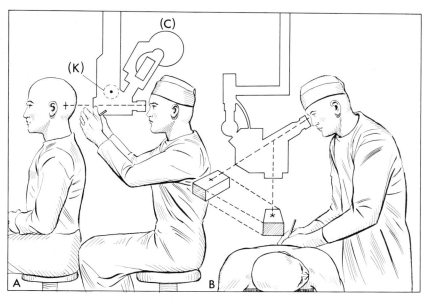

FIGURE 22–1 *A.* The most efficient and advantageous use of the straight eye piece (c). The weight of the camera may require excessive tightening of friction clutch (K) and cause an awkward reduction of maneuverability in this axis. *B.* The "cerebral" image conversion required of the surgeon with the angled scope, and one position (prone laminectomy) in which the angled eye piece is superior.

however, for the beginner enough adaptation is required in going to microtechniques without unnecessarily adding to it. In addition, the straight tube can be brought into all surgical fields, whereas the angled tube can be used in the posterior fossa and tic positions only with awkward and impractical adjustments. The angled eyepiece, however, is clearly most advantageous for laminectomy in the prone position. The observer's tube may be turned 90 degrees for the first assistant across the table.

There is no doubt that the ceiling mounted system is far superior to one that is mounted on the floor (Fig. 22-1). One of the problems of preparing for microneurosurgery is introducing the instrument into the operative field, particularly if the operating team has only limited experience. The overhead mount simplifies introduction of the instrument and provides increased maneuverability and stability. The expense and technical difficulties associated with its installation, however, may preclude its use.

The floor stand system can be effectively introduced if the tallest floor stand available is obtained. A stand 2200 mm or 2000 mm high is important for operations in the upright and sitting positions.

A variety of carrying arms between the stand and microscope is available. The system of arms should be carefully selected by the surgeon after demonstration and testing in his own operating room. The commercial exhibit of a convention hall offers neither realistic conditions nor insight into the surgeon's specific needs.

The ideal supporting stand and carrying arm combination should provide unlimited maneuverability (e.g., 120 degrees horizontal, 90 degrees sagittal) and instantly lock into a stable system that is controlled by the surgeon. The technology for this simple engineering feat exists but unfortunately is not available because adequate financial incentive is lacking. Because of the limitations imposed by the present equipment, adaptation of the zero point concept commonly used in stereotaxic systems is useful. Briefly, this involves predetermining the point in the operating room that is most desirable for the surgical field from the standpoint of the overhead light system; accessibility to suction, compressed air, electrical outlets, anesthetic gases, leads to monitoring equipment, and the like; and customary table height for both horizontal and sitting posture. Once this point has been determined, the floor stand or overhead arm attachments should be selected to match the desired function.

The next step is to select the viewing arms and photographic and television accessories. Each of these items influences the weight of the total assembly. Counterbalances must be made accordingly. With them the instrument may be elevated or lowered within the range required without locking in place. This is a most important step that can best be appreciated during the operative procedure.

Adjustment of the friction locks on the instrument and the supporting arms is essential to both mobility and stability. The instrument should not wander off the target under the slight pressure exerted by the contact of the surgeon and the assistants with the eyepieces. Adjustments of the friction locks are made by unsterile operating room personnel. They should be cautioned against tightening these locks excessively, since it will reduce the mobility of the instrument and damage the locks so that fine adjustment is no longer possible.

Selection of photographic and television display equipment is a highly individual matter. To date, because of the limited view afforded to assistant surgeons and other operating room personnel during the operation, motion pictures are the best means for recording and showing microneurosurgical procedures. However, film and processing are expensive. Still films are less expensive but do not record the dynamics of the surgical procedure.

OPERATIVE SET-UP

The operating microscope cannot be sterilized. Two methods to prevent contamination of the operative field are available. Most surgeons prefer covering the microscope with a tailored stockinet or plastic bag. This method is satisfactory. Its prime disadvantages are the additional effort required to prepare the instrument for the operation and retention of heat from the lamp. The latter is significant only when the plastic covering is used. It can be circumvented by a suction air pump, which adds another set of tubes and impediments to the conglomeration already present for the procedure. The technique preferred by the author is to place sterilizable rubber covers on the focus and magnification adjustments. With a little practice, the surgeon can learn to maneuver the instrument with these covers and not contaminate his gloved hands.

Detailed instructions for focusing the instrument accompany the microscope and should be followed. Before scrubbing for the operation, the surgeon should focus the instrument on some print. If photography is to be used, taking a picture of the patient's name and hospital file number serves a dual purpose. The human's ability to accommodate the variance in interpupillary distance is ordinarily quite a bit greater than is generally appreciated. Therefore, if the surgeon has difficulty with image fusion, it is most likely caused by a focus discrepancy in either of the eyepieces.

INSTRUMENTS

A large variety of microneurosurgical instruments are now available. As the surgeon's experience increases in micro-

surgery, the number of essential instruments will progressively decrease.

For cutting, scissors are the best choice for most microneurosurgical purposes. They provide tissue stability by their action, and the edges are more readily preserved. The small Metzenbaum type with a pistol grip is preferable (Fig. 22–2).

For dissection, a curved semisharp dissector, a cerumen curet, and a Sheehy canal knife will be needed.

Devices for suction and irrigation are essential parts of the microneurosurgical armamentarium. The presence of irrigating fluid in the microsurgical field assures continuous moistening of the cranial nerves and blood vessels, reduces the formation and adherence of small blood clots to the dissecting surfaces, and increases the effectiveness of the bipolar coagulation by reducing sticking of the forceps to the coagulated tissue. A continuous stream of irrigation fluid is necessary during drill dissection of bone. The Adson type of suction with the curve close to the tip of the instrument is preferable. Its configuration increases the number of angles at which the suction orifice can be applied to tissue, and has distinct advantages over the Frazier type of suction with the bend in the instrument above the wound edge.

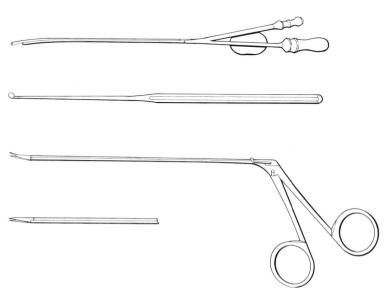

FIGURE 22–2 *Top to bottom:* suction irrigation tip, Sheehy canal knife, Kurze scissors (curved right), Kurze scissors (curved left). See text for discussion.

A system of self-retaining retractors is fundamental to neurological surgery. The Dott or Edinburgh retractor has given satisfactory performance for the past 10 years. However, the Leila cable retractor introduced by Yasargil appears to be superior from the standpoint of maneuverability and fixation.

Bipolar coagulation with forceps is the best method available for the meticulous hemostasis that is fundamental to microneurosurgery. A wide selection of forceps is available. Selections of forceps should be made with care. The surgeon should heft the instrument and check its balance with cord attached. He should also note whether he has position control over the distance between the points, since when used properly, the tips are not approximated during coagulation. Also there should be enough resistance to compression to activate his own feedback mechanism. Some of the forceps that are available are attractive for their delicacy, but compress with so little pressure that the surgeon cannot avoid completely closing them during coagulation. Bayonet forceps are preferred for obvious reasons. The very narrow tips are attractive for developing tissue planes around small blood vessels; they are, however, useless for grasping tissue.

Frequent exchange of equipment for coagulation and dissection are necessary. A forceps that has a relatively fine tip but a grasping surface with some traction is preferable. By using these instruments one can reduce the required number of forcep exchanges.

Surgeons, with long experience in conventional (anodal) coagulation are conditioned to acquire maximum dryness at the surface of application. They must remember that the reverse is true with the bipolar unit. To avoid tissue adherence, the field should be wet with irrigation fluid during coagulation. Despite this precaution the forceps still will stick to the tissue quite often.

Microdrilling is usually limited to enlargement of the foramina at the base of the skull. Both air and mechanical drills are available. The drills should have angled shafts, minimal oscillation at high speed, and a wide variety of cutting and diamond burrs.

A large selection of clips of all the types used for intracranial aneurysm should be available in the operative set-up at all times.

The authors do not have a preference for a particular suture.

Adaptation to manipulation of instruments and tissues under magnification is the easiest part of microsurgery. A conscious effort must be made to reduce the number of times the surgeon looks away from the microscope. One of the most common causes for this is the difficulty in getting instruments to where they are visible in the microscopic field. This difficulty can be avoided by always keeping one instrument in the field during instrument changes. Then the surgeon merely has to bring his right hand to his left hand or vice-versa. At present there is very little the first assistant can do in the microscopic field; however, his role as monitor of macroscopic events in and beyond the surgical exposure assumes enormous importance.

The surgeon should learn to manipulate his retractor while looking through the scope. His assistant must become expert in releasing and locking the retractor. A protective covering for the entire surface of the exposed brain is further insurance against inadvertent retractor damage to brain surfaces not in the microscopic view.

The role of the nurse cannot be overemphasized.[2] For example, the points of the coagulating forceps must be cleaned after each application to the tissue to avoid sticking after coagulation. The irrigation of the suction should be regulated so that the irrigating solution does not enter the surgical field unless the surgeon removes his finger from the suction release hole. The nurse should place the patties in the surgeon's forceps without his looking away from the microscope. In order to anticipate the surgeon's needs, she must have a thorough knowledge of the various phases of the procedure. She should be encouraged to leave her post whenever practical to observe the microsurgical field, and should be briefed on the strategy for the operation.

The endurance of the surgeon is a topic seldom discussed by neurosurgeons. There is little doubt that fatigue of the surgeon increases the hazards of the operation. Microsurgery extends tissue tolerance to surgical manipulation and permits safer access to otherwise precarious areas. However, it does not reduce the duration of operation. The surgeon, therefore, must consider his own endurance and plan so that he will be at his peak during the critical phase of the procedure. This may require that certain portions of the procedure be accomplished by his associates. If these require microtechniques, his assistants must be thoroughly prepared for them.

REFERENCES

1. Kurze, T.: Microtechniques in neurological surgery. Clin. Neurosurg., *11*:128–137, 1964.
2. Rand, R. W.: Microneurosurgery. St. Louis, C. V. Mosby Co., 1969.
3. Taylor, D.: The operating-room nurse's role in microneurosurgery. J. Microsurgical Nursing, *3*:51–58, 1971.
4. Yasargil, M. G.: Microsurgery. Stuttgart, Georg Thieme Verlag, 1969.

VI

Developmental and Acquired Anomalies

23

HYDROCEPHALUS

The term hydrocephalus, although technically including an accumulation of fluid anywhere within the cranium, commonly implies only internal hydrocephalus or the progressive dilatation of the ventricular system due to an excess of cerebral spinal fluid production over its absorption.

CEREBROSPINAL FLUID CIRCULATION

Normal

Cerebrospinal fluid normally is produced at the rate of from 0.3 to 0.35 ml per minute or about 432 to 504 ml per day.[10, 36] It is probably produced principally by the choroid plexus of the ventricular system, the greatest bulk of which lies in the two lateral ventricles. There is a smaller transependymal component.[6] The fluid occupies the ventricular system, from which it circulates caudally to the outlets of the fourth ventricle, the foramina of Megendie and Luschka. Impetus for this circulation is in part derived from its ventricular site of greatest production and possibly from the pulsatile action of the choroid plexus.[8] At the fourth ventricle it passes either into the spinal subarachnoid space via the foramen of Magendie or out the two foramina of Luschka at the lateral angles of the fourth ventricle, entering the cranial subarachnoid pathways and the large basal cisterns. Prin-cipal absorption occurs at the parasagittal sites of arachnoid granulations, which are socklike structures that allow cerebrospinal fluid to pass into the venous blood within the sagittal sinus (Fig. 23–1).[63] It has been postulated that this "third circulation" of the brain begins to form in embryo with the appearance of the choroid plexus tufts.[22] The ventricular system and central canal of the spinal cord form first, enlarge, and then, by rupture of the rhombic roof over the fourth ventricle, the cerebrospinal fluid escapes from within the neural axis and spreads over the brain developing the plane that will become the subarachnoid space.

Abnormal

Hydrocephalus can develop antenatally if any part of the cerebrospinal fluid pathways fails to develop adequately. Thus, obstruction at the aqueduct due to stenosis or forking of this tiny channel will lead to gross dilatation of the lateral and third ventricles and underdevelopment of the fourth ventricle and subarachnoid pathways.[53] Failure of the rhombic roof to rupture will cause persistent hydrocephalus and hydromyelia.[22] Congenital absence of the foramina of Magendie and Luschka will cause enlargement of all the cerebral ventricles.[3] A blood clot or tumor in or adjacent to the ventricular system may obstruct the flow at any age. All such conditions are termed obstructive, or noncommunicating, hydrocephalus because the cerebrospinal fluid in the ventricular system does not com-

J. SHILLITO, JR.

R. G. OJEMANN

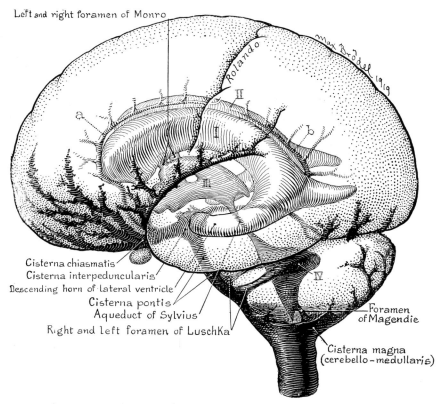

Left and right foramen of Monro

Rolando

Cisterna chiasmatis
Cisterna interpeduncularis
Descending horn of lateral ventricle
Cisterna pontis
Aqueduct of Sylvius
Right and left foramen of Luschka

Foramen of Magendie

Cisterna magna
(cerebello-medullaris)

FIGURE 23-1 The ventricular system. (From Dandy, W. E.: Surgery of the brain. *In* Lewis' Practice of Surgery. Vol. XII, Chap. 1. Hagerstown, Md., W. F. Prior Co., Inc., 1932.)

municate properly with the subarachnoid spaces.[26]

Communicating hydrocephalus will occur if the arachnoidal granulations along the sagittal sinus are insufficient or are kept from fulfilling their normal function as one-way valves.[24] Sufficient subarachnoid hemorrhage can plug the villi and produce transient or lasting hydrocephalus.[59] Thus, birth trauma with attendant intracranial bleeding can cause neonatal hydrocephalus. This type of communicating hydrocephalus can undergo spontaneous arrest just as it may in adults following trauma or rupture of an aneurysm.[18] Such a favorable resolution usually is evident within a few weeks if it is going to occur. Meningitis may so thicken the meninges that the large basal subarachnoid cisterns are occluded.[53] Tuberculous meningitis is a severe offender in this regard. Although the cerebrospinal fluid may reach the subarachnoid space of both spinal cord and brain, it cannot reach its principal absorption sites in adequate amount.

The knowledge of the site and nature of an obstruction, and of whether the obstructed fluid is present in the spinal subarachnoid space, as in communicating hydrocephalus, is necessary in order to judge whether a direct surgical attack upon the obstruction is justifiable, and, if not, into what portions of the cerebrospinal fluid pathways a tube may be placed to shunt the accumulating fluid elsewhere.

The symptoms and signs and causes of hydrocephalus vary with the age of the patient, as does the suitability of various operative techniques. For example a shunting technique that may work well either in infancy or adulthood may be rendered inadequate by growth of the young patient. For clarification of the problems peculiar to each extreme of age, the hydrocephalus of infancy and childhood, and that of adulthood, are dealt with separately.

HYDROCEPHALUS OF INFANCY AND CHILDHOOD

In dealing with active hydrocephalus, the goal of the neurosurgeon should be to establish the diagnosis as promptly as possible, using a minimum of clinical diagnostic criteria; to confirm his impression by appropriate tests; and to institute therapy specifically designed to be optimum for that patient before irreversible changes have occurred.

Diagnosis

Infantile Hydrocephalus

In advanced cases of infantile hydrocephalus, the head may be so grossly enlarged that the diagnosis is obvious (Fig. 23–2). Cephalopelvic disproportion may have led to the diagnosis even before birth. In such cases the problem is not the diagnosis but rather whether the degree of damage precludes the necessity for further diagnostic study and treatment. Differential diagnoses should include hydranencephaly, in which no cortical mantle has developed, and subdural hematomas.

In less obvious degrees of infantile hydrocephalus several signs aid in the diagnosis. (Fig. 23–3).

Head size should be established by taking the maximum obtainable circumference of the head, using a narrow steel or plastic

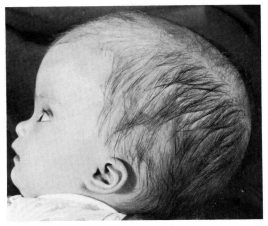

FIGURE 23–2   Marked untreated hydrocephalus in a 6-month-old child.

tape. Use of the maximal obtainable circumference, rather than specific landmarks on the skull, allows standardization of technique and facilitates meaningful comparison with one's own records, and with the records of other physicians. Finer changes can be noted between successive measurements if the metric system is utilized. The head circumference should be recorded with the patient's exact age, and plotted on an accepted growth curve chart (Fig. 23–4). The growth chart is invaluable in depicting abnormalities of rate of growth. This chart also brings inaccurate measurements to the attention of the physician since they will not fit into a proper curve of any growth rate.

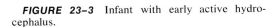

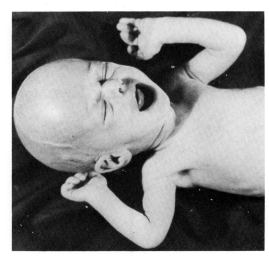

FIGURE 23–3   Infant with early active hydrocephalus.

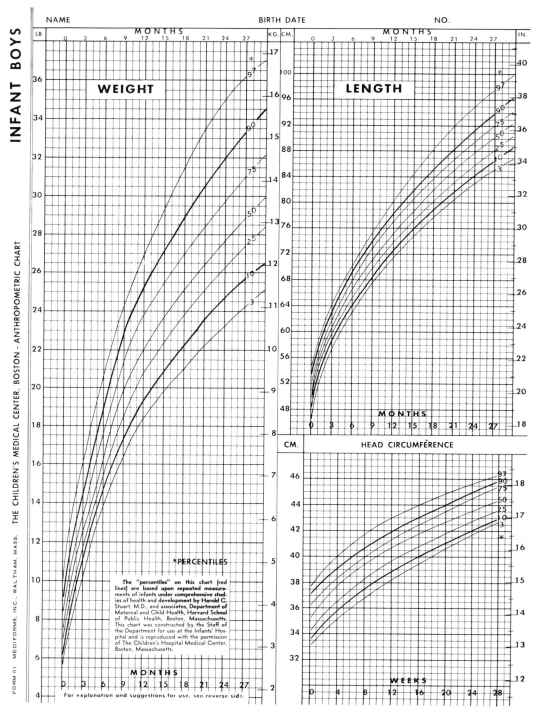

FIGURE 23–4 *A*. Normal head growth curves for a male infant. (The Children's Medical Center, Boston — Anthropometric Chart.)

Illustration continued on opposite page.

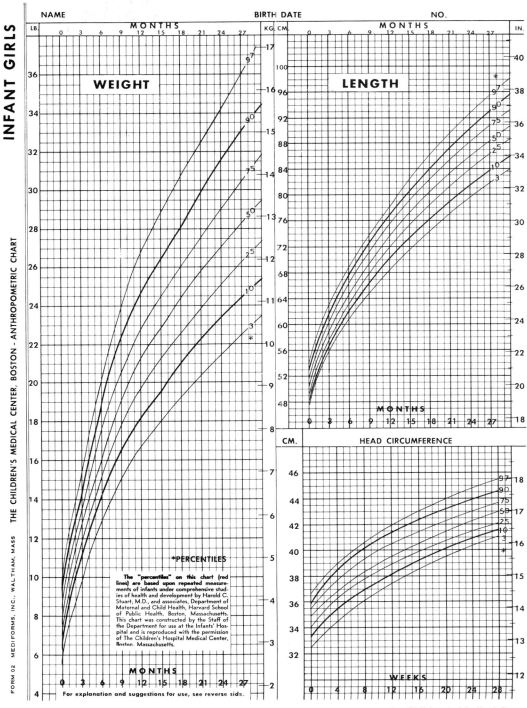

FIGURE 23–4 *Continued* *B*. Normal head growth curves for a female infant. (The Children's Medical Center, Boston—Anthropometric Chart.)

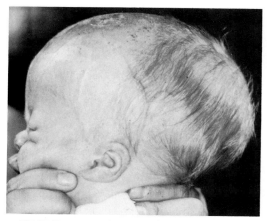

FIGURE 23-5 Infant with aqueduct stenosis. The supratentorial portion of the skull has enlarged while the posterior fossa remains small.

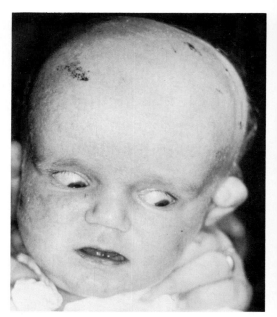

FIGURE 23-7 Infant with chronic bilateral subdural hematomas. The head is more globular than in cases of internal hydrocephalus, and does not show the prominence of the frontal areas seen in marked internal hydrocephalus.

Having recorded the initial circumference, the physician should assess the configuration of the head. Aqueduct stenosis, for example, causes enlargement of the supratentorial portion of the cranium at the expense of the posterior fossa (Fig. 23–5). Congenital atresia of the foramina of Magendie and Luschka, the Dandy-Walker syndrome, leads to prominence of the posterior fossa (Fig. 23–6).[3] Elevation of the tentorium may be demonstrated by transillumination (cf. Fig. 23–10). Asymmetery of the skull may be indicative of underlying porencephaly with enlargement of one hemicranium. Bilateral subdural hematomas cause globular enlargement of the skull with prominent parietal areas (Fig. 23–7).

The anterior fontanelle will be larger than usual and its turgor can reflect intracranial pressure. It should be evaluated when the child is held upright and is relaxed. If horizontal or if straining, even the normal child will have a bulging fontanelle. In infancy the cranial sutures are quite pliable. As a result, the intracranial pressure can be normal in mild cases of hydrocephalus. In these, the tenseness of the fontanelle will not be as helpful in diagnosis as the width of the cranial sutures, which may be as wide as a fingertip. Papilledema is uncommon in infancy. The percussion note of an infant skull, normally that of a "cracked pot," comes to resemble that of a filled hotwater bottle when hydrocephalus is present.

If intracranial pressure is high the scalp veins become prominent. The intracranial venous channels are compressed by increasing intracranial pressure and shunt their contents through valveless collateral systems into easily distended scalp veins. These will be particularly obvious when the infant cries or strains. As the head enlarges further the scalp begins to appear stretched

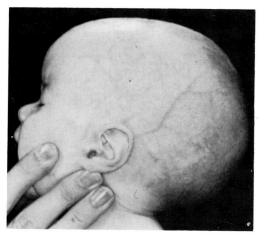

FIGURE 23-6 Infant with the Dandy-Walker syndrome. The posterior fossa is prominent and extends higher than in the normal cranium.

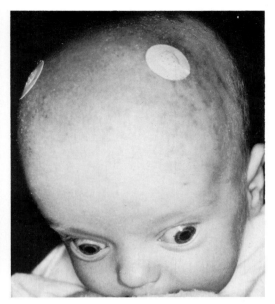

FIGURE 23-8 "Setting sun" eyes; apparent downward displacement of the eyes seen in a child with hydrocephalus. This can also be seen in infants with chronic increased intracranial pressure from other causes (see Fig. 23-7).

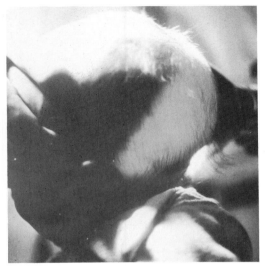

FIGURE 23-10 Infant with Dandy-Walker syndrome. Transillumination of the posterior fossa demonstrates the elevated position of the tentorium and the extent of the cyst. Degree of supratentorial hydrocephalus did not permit transillumination.

and shiny. Quite probably because of continued intracranial pressure upon the soft orbital roofs, the hydrocephalic infant's eyes are pushed downward until one sees only the upper part of the pupils, and can see sclera above the pupils (Fig. 23-8). This "setting sun appearance" is characteristic of moderate or advanced hydrocephalus.

If a significant collection of fluid displaces or replaces the brain and lies within a few millimeters of the skull, it may be possible to transilluminate the skull. Testing for

transillumination of the skull should be made in total darkness. A strong flashlight that has been fitted with an opaque rubber cuff to prevent leaks of light should be used. A cap from a fluid dispensing bottle may be used as the rubber cuff for the flashlight (Fig. 23-9).

All parts of the skull including the posterior fossa should be tested by transillumination (Fig. 23-10). Subdural hematomas in the frontal area may be transilluminated; this should not be misconstrued as hydro-

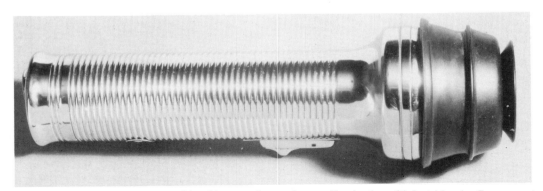

FIGURE 23-9 Flashlight fitted with rubber cap for use in transillumination of infants' heads. Cap prevents light leaks at scalp.

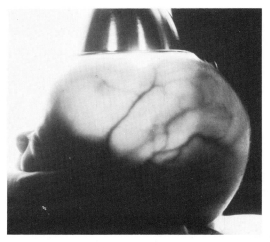

FIGURE 23-11 Transillumination of the left hemicranium in an infant with subdural hematoma. Effect is more pronounced anteriorly, where fluid usually tends to accumulate in greater quantity.

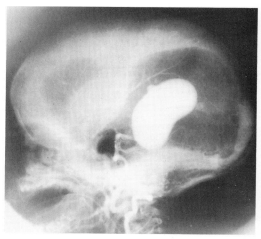

FIGURE 23-13 Angiographic demonstration of an arteriovenous malformation involving the vein of Galen, enlargement of which causes occlusion of the aqueduct of Sylvius and hydrocephalus.

cephalus (Fig. 23–11). Hydrocephalus usually thins the occipital more than the frontal mantle. Hence with marked hydrocephalus, transillumination should be greater in the occipital area (Fig. 23–12). Scalp edema, subgaleal fluid, and even normal subarachnoid pathways, may give false positive results. If so, other studies will be necessary for clarification.

Hydrocephalus may be secondary to vascular abnormalities, such as those of the vein of Galen (Fig. 23–13). Auscultation of

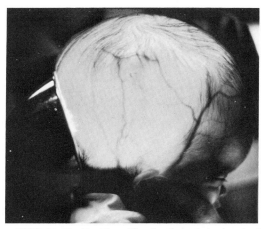

FIGURE 23-12 Transillumination of the head of an infant with marked hydrocephalus secondary to aqueduct stenosis. The occipital horns dilate more readily than the frontal horns; transillumination is more pronounced posteriorly.

the head for bruits should be performed in all patients. The presence of a bruit should lead directly to arteriography.

In mild but active hydrocephalus, only the head circumference may be abnormal. Even a head that measures larger than the ninety-seventh percentile may be normal since, by definition of such growth curves, 3 per cent of normal patients may have measurements that lie above this percentile. Some indication of the significance of the large head can be gained by also plotting the infant's weight and length. Consistency between these criteria may be reassuring (Fig. 23–14).

Only the rate of growth of the head can establish the activity of mild hydrocephalus. Thus serial head circumference determinations can demonstrate that active hydrocephalus exists even in a child born with a normal head size (Fig. 23–15). Before any but the slightest clinical features are evident, and well before any neurological abnormalities develop, appropriate contrast studies can demonstrate enlarged ventricles. If treatment is instituted promptly, the outcome should be excellent.

If hydrocephalus is advanced at birth, or has been allowed to progress too long before the diagnosis is made, neurological changes may be evident. Increased intracranial pressure may cause the infant to exhibit irritability. Later somnolence will

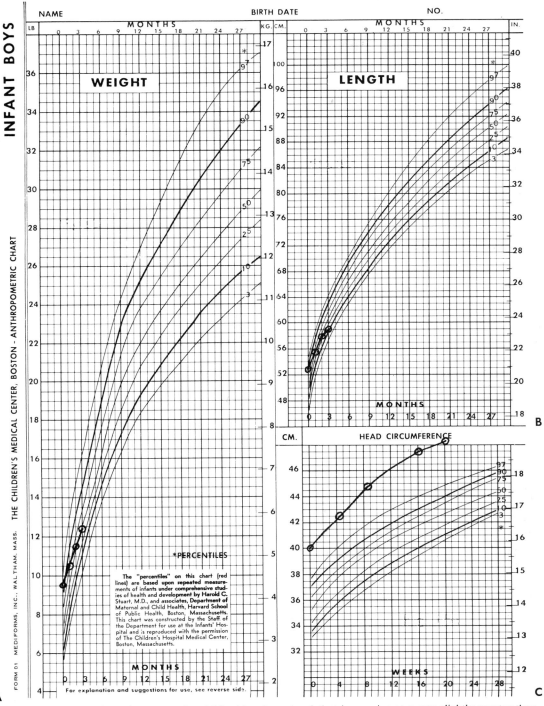

FIGURE 23–14 Growth curves of a child with a large head that is growing at a rate slightly greater than normal. Comparison with child's normal parameters of weight and length emphasizes the abnormality of the head. *A.* Weight curve of the child. Values are in normal range. *B.* Length curve of same child. Values are in normal range. *C.* Child's head growth curve.

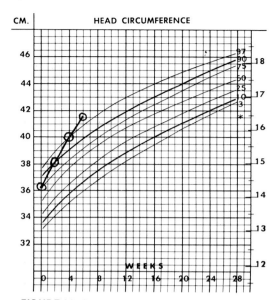

FIGURE 23–15 Head growth curve of a child with active hydrocephalus.

supervene. Deep tendon reflexes in the legs become hyperactive before any changes in the upper extremities appear. Presumably the reflex changes are due to the greater stretching of leg fibers as they course around the dilated lateral ventricles. The child may suck poorly. Its reaction to its environment may be dulled. Vision can be reduced or absent either because of damage to the occipital cortex by grossly enlarged occipital horns or because of the pulsatile pressure of the enlarged third ventricle on the underlying optic chiasm. If the third ventricle is pressing on the optic chiasm, pupillary reaction as well as apparent light perception will be reduced or abolished. Regurgitation of food and fluids will become frequent as the intracranial pressure increases. As the terminal stage approaches, the respirations become shallow and irregular and finally cease.

Hydrocephalus in Older Children

In older children, in whom hydrocephalus has either been active but very mild since birth or in whom acquired hydrocephalus appears, as in postinfectious aqueduct stenosis, a different constellation of symptoms and signs appears.

The milder cases may be diagnosed only because of the deviation from normal of the growth rate of the head. Alert pediatricians who keep graphic records of the head growth curve are apt to detect the abnormality early. The neurosurgeon can follow the child's growth curve with the pediatrician, and observe for other signs that aid in the diagnosis. Close observation of the growth curve should be continued until it becomes clearly normal or abnormal (Fig. 23–14 *A*). Again weight and length curves, by their variance from the head growth curve, may be of value (Fig. 23–14 *B* and *C*).

After the fontanelle and sutures have closed, the appearance of the eyegrounds can be helpful. The physiological cupping of the optic discs may be absent and the discs flat. Venous pulsations at the nerve head, so common in childhood, will not be present with mild elevation of intracranial pressure. The veins may appear tortuous. Ultimately, papilledema will appear. The percussion note of the skull may be cracked, which suggests early splitting of the cranial sutures. Splitting of the sutures can be assessed further by radiological examination of the skull.

Extraocular palsies, if new, may be significant. In slowly progressive hydrocephalus, weakness of abduction first of one and later possibly of both eyes indicates stretching of one or both sixth cranial nerves owing to downward displacement of the brain stem and traction upon these nerves as they traverse the dura. Asymmetrical involvement is not of lateralizing significance.

Hyperactivity of knee and ankle jerks may become evident as the hydrocephalus progresses. As it does, a child may show regression in motor ability. Newly-acquired skills such as walking may be abandoned. A general reduction of physical activity may indicate awkwardness or simply not feeling well. Mental retardation is a late sign, and in mild cases, it may not be apparent until the child is in high school.

Irritability may herald an intracranial pressure level that is incompatible with normal activity. If a partial obstruction is the cause of the hydrocephalus, headache is often present after prolonged rest in the recumbent position. Morning headache, relieved by activity, is a common feature in the history of children with hydrocephalus due to incomplete obstruction of the ventricular system. Presumably, the frequent transient increases of intracranial pressure caused by diurnal exertions help squeeze cerebrospinal fluid past the obstruction. During sleep no such variations occur and ventricular fluid accumulates. Such a story is most common in children with cerebellar or fourth ventricular tumors; it can, however, occur in benign conditions as well. When a child has a history of this type of headache, a tumor must be considered in the list of differential diagnostic conditions.

Vomiting, when it occurs, usually follows a morning headache. It is usually more frequent before or just after arising from bed. Initially, at least, it relieves the headache.

When ventricular enlargement becomes marked, signs of cerebellar dysfunction and brain stem involvement may appear. The truncal ataxia and broad-based stance and gait suggest a midline cerebellar tumor. Loss of upward gaze mimics the Parinaud's syndrome that is associated with tumors of the pineal region. Long-tract signs can progress to spastic paraparesis. The clinical appearance thus begins to resemble that of adult hydrocephalus.

Diagnostic Studies

Indications

If the growth curve of the patient's head, alone or with the support of other clinical clues, indicates the possibility of hydrocephalus, confirmatory tests are indicated. How long an excessive growth curve should be watched depends upon its rate and other findings. For example, a rapid enlargement of the head and a skull configuration that suggests aqueduct stenosis demands prompt investigation, even though the head may still be within the normal range (Fig. 23–16). Mild asymptomatic cases warrant follow-up long enough to establish, by repeated personal measurements, an accurate growth curve. If this demonstrates continued deviation away from the normal, that is, a large head that is growing too fast, further tests are indicated. Except in flagrantly abnormal cases, the importance of establishing the growth curve before contrast studies are done cannot be

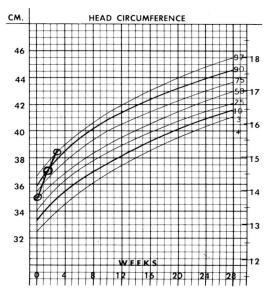

FIGURE 23–16 Head growth curve of a child with clinical hydrocephalus and prominence of the supratentorial portions of the skull suggesting aqueduct stenosis.

overemphasized. A child with slightly or moderately enlarged ventricles does not necessarily require a shunting procedure; it is, however, necessary to establish that the hydrocephalus is active and has not been spontaneously arrested before proceeding to operative treatment.

Selection of Studies

Skull Films

Skull films define the cranial landmarks and may give a more accurate indication of the location of an obstruction than the clinical examination. For example, in aqueduct stenosis, a tiny posterior fossa will be apparent from the low position of the lamboid sutures on the roentgenograms (Fig. 23–17).

The width of all the sutures may suggest increased intracranial pressure, and their pattern may, in older children, be a clue to the rapidity of the process. Elongated interdigitations imply chronicity. Figure 23–18 shows a 2¼-year-old child who had a history of many months of symptoms related to obstructive hydrocephalus secondary to a posterior fossa tumor. The classic changes of the sella turcica are not apparent in infancy when splitting of the sutures will allow reduction of the intracranial pressure.

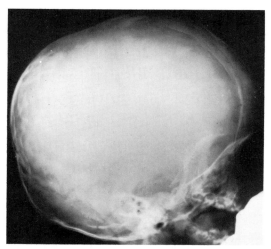

FIGURE 23–17 Skull film of a child with aqueduct stenosis. Note small posterior fossa.

Certain surprises may alter the diagnosis; an unsuspected fracture makes the possibility of subdural hematomas more likely; calcification may be apparent in tumors such as craniopharyngiomas, gliomas, or teratomas. Later in childhood a circular ring of calcium can be seen in the wall of vein of Galen aneurysms.

Scanning Techniques

Unless the presence of a tumor is suspected, electroencephalography and isotope scanning usually are not helpful. Sonar scanning, particularly a good "B-scan," may give a fairly accurate estimate of ven-

tricular size, but should be used in close conjunction with, rather than to the exclusion of, more definitive tests.[21]

Radioiodinated serum albumin (RISA) cisternography, which is very helpful in adult hydrocephalus, has not been widely used in pediatrics. Undoubtedly this is, in part, because during the first two years of life, the appearance of the head growth curve provides more quantitative information than the RISA scan. The scan is, however, helpful in evaluating borderline cases of communicating hydrocephalus in older children.

Ventriculography

Unless tumor is suspected, ventriculography ordinarily follows assessment of the plain skull films. In infancy, a "bubble study" is performed through a thoroughly prepared scalp (Fig. 23–19). The ventricular needle is placed in the coronal suture well away from the midline. Usually a No. 18 styletted needle is used. If significant subdural fluid is present, it can be detected by pausing with the tip of the needle in the subdural space and momentarily removing the stylet. Estimation of ventricular size can be made by removing the stylet after each 1-cm. advance of the needle. After encountering the ventricle, 5 to 40 cc

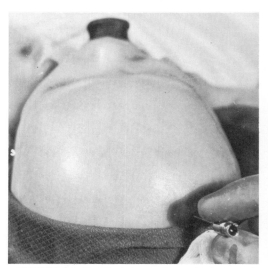

FIGURE 23–19 Technique of ventricular or subdural tap. Entire frontal scalp has been shaved to well behind coronal suture. Styletted needle is inserted through coronal suture as far from the midline as the pupil to avoid bridging cortical veins.

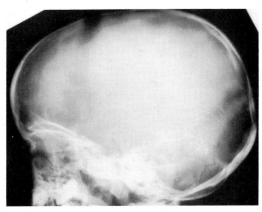

FIGURE 23–18 Skull film of a child with obstructive hydrocephalus. Cranial sutures are widely separated.

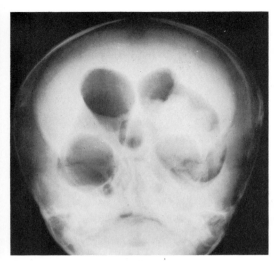

FIGURE 23–20 Ventriculogram demonstrating asymmetrical communicating hydrocephalus caused by a choroid plexus papilloma of the left lateral ventricle.

of air should be introduced slowly in increments of 5 cc with alternate withdrawal of 5 cc of cerebrospinal fluid. This amount of air should provide sufficient volume to outline the entire ventricular system of most hydrocephalic infants provided there is proper positioning and manipulation of the bubble. Views of the skull should include anteroposterior and lateral films with the brow up, the posteroanterior and lateral films with the brow down, and a lateral film with the child prone and his head hanging over the table edge at an angle of about 60 degrees from the horizontal. The latter position will demonstrate the posterior fossa and cervical spinal canal. In communicating hydrocephalus, a lateral view of the caudal sac that is taken with the buttocks up and the head down will confirm the presence of air in the lumbosacral spinal subarachnoid space.

If more air is required because of the large ventricles, it can be added cautiously. If asymmetrical communicating hydrocephalus is found, the larger lateral ventricle should be assessed thoroughly by lateral views utilizing sufficient air to rule out a choroid plexus papilloma at the glomus (Fig. 23–20).

Air ventriculography can outline the entire ventricular system and indicate not only its size, contents, and continuity, but also its position. As a result it has been and probably will remain the most valuable contrast study for the neurosurgeon who must deal with hydrocephalus. If desired, a simultaneous combined tap of the ventricular system and the lumbar subarachnoid space can be made to assess the communication between the two areas.[7] Instilling 1 ml of indigo carmine into one ventricle and noting the interval until its first appearance in the lumbar spinal fluid is valuable if the air study has been equivocal. If free communication between the ventricular and lumbar subarachnoid spaces exists, the dye will be visible in four or five minutes. Intervals over 10 to 15 minutes indicate poor flow or great dilution in grossly enlarged ventricles.

Iophendylate (Pantopaque) ventriculography is rarely necessary. It is most valuable in defining details around the aqueduct of Sylvius when attempting to differentiate between aqueductal stenosis and tumor. The risks involved with the use of other positive contrast materials are not justified by any advantage over a thorough and safe air study.

Angiography

Although thorough arteriography of both supratentorial and infratentorial areas can give valuable clues to the cause of hydrocephalus, it is felt that direct study of the ventricular system is much more satisfactory than opacification of the vessels that it displaces. Angiography does offer the advantage of leaving the ventricular system unmolested. In older children this is a very important consideration. Even small bubble studies may upset the delicate balance between production and absorption in a patient with mild active chronic hydrocephalus. Such studies have led to severe decompensation and even death.

If the patient is suspected of having a tumor, angiography may be diagnostic and will permit more leisurely plans for operative therapy. The operation, either to excise the tumor or to provide ventricular decompression by shunt or external drainage, should immediately follow ventriculography if the obstructive hydrocephalus is due to a tumor. In markedly hydrocephalic children of any age, angiography may be safer, since ventriculography, by its substitution of compressible air for incompressible fluid, may permit a thinned cortical mantle to collapse away from the dura, rupturing bridging veins and causing subdural hemorrhage.

Pneumoencephalography

Pneumoencephalography is not recommended in infantile hydrocephalus. Ventriculography is easier to perform, is more likely to succeed, and entails less risk. Subarachnoid air is more painful, and an infant in the upright position is more difficult to immobilize than one who is supine. Subdural hemorrhage caused by lumbar pneumography in a hydrocephalic child has occurred. In obstructive hydrocephalus the study cannot be definitive. It has been useful in delineation of the fourth ventricle after ventriculography has suggested aqueduct stenosis, and in the confirmation of the diagnosis of pseudotumor cerebri. Pneumography should not be used if an obstructing tumor of the posterior fossa is considered to be the cause of the hydrocephalus.

Indications for Treatment

When the growth rate of a child's head has been established as excessive and an enlarged ventricular system has been shown to be the cause of the excessive growth rate, a diagnosis of active hydrocephalus can be made and treatment recommended.

In mild cases, two questions plague the neurosurgeon who must make the decision to intervene. First, will arrest of the hydrocephalus occur spontaneously and soon? Second, is the condition severe enough to warrant shunting?

The hydrocephalic process does undergo spontaneous arrest on occasions; this may be seen at a few weeks of age in a child whose traumatic birth produced an intracranial hemorrhage. Excessive head growth may follow, change first to a normal rate, then to a less than normal rate, until the head ultimately falls again within the normal range and grows at a normal rate (Fig. 23–21). Spontaneous arrest may also

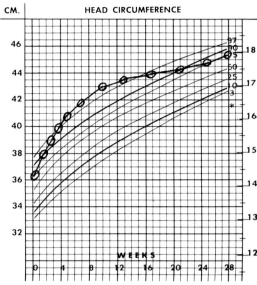

FIGURE 23–21 Head growth curve illustrating spontaneous arrest of hydrocephalus. Infant was delivered with considerable difficulty and had grossly bloody spinal fluid.

occur after acquired hydrocephalus following head injury or spontaneous subarachnoid hemorrhage.[18, 27, 59] All these conditions are instances of acquired communicating hydrocephalus. Arrest of congenital obstructive hydrocephalus is rare. One way in which it may occur is when a dilated third ventricle ruptures into the subarachnoid space in a patient who has aqueductal stenosis.

Hydrocephalus can be accepted as spontaneously arrested only when a child's head that is too large because of enlargement of the ventricular system assumes a rate of growth that is less than normal. The process is optimally arrested only if the reduced growth rate is achieved early enough in life to permit the child's head to come eventually within the normal range.

Courage to act promptly in cases of mild hydrocephalus can be gained by projecting the head growth curve forward a few years to appreciate what a child's head will be like without intervention, and from experience gained by following of patients with unshunted hydrocephalus. Asymptomatic but still active, hydrocephalus may exist well into the teens and beyond. Accurate head measurements will show that the head does not cease enlarging. Notorious for this

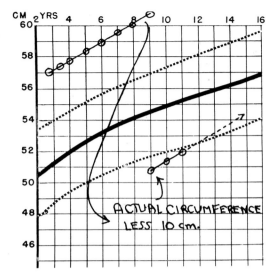

FIGURE 23-22 Head growth curve of a myelodysplastic child with a large head. Growth rate is close to normal, but slightly excessive. Hydrocephalus is *not* arrested. If it were, growth rate would be less than normal, or there would be no growth at all. (Graph from Pediatric Neurology Service Research and Educational Hospitals, Chicago, Ill.)

mild, active condition are children who are born with a myelomeningocele and the Arnold-Chiari malformation. If the patient is first seen at several years of age and is asymptomatic except for mental retardation and an obviously large head, it may take many months to establish that the head is still growing. This difficulty is due to the fact that the normal rate of growth at this age is very slight (Fig. 23-22). Nevertheless, a head that is too large because of hydrocephalus, and that is still growing, is not compatible with a diagnosis of arrested hydrocephalus; the child is simply living with mild progressive hydrocephalus. Were it truly arrested, the head should not be growing and the ventricles should be returning to normal size.[56]

If the head size of such a child is followed accurately from birth, activity of the hydrocephalus can usually be detected more easily and appropriate action taken during the period of rapid normal brain growth. Intervention at several years of age, when the head may be 10 cm larger than the normal circumference and the cortical mantle quite thin, may entail greater risk of complications such as subdural hemorrhage. The decision to shunt is then much more difficult to make and must be guided by all other factors pertinent to that child's future, including his mental and motor ability, other physical abnormalities, and the likelihood that shunting can still favorably alter his life.

Megalencephaly due to other conditions must be ruled out before shunting.[64] Inborn errors of metabolism may cause a mild excess in the growth rate of the head owing to brain enlargement. Seizures may occur, and mental retardation will be out of proportion to ventricular enlargement, if any exists at all. The condition may mimic mild, active communicating hydrocephalus. Treatment is unrewarding.

Familial large heads occasionally confuse the issue. Since no growth curve of either parent's head will be available, comparison of the head growth curve with the weight and length curves (see Fig. 23-14 *B* and *C*), examination of siblings, and ultimately even serial ventriculography, may be necessary. An elongating head, such as in untreated sagittal synostosis, will have a greater circumference than a spherical head of the same volume, and a growth rate greater than normal.[58]

Surgical Treatment

Operative treatment remains the only successful one for hydrocephalus. If the condition can be relieved by a single operative procedure, that procedure should be used. Preferably, the procedure will be one that does not make the child forever dependent on the continued patency and proper position of a tube or the functioning of a mechanical device. If a shunt is necessary, the simplest device that is least likely to be outgrown or suffer mechanical failure should be selected.

Direct Approach

Choroid Plexectomy

This procedure was used before adequate shunts were available.[11, 12] It can reduce the amount of cerebrospinal fluid that is produced. However, since only that choroid plexus in the lateral ventricles is easily accessible, the resultant lessening of production of fluid usually is inadequate to effect a balance between its formation and absorption. The operation is difficult unless ventricular enlargement is marked, as is seen with aqueduct stenosis. Therefore, it usually is not available to the patient with mild hydrocephalus and minimal ventricular enlargement that might well be controlled by a relatively minor change in rate of production. Shunting is easier to perform and supplanted choroid plexectomy long ago. As neurosurgeons become disenchanted with the long-term maintenance of shunts, however, this technique may regain some appeal.[54, 55]

Excision of Papillomas of the Choroid Plexus

The only circumstance known in which overproduction of cerebrospinal fluid is the sole cause of hydrocephalus is the presence of a papilloma of the choroid plexus. In childhood, most papillomas occur in a lateral ventricle and can be excised through a parietal transcortical approach to the atrium of the ventricle where the tumor lies. Excision cures the hydrocephalus.[9, 40]

Removal of Obstruction

Thorough ventriculography may indicate not only the site of obstruction, but by its appearance suggest veils or cysts that warrant exploration.[37, 53] Preoperatively some posterior fossa arachnoid cysts may be in-

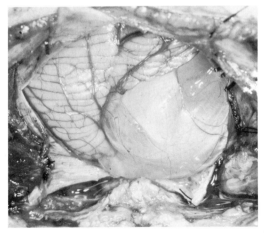

FIGURE 23–23 Arachnoid cyst of the posterior fossa. Presenting symptoms and signs were consistent with hydrocephalus and a right cerebellar tumor.

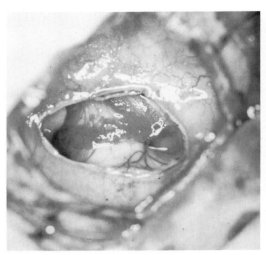

FIGURE 23–24 Porencephalic cyst of left posterior parietal area. Cyst presented at surface of brain, was entered, and its inner wall was then fenestrated into lateral ventricle. Glomus of choroid plexus lies at depth of exposure.

distinguishable from tumors (Fig. 23–23). Others, such as Blake's pouch cysts, communicate with the fourth ventricle, but partially obstruct it, thus producing hydrocephalus.[25] Direct operative treatment alone has succeeded in relieving hydrocephalus in 5 of 21 cases of Dandy-Walker syndrome.[42]

Noncommunicating porencephalic cysts may cause obstruction by extrinsic pressure on part of the ventricular system, which often can be corrected by fenestration of the cyst into the ventricular system (Fig. 23–24).

Occasionally children with the Arnold-Chiari malformation may be relieved of mild hydrocephalus by a posterior fossa decompression, which allows more room for circulation of fluid into the subarachnoid space. This procedure should be considered only after ventriculography has ruled out aqueduct stenosis and has indicated that the only obstruction lies in this area.

Brain tumors in infancy and childhood so often either occur in the posterior fossa or involve the ventricular system in the midline in some way that symptoms of acute hydrocephalus may be the presenting complaint.[42] Some surgeons believe that in certain cases the child should have a shunt prior to operation for definitive tumor excision, so that he can recover from the effects of the hydrocephalus. Other surgeons utilize drainage for a few days preoperatively.[5] In cases of deep-seated, poorly accessible malignant tumors, shunting and radiation therapy offer the most palliation and the least discomfort to the patient.

Third ventriculostomy, the operative fenestration of the dilated third ventricle into the basal cisterns, has recently received renewed attention.[54] One factor in determining its success is the ability of the subarachnoid space to handle the unaccustomed load of cerebrospinal fluid. Radioiodinated serum albumin studies suggest that the subarachnoid space not only is patent, but may increase its capacity when obstruction of the ventricular system is relieved and compression of the subarachnoid space is lessened.[44]

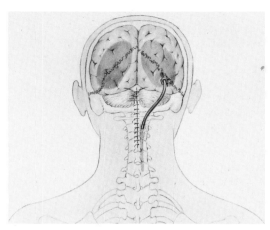

FIGURE 23–26 A ventriculocervical shunt. This variation of the Torkildsen procedure makes posterior fossa craniectomy unnecessary, and is useful when the cisterna magna is obliterated or inadequate.

Indirect Approach — Shunting Procedures

The shunt that best fits a patient's problem may be selected from an armamentarium of about eight commonly-used types. A catheter in the cerebrospinal fluid above the obstruction delivers accumulating fluid either (1) directly to the cerebrospinal fluid pathways below the obstruction, as in the Torkildsen procedure (Fig. 23–25) or the ventriculocervical shunt (Fig. 23–26);[42] (2) to a body cavity from which fluid is readily absorbed, as in pleural and

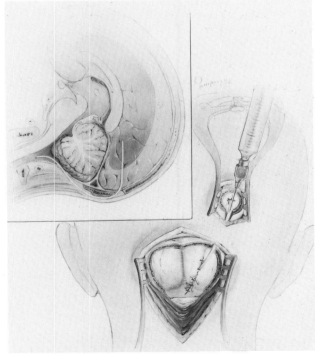

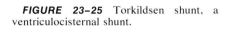

FIGURE 23–25 Torkildsen shunt, a ventriculocisternal shunt.

peritoneal shunts;[14,50,52,57] (3) to the blood-stream itself, with an appropriate intervening valve system, as in atrial shunts;[45,46,49,62] or (4) to the urinary bladder, for elimination from the body completely.[38,39,41]

Each method has some advantages over the others and its own particular disadvantages. Appreciation of these problems helps one to select the shunt best suited for each patient, and to inform the parents honestly at the outset what the future may hold in store.

Failings and advantages depend upon problems at the inflow end, problems at the outflow end, and the length and nature of the tubing and the anatomical area that lies between.

Ventricular Shunt

Any ventricular shunt must be positioned properly to avoid the ventricular wall and the choroid plexus, and to remain in adequate position as the shunted ventricle assumes a more normal size. Placement of such a catheter is relatively simple and its use is applicable to all hydrocephalics. The frontal horn, which is free of choroid plexus, is used by most surgeons, either via the posterior parietal or frontal approach. Lateral approaches to the ventricle may fail with time, as the change in ventricular size effectively shortens the catheter.

Lumbar Shunt

Lumbar shunts are available only to patients with communicating hydrocephalus. In some patients, obstructed hydrocephalus has first been converted into the communicating type by ventriculocervical shunts in order to avoid growth problems and utilize the lumbar shunt. Although the necessary hemilaminectomy is a little more work than a burr hole, and correct positioning in the subarachnoid space may be tricky, the use of this shunt has two major advantages: (1) growth is not a problem since the shunt runs at right angles to the direction of the body's greatest growth, and (2) the problem of small ventricles in later life is avoided. Such shunts cannot easily be tested, unless positioned subcutaneously somewhere along their course. Late scoliosis and kyphosis have been reported, but

should be avoidable with small, soft, correctly positioned tubes.[14,33]

Cisternal or Cervical Subarachnoid Shunt

Cisternal or cervical subarachnoid shunts are applicable only to patients with acquired obstructive hydrocephalus. The adequacy of the subarachnoid space in handling the load of fluid delivered to it appears to be dependent upon the duration and completeness of the obstruction. In late aqueduct stenosis or in tumor obstruction this method will work very well. It may take several weeks for spinal fluid pressure to come to normal after shunting; this can be followed by periodic lumbar punctures. Positioning of the tube is critical. In the cervical shunt, it should be placed well down the spinal canal anterior to the dentate ligament to avoid irritation of cervical sensory roots. Growth of the patient presents no problem, and no intervening absorptive surface is involved.

Pleural Shunt

Pleural shunts are simple to place and their positioning is not critical. The growth problem is reduced by putting extra tubing in the pleural space. The ability of the pleural space to absorb fluid may be inadequate, however, and in severe degrees of obstructive hydrocephalus, particularly in small infants, hydrothorax is excessive and defeats this method of treatment.

Peritoneal Shunt

Peritoneal shunts are simple to establish, their positioning is not critical, and using greater lengths of tubing can defer revision that is made necessary by growth of the patient. Absorptive capacity of the peritoneum is usually more than adequate, except possibly in some tiny infants with aqueduct stenosis. The reaction of mesentery or viscera to abrasion has occluded such tubes, but with tubes of silicone rubber this complication is less frequent. Suprahepatic location avoids the mesentery, but by simply introducing several inches of tubing into the general abdominal cavity, patency is apparently assured by the motion of the intestines, which sweeps the tubing from place to place, avoiding obstruction or loculation of fluid.[51]

Previous abdominal surgery may reduce the effectiveness of peritoneal shunts, but does not contraindicate them by any means.[17] For instance, myelodysplastic children with ileal loop bladders can enjoy good peritoneal shunt function. Occasionally congenital inguinal hernias or hydroceles will become apparent after shunting. Several appendectomies have permitted inspection of the lower end of such shunts and have not disturbed their function.

Atrial Shunt

Atrial shunts came into being after trials in the jugular vein failed because of venous thrombosis. The churning action of the heart must prevent thrombus formation from occluding the catheter, and the scar tissue sheath that surrounds the tubing elsewhere cannot seal its tip while it is in the right atrium. Significant pulmonary emboli are infrequent.[15, 16, 19] Proper positioning of the shunt is important. There is some evidence that if the shunt tip is low, it will be more apt to facilitate recalcitrant sep-

ticemia.[45] Shorter catheters will come out of position sooner as the patient grows.

Septicemia occurs in 20 to 30 per cent of such patients, with the initial insertion or after one of the several revisions made necessary by growth. The source of infection is not usually clear, but the time relation between onset of symptoms and the operation usually suggests that it is due to intraoperative contamination. Symptoms and signs of the infection may be insidious. Chronic problems can arise if it is not corrected, and ultimate removal or renewal of the shunt apparatus is usually necessary.[60]

The prevention of reflux of blood requires a one-way valve, and this introduction of moving parts and small orifices adds another possible point of failure to the system. The various types of apparatus are palpable beneath the skin. They can be tested and even cleared by pumping. They may be tapped percutaneously, for both diagnostic and therapeutic purposes.

Adequate care is more assured if the atrial shunts are revised prophylactically when chest x-rays indicate that the tip of the catheter has reached the superior vena cava. The tragic and unnecessary loss of children whose shunts become obstructed suddenly attests to the continued function

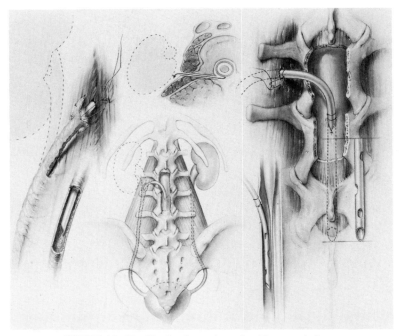

FIGURE 23–27 The lumbar subarachnoid-ureteral shunt.

and need of such shunts long after observers have wrongly assumed that they are occluded and the hydrocephalus arrested. Even with all their idiosyncracies, ventriculoatrial shunts are the most popular now in use, because if properly inserted and maintained they work well.

Ureteral Shunt

The late Dr. Donald Matson popularized the ureteral shunt. The proximal end of this shunt may be in either of the lateral ventricles or the lumbar subarachnoid space. After a nephrectomy, the distal end is inserted into the ureter.[38,39] Care should be taken to leave several centimeters of ureter that, with a competent ureterovesicle junction, can act as a valve, both to prevent reflux of urine and to maintain some pressure in the cerebrospinal fluid (Fig. 23–27). Unlike other shunts, the ureteral shunt discharges cerebrospinal fluid from the body. In infancy, temporary dehydration from other causes can be disastrous if not corrected immediately by intravenous saline.

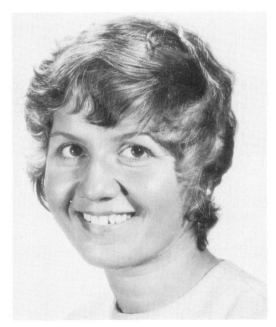

FIGURE 23–28 This 23-year-old girl has had her lumbar-ureteral shunt since 4 months of age, at which time she had about 2 cm of frontal cortical mantle. The shunt has never been revised. Its continued patency is demonstrable by significant amounts of cerebrospinal fluid protein in the urine.

Extra salt must be given daily to compensate for the salt lost in the cerebrospinal fluid that is excreted with the urine. As the child grows larger, the danger of dehydration decreases. If severe dehydration or meningitis, either sterile or septic, occurs more than twice, it may be necessary to remove the ureteral shunt. If the cerebrospinal fluid is chronically infected or contains tumor cells, the ureteral shunt has the advantage of excreting and not recirculating the fluid.

The lumbar-ureteral shunt has the most remarkable record for longevity of any type of shunt. Some of the first children who were treated by this method are now in their twenties and are perfectly normal in all ways, except for one missing kidney. Furthermore, they still show evidence of shunt patency by excreting measurable albumin from cerebrospinal fluid in their urine. One patient plans marriage within the year (Fig. 23–28). One of the reasons for the remarkable longevity of this shunt is that its position and direction effectively avoid the problem of growth.

Fewer lumbar-ureteral shunts are being done in recent years. Great efforts are being made to perfect the lumbar peritoneal shunt in the hope of avoiding nephrectomy and the problems of fluid loss.[14]

Continued Care

It should be assumed that a child with bona fide active hydrocephalus, who has been treated by an effective shunting procedure, will be thereafter shunt dependent. Exceptions are few. An obstructing tumor may shrink after irradiation and the cerebrospinal fluid circulation be re-established. Severe episodes of ventriculitis may so damage the choroid plexus that mild active hydrocephalus is arrested.

If it has been well documented prior to shunting that a child has active hydrocephalus that shows no tendency toward spontaneous arrest, the likelihood is not great of such arrest occurring after a functioning shunt has lowered the cerebrospinal fluid pressure. Careful investigations of children whose shunts have been removed may indicate either that the indications for shunting were questionable in the first place, that the shunt never altered the course of the hydrocephalus and could not have been functioning properly, or that the hydrocephalus became active again after shunt removal—without symptoms.

The neurosurgeon who deals with pediatric hydrocephalus would do well to adopt the philosophy "once a shunt, always a shunt." He will then make every effort to relieve hydrocephalus by a direct approach whenever possible. He will keep his patients' shunts in good repair at all times, anticipating troubles and avoiding them. He will follow closely the child's head circumference curve, state of the cranial sutures, eyegrounds, and neurological status. Thus, perhaps, he will avoid the sudden, unexpected tragedy many years later when a shunt malfunctions in a then otherwise normal youngster.

NORMAL-PRESSURE HYDROCEPHALUS

Neurological symptoms in adults can be due to enlarged ventricles compressing cerebral tissue but associated with normal cerebrospinal fluid pressure. The syndrome is called normal-pressure hydrocephalus, but has also been termed occult hydrocephalus, low-pressure hydrocephalus, normotensive hydrocephalus, and hydrocephalic dementia.[1,28,47]

Etiology and Pathology

Mechanisms for development of this syndrome are not fully known, but a number of theories have been proposed.[23,29,47] The underlying pathological process appears to be obliteration of the subarachnoid pathways in the region of the tentorium and base of the brain.[47]

This pathological change may be due to subarachnoid hemorrhage from aneurysm, vascular malformation, cerebral trauma, or intracranial operation (most frequently associated with posterior fossa surgery). Obliteration of the subarachnoid space may also be due to meningitis. In some patients, particularly in the sixth and seventh decades, the history does not reveal a specific etiological process, and these cases are termed idiopathic. Pathological study in one such case has shown dense scarring in the subarachnoid space around the brain stem.[47]

Neurological Symptoms and Signs

Cardinal symptoms are mental change and disturbance of gait.[1,47,48] Changes in mentation usually appear first, but, at times, gait disturbance is the earliest and most prominent symptom. Headache is not present. Urinary incontinence is usually not present in the early stages, but appears as the illness progresses.

Mental changes usually develop slowly over a period of weeks or months. Initially, there is a mild forgetfulness combined with a slowing-up of mental processes and physical activity. Less spontaneous action and conversation is noted. Aberrant behavior, delusions, hallucinations, paranoia, irrational speech, and dysphasia are not part of the picture. Calculations are frequently slow and inaccurate. In advanced cases, mutism, severe hypokinesia, and abulia may develop.

The gait disturbance is difficult to describe. Initially, it is usually slow with a wide base and zigzag steps. In more advanced cases, ambulation is difficult or impossible because of unsteadiness and slowing of activity. There are usually no clear cerebellar signs.

Neurological examination reveals no papilledema. The extraocular movements are full, but nystagmus may be present. Movement of limbs is slow. Tendon reflexes may be increased, especially in the lower extremities, and plantar responses are often extensor. Sucking and grasping reflexes appear in the late stages.

In some cases in which there has been brain damage from one of the disease processes mentioned earlier, it may be difficult to recognize the onset of symptoms. In such cases, there may also be focal neurological signs. An enlarging porencephalic cyst with or without ventricular enlargement may occur with normal cerebrospinal fluid pressure. Symptoms of normal-pressure hydrocephalus may be combined with focal neurological signs in these patients.

Diagnostic Studies

Skull Films

These are usually normal with no evidence of changes characteristic of chronic increased intracranial pressure.

Pneumonencephalography

This study will demonstrate enlargement of the ventricular system similar to that in patients with hydrocephalus that is accompanied by elevated pressure (Fig. 23–29). The increase in ventricular size is most prominent in the frontal horns, although the entire system may be enlarged. The ventricular span of the frontal horns is usually greater than 50 mm on the brow-up anteroposterior films. In the typical case, there is a complete obstruction to the passage of air through the basal cisterns. In some patients, a small amount of air may enter the frontal subarachnoid space or syl-vian cisterns, but no air is seen over the convexity of the cerebral hemispheres.[47] Findings on the pneumoencephalogram that may be characteristics of normal-pressure hydrocephalus have been reviewed in the literature.[34]

Marked deterioration in neurological symptoms and signs occurs in some patients after a pneumoencephalogram. When this happens, it helps to confirm the diagnosis of normal-pressure hydrocephalus, but an absence of worsening in the patient's condition does not exclude the syndrome. A few patients have shown temporary elevation of cerebrospinal fluid pressure after the pneumoencephalogram.

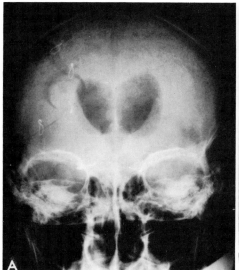
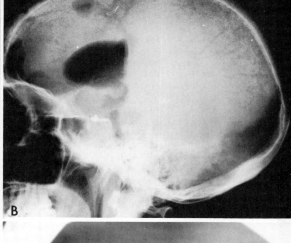
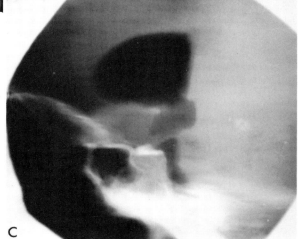

FIGURE 23–29 Pneumoencephalogram of a 70-year-old woman who developed symptoms and signs of normal-pressure hydrocephalus two weeks after successful clipping of an internal carotid aneurysm. *A* and *B*. Anteroposterior and lateral views. *C*. Midline tomographic cut in brow-up position. There is marked ventricular enlargement with span of lateral ventricles measuring 56 mm (upper limit of normal = 40 mm) on anteroposterior view. There is no air over the cerebral convexity; air does not ascend beyond the basal cisterns.

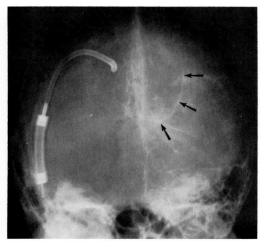

FIGURE 23–30 Anteroposterior view from venous phase of angiogram in a patient with hydrocephalus and a nonfunctioning shunt. The arrows outline the course of the thalamostriate vein, indicating size and configuration of the body of the lateral ventricle. The distance from the midline to the lateralmost part of this vein (*upper arrow*) is used to record the ventricular span. The upper limit of normal is 20 mm; in this case the measurement is 28 mm. In most cases of normal-pressure hydrocephalus this value is 25 mm or more.

Angiography

By noting the position of the subependymal veins, an accurate estimation of the ventricular size can be made from the anterior-posterior view of the venous phase of the carotid angiogram (Fig. 23–30). However, this is not the primary diagnostic procedure since a detailed view of the subarachnoid space and ventricles with oxygen or air gives much more diagnostic information.

Some patients are quite ill with symptoms of hydrocephalus after subarachnoid hemorrhage, trauma, or an intracranial operation. In these patients angiography confirms the suspicion of enlarged ventricles, excludes other pathological conditions, and is associated with less morbidity than ventriculography or pneumoencephalography. In such patients, the angiographic findings taken in combination with the results of the radioiodinated serum albumin flow study may establish the diagnosis.

Lumbar Puncture

The cerebrospinal fluid pressure from the lumbar subarachnoid space, with the patient in the lateral recumbent position, is usually less than 180 mm of water. Protein and cell count are normal unless altered by the basic disease process that is causing the hydrocephalus.

An attempt has been made to predict the results of a shunt operation by lowering cerebrospinal fluid pressure at the time of lumbar puncture. This has not proved reliable, and failure to improve after such a test should not exclude the patient from treatment. Sustained reduction of cerebrospinal fluid pressure for several days or weeks may be required before improvement is seen in some cases.

Cerebrospinal Fluid Absorption Test

Measurement of cerebrospinal fluid absorption by a constant-infusion manometric test has been reported.[31, 32] Saline infused at a rate of approximately twice the normal rate of cerebrospinal fluid formation in patients with normal absorption capacity produces a predictable rise in the cerebrospinal fluid pressure, while in abnormal situations the pressure rises abruptly. In adults with occult hydrocephalus due to specific etiological factors, the capacity to absorb added fluid is reduced, but in 13 of 14 patients with Alzheimer's disease, the infusion test was normal.

Isotope Cerebrospinal Fluid Flow Study

This study is performed by injecting radioiodinated serum albumin with high specific activity into the lumbar subarachnoid space.[13, 43] The usual adult dose is 100 microcuries. In some cases, cisternal injection may be used.[61] Normally, the isotope reaches the posterior fossa and basal cisterns by 4 hours after injection. At 24 hours, the isotope has moved over the cerebral convexity, and by 48 hours is diffused over both cerebral hemispheres. Normally, there is little or no activity in the ventricular system. (Fig. 23–31).

Abnormal studies are usually characterized by one of the following features: persistent ventricular filling with delayed clearance and reduction or absence of flow in the cerebral subarachnoid space, transient ventricular filling with delayed or normal convexity flow, no ventricular filling but de-

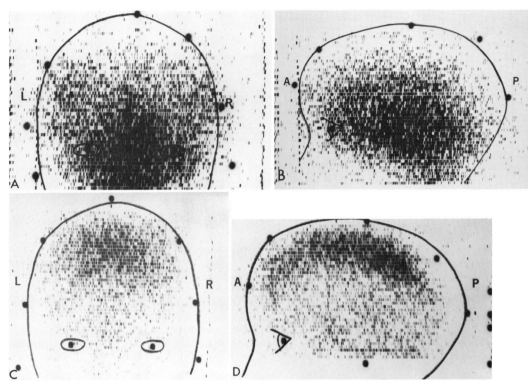

FIGURE 23–31 Normal radioiodinated serum albumin (RISA) cerebrospinal fluid flow study. Injection of 100 mc of high specific activity RISA in the lumbar subarachnoid space. *A* and *B*. Anteroposterior and lateral views 4 hours after injection. Concentration is maximum in the basal cisterns and in the subarachnoid space around the temporal lobes. *C* and *D*. Anteroposterior and lateral views 24 hours after injection. The concentration of RISA is now noted over the superior cerebral convexity, particularly in the parasagittal region. At 48 hours, the same pattern was noted with less activity.

layed flow over the cerebral surface, and abnormal concentration in cystic areas of disease.[47]

In the typical case of normal-pressure hydrocephalus, this isotopic study will show essentially all the activity in the ventricles with very little reaching the cerebral convexity even 48 hours after injection (Fig. 23–32).[2, 4, 47] When the other types of scan abnormalities are noted, correlation with clinical symptoms has not been consistent. The results of other diagnostic studies and treatment in such cases have also been variable.

Differential Diagnosis

The chief problem in differential diagnosis in cases without a specific etiological factor has been to distinguish those patients with dementia due to Alzheimer's or related diseases. Most reports indicate that the latter group does not benefit appreciably from operative treatment.[47]

In typical cases of Alzheimer's or degenerative disease, the history, pneumoencephalogram, and RISA cerebrospinal fluid flow study will establish the diagnosis. The principal symptom is loss of memory to which are later added defects in calculation, speech, and thinking. Slowing of mental and physical activity and gait disturbance are rarely early manifestations. Deficits usually develop over several years. The pneumoencephalogram shows dilated ventricles and large pools of the air in widened sulci in the cerebral subarachnoid space. The RISA cerebrospinal fluid flow test will be normal or show only transient ventricular filling.

There is, however, a small group of patients who are difficult to characterize. Their history is not typical, but it suggests the possibility of normal-pressure hydroce-

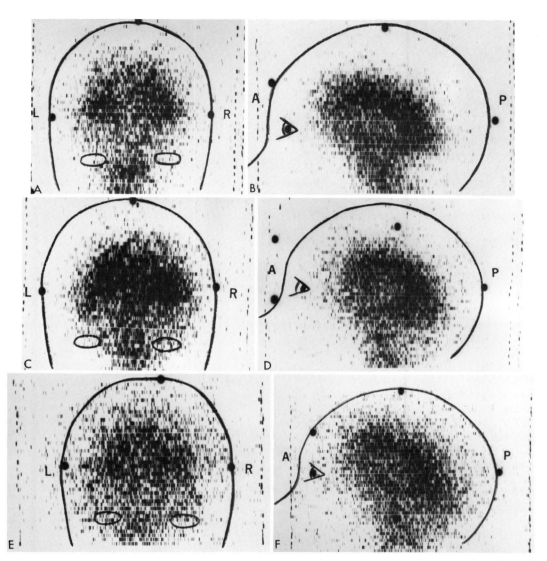

FIGURE 23-32 Abnormal radioiodinated serum albumin (RISA) cerebrospinal fluid flow study. This study was done on a 55-year-old woman who developed symptoms and signs of normal-pressure hydrocephalus several weeks after a subarachnoid hemorrhage. Injection of 100 mc of high specific activity RISA in the lumbar subarachnoid space. *A* and *B*. Anteroposterior and lateral views 4 hours after injection. The isotope is outlining the enlarged lateral ventricles. Some concentration remains in the basal cisterns. *C* and *D*. Anteroposterior and lateral views 24 hours after injection. Increased isotopic concentration is present in the ventricular system. The isotope does not ascend into the cerebral subarachnoid space. *E* and *F*. Anteroposterior and lateral views 48 hours after injection. The RISA remains in the enlarged ventricular system.

phalus. Their pneumoencephalograms show large ventricles, but some air enters portions of the cerebral subarachnoid space; and their RISA scans show an atypical abnormality. Some of these patients benefit from surgical treatment. In some cases, improvement may be temporary, lasting only several months before progressive deterioration resumes. It is postulated in such cases that an element of normal-pressure hydrocephalus is present in addition to an underlying degenerative disease.[47]

There is no doubt that an intracranial tumor can partially obstruct the flow of cerebrospinal fluid and may produce the syndrome of normal-pressure hydrocephalus without any focal sign of the tumor.[47] This is another reason why it is important to do a pneumoencephalogram in these patients.

Surgical Treatment

The majority of patients are treated with a ventriculovenous shunt. In most patients the authors have used a medium-pressure (40 to 70 mm) Hakim valve. Following insertion of a shunt, the most rapid improvement usually is in the mental sphere. Incontinence also clears, but gait is usually slow to improve, and some residual deficit may persist. Improvement may be seen almost immediately in some cases, but in others it is more gradual, occurring over several days to weeks.

In Figure 23–33, one method of placing a ventriculovenous shunt is illustrated. The entire right side of the head and neck is prepared, utilizing some type of adherent drape so that no skin is exposed. Three incisions are made. The frontal burr hole is placed behind the anterior hairline approximately 10 to 12 cm from the glabella and 2.5 to 3 cm from the midline. A catheter is inserted into the anterior horn of the right lateral ventricle. The landmark for this insertion is the inner canthus of the eye in the frontal plane and a point 1 to 2 cm anterior to the external auditory meatus in the lateral plane. At a depth of approximately 5.5 cm, the catheter will lie in the midportion of the frontal horn in the adult. The figure illustrates the J-shaped Hakim catheter, but any type of catheter may be used.

The second incision is in the postauricular region. A reservoir, if desired, and valve are attached to the ventricular catheter. The system is brought through a subgaleal tunnel from the frontal to the postauricular incision. Its placement is determined by the type of valve and reservoir that are to be used.

The third incision is made in line with a skin crease centered over the upper portion of the sternocleidomastoid muscle. The common facial vein is identified and ligated, and a small silicone radiopaque catheter is inserted through this vein into the jugular vein. If a good branch of the jugular vein is not available, the catheter may be inserted directly through a purse-string suture. Depending on the size of the individual, insertion of 20 to 23 cm of catheter usually places the cardiac end in proper position in

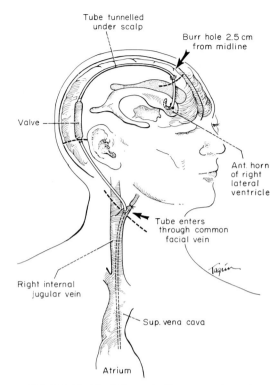

FIGURE 23–33 Schematic diagram to show placement of the ventriculovenous shunt for hydrocephalus. In the adult, the frontal burr hole on the right side is usually just behind the anterior hair line, 10 to 12 cm from the glabella, and 2.5 cm from the midline. The average depth for the catheter to lie in the frontal horn of the lateral ventricle is 5.5 cm. External landmarks for placement of the ventricular catheter are the inner canthus of the eye in the frontal plane, and approximately 1 to 2 cm anterior to the external auditory meatus in the lateral view. The neck incision is made in a skin crease centered over the upper portion of the sternocleidomastoid muscle. Usually, the catheter can be inserted through the common facial vein. Under x-ray control, the distal end of the catheter is placed at approximately the level of the sixth thoracic vertebra. The scalp incisions depend on the type of valve and reservoir used.

the adult. An x-ray is taken and the catheter is positioned at about the level of the body of the sixth thoracic vertebra. The catheter is then tied in place and the proximal portion brought through a subgaleal-subcutaneous tunnel to the postauricular incision and attached to the valve.

Characteristics of Clinical Groups

Idiopathic

In this group are those patients who have the onset of symptoms suggestive of normal-pressure hydrocephalus in the sixth to seventh decades with no history of a specific etiological factor. Evaluation of these patients has revealed two subgroups: a small group with typical clinical and radiographic features of normal-pressure hydrocephalus usually having good response to treatment; and a larger group with some clinical features suggesting the diagnosis but some atypical symptoms, enlarged ventricles with partial obstruction of subarachnoid space on the pneumoencephalogram, and an abnormal but not typical RISA cerebrospinal fluid flow study.[47] Some of the patients respond to treatment, at times only temporarily, while others derive no benefit from surgery. Evaluation and selection of these cases continues to be a problem.

Patients with enlarged subarachnoid spaces over the cerebral convexity secondary to atrophy do not improve following placement of a ventriculovenous shunt.

Subarachnoid Hemorrhage

Enlargement of the ventricular system occurs in over 30 per cent of patients following subarachnoid hemorrhage, and about half of these will have some symptoms referable to hydrocephalus.[20] Initially, there may be a temporary increase in cerebrospinal fluid pressure, but in most cases, symptoms of hydrocephalus develop when the pressure has returned to or has been persistently normal.

Symptoms may begin almost immediately, but more commonly there is a delay in onset of one to several weeks.[47] Typical abnormalities on pneumoencephalogram and RISA cerebrospinal fluid flow study are usually found. In some cases, the syndrome is temporary, and spontaneous improvement occurs. If a ventriculovenous shunt is required, improvement is evident within a few days, and over one to three weeks, the hydrocephalic symptoms gradually subside.[18, 47]

Trauma

The natural history of patients who develop enlarged ventricles after head trauma has not been fully studied. The obstruction of cerebrospinal fluid flow is usually due to scarring and obstruction of the basal cisterns and subarachnoid space from subarachnoid hemorrhage. On rare occasions, there may be obstruction of a major venous sinus or block in the third ventricle and aqueduct. As with spontaneous subarachnoid hemorrhage, symptoms may be associated with mildly elevated or normal cerebrospinal fluid pressure, and the onset may be delayed for a period of up to several weeks or even months after the trauma.[47]

In many cases, it is difficult to separate the direct effects of the brain injury and those secondary to obstruction of cerebrospinal fluid flow. Lewin has reported the largest series.[35] In 59 cases of severe head injury with generalized ventricular enlargement, 20 had obstruction of cerebrospinal fluid flow. Eight of the twenty had increased cerebrospinal fluid pressure, and six of them were treated with a shunt, with good recovery in two. Of the 12 who had an obstruction to cerebrospinal flow and a normal cerebrospinal fluid pressure, 6 recovered spontaneously.

In another report of 11 patients with normal-pressure hydrocephalus, improvement in symptoms was striking in some cases, but did not occur in others.[47] In those who did not improve, the underlying brain injury was so severe that recovery did not take place despite the radiographic and isotopic findings being typical for the syndrome.

Intracranial Operations

Several days or weeks after an intracranial operation, particularly a posterior fossa exploration, symptoms of normal-pressure hydrocephalus may develop. Typical pneumoencephalogram and isotope cerebrospinal fluid flow study abnormalities are found. If the symptoms do not improve spontaneously, a ventriculovenous shunt is indicated.[47]

Meningitis

On rare occasions, obliteration of the subarachnoid space develops following meningitis. Symptoms of normal-pressure hydrocephalus may follow immediately or may not develop for several months. Pneumoencephalogram and cerebrospinal flow abnormalities are typical.[47] There is a good response to placement of the ventriculovenous shunt.

Intracranial Tumors

The importance of complete radiographic studies in patients presenting with symptoms of normal-pressure hydrocephalus only has been illustrated in two such cases in which partial obstruction of cerebrospinal fluid pathways was found to be due to intracranial tumor. In one there was a third ventricular mass, and in the other a pineal tumor.[47] All the presenting symptoms were relieved by placement of a shunt.

REFERENCES

1. Adams, R. D., Fisher, C. M., Hakim, S., Ojemann, R. G., and Sweet, W. H.: Symptomatic occult hydrocephalus with "normal" cerebrospinal-fluid pressure: a treatable syndrome. New Engl. J. Med., 273:117-126, 1965.
2. Bannister, R., Gilford, E., and Kocen, R.: Isotope encephalography in the diagnosis of dementia due to communicating hydrocephalus. Lancet, 2:1014-1017, 1967.
3. Benda, C. E.: Dandy-Walker syndrome or the so-called atresia of the foramen of Magendie. J. Neuropath. Exp. Neurol., 13:14-29, 1954.
4. Benson, D. F., LeMay, M., Patten, D. H., and Rubens, A. B.: Diagnosis of normal-pressure hydrocephalus. New Engl. J. Med., 283:609-615, 1970.
5. Bering, E. A., Jr.: A simplified apparatus for constant ventricular drainage. J. Neurosurg., 8:450-452, 1951.
6. Bering, E. A., Jr.: Water exchange of central nervous system and cerebrospinal fluid. J. Neurosurg., 9:275-287, 1952.
7. Bering, E. A., Jr.: The use of phenolsulphonphthalein in the clinical evaluation of hydrocephalus. J. Neurosurg., 13:587-595, 1956.
8. Bering, E. A., Jr.: Circulation of the cerebrospinal fluid, demonstration of the choroid plexus as the generator of the force for flow of fluid and ventricular enlargement. J. Neurosurg., 19:405-413, 1962.
9. Crofton, F. D. L., and Matson, D. D.: Roentgenologic study of choroid plexus papillomas in childhood. Amer. J. Roentgen., 84:479-487, 1960.
10. Cutler, R. W. P., Page, L. K., Galicich, J., and Watters, G. V.: Formation and absorption of cerebrospinal fluid in man. Brain, 91:707-720, 1968.
11. Dandy, W. E.: Extripation of the choroid plexus of the lateral ventricles in communicating hydrocephalus. Ann. Surg., 68:569-579, 1918.
12. Dandy, W. E.: Cerebral ventriculoscopy. Bull. J. Hopk. Hosp., 33:189, 1922.

13. DiChiro, G.: New radiographic and isotopic procedures in neurological diagnosis. J.A.M.A., 188:524-529, 1964.
14. Eisenberg, H. M., Davidson R. I., and Shillito, J.: Lumbar-peritoneal shunts: A review of 34 cases. J. Neurosurg., 35:427-431, 1971.
15. Emery, J. L., and Hilton, H. B.: Lung and heart complications of the treatment of hydrocephalus by ventriculoauriculostomy. Surgery, 50:309-314, 1961.
16. Erdohazi, M., Eckstein, H. B., and Crome, L.: Pulmonary embolism as a complication of ventriculoatrial shunts inserted for hydrocephalus. Devel. Med. Child Neurol. (suppl.), 11:36-44, 1966.
17. Fischer, E. G., and Shillito, J.: Large abdominal cysts: A complication of peritoneal shunts. Report of three cases. J. Neurosurg., 21:441-444, 1969.
18. Foltz, F. I., and Ward, A. A., Jr.: Communicating hydrocephalus from subarachnoid bleeding. J. Neurosurg., 13:546-566, 1956.
19. Friedman, S., Zita-Gosum, C., and Chatten, J.: Pulmonary vascular changes complicating ventriculovascular shunting for hydrocephalus. J. Pediat., 64:305-314, 1964.
20. Galera, R., and Greits, T.: Hydrocephalus in the adult secondary to the rupture of intracranial arterial aneurysms. J. Neurosurg., 32:634-641, 1970.
21. Galicich, J. H., Lombroso, C. T., and Matson, D. D.: Ultrasonic B-scanning of the brain. J. Neurosurg., 22:499-510, 1965.
22. Gardner, W. J.: Myelocele: Rupture of the neural tube. In Ojemann, R. G., ed.: Clinical Neurosurgery. Baltimore, Williams & Wilkins Co., 1968, Vol. 15, pp. 57-58.
23. Geschwind, N.: The mechanism of normal pressure hydrocephalus. J. Neurol. Sci., 7:481-493, 1968.
24. Gilles, E. H., and Davidson, R. L.: Communicating hydrocephalus associated with deficient dysplastic parasagittal arachnoidal granulations. J. Neurosurg., 35:421-426, 1971.
25. Gilles, F. H., and Rockett, F. X.: Infantile hydrocephalus: Retrocerebellar "arachnoidal" cyst. J. Pediat., 79:436-443, 1971.
26. Gilles, F. H., and Shillito, J.: Infantile hydrocephalus: Retrocerebellar subdural hematoma. J. Pediat., 76:529-537, 1970.
27. Gurdjian, E. S., and Fishman, R. A.: Posttraumatic hydrocephalus in head injury. In Caveness, W. E., and Walker, A. E., eds.: Head Injury: Conference Proceedings. Philadelphia, J. B. Lippincott Co., 1966, pp. 550-551.
28. Hakim, S.: Algunas observaciones sobre la presion del L. C. R. sindrome hidrocefalico en el adulto con "presion normal" del L. C. R. Tesis de grado. Universidad Javeriana, Bogotá, Colombia, 1964.
29. Hakim, S., and Adams, R. D.: The special clinical problem of symptomatic hydrocephalus with normal cerebrospinal fluid pressure: Observations on cerebrospinal fluid hydrodynamics. J. Neurol. Sci., 2:307-327, 1965.
30. Hill, M. E., Lougheed, W. M., and Barnett, H. J. M.: A treatable form of dementia due to nor-

mal-pressure, communicating hydrocephalus. Canad. Med. Ass. J., 97:1309-1320, 1967.

31. Hussey, F., Schanzer, B., and Katzman, R.: A simple constant-infusion manometric test for measurement of CSF absorption. II. Clinical studies. Neurology (Minneap.), 20:665-680, 1970.

32. Katzman, R., and Hussey, F.: A simple constant-infusion manometric test for measurement of CSF absorption. I. Rationale and method. Neurology (Minneap.), 20:534-544, 1970.

33. Kushner, J., Alexander, E., Jr., Davis, C. H., and Kelley, D. L., Jr.: Kyphoscoliosis following lumbar subarachnoid shunts. J. Neurosurg., 34:783-791, 1971.

34. LeMay, M., and New, P. F. J.: Radiological Diagnosis of occult normal-pressure hydrocephalus. Radiology, 96:347-358, 1970.

35. Lewin, W.: Preliminary observations on external hydrocephalus after severe head injury. Brit. J. Surg., 55:747-751, 1969.

36. Lorenzo, A., Page, L. K., and Watters, G. V.: Relationship between cerebrospinal fluid formation, absorption, and pressure in human hydrocephalus. Brain, 93:679-692, 1970.

37. Lourie, H., and Berne, A. S.: Radiological and clinical features of an arachnoid cyst of the quadrigeminal cistern. J. Neurol. Neurosurg. Psychiat., 24:374-378, 1961.

38. Matson, D. D.: A new operation for the treatment of communicating hydrocephalus. Report of a case secondary to generalized meningitis. J. Neurosurg., 6:238-247, 1949.

39. Matson, D. D.: Ventriculo-ureterostomy. J. Neurosurg., 8:398-404, 1951.

40. Matson, D. D.: Hydrocephalus in a premature infant caused by papilloma of the choroid plexus, with report of surgical treatment. J. Neurosurg., 10:416-420, 1953.

41. Matson, D. D.: Hydrocephalus treated by arachnoid-ureterostomy; report of 50 cases. Pediatrics, 12:326-334, 1953.

42. Matson, D. D.: Neurosurgery of Infancy and Childhood. Springfield, Ill., Charles C Thomas, 1968, pp. 8, 259-268.

43. McCullough, D. C., Harbert, J. C., DiChiro, G., and Ommaya, A. K.: Prognostic criteria for cerebrospinal fluid shunting from isotope cisternography in communicating hydrocephalus. Neurology (Minneap.), 20:594-598, 1970.

44. Milhorat, T. H., Hammock, M. K., and DiChiro, G.: The subarachnoid space in congenital obstructive hydrocephalus: Part 1: Cisternographic findings. J. Neurosurg., 35:1-6, 1971.

45. Nulsen, F. E., and Becker, D. P.: Control of hydrocephalus by valve-regulated shunt. J. Neurosurg., 26:362-274, 1967.

46. Nulsen, F. E., and Spitz, E. B.: Treatment of hydrocephalus by direct shunt from ventricle to jugular vein. Surg. Forum, 2:399-403, 1951.

47. Ojemann, R. G.: Normal pressure hydrocephalus. In Tindall, G. T., ed.: Clinical Neurosurgery. Baltimore, Williams & Wilkins Co., 1971, pp. 337-370.

48. Ojemann, R. G., Fisher, C. M., Adams, R. D., Sweet, W. H., and New, P. F. J.: Further experience with the syndrome of "normal" pressure hydrocephalus. J. Neurosurg., 31:279-294, 1969.

49. Pudenz, R. H., Russell, F. E., Hurd, A. H., and Shelden, C. H.: Ventriculo-auriculostomy: A technique for shunting cerebrospinal fluid into the right auricle. Preliminary report. J. Neurosurg., 14:171-179, 1957.

50. Ransohoff, J.: Ventriculo-pleural anastomosis. J. Neurosurg., 11:295-298, 1954.

51. Ransohoff, J., and Hiatt, R.: Ventriculoperitoneal anastomosis in the treatment of hyrdocephalus: Utilization of the suprahepatic space. A preliminary report. Trans. Amer. Neurol. Ass., 77:147-151, 1952.

52. Ransohoff, J., Shulman, K., Fishman, R. A.: Hydrocephalus. A review of etiology and treatment. J. Pediat., 56:399-411, 1960.

53. Russell, D. S.: Observations on the Pathology of Hydrocephalus. Med. Res. Council Spec. Report Series No. 265: His Maj. Stationery Office, 12-21, 1949.

54. Sayers, M. P.: The treatment of hydrocephalus. Trans. Latin American Congress of Neurosurgery. In press.

55. Scarff, J.: Treatment of hydrocephalus: A historical and critical review of methods and results. J. Neurol. Neurosurg. Psychiat., 26:1-26, 1963.

56. Schick, R. W., and Matson, D. D.: What is arrested hydrocephalus? J. Pediat., 58:791-799, 1961.

57. Scott, M., Wycis, H. T., Murtagh, F., and Reyes, V.: Observations on ventricular and lumbar subarachnoid peritoneal shunts in hydrocephalus in infants. J. Neurosurg., 12:165-175, 1955.

58. Shillito, J., and Matson, D. D.: Craniosynostosis: A review of 519 surgical patients. Pediatrics, 41:829-893, 1968.

59. Shulman, K., Martin, B. F., Popoff, N., and Ransohoff, J.: Recognition and treatment of hydrocephalus following spontaneous subarachnoid hemorrhage. J. Neurosurg., 20:1040-1049, 1963.

60. Stickler, G. B., Shin, M. H., Burke, E. C., Holley, K. E., and Miller, R. H.: Diffuse glomerulonephritis associated with infected ventriculoatrial shunt. New Eng. J. Med., 279:3:1077-1082, 1968.

61. Tator, C. H., Fleming, J. F., Sheppard, R. H., and Turner, V. M.: A radioisotopic test for communicating hydrocephalus. J. Neurosurg., 28:327-340, 1968.

62. Weinman, D., Paul, A. T. S.: Ventriculoauriculostomy for infantile hydrocephalus using a direct cardiac approach. J. Neurosurg., 24:471-474, 1967.

63. Welch, K., Friedman, V.: The cerebrospinal fluid valves. Brain, 83:454-469, 1960.

64. Wilson, S. A. K.: Megalencephaly. J. Neurol. Psychopath., 14:193-216, 1934.

24

MIDLINE FUSION DEFECTS AND DEFECTS OF FORMATION

The clinical management of infants born with major central nervous system defects and anomalies presents a challenge that is perhaps unsurpassed in the field of pediatric neurosurgery. Previous concepts have had to undergo radical revision and re-evaluation as new experience and the knowledge constantly being amassed have provided fresh motivation for pediatricians, neurologists, and neurosurgeons to offer as much scientific medical assistance to these unfortunate children as contemporary methods will allow. The responsibility of directing the clinical therapeutic efforts involving many disciplines is one of awesome magnitude and requires dedication and perseverance that is demanding. The course is punctuated by periods of frustration, failure, and vicissitudes; success is often measured in terms of a surviving severely crippled child with many handicaps and problems, who can nevertheless be considered educable and, to some degree, competitive. To achieve this end-result in a child with a major central nervous system defect, such as commonly occurs in the myelodysplastic child, requires the concerted efforts of a team of experts in several specialty areas, often working simultaneously or nearly so to stay the ravages of infection, musculoskeletal deformities, meningitis, ventricular enlargement, and urinary tract complications. No longer is it feasible for a single person to direct such a complex procedure or to attempt to decide the issues without multidisciplinary consultation.[6, 12]

Defects that embrace the clinical gamut from simple spina bifida occulta to the devastating spinal dysrhaphic state with associated hydrocephalus can indeed tax the knowledge and technical ingenuity of every physician willing to become involved in such cases. The "new look" in the management of these disorders must discard the axiomatic recipe-type decisions employed in the past and based on unfounded clinical judgment. In its place, one must adopt an aggressive approach to a problem beset with difficulties, to be sure, but one in which a human intellect and a handicapped but competitive personality may possibly be salvaged. To attain this degree of success will require the patience and understanding of the parents and other family members with whom rapport must be established and whose support must be enlisted from the outset.

EPIDEMIOLOGY

Until very recently little has been known concerning the statistical frequency of major birth defects on a world-wide basis. Through studies conducted under the auspices of the World Health Organization some meaningful data have been gathered from studies of consecutive births in 24 areas throughout the world. The major defects in these studies included anencephaly, hydrocephalus, spina bifida cystica, and encephalocele, each of which can be

W. F. MEACHAM
R. D. DICKINS, JR.

detected easily and without diagnostic difficulty in early life. The majority of such defects occur in the hospital where pregnancies complicated by toxemia, malpresentations, and hydramnios are usually managed. In such situations, 30 to 50 per cent of the defective children are born of mothers with hydramnios.

Anencephaly, peculiarly, is found commonly in Ireland and Wales (4:1000) and infrequently in South America and the United States and Africa. With or without spina bifida, anencephaly occurs slightly more than once per thousand live births with a preponderance occurring in female children (two thirds). Hydrocephalus, alone or with spina bifida, likewise occurs most frequently in Ireland (Belfast) as well as in Egypt (Alexandria). There is no known reason for the geographical preponderance in some areas of these defects that are considered rare in others.

Environmental and cultural differences play no known part in the development of birth defects, nor has there been plausible evidence of specific prenatal factors exerting any influence. Yet it is difficult to assign such cases to "bad luck" or to the laws of chance. More sophisticated studies and investigation into social and environmental influences on the course of gestation and fetal development may shed light on these events in the future. The months of November and December are known to yield the highest number of neural defective births — a minor mystery itself. Sporadic accounts of "epidemics" of birth defects (spina bifida) have been reported in Atlanta, Philadelphia, and Vermont. Since birth defects rank high as a cause of death, it is obviously necessary to rekindle interest in the causes and prevention of these disorders. Few valid statistical studies relating to frequency have appeared in the past, but currently interested epidemiologists have provided data suggesting that all forms of malformations (anatomical and metabolic) affect some 15 million persons in the United States, accounting for over 62,000 deaths in 1965, of which 19,000 were congenital malformations. There is an urgent need for a uniform nomenclature, a standardization of diagnostic criteria, and accurate statistical recordings to allow meaningful epidemiological studies to be made.[20, 38]

ETIOLOGY

No single factor or group of factors has yet been found to be responsible for the occurrence of birth defects of the central nervous system. In these cases, unlike those of the babies deformed by the toxic effects of thalidomide, no drug or other agent (including radiation exposure) has been indicted as a possible etiological factor. It is true that a high percentage of babies live born or stillborn from mothers with hydramnios have shown birth defects (68 of 145 in Boston). Age, family history, infections, diet, and other environmental factors have been studied in the authors' clinic as in others, but no common factor has yet emerged that can offer a valid clue to etiology.[24, 25]

In some families an undesirable family trait has emerged as a possible inheritable feature — a gloomy prospect for prospective parents to consider. Furthermore, the likelihood of additional neural defects occurring in subsequent siblings is estimated at 1:30, a degree of chance high enough to dissuade many from risking another pregnancy. A family whose first and twelfth children were born with myelomeningocele, all the intervening children being normal, is known to the authors.

It is hoped that the increasing interest in this problem throughout the world will result in sufficient statistical data on all aspects of these defects to, when pooled, make some significant correlation of common features apparent and give some hint regarding the possible etiology. Whatever causative factors exist must obviously come into play in the early weeks of pregnancy since the neural tube is complete by the fourth or fifth week. Prior to this, any noxious influence conceivably could create a defect at a precise time in the development of the spine and neural elements. Experimentally it is known that dissimilar agents produce the same effects in embryos if applied at the identical gestational period.[8, 38]

From the embryological viewpoint, most cases of spinal dysrhaphism, as well as some other central nervous system defects, have been thought to occur as the result of failure of the vertebral posterior arches to fuse, allowing for a herniation of the meningeal-neural elements; of failure of the neural tube to develop progressively and to fuse along its length to form a complete tube; of rupture of the sac in hydromyelia secondary to delay in the establishment of the cerebrospinal fluid circulation by failure of patency of the roof of the fourth ventricle; and finally, of possible excessive growth of the neural tissue in the area of the spina bifida. These theoretical possibilities have been scrutinized in great detail by embryologists and pathologists, but there is no general agreement yet forthcoming regarding the true cause of these developmental defects. Defects of notochordal development such as failure of segmentation, hemivertebra, and congenital absence of vertebrae are equally mystifying from the etiological standpoint.

SPINA BIFIDA OCCULTA

As the term indicates, the defect of the vertebral arches is not obvious and is unassociated with herniation of the meninges. This common condition may exist throughout life without producing any clinical signs or symptoms, since the defect usually involves only the bony elements, and only rarely is there a neural deficit that can be related directly to the vertebral level involved.

Even though the bony defect is occult, there may be one or more surface clues suggesting the presence of the underlying defect. These include lipomas, skin dimples, patches of excessive hair, and portwine staining or pigmentation of the overlying skin. Such lesions may constitute the only reason for surgical consideration in the asymptomatic spina bifida and should be operated on only for cosmetic correction of an unsightly back. Since spina bifida occulta occurs most frequently at the lower lumbar—upper sacral level, it is rare for the cosmetic disturbance to be severe enough to justify correction in an area ordinarily hidden by clothing.

The presenting signs of spina bifida occulta may relate solely to a maldevelopment of one or both feet. This may be a "clubbed foot," or a variant of it, and may be so mild as to escape notice until some abnormality of gait is noted after the child becomes ambulatory. There may also be present a degree of scoliosis noted when erect posture is assumed. It is significant that scoliosis associated with the cutaneous stigmata is almost pathognomonic of an underlying spinal defect. Approximately 10 per cent of those individuals with symptoms relating to spina bifida occulta will have enuresis or some form of sphincter incontinence. Anatomical and radiographic studies indicate that approximately 1.2 per cent of the adults so studied had spina bifida occulta, 6 per cent of them had the defect at the fifth lumbar lamina, and 11 per cent at the first and second sacral levels.

Attempts to correlate spina bifida occulta with a variety of clinical conditions have not been generally rewarding. It is difficult to relate this lesion with any degree of certainty to the problem of low back pain, the "unstable back" rupture of lumbar discs, sphincter incontinence, enuresis in children, and other neurological abnormalities involving the lower extremities. Since fusions of the posterior arches may continue to occur throughout early childhood, the presence of one or more deficient arches disclosed by x-ray in infancy may disappear by the age of puberty. If, however, neurological signs develop and are progressive in a child with spina bifida occulta, a myelographic study should be carried out before operative treatment is recommended, and the presence of an intraspinal mass, usually a lipoma, is sufficient justification for an exploration. A normal myelogram would indicate that an exploration was entirely unjustified and undesirable. The loss of sphincter control or impairment of sensory and motor function in the feet and legs and other disturbances of posture and gait may make a myelographic study advisable, particularly if the neurological deficits are advancing. It should never be assumed that such symptoms are the result of the spina bifida occulta, since other intraspinal lesions may be present (e.g., neoplasms, diastematomyelia) and can only be confirmed by myelography.[3, 14, 16, 19]

It is the authors' opinion that operations on spina bifida occulta are indicated only when a neurological and myelographic deficit that correlates with the level of spina bifida justifies an operative exploration. Similarly, operations on the spina bifida for enuresis without a myelographic defect are useless and unjustified.

SPINA BIFIDA CYSTICA

Meningocele

One of the rare forms of spinal dysrhaphia is a true meningocele (Fig. 24–1). Although the term is commonly employed when referring to all forms of spina bifida cystica, this is technically erroneous, since, as the name implies, it is a herniation of the meninges through the defect of the posterior arches. It is important that meningoceles be differentiated from myelomeningocele, since the prognosis in the former is infinitely better; yet death can ensue from a neglected meningocele that has become infected, leading to leakage of spinal fluid and meningitis. The majority occur in the lumbar area, and in many respects they may resemble myelomeningocele. Often, however, they are covered by skin rather than by translucent membrane. They are more often pedunculated than sessile, neurological deficit in the sphincters and lower extremities is not present, and there are usually no neural elements present in the sac. Occasionally one finds nerve fibers trav-

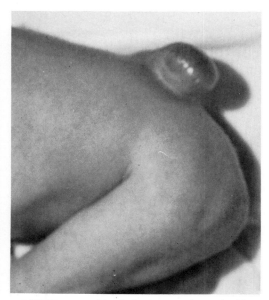

FIGURE 24–1 Simple lumbar meningocele. Neurological status normal. Prognosis excellent.

ersing the wall of the sac at operation, but there is lacking the usual fixation by neural plaque at the dome or apex of the herniation. Where the integumentary covering is deficient, the usual chance of rupture, spinal fluid leakage, and infection exists. Some meningoceles, apparently voluminous but covered with healthy skin, are in actuality small meningocele pockets contained in a mass of lipomatous tissue; they are often referred to as lipomatous meningoceles. When no neurological deficit is present, there is no reason to consider operative correction of this lesion except for cosmetic reasons. This can be done as an elective procedure at any time and preferably after a certain degree of maturity has been attained rather than in early infancy. When operating upon these fatty masses, great care must be taken to identify and preserve for adequate closure the herniated dura hidden in the lipoma.

It is fortunate that infants born with meningoceles not only escape the crippling effects of the segmental neural deficits but also are usually spared the vicissitudes and ravages of progressive hydrocephalus. In the average case, some degree of hydrocephalus may be present, but unless air contrast ventriculograms are made, this cannot be stated with certainty. It is likely that minimal hydrocephalus, spontaneously arrested, is present and is sufficiently subtle so that head enlargement is not recognizable. The majority of the lesions that constitute the conditions of spina bifida cystica are myelomeningoceles, only about 4 per cent representing the true meningocele. The simple meningocele is less apt to be associated with progressive hydrocephalus, and those that do so are usually located at the cranial cervical or upper dorsal levels (15 per cent). It is almost axiomatic, therefore, that the lower the level of the meningocele, the less the likelihood of developing hydrocephalus. Hydrocephalus can be expected to occur in 60 to 70 per cent of all cases of spina bifida cystica, in 65 per cent of all cases of myelomeningocele, and in 9 per cent of the true meningoceles.

One of the unscheduled joys of pediatric neurosurgery is the discovery of a relatively harmless meningocele in a newborn child whom one has been called to see because of spina bifida cystica. Not only is the prognosis excellent for a normal and active life, but in the event that operative treatment is required, the anticipated hydrocephalus and the entire galaxy of clinical problems that so often follow fail to materialize.[6, 18]

It should be re-emphasized that the infant with a lumbar mass who shows no neurological deficit and who is otherwise normal probably harbors a meningocele, especially if the mass is pedunculated, covered by skin, and has a narrow neck. If the covering is membranous or ulcerative in the newborn, it is preferable to perform immediate operative repair of the defect rather than subject the infant to the risks of an infected granulating surface from which serious meningeal infection might ensue. The operative repair on such infants should be performed on the first or second day of life; beyond that time the nonepithelialized surfaces are probably heavily contaminated.

The operative excision of a meningocele is not a complicated procedure. Excision of the redundant skin, membrane, and meninges can easily be accomplished with sufficient tissue remaining to effect a layer closure without suture line tension. The interior of the sac may be multiloculated or, more often, a single cavity in free communication with the subarachnoid space of the spinal canal. The neck of the herniation may vary in size from a wide yawning opening bridging several segments to a small narrow neck requiring only a stitch or two to close it. The spinal cord and nerve roots remain in the spinal canal and do not, except in rare instances, intrude into the sac. Inspection of the neural elements will reveal no evidence of myelodysplasia. A watertight dural closure is recommended, followed by imbrication of flaps of lumbosacral aponeurosis across the defect. The skin and subcutaneous tissues are closed as one layer after being mobilized by undermining sufficiently to allow superficial closure without tension. The skin sutures must be tied with strict attention to the preservation of capillary circulation in the skin margins. Blanching or discoloration of the skin between sutures signals an ischemic capillary bed; such sutures must be removed and retied to insure a viable

skin margin, particularly if extensive undermining was necessary.

From this point on, these infants may be treated in every way like normal infants. No special care is required for the spine or back; in essence the surgeon has converted a meningocele into a spina bifida occulta. In such cases there is no need to consider stabilization procedures on the spine or to attempt a spinal fusion at the time of operation. A simple dressing is all that is required until wound healing has taken place, during which time the child can be nursed and handled in a normal fashion, care being exercised to avoid urinary and fecal contamination of the fresh operative wound.

Myelomeningocele

Unfortunately this form of spina bifida cystica represents a common variety of birth defect, one that is devastatingly crippling, and one that presents difficult and perplexing problems to the clinician. These lesions, containing compromised neural tissue in the herniated sac with a myelodysplastic cord segment, may on casual inspection resemble a simple meningocele.

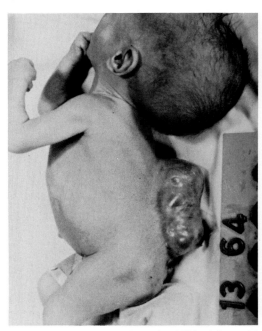

FIGURE 24–2 Extensive spina bifida defect with massive myelomeningocele, hydrocephalus, paralysis of sphincters and lower extremities.

The similarity, however, is only superficial, for these unfortunate infants commonly have paralyzed lower extremities and paralyzed anal and bladder sphincters and in addition are prone to develop progressive hydrocephalus (Fig. 24–2). The awesome problem of caring for them has been of such magnitude and so disappointing in terms of physical and intellectual salvage that for many years most were given no treatment whatsoever. In fact, death of the infant was secretly felt preferable to survival. In many clinics parents were advised to offer only nursing care at home for such children, and no hope was held out for any type of professional assistance. Nash has described such a child as a "paraplegic incontinent cripple, who may be snatched from the jaws of death in the neonatal months, only to be delivered over to the tragedy of an expanding head, or to a life of social exclusion amid the fumes and filth of double incontinence and trophic ulcers."[29] A more dramatic description could not be made! In more recent times, challenging aspects of this common malady have stimulated many centers to bring into play every possible therapeutic advantage for such children in the hope that an educable, and possibly a competitive, individual would result. This can be accomplished only by the combined and energetic efforts of a team involving pediatricians, neurosurgeons, orthopedists, urologists, physical therapists, nurses, social service workers, and speech and audiology representatives. Failures and poor results and complications continue, but the score is gradually improving. The clinical goal of a child who can walk with crutches and braces, who can attend school, who is free of urinary and fecal soilage, and whose hydrocephalus is controlled or arrested is being attained with increasing frequency.

Since there are many variations of myelomeningocele, it is impossible to devote attention to all.[40] Typically such a lesion will involve a spina bifida of from one to four segments, usually in the lumbar area, seldom completely covered by normal skin, usually sessile, and containing a midline neural "plaque" representing the fixation of the spinal cord to the dome or apex of the sac (Fig. 24–3). This portion of the spinal cord represents a local myelodys-

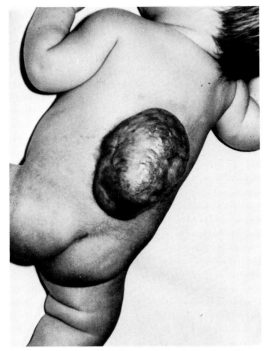

FIGURE 24–3 Sessile myelomeningocele with severe myelodysplasia.

plasia that may be cystic, degenerative, or hypertrophied (by excessive proliferation of neuroglia). In any event, neural function distal to the lesion is ordinarily absent or severely compromised. Clubfoot deformities, a patulous anal sphincter, urinary incontinence, and an oversized head complete the picture of the "typical" case. Those who will contend with these problems have in truth accepted a real challenge.[1, 5, 13, 22, 23, 28, 29, 35, 41]

The neurosurgeon who is called to consult on a newborn of the type just described is compelled to make an important decision. Several options are available:

1. He can recommend that nothing be done, that the prognosis is too poor to justify therapy other than the humanitarian measures of feeding and the usual infant care.

2. He can recommend operative closure and repair of the myelomeningocele at a later date depending on the satisfactory growth and development of the infant and the arrest of hydrocephalus (Fig. 24–4).

3. He can recommend that first priority

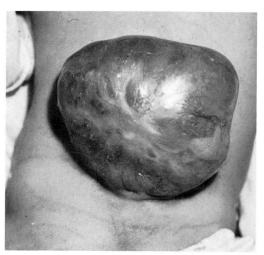

FIGURE 24–4 Typical spina bifida cystica covered by thin squamous epithelium. Danger of ulceration and leakage is constantly present.

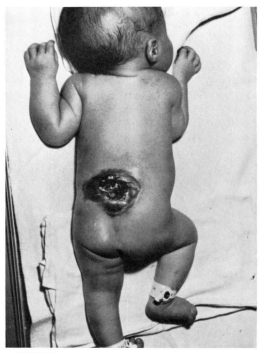

FIGURE 24–5 Myelomeningocele ruptured at birth. Prompt definitive closure is indicated.

be given to the problem of hydrocephalus with appropriate shunting procedures if necessary and ultimately a tardy repair of the myelomeningocele.

4. He can recommend immediate repair and closure of the spinal defect within the first 72 hours of neonatal life, followed by other corrective measures for hydrocephalus, foot deformities, and urinary sphincter incontinence as indicated (Fig. 24–5).

There are good and valid reasons that can be presented in favor of each of the options just presented, and each physician must decide on the basis of his personal preference and conviction so long as any decision can be considered controversial.

For several reasons, the preferable one seems to be to advocate an early and aggressive approach to this problem if the infant's condition will permit. Closure of myelomeningocele should be carried out on the first or second day of life. By so doing, it is felt, the problem of the denuded, weeping, granulating, and contaminated sac can be avoided and the likelihood of meningitis can be to a large extent obviated. In

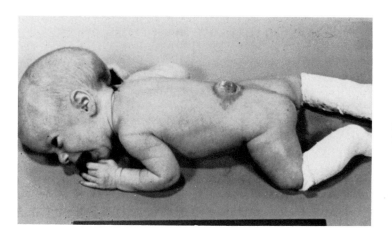

FIGURE 24–6 Small myelomeningocele. Closure should have been performed during first day of life. Casts for correction of clubfoot deformities were instituted early. Hydrocephalus is present.

addition, the closure of the sac facilitates the normal handling of the infant and is of great psychological help to the parents as well as shortening the period of necessary hospitalization of the infant. If one accepts the premise that all clean wounds should be closed, there appears to be no conflict in applying this philosophy to this particular situation (Fig. 24–6).

In the authors' experience, early closure of the defect has not resulted in detectable improvement in the neurological deficits as some have reported. Care should be taken to avoid generating false hopes in the minds of the parents in this regard. The danger of promoting the advance of hydrocephalus, except temporarily, by early operative repair is yet to be firmly established and is a debatable issue at present.

Nothing could be more erroneous than to assume that a blanket policy could be adopted that would apply to all cases. Good clinical judgment would dictate against an operative procedure of such magnitude that it would jeopardize the infant's chance of survival. If the sac is not excessively large and sessile, and if it can be repaired with operative ease, it should be done. If the defect is flat and extensive as in the case of a large rachischisis, operation is not indicated, and such lesions are better left undisturbed (Fig. 24–2). Those masses that are covered by normal skin require no operative consideration until later when cosmetic considerations and possible intraspinal masses indicate the need for surgical investigation.[37]

The frankly ruptured sac or one that is leaking cerebrospinal fluid from a minute perforation or area of distention should be closed if infection is not already present. When the child is seen several days after birth and the surface of the sac cannot be considered clean, there is no reason to consider operative closure, since meningitis will almost certainly ensue and a breakdown of the wound with cerebrospinal fluid leakage is virtually unavoidable (Fig. 24–7). In such cases it is preferable to attempt to promote the growth of healthy granulation tissue over the membranous portion of the sac and then to promote epithelialization by applying pinch grafts or small split grafts to the area. This may save weeks of waiting for epithelium to progress from the edges

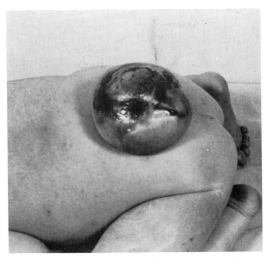

FIGURE 24–7 Sacral myelomeningocele. Ulceration and infection are present. Sphincter function is impaired.

of the defect. In male infants we have obtained excellent skin covering by the simple expedient of circumcision, using the stretched and split prepuce as a useful skin graft that remains soft and pliable and has prevented excessive scarring and fibrosis of the sac.

The development of hydrocephalus is an indication of the need for early shunting of the ventricular fluid, and in conformity with the principle of early closure of the back, early operation for the hydrocephalus is recommended, understanding full well that failures and problems are inherent in a certain proportion of cases so treated. In fact, some will prove to be hopelessly complicated, and the patient will succumb to infection, increased intracranial pressure, or the like. However, no apology need be made for any failure in this field of endeavor, since every practical alternative of treatment may present a similarly disappointing result.

If infection is avoided and the child's condition is otherwise satisfactory, attention is diverted from the dysrhaphic defect to the problem of hydrocephalus. It is apparent that if ventricular dilation continues unchecked, cerebral damage will result that can be irreversible; it is advisable in this instance to perform a shunting procedure before the back lesion is repaired. In some cases in which this reversed order was carried out, there was sufficient collapse and shrinkage of the sac that operative repair has been indefinitely deferred. Decisions regarding the concomitant treatment of hydrocephalus must be made on the basis of circumferential head measurements, ventricular size, and cortical mantle thickness plus other signs of increasing cranial pressure. It is hoped that more sophisticated studies employing radioactive iodinated serum albumin scanning techniques will offer some help in making these clinical judgments in the future.

The association of hydrocephalus with myelomeningocele occurs peculiarly with spinal lesions in the thoracolumbar and upper sacral areas and with diminishing frequency as the higher levels of the vertebral segments are involved (Fig. 24–8). The reason for this is not known. The contributing features that produce hydrocephalus in spina bifida cystica in the majority of cases relate to the associated Arnold-Chiari malformation, producing an obstruction at the foramen magnum by virtue of cerebellar and hindbrain herniation and by obliteration of the subarachnoid spaces at the tentorial incisura. The association of this malformation with stenosis, atresia, or forking of the cerebral aqueduct is well established and represents a partial explanation for the progressive ventricular dilatation. Atresia of the foramina of Luschka and Magendie (Dandy-Walker syndrome) may also occur in conjunction with myelomeningocele.[2, 4, 9, 10, 32, 33, 39] The occurrence of hydrocephalus shows some peculiar differences when related to the segmented levels involved. Since about 75 per cent of all cases of spina bifida cystica develop hydrocephalus to some degree, usually related to the Arnold-Chiari malformation, it is surprising that such differences should relate to the vertebral levels at all. Yet it is true that, of those patients whose lesions occupy the thorocolumbar area, the highest percentage (89 per cent) develop hydrocephalus; of those with lesions occurring at a low sacral level, the lowest percentage (36 per cent); and of those with lesions of the cervical and lumbar areas, 65 to 70 per cent each.

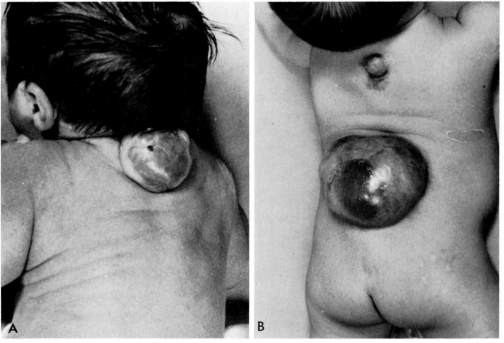

FIGURE 24–8 *A.* Upper thoracic meningocele. No neurological deficit or hydrocephalus. *B.* Multiple dysrhaphic defects. Small thoracic and large lumbar myelomeningoceles.

The operative repair of a myelomeningocele may prove to be a simple uncomplicated undertaking when the defect is small and the neural tissue can be reposited easily within the spinal canal and when there is sufficient dura and cutaneous tissue for adequate closure. In some instances, the operation can tax the surgical ingenuity of the most accomplished surgeon. In large lesions with large defects, adequate shifting of skin flaps must be planned to allow for the superficial closure, requiring undermining for considerable distances laterally as well as above and below the defect; in the occasional case, relaxation incisions may be required. Inspection of the sac contents should be made early in the operation by opening the sac widely and excising the redundant membranous covering, but preserving as much as possible of the dura, which usually terminates at the margin of the skin edge where it is fused, the remainder of the sac being composed of arachnoidal membrane. It is unwise to attempt a meticulous dissection of the neural plaque from the adherent sac. The entire neural mass is preserved and placed within the spinal canal, leaving the attenuated nerve roots undisturbed but enclosed in the enfolded dural sac, which is closed loosely over the plaque within the reconstructed spinal canal. If the canal is shallow or the neural mass is too large to lie in the canal, it should be left outside the canal, and the dura should be reconstructed over it and closed with interrupted silk sutures. The association of diastematomyelia with spina bifida cystica must be kept in mind and looked for while the dural compartment is open. If it is advisable to obtain a more generous exposure during the procedure of repair, a one-segment laminectomy above or below the dural opening will usually suffice. This is especially necessary if the spur of an associated diastematomyelia is to be removed. To persist in performing a tight and constricting closure over a small and shallow canal will only create an ischemic compression necrosis of the tissues one is trying to preserve. The procedure is completed by approximating or imbricating reflected flaps of lumbodorsal aponeurosis over the dural repair and then approximating the skin flaps. The wound must be kept free of urinary and fecal soilage by a sealed dressing and prone positioning until epithelial healing at the suture line has occurred.

The postoperative care is not associated with any particular problems, barring the development of wound infection, dehiscence, or cerebrospinal fluid leakage. Constant attention must be paid to the possibility of developing hydrocephalus and the appearance of a tense fontanelle, dilated scalp veins, and frank cranial enlargement; opisthotonos may signal the beginning of serious intracranial hypertension requiring measures to alleviate this life-threatening complication. As already mentioned, a ventricular shunting procedure may be necessary, and in some a decompression of the occipitocervical region may be required when the Arnold-Chiari malformation is producing signs of local compression of the bulbar mechanism.

The common deformities of the lower extremities relating to the myelomeningocele are congenital dislocation of the hips and, more frequently, the clubfoot deformity of talipes equinovarus. These are most certainly distinct and separate deformities and are not the result of the paralytic state, although dislocation of the hips may later appear as the result of the paralysis. Early corrective molding of the feet is carried out by our orthopedic colleagues concurrently with other therapeutic measures being undertaken. Abduction splinting for the congenital hip dislocation lends itself quite well to the management of the other problems, and on a daily basis, passive manipulations by physical therapists aid in reducing the abnormal postures and contractures that may occur in the paralytic limbs. It is anticipated that every child will have the potential capacity to walk with appropriate bracing and other mechanical aids. If this fails to materialize, it should not be because of failure to begin corrective measures early. Later the child may require various forms of corrective operative treatment to improve performance in ambulation, but these issues have to be met on an individual basis and may in part be influenced by factors difficult to quantitate, such as personal motivation of the child and the parents, home environment, intellectual capacity, and educability. Of particular importance is the regular periodic evaluation of the child's intellectual potential. This quantitative estimate of the mental capabilities serves as an extremely valuable aid in forecasting his educational future. Furthermore, such information may play an important role in future clinical decisions relating to further efforts toward ambulation and other aspects of developmental training.[36]

A particularly distressing spinal deformity may exist in which the dysrhaphic lesion takes the form of a severe local kyphosis, often so prominent that the anterior faces of the involved vertebrae are opposite each other. This drastic deformity not only makes adequate closure of the lesion difficult, but the bony prominences thus produced are certain to become the site of pressure decubiti and present a recurrent problem of healing and prevention. In a few selected children whose outlook is favorable in other respects, correction of this kyphotic deformity may be undertaken by removal of the appropriate vertebral bodies in conjunction with a spinal fusion.

One of the most prominent causes of continued morbidity and death in the child who has survived the early problems of major dysrhaphism is urinary tract infection and renal failure. The social problem associated with the malodorous urinary incontinence is itself a distressing and compelling reason for seeking relief, but of great importance is the insidious damage that may ensue from recurrent infections, ureteral reflux, pyelectasia, and renal failure. The neurogenic bladder associated with myelomeningocele is usually of the flaccid atonic type, the segmental nerve supply being compromised at the level of the lumbar or sacral myelodysplasia. There is, therefore, a relatively complete denervation of the bladder without the likelihood of any of the spinal reflex arcs influencing bladder or sphincter muscle. The relaxed voluminous bladder without sphincteric resistance may always contain urine, always be dribbling, and allow for ureteral distention and reflux, which increases intrapelvic pressure and dilation of the calyces and can finally lead to uremic coma and death. Stated simply, it is imperative that these infants from the outset have the constant attention of an interested urologist who can evaluate the urological status on a continuing basis and

is prepared to carry out diversionary measures when indicated. Of the greatest help is the voiding cinecystourethrogram and the evaluation of bladder and ureteral behavior at varying levels of intravesical pressure.

The use of ileal loop conduits has been of particular value in those cases in which preservation of renal function demands some type of diversion as well as in those in which relief is sought for social reasons and the avoidance of constant wetness. This has been particularly effective in female children who cannot be kept dry by the wearing of an external vulvar appliance.[30, 38]

Finally, some degree of clinical success can be conceded in the severe case of a child who has weathered (1) an operative repair of his myelomeningocele; (2) control of hydrocephalus by ventricular shunt; (3) operative or manipulative correction of clubfeet and dislocated hips; and (4) the establishment of an ileal conduit for urinary diversion. Such a child, who has learned to walk with aid of crutches and braces, and who is demonstrating that he is edu-

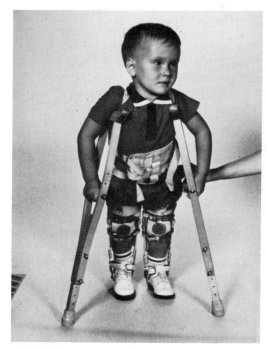

FIGURE 24–9 Lumbar myelomeningocele repaired early. Ventriculoatrial shunt functioning. Urinary diversion by ileal conduit. Ambulation with crutches and braces. Child is educable.

cable and is motivated to continue an increasingly independent existence, can be considered to have been clinically salvaged (Fig. 24–9). Obviously this is a large order and it can be achieved in only a few; varying levels of success must be accepted by parents and physicians when the child's potentials for development and training have been reached. It is of paramount importance that rapport and mutual sharing of responsibilities among the professional persons involved and the child and its parents be maintained.

ENCEPHALOCELE

Cranial defects through which meningeal herniations occur are by common usage termed encephaloceles. Properly, cranium bifidum with a meningeal sac containing only cerebrospinal fluid is a cranial meningocele. A similar lesion containing neural tissue is more accurately a true encephalocele. The embryological reasons for the development of these defects is similar to that alluded to in relationship to other forms of dysrhaphism. Encephalocele is less common than the spinal forms, but it occurs frequently enough to constitute a problem in pediatric management in all large centers. In contradistinction to myelomeningocele, encephalocele is not associated with the gloomy prognosis attached to spina bifida cystica. Cranial meningocele, like spinal meningocele, requires only careful operative removal and cosmetic restoration to make for a successful result. In some instances the sac is huge and may equal or surpass the infant's head in size, but when the base is narrow and the sac is pedunculated, the cranial defect is usually small and the operative excision of such a massive lesion is quite simple.

Encephaloceles may occur at any point along the cranial midline. The most common site is the occipital area, where the protruding pendulous appendage is sufficiently deforming and grotesque to create consternation in all concerned (Fig. 24–10). Such children, because of the great disfigurement are often referred promptly for cosmetic correction. Unless rupture is imminent, or unless leakage has already occurred, there is no reason for great haste in the repair of encephaloceles, and it is

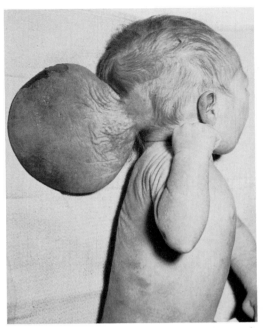

FIGURE 24–10 Pedunculated occipital encephalocele containing cerebrospinal fluid and cerebellar tissue. Easily repairable.

usually recommended that the infant be progressing satisfactorily in his early development before operative repair is performed. Small encephaloceles may be hidden by a generous growth of hair and do not create the cosmetic problem of the large lesion; they are thus apt to be neglected until ulceration and infection occur, presenting then the same problem as the myelomeningocele with inadequate skin covering. Occasionally the small anteriorly placed encephalocele is mistaken for a sebaceous or dermoid cyst, and removal is attempted as an office procedure, a mistake that could be costly.[7, 11, 17]

Encephaloceles that present as facial masses through the nasofrontal area are very disfiguring and can only effectively be repaired transcranially with dural reinforcement by fascia or by dural imbrication and suture after the meningeal sac and its contents have been excised or reposited within the cranium (Fig. 24–11). The presence of a mass occluding the nasal passages in an infant or child should always arouse the suspicion of an intranasal encephalocele. Careful examination for pulsation, for increased tension by Valsalva maneuver,

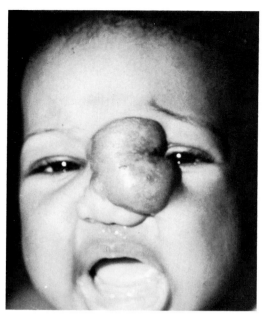

FIGURE 24–11 Frontonasal encephalocele. Transcranial repair is indicated.

and for defects in the bony anterior fossa by tomography may be of aid in the diagnosis. Encephaloceles so located have been "snared" by the wire loop technique of removing nasal polyps by mistake.

When the operative removal of an encephalocele is undertaken, the sac should first be opened for inspection of the contents and to evacuate the fluid compartment, allowing for ease in handling the collapsed mass. If cerebral or cerebellar tissue is present, it can usually be reintroduced within the cranium, but in a few instances the mass of tissue present precludes this possibility, and sacrifice of the neural tissue is necessary. Such tissue is often atrophic and gliotic and may be without function. The dura should be excised near the cranial defect, care being taken to preserve sufficient dura to allow an imbrication type closure for additional strength. Fortunately there is rarely a paucity of skin, the cutaneous closure being performed in a way best designed for acceptable cosmetic results. No attempt is made to cover the cranial defect with bone, plastic, or metal.

Hydrocephalus is not as frequently associated with cranial meningoceles and en-cephalocele as with the spinal variant of these dysrhaphic states, occurring in about one fourth of occipital meningoceles and in two thirds of occipital encephalocele, and rarely, if ever, in the frontal, nasal, or orbital defects. If obstruction of the fourth ventricle or the foraminal outlets occurs or if there are associated malformations of the cerebral aqueduct or hindbrain, the problem of progressive ventricular enlargement will have to be met by the same techniques described elsewhere. This is not likely to occur with encephaloceles located anywhere except in the occipital or occipitocervical area. The repair of occipital encephaloceles must be done with the possibility of a posterior fossa exploration kept in mind. If septa, blind compartments, adhesions, and deformities of this intracranial area are present, the excision and repair of the encephalocele may not be successful, and a secondary procedure will be necessary. It is preferable to carry out an appropriate craniotomy with a careful inspection of the area to insure patency of fluid pathways if possible.

The contents of an encephalocele sac cannot be precisely determined except by direct inspection during the operation. However, the presence of neural tissue within the sac may be detected by palpation, by air contrast studies, or (recently) by arteriography. It is not essential that these studies be carried out unless there is reason to suspect other major intracranial malformations that might preclude the consideration of operation for the encephalocele.

SPINA BIFIDA WITH ANTERIOR MENINGOCELE

These rare lesions have been reported sporadically and may occur most often as meningeal herniations into the pelvis, vagina, rectum, or gluteal areas from defects in the anterior sacrum. Some have attained massive proportions, interfering with parturition, bladder and bowel function, and ambulation. Anterior meningoceles may occur in the thoracic area and be confused with mediastinal or lung lesions. Generally they are best treated conservatively unless there are compelling reasons for operative correction.[1, 40]

DIASTEMATOMYELIA

One of the varieties of occult dysrhaphism that is productive of severe neurological handicap is the peculiar disorder known as diastematomyelia. In this condition the normally low-lying spinal cord is prevented from making its growth ascent by a transfixing cartilaginous or bony spur or septum. The cord is insidiously split as axial growth occurs, and progressive neurological dysfunction may ensue. The frequency with which the anomaly occurs in conjunction with other vertebral defects, such as hemivertebra, failure of segmentation, spina bifida occulta, and myelomeningocele, suggests that some basic fault of the mesenchymal cells occurred during the early period of neural tube development.

Like spina bifida cystica, diastematomyelia is found most often in the lumbar segment of the spinal canal, but it can occur in the thoracic area as well. The cervical area is apparently involved only rarely.

Clinical clues suggesting the presence of this lesion are similar to those described for spina bifida occulta: an area of localized hypertrichosis, a lipomatous mass, a cutaneous dimple, a vascular nevus, or a sinus tract opening. There may be weakness or paralysis and atrophy of the lower extremities, deformities of the feet, saddle area sensory loss, and disturbance of sphincter control. Since these clinical abnormalities may occur with other intraspinal disorders, there is no certain method of identifying the presence of diastematomyelia on neurological examination alone. The disclosure of the calcific spur by radiographic examination is, of course, diagnostic, but in many instances this cannot be ascertained by plain film techniques, since the septum or spur may be cartilaginous or insufficiently calcified to be detected by the usual anteroposterior views of the spine. A characteristic deformity is always present on myelographic study and consists of a central defect in the oil column, which clearly delineates the exact location of the transfixing spur. A myelographic study is recommended for all infants and children who have the superficial signs of an occult form of dysrhaphism and who in addition have major neurological deficits, either stationary or progressive, or who reveal a neurological difficulty when learning to walk.

Examination of the cerebrospinal fluid is not helpful in this condition, since there is no subarachnoid block present and the chemical constituents of the fluid are not altered. Therefore, lumbar puncture should be performed only to introduce the myelographic dye several segments above or below the suspected site of abnormality.

When the diagnosis of diastematomyelia has been confirmed, operative removal of the spur should be advised. There is no assurance that correction of the existing neurological deficits will occur, but the prevention of additional damage to the spinal cord as further growth occurs can be anticipated.[16, 27, 34]

The operation should be initiated with a generous exposure utilizing a laminectomy above and below the lesion for at least one or two segments. The abnormally wide spinal canal at the spur site facilitates the exposure once the posterior arches have been removed. The procedure of choice is to open the dura longitudinally above and below the spur and then to incise the dura adjacent to the spicule in an elliptical fashion so that this medial dura can be excised until it is flush with the anterior dural layer. Resection of the spur is done by careful piecemeal nibbling with a small rongeur until the base is flush with the anterior spinal canal wall. By carefully retracting each segment of the split cord, access to the spur is enhanced. Adhesions between the halves of the cord and the medial dura may require division before mobilization of the cord is feasible. The entire procedure is greatly simplified by the use of a magnifying loupe or the low-power microscope. Occasionally the cord will have been transfixed eccentrically and the two "halves" will be unequal in size, but this does not alter the operative method in any way. Rarely, the transfixion will have occurred just at the conus medullaris with cauda equina rootlets and terminal cord contained within the two dural compartments. The filum terminale should be identified and sectioned to lessen any "tethering" effect on the cord, particularly where it is adherent to the spicule itself.

When the spur and the medial dural leaves have been excised, the medial surfaces of the split cord will be juxtaposed and the posterior dura will close easily, without tension or compression. No attempt at closure of the anterior dura should be made. The postoperative management does not differ from that of any intraspinal operative procedure.

Diplomyelia, a term used to denote a true duplication of the spinal cord, is sometimes used interchangeably with diastematomyelia. Unless one can demonstrate by histological study that each cord is complete and has appropriate anterior and posterior roots, it is difficult to justify this designation. If nerve rootlets are seen emerging from the medial surfaces of the cords, there is strong likelihood that a diplomyelia exists, or perhaps an imperfect variant of it. This condition is thought to represent a form of incomplete twinning.

CONGENITAL DERMAL SINUS

One of the most benign-appearing but potentially lethal congenital lesions is the congenital dermal sinus. This apparently inoffensive lesion may exist on the surface as a simple pit or depression, which may be surrounded by an area of port-wine skin blemish or hair tufts in and around the dimple. In some cases a small lumpy mass can be palpated at the opening. When infection is present, there is edema, redness, and tenderness of the local area. These sinus tracts can occur at any level of the cerebrospinal axis but are most common in the occipital and the lumbar areas. Since these sites represent the polar aspects of the neural tube, it is logical for them to occupy more frequently the areas corresponding to the anterior and posterior neuropores—those segments lying between being the first to close and to separate from the superficial ectoderm.

The sinus tract is lined with stratified squamous epithelium and extends from the surface through the deeper tissues into the cranial or spinal cavity, usually ending on the dura or within the dura in conjunction with a terminal epidermoid or dermoid cyst. In the spinal canal, the tract may extend through a lamina; or if spina bifida is present, it may enter the spinal canal through the bony defect; or it may penetrate the interlaminar ligaments without relationship to the posterior bony arches. Localized cystic expansions may occur along the course of the tract, suggesting termination of the sinus, but a deeper extension must be expected and followed to its true terminus.

In the cranium, the tract will penetrate the skull and end blindly on the dura, or it will penetrate the dura and end in a cystic expansion within the substance of the cerebellum or fourth ventricle.

The apparently healthy child harboring such a lesion is in jeopardy because of the possibility of acute meningeal infection and subdural abscess. In most instances, an unexplained pyogenic meningitis may be the first clue suggesting the presence of the lesion, which may elude any but the most minute inspection. It should be routine to inspect the midline scalp and spine in all newborn infants for the telltale signs of the sinus opening. When abundant hair covers the scalp, parting the moistened hair along the midline may aid in identifying the lesion. Recurrent staphylococcal meningitis in an infant or child is very likely due to the presence of a cranial dermal sinus, whereas meningitis due to the coliform bacillus is more likely related to a spinal dermal sinus.

A second cause for concern about the presence of a dermal sinus is the possibility of progressive neurological damage due to the compression effects of the mass cystic lesion at the intradural terminus of the tract. Compression of the cauda equina, spinal cord, cerebellum, and lower brain stem may occur. In the posterior fossa, obstruction of the ventricular system will create the additional problem of obstructive hydrocephalus.

It is important to emphasize that the diagnosis of this disorder is dependent more upon the clinical examination of the patient than upon x-ray confirmation. It is true that the sinus tract may produce an identifiable skull defect or spina bifida, but the detection of small bony defects may be impossible in infants and younger children. The failure of such defects to appear on the x-ray film does not militate against the diagnosis. Similarly, since all sinus tracts should be operatively excised, there is little reason for performing routine myelography or air contrast ventriculography in these children unless there are some special reasons for doing so. In the low lumbar and sacral areas, some confusion might exist because of the commonly occurring pilonidal sinus. These tracts end blindly at the sacral fascia, may branch complexly, and are often the source of recurrent local infection, but they cause no neurological damage and do not cause infection of the meninges.

Treatment for congenital dermal sinus is essentially that of operative removal, preferably before infection has occurred, but if not, then certainly when infection has been controlled. When neurological function is being progressively compromised, the operation may become a matter of urgency; otherwise it is preferable to wait until all clinical and bacteriological evidence of infection has subsided. Appropriate antibiotics are continued throughout the immediate postoperative period until complete wound healing has occurred.

The essential features of the operation consist of adequate exposure, preservation of the dissected sinus tract throughout its course, and removal of laminae or skull sufficient to allow intradural exploration of the spinal canal or posterior fossa as the case may be. If mass cystic lesions are present at the central end of the tract, they are removed, piecemeal if necessary, to avoid damage to cord or brain. If the tract ends by attenuation on the dura or pia, it is simply excised. The wound is closed without drainage. When an adherent capsule of an epidermoid or dermoid cyst cannot be easily separated from neural parenchyma, sharp dissection and removal of the capsule is to be avoided. Better to leave some capsule remnant than to risk damage to the brain or spinal cord. This situation is apt to occur following infection resulting in the usual proliferative inflammatory reaction and the subsequent formation of dense adhesions about the infected cyst wall. Failure to relieve obstructive hydrocephalus by excising the sinus tract and its intracranial cyst implies that subarachnoid pathways have been obliterated by postinfection arachnoidal adhesions and it will probably be necessary to consider a ventricular shunting procedure.

The early detection and successful treatment of congenital dermal sinus is a rewarding area in the field of pediatric neurosurgery.[16, 42]

CONGENITAL ABSENCE OF SCALP AND SKULL

The cause of congenital absence of portions of the scalp is obscure, but a familial factor has been prominent in some cases, involving twins, siblings, and members of several generations of the same family.

Absence of the scalp usually occurs over the vertex, the fontanelle areas, and the inferior parietal sites. Some predilection is shown for the areas of the suture lines. Since one fifth of the defective scalp areas occur well away from the midline, it is doubtful that this can be considered a true dysrhaphism (congenital absence of skin also occurs in other nonmidline areas of the body). The lesions may be small punched-out defects, or they may be extensive long defects occupying the entire vertex. There may be normal bone and dura beneath, or one or both may be absent.

In the place of normal scalp, a thin transparent membrane is present through which the underlying skull, dura, or brain can be seen in the newborn. It soon converts to an opaque granulating or darkened exudative eschar. Histologically, the membrane consists of a flattened layer of epithelial cells with absence of sweat glands, sebaceous glands, and hair follicles. The membrane merges gradually at the borders of the defect into normal scalp. Small lesions, amenable to excision and plastic closure, should be repaired early before infection and eschar formation occurs. A simple moist dressing should be applied to prevent drying until the operation has been accomplished. Extensive lesions may require complicated plastic repairs, and the advice of a plastic surgeon is desirable before and during the operation.

Congenital absence of scalp and underlying areas of skull requires primary closure of the scalp defect by scalp or pedicle flap rather than by split graft since cranioplasty may be required later. It cannot be anticipated that spontaneous growth of bone will ultimately cover the defect; therefore, with cranioplasty an expected future necessity, it is advisable to cover the scalp defect with full-thickness skin.

In those instances in which the dura is defective and the vertex surfaces of the brain are exposed, meticulous attention is paid to the prevention of the exudative eschar. Constant wet dressings are required if primary plastic closure with full-thickness flaps or pedicle cannot be done. Eschar formation may result in mechanical tearing of surface vessels with serious hemorrhage. Excision of the eschar must be undertaken as a major operative procedure employing blood replacement and stringent hemostasis. Under conditions of appropriate care with moist dressings, gradual complete epithelialization may occur.

Congenital defects of the skull without overlying scalp defects occur frequently. Some are extensive, and since they are not apt to close spontaneously, they may require a cranioplasty at an older age (3 to 5 years) after head growth has progressed past the stages of rapid development. Smaller defects require no treatment when they occupy the convexity surfaces. Congenital absence of the orbital roof may produce an unsightly pulsating progressive exophthalmos and require a plastic reconstruction interposing a rigid material (bone or tantalum) between the dura and the orbital contents. Similar reparative measures can be employed to correct defects in the greater wing of the sphenoid.[26, 31, 43]

ANOMALIES INVOLVING BRAIN PARENCHYMA

Anencephaly, Cyclopia, and Hydranencephaly

The severest forms of anomalous brain involvement occur in anencephaly, cyclopia, and hydranencephaly. Anencephalic infants do not survive; the brain is rudimentary or absent, usually a large portion of scalp and cranium is absent, and often an extensive spinal rachischisis is present. Cyclopian monsters also have a severely deformed or rudimentary brain, absence of the corpus callosum, a single ventricle, and a midline orbit containing various component parts of an incompletely formed globe. Survival is mercifully not likely. Hydranencephaly occurs in the viable infant and may be present without noticeable enlargement of the head at birth. Presumably, due to circulatory interference to the brain, the cerebral hemispheres are replaced by a sac of fluid contained within a thin gliotic vestige of cortex with only basal ganglia, brain stem, and cerebellum remaining. Cranial transillumination performed after rapid head growth is noted suggests the presence of this disorder. There is no treatment that is effective, although shunting operations have been carried out for purely social reasons and to facilitate home care.

Agenesis of Corpus Callosum

Agenesis of the corpus callosum may occur in relationship to other severe cerebral anomalies or it may exist asymptomatically in an otherwise normal and healthy person. In clinical practice it is usually found by pneumoencephalography as part of an investigation of convulsive seizures or mental retardation. Failure of the commissural fibers of the corpus callosum to cross the midline in whole or in part results in absence of the septum pellucidum and an abnormal arrangement of the convolutions on the medial surface of the hemispheres. No specific neurological deficits are associated with this anomaly, which cannot be blamed for epilepsy or mental retardation.

Agenesis of Cerebellum

Agenesis of the cerebellum may be virtually complete with only the tiniest cerebellar remnant detectable. This may occur bilaterally or it may be confined to one cerebellar hemisphere, in which case the contralateral olivary nucleus may be vestigial.

Arnold-Chiari Malformation

Arnold-Chiari malformation occurs commonly in association with myelomeningocele and is an important contributing factor in the development of hydrocephalus in these children. The malformation involves the cerebellum and lower brain stem, occurring commonly as a downward displacement of the medulla into the spinal canal along with elongated tongues of cerebellar tissue (Type I); or in addition, the medulla may be entirely within the spinal canal, nodular, and widened at its junction with the cervical cord, which is abnormally shortened (Type II). Almost invariably Type II is found associated with myelomeningocele, while Type I is rarely present in these infants and may be found as the cause of obstructive hydrocephalus in older children and adults or as an isolated finding at autopsy. It has also been reported in association with platybasia.

The cause of this deformity is not known, and for years it was assumed that fixation of the cord at the site of a spina bifida resulted in a traction deformity of the medulla and cerebellum as axial growth occurred. This premise is no longer deemed tenable, the more rational explanation being that existing hydrocephalus and an obstructed outlet "pushes" the structures into the abnormal situation, explaining the upward direction taken by the cervical nerve roots in this deformity.

The operative procedure for Arnold-Chiari malformation consists of a generous cervical laminectomy and suboccipital craniectomy. The dura is opened and the cerebellar tissue overlying the medulla and cervical cord carefully teased away or, occasionally, excised to allow for decompression of the cervical canal and cerebellar areas. The vermis should be resected at the apex to relieve obstruction at the terminal fourth ventricle. No cisterna magna is present in these cases, the herniated tissue filling this space completely. The primary purpose of the operation is to relieve the compression in the critical areas involved, to relieve the obstructive hydrocephalus, and to promote communication of the ventricular cerebrospinal fluid with the spinal subarachnoid fluid. It has not been possible to attain these goals uniformly. In particular, infants with myelomeningocele and Arnold-Chiari malformation have, in many instances, still required shunting operations for better control of progressive hydrocephalus even though an adequate operative procedure was carried out for the malformation. This failure must relate to inadequacies of the absorptive mechanism and to failure of cerebrospinal fluid to reach efficient absorptive areas. Currently, unless bulbar decompression is required, the op-

eration for Arnold-Chiari malformation is no longer routinely recommended in the infant with myelomeningocele. Ventriculoatrial shunting is the safest and most expedient way to benefit the ventricular obstruction.

MISCELLANEOUS ANOMALIES OF THE VERTEBRAL COLUMN

While no pretense of complete cataloguing of the vast subject of congenital defects and anomalies has been made, there remain some that are seen with sufficient frequency in pediatric and neurosurgical clinics to justify inclusion in this chapter.

Existing alone or in conjunction with spina bifida and other defects, one may encounter various forms of failure of vertebral segmentation ("congenital fusion"), single or multiple hemivertebrae, or total absence of one or more vertebrae. Coexisting with such defects are kyphoscoliosis, deformities of the chest and ribs, impaired vital capacity, umbilical and lateral flank

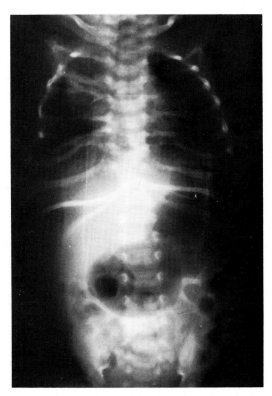

FIGURE 24-12 Hemivertebra. Associated spina bifida.

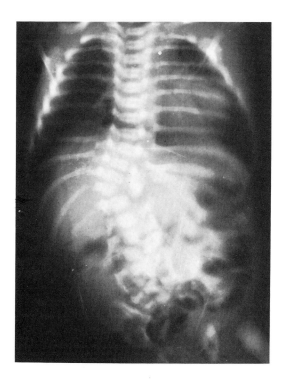

FIGURE 24–13 Hemivertebra. Associated rib anomalies.

FIGURE 24–14 Congenital absence of lumbar vertebra and sacrum.

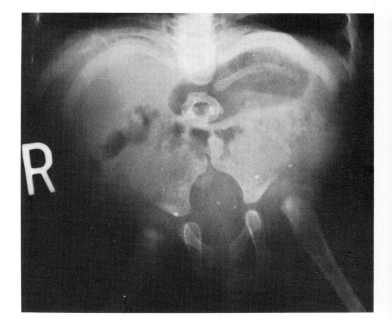

hernias, and various degrees of neurological impairment of function of the lower extremities and bowel and bladder sphincters. Unfortunately, no specific treatment can be recommended for these anomalies (Figs. 24–12, 24–13, 24–14).

REFERENCES

1. Adson, A. W.: Spina bifida cystica of the pelvis. Minn. Med., *21*:468, 1938.
2. Alexander, B., Patten, B. M., and Stewart, B. H.: Possible factors in the development of the Arnold-Chiari malformation. J. Neurosurg., *14*:285, 1957.
3. Anderson, F. M.: Occult spinal dysraphism. J. Pediat., *73*:163, 1968.
4. Chorobski, J., and Stepien, L.: On the syndrome of Arnold-Chiari. Report of a case. J. Neurosurg., *5*:495, 1948.
5. Coller, F. A., and Jackson, R. G.: Anterior sacral meningocele. Surg. Gynec. Obstet., *76*:703, 1943.
6. Doran, P. A., and Guthkelch, A. N.: Studies in spina bifida cystica: I. General survey and reassessment of the problem. J. Neurol. Neurosurg. Psychiat., *24*:331, 1961.
7. Fisher, R. G., Uihlein, A., and Keith, H. M.: Spina bifida and cranium bifidum: Study of 530 cases. Proc. Mayo Clin., *27*:33, 1952.
8. Gardner, W. J: Anatomic anomalies common to myelomeningocele of infancy and syringomyelia of adulthood suggest a common origin. Cleveland Clin. Quart., *26*:118, 1959.
9. Gardner, W. J.: Myelomeningocele, the result of rupture of the embryonic neural tube. Cleveland Clin. Quart., *27*:88, 1960.
10. Gardner, W. J., and Goodall, R. J.: The surgical treatment of Arnold-Chiari malformation in adults. J. Neurosurg., *7*:199, 1950.
11. Gross, S. W., and Sachs, E.: Spina bifida and cranium bifidum. Arch. Surg., *28*:874, 1934.
12. Guthkelch, A. N.: Discussion on the problems of spina bifida cystica. Proc. Roy. Soc. Med., *50*:738, 1957.
13. Guthkelch, A. N.: Studies in spina bifida cystica. II. When to repair the spinal defect. J. Neurol. Neurosurg. Psychiat., *25*:137, 1962.
14. Hamby, W. B.: Pilonidal cyst, spina bifida occulta, and bifid spinal cord. Arch. Path., *21*:831, 1936.
15. Hoffman, E. P.: The problem of spina bifida and cranium bifidum. Clin. Pediat., *4*:709, 1965.
16. Ingraham, F. D., and Matson, D. D.: Neurosurgery of Infancy and Childhood. Springfield, Ill., Charles C Thomas, 1954.
17. Ingraham, F. D., and Scott, H. W., Jr.: Spina bifida and cranium bifidum. V. The Arnold-Chiari malformation: A study of 20 cases. New Eng. J. Med., *229*:108, 1943.
18. Jackson, I. J., and Thompson, R. K.: Pediatric Neurosurgery. Springfield, Ill., Charles C Thomas, 1959.
19. Jelsma, F., and Ploetner, E. J.: Painful spina bifida occulta. J. Neurosurg., *10*:19, 1953.
20. Kennedy, W. P.: Epidemiologic Aspects of the Problem of Congenital Malformations. Birth Defects—National Foundation, Vol. III, No. 2, 1967.
21. Lawrence, K. M.: Natural history of spina bifida cystica. Arch. Dis. Child., *39*:41, 1964.
22. Lichtenstein, B. W.: Spinal dysraphism. Arch. Neurol. Psychiat., *44*:792, 1940.
23. Lichtenstein, B. W.: Distant neuroanatomic complications of spina bifida (spinal dysraphism). Arch. Neurol. Psychiat., *47*:195, 1942.
24. Lichtenstein, B. W.: Cervical syringomyelia and syringomyelia-like states associated with the Arnold-Chiari deformity and platybasia. Arch. Neurol. Psychiat., *49*:881, 1943.
25. Lichtenstein, B. W.: A Textbook of Neuropathology. Philadelphia, W. B. Saunders Co., 1949.
26. List, C. F.: Neurologic syndromes accompanying developmental anomalies of occipital bone, atlas and axis. Arch. Neurol. Psychiat., *45*:577, 1941.
27. Maxwell, H. P., and Bucy, P. C.: Diastematomyelia: Report of clinical case. J. Neuropath. Neurol., *5*:165, 1946.
28. Merrill, R. E., McCutcheon, T., Meacham, W. F., and Carter, T.: Myelomeningocele and hydrocephalus. J.A.M.A., *191*:21, 1965.
29. Nash, D. F. E.: Congenital spinal palsy. Brit. Med. J., *2*:1333, 1956.
30. Nash, D. F. E.: Ileal loop bladder in congenital spinal palsy. Brit. J. Urol., *28*:387, 1956.
31. O'Brien, B. McC., and Drake, J. E.: Congenital defects of skull and scalp. Brit. J. Plas. Surg., *13*:102, 1960.
32. Parker, H. L., and Kernohan, J. W.: Stenosis of the aqueduct of Sylvius. Arch. Neurol. Psychiat., *29*:538, 1933.
33. Penfield, W., and Coburn, D. F.: Arnold-Chiari malformation and its operative treatment. Arch. Neurol. Psychiat., *40*:328, 1938.
34. Pickles, W.: Duplication of spinal cord (diplomyelia). J. Neurosurg., *6*:324, 1949.
35. Russell, D. S., and Donald, C.: The mechanism of internal hydrocephalus in spina bifida. Brain, *58*:203, 1935.
36. Sharrard, W. J. W.: Congenital parlytic dislocation of the hip in children with myelomeningocele. J. Bone Joint Surg., *41-B*:622, 1959.
37. Sharrard, W. J. W., Zachary, R. B., Lorber, J., and Bruce, A. M.: A controlled trial of immediate and delayed closure of spina bifida cystica. Arch. Dis. Child., *38*:18, 1963.
38. Smith, E. D.: Spina Bifida and the Total Care of Spinal Myelomeningocele. Springfield, Ill., Charles C Thomas, 1965.
39. Steele, G. H.: The Arnold-Chiari malformation. Brit. J. Surg., *34*:280, 1947.
40. Thomas, T. G.: Pelvic spina bifida. Gaillard's Med. J., *40*:237, 1885.
41. Von Recklinghausen, F. D.: Untersuchungen über die Spina bifida. Virchow Arch. Path. Anat., *105*:243, 1882.
42. Walker, A. E., and Bucy, P. C.: Congenital dermal sinuses: A source of spinal meningeal infection and subdural abscesses. Brain, *57*:401, 1934.
43. Walker, J. C., Koenig, J. A., Irwin, L., and Meijer, R.: Congenital absence of skin. Plast. Reconstr. Surg., *26*:209, 1960.

25

CRANIOSYNOSTOSIS

DEFINITION OF TERMS

Abnormal fusion of various membranous bones of the skull will cause deformities to develop by limiting the ability of the skull to expand in a direction perpendicular to the involved suture. For example, an abnormal adherence between the parietal bones prevents widening of the skull except as the squamosal sutures may permit (Fig. 25–1). The untreated child will develop an elongated upside-down-canoe-shaped head to which the term scaphocephaly ("boat-head") has been applied. Since this condition is due to absence of at least a part of the sagittal suture, the anatomical term "sagittal synostosis" more clearly defines the condition and its cause.

Similarly, all abnormalities of skull contour caused by absence of all or part of a cranial suture or sutures, may be so defined.

Multiple or *total synostosis* indicates involvement of several or all the cranial sutures.

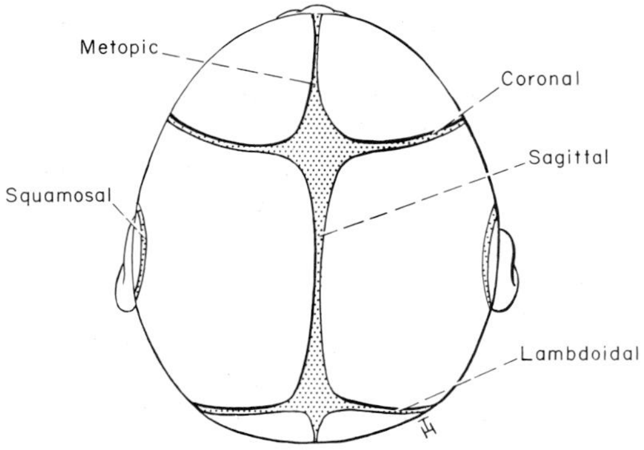

As is illustrated later, absence of only part of the length of a suture will permit variation in the appearance of children with involvement of identical sutures, and will cause the patent portion of the involved suture to be obliterated progressively and prematurely. This may make early diagnosis difficult since routine x-ray projections may not adequately show the synostotic area.

Primary craniosynostosis implies a spontaneous failure of development of all or part of one or more cranial sutures.

Secondary synostosis indicates obliteration of one or more sutures prematurely.

Secondary sagittal synostosis may occur in a hydrocephalic child after shunting, which so collapses the ventricular system that the parietal bones override and fuse.[11] Only primary synostosis is discussed in this chapter.

SIGNIFICANCE

Since deformity of the skull is produced by its inability to respond to the growth of the brain at involved sites, the condition worsens with time during the period of brain growth, which is particularly rapid during the first several months of life (Fig. 25–2).[5] Timely surgical intervention will permit an improvement of the appearance of the skull. It must be stressed that there will be worsening of the deformity if nothing is done.

Constriction of the brain and interference with its function can occur if many or all sutures are involved.[14] X-ray examination should easily rule out total primary cranio-

FIGURE 25–1 Normal sutures, infant's skull. (From Shillito, J., and Matson, D. D.: Pediatrics, *41*: 829–853, 1968. Reprinted with permission.)

J. SHILLITO, JR.

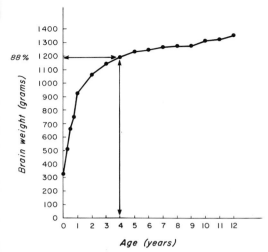

FIGURE 25-2 Growth curve of brain. By 4 years of age, 88 per cent of the weight of a 12-year-old brain has been achieved. During this period of rapid growth, cosmetic improvement will be most rewarding following craniectomy. Operation carried out during first few weeks of life permits greatest change in appearance. (From Shillito, J., and Matson, D. D.: Pediatrics, *41*:829–853, 1968. Reprinted with permission.)

In all cases, adequate operative treatment can permit return to, or toward, a normal appearance of the skull, depending on age at operation, degree of deformity, and the sutures involved. With operation, the threat, however small, of subsequent brain damage can simultaneously be removed. This combination of indications warrants intervention except when age precludes cosmetic improvement and no evidence of increased intracranial pressure exists. The aforementioned 8-year-old boy would fall in this category. Little, if any, cosmetic change can be expected after 4 years of age.

ETIOLOGY

The cause of primary craniosynostosis is not known.[12] There is no evidence that it is caused by deficiency of brain underlying the involved suture. The condition is known to occur in utero, and probably always does begin there. Delay in making the correct diagnosis leads to the false impression that primary craniosynostosis develops after birth.

The defect is presumed to be one of membranous bones or their anlage. Operative findings indicate that very often only part of the involved suture is missing, suggesting that a short area of stenosis is adequate to prevent separation of the adjacent bones, and giving to the remaining patent portion of the suture the false signal that it is no longer needed.[3] This allows progressive obliteration of that suture only, just as obliteration of all sutures occurs after brain growth ceases in normal individuals.

The importance of mechanical factors in maintaining patency of cranial sutures has been noted when on occasion an artificial suture has developed and persisted in a craniectomy site, even when the craniectomy has been made in an unnatural parasagittal position.[15] Such iatrogenic sutures have been seen, unpredictably, on many postoperative films. They do not necessarily occur at the site of the old bone edge, but may be anywhere in the new bone formation. As yet, none have been explored surgically, for their presence seems to guarantee a functional craniectomy.

Histologically, there is nothing remark-

synostosis as the cause of inadequate skull growth. Fortunately, total synostosis is rare, and the asymmetry of the skull produced by the more common subtotal synostosis quickly draws attention to the problem.

The effect upon brain function of synostosis of a single suture is questionable.[16] It is clear, however, that the psychological effect of a noticeably misshapen head is important, and its prevention is in itself an indication for operation. An example is an 8-year-old boy who required neurosurgical consultation because his elongated head, the result of untreated sagittal synostosis, had marked him as unusual and he had become the target of jokes and taunts from his second-grade classmates. He had developed a duodenal ulcer. Thorough testing revealed normal intelligence and no evidence of increased intracranial pressure, but only emotional problems caused by the appearance of his head.

Documentation of increased intracranial pressure is difficult in infants with synostosis involving one or two sutures; normal sutures widen as brain growth demands, and x-ray changes alone may indicate adaptation rather than intracranial hypertension.

able about a suture that is partially obliterated, nor is the bone that occupies the suture's normal position characteristic except that it is apt to be unusually thick. A normal suture consists of fibrous tissue to which adhere both pericranium and dura. The synostosis in serial section shows the gradual narrowing and ultimate disappearance of the fibrous tissue.[12] There are no changes in either the adjacent pericranium

or the dura that might explain the formation of a suture or the reason for its absence.

DIAGNOSIS

Craniosynostosis of one or several cranial sutures can be suspected, and in some cases confirmed, by observing the shape and symmetry of the vault, the presence of a ridge of bone replacing the involved

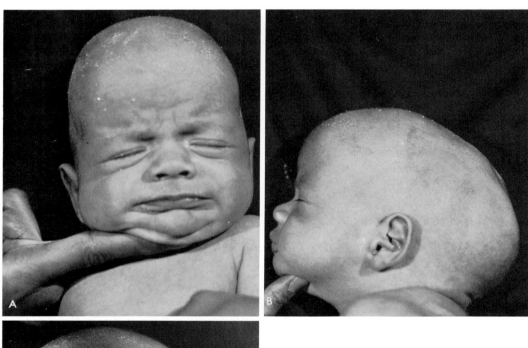

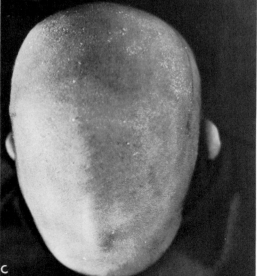

FIGURE 25–3 Sagittal synostosis. *A.* Except in frontal area, widest portion of skull is at or just above squamosal sutures. *B.* Note elongation of head, particularly noticeable after it has been shaved. *C.* Child is face up; elongation of head is much more noticeable. Note presence of ridge in sagittal region posteriorly where head is also narrowest. In this case, the anterior few centimeters of sagittal suture were patent, as was the anterior fontanelle. (From Shillito, J., and Matson, D. D.: Pediatrics, *41:*829–853, 1968. Reprinted with permission.)

suture, clues about the orbits and face, and mobility of cranial bones under palpation adjacent to the sutures. Appropriate x-rays will establish the diagnosis.

Sagittal Synostosis

The width of the skull in sagittal synostosis is as significant as the presence or absence of a ridge. The anterior fontanelle is patent in over half of such patients. One third will show closure of only part of the suture, usually the posterior two thirds.[17] A sagittal ridge is also found where the head is most narrow (Fig. 25–3). These findings are common in infants of a few weeks of age, suggesting that the initial site of fusion is posterior and obliteration progresses anteriorly with age.

Radiographic findings clarify the length of the parietal bones; may indicate excessive separation of the coronal, lambdoid, and squamosal sutures; and in anteroposterior view may reveal thickening of bone in the sagittal area (Fig. 25–4). A straight crack may replace the suture in this thickened bone; this is usually adjacent to the fused area. It must be appreciated that a true anteroposterior view projects the profile of the anterior portion of the sagittal suture. A Towne's view (anteroposterior projection 30 degrees above the orbito-meatal line) will be tangent to and illustrate better the part of the suture more usually involved. The "beaten silver" appearance of the skull due to increased intracranial pressure is not present in infancy, and its absence is not significant. The sagittal suture is by far the most commonly involved, with about five times the frequency of the next most commonly affected single suture, the coronal.[16] The male is predominantly involved in a ratio of 3.6 males to 1 female.

Unilateral Coronal Synostosis

Unilateral coronal synostosis prevents development of the ipsilateral frontal boss, giving a flattened appearance to the forehead on that side. The brow ridge is less well developed, and in sighting over the infant's head from above, one sees the upper eyelid rather than the brow. The anterior fontanelle, present in 55 per cent of cases, is not in the midline, but will be drawn *toward the normal side*. The ridge may be present in about one quarter of these children, but it is less prominent and of less help clinically. Discrepancy in the ease of producing motion by pressure along the bone edges on each side is of help if the involvement includes the medial part of the suture. Laterally motion is harder to

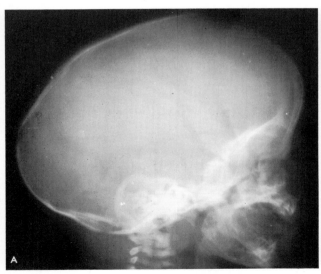
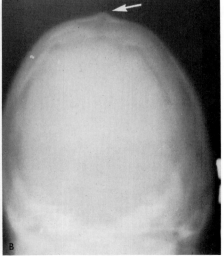

FIGURE 25–4 Sagittal synostosis, same patient as shown in Figure 25–3. Note widening of uninvolved coronal, lambdoid, and squamosal sutures, *A,* and the sagittal ridge in the Towne's view, *B.* (From Shillito, J., and Matson, D. D.: Pediatrics, *41*:829–853, 1968. Reprinted with permission.)

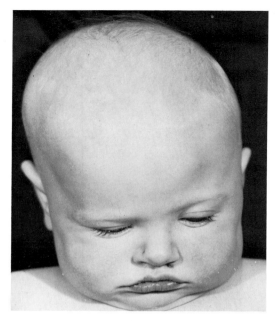

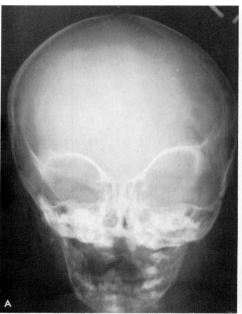

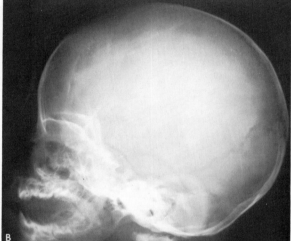

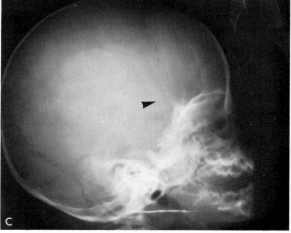

FIGURE 25–5 Unilateral coronal synostosis, left, 5-month-old girl. There is flattening of left frontal area and relative prominence of right frontal boss. Involvement of left orbit, which is shallower and more oblique, may produce apparent slight proptosis on the involved side, for there is little, if any, overhanging brow ridge. (From Shillito, J., and Matson, D. D.: Pediatrics, *41*: 829–853, 1968. Reprinted with permission.)

FIGURE 25–6 Unilateral coronal synostosis, same girl as in Figure 25–5. *A*. Note obliquity of left orbital rim on involved side. Normal lambdoid sutures may be seen on this view. Comparing lateral x-ray on the involved side, *B*, with normal side. *C*, one can see the patent right coronal suture more clearly in the right lateral view (*arrow*). The frontal fossa on the involved side is smaller and its base steeper. Lambdoid and squamosal sutures are clearly patent. (*A* and *B* from Shillito, J., and Matson, D. D.: Pediatrics, *41*:829–853, 1968. Reprinted with permission.)

demonstrate, even in a normal individual (Fig. 25–5).

The orbit gives a nice clue due to an elevated sphenoid wing, which gives an obliquity to that orbital rim reminiscent of the fancy sunglasses popular a decade ago (Fig. 25–6A). X-rays show a discrepancy in the clarity of the coronal sutures when one compares the left and right lateral views (Fig. 25–6B and C). The involved suture shows a greater density, particularly near the pterion, and lies more anteriorly than its opposite, the frontal fossa appearing smaller and its floor steeper on the abnormal side.

Bilateral Coronal Synostosis

Bilateral coronal synostosis presents most of the foregoing findings, but the symmetrical flattening of the forehead may not as readily draw attention as will the unilateral condition (Fig. 25–7).

The fontanelle, if present, will be in the midline, but far anterior. There may be actual depressions just above the lateral brow areas.

Proptosis may be marked, especially in children with Crouzon's syndrome (hereditary craniosynostosis and facial deformities).[6] This can be so severe that the lids may, on occasion, close behind the globe, necessitating canthorrhaphy.[14] Some of the circus freaks who can pop their eyes out show characteristics of bilateral coronal synostosis. This condition may coexist with other congenital anomalies, as in Apert's syndrome (craniosynostosis and syndactyly).[4]

X-rays show obliquity of both orbital rims and a short shallow frontal fossa (Fig. 25–8). If any part of the coronal suture is still patent, usually near the fontanelle, its position will appear displaced anteriorly. Increased density of the coronal areas may be present more laterally.

Metopic Synostosis

Metopic synostosis draws attention because of a midfrontal ridge extending from the fontanelle down toward the nasion (Fig. 25–9). In extreme degrees, this deformity also shows pinching of the forehead

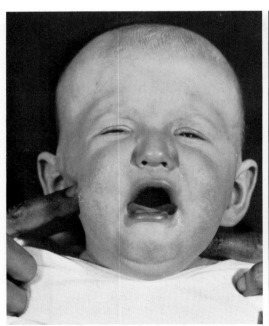 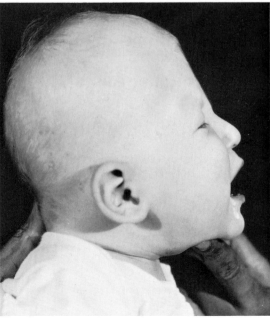

FIGURE 25–7 Bilateral coronal synostosis, 5-month-old boy. There is flattening of the forehead bilaterally, slightly pinched appearance of the frontal bones, absence of brow ridges. (From Shillito, J., and Matson, D. D.: Pediatrics, *41*:829–853, 1968. Reprinted with permission.)

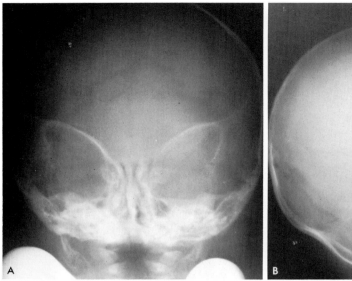
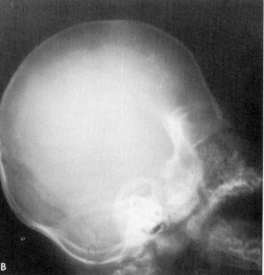

FIGURE 25–8 Bilateral coronal synostosis, same child as in Figure 25–7. *A.* Note obliquity of both orbits, and normal lambdoid sutures. *B.* Frontal fossa is very small with a steep floor, and no coronal sutures can be seen. (From Shillito, J., and Matson, D. D.: Pediatrics, *41*:829–853, 1968. Reprinted with permission.)

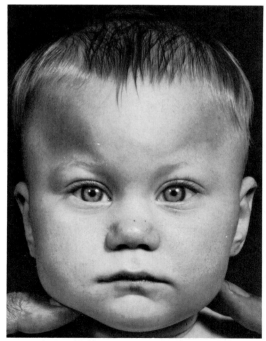

FIGURE 25–9 Metopic synostosis, 8-month-old boy. Prominent ridge in midforehead extends down to nasion. Frontal bones appear pinched in on each side of this ridge. Palpation behind the hair line will indicate full extent of metopic ridge. (From Shillito, J., and Matson, D. D.: Pediatrics, *41*:829–853, 1968. Reprinted with permission.)

on either side of the ridge, giving the child's head an appearance resembling the bow of a fisherman's upside-down dory.

The usual x-ray views may show excessive separation of the other cranial sutures and a small frontal fossa, but the ridge can only be appreciated by a properly angled submentovertex view, which throws the metopic area in profile anterior to the facial bones and teeth (Fig. 25–10).

Lambdoid Synostosis

Less frequent in large series, lambdoid synostosis presents in unilateral form as a flattening of one side of the occiput.[1, 17] This may closely resemble positional molding clinically, but by history and x-ray, the diagnosis can be made. In marked deformity due to positional molding there may also be a secondary slight prominence of the ipsilateral frontal area. This is not seen in primary lambdoid synostosis. X-rays will clearly show both lambdoid sutures in cases of positional molding; a synostotic suture will be replaced by denser bone and will be visible over only a part of its length at best (Fig. 25–11).

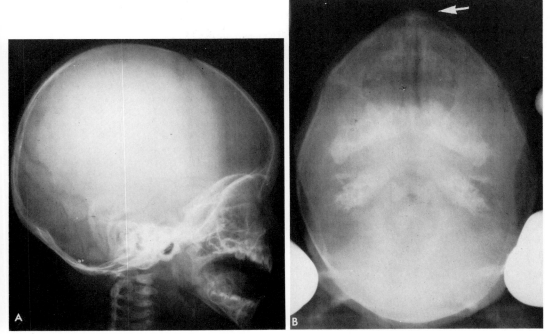

FIGURE 25–10   Metopic synostosis, same child as in Figure 25–9. *A.* Lateral view often shows splitting of coronal and lambdoid sutures. *B.* Standard views do not always allow one to appreciate the ridge, which may best be seen in a submentovertex view angled so that the ridge (*arrow*) is projected anterior to the facial bones. (From Shillito, J., and Matson, D. D.: Pediatrics, *41*:829–853, 1968. Reprinted with permission.)

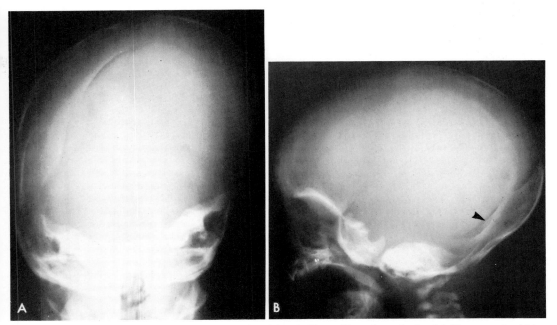

FIGURE 25–11   Unilateral lambdoid synostosis, right. *A.* Note ridge where the lambdoid suture should be and asymmetry of skull. *B*, In the lateral view one can see only one lambdoid suture and thicker bone in lieu of the other (*arrow*). (From Shillito, J., and Matson, D. D.: Pediatrics, *41*:829–853, 1968. Reprinted with permission.)

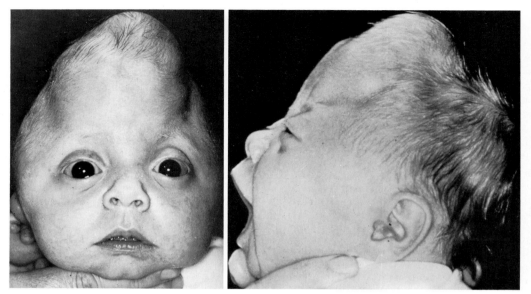

FIGURE 25–12 Multiple synostosis; sagittal, bilateral coronal, bilateral lambdoid; 1 week old. Brain is protruding through site of anterior fontanelle and also slightly through posterior fontanelle. Widest part of skull is at the squamosal suture level. (From Shillito, J., and Matson, D. D.: Pediatrics, *41*:829–853, 1968. Reprinted with permission.)

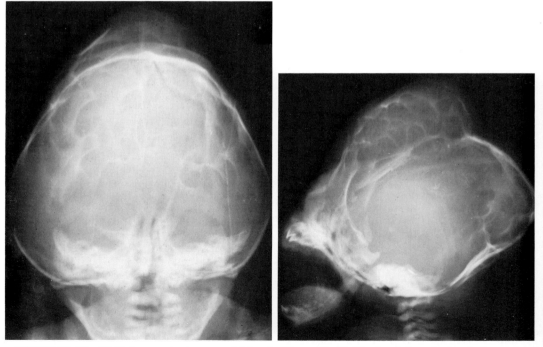

FIGURE 25–13 Multiple synostosis, same child as in Figure 25–12. The loculations in the skull contained cranial contents, making craniectomy difficult. (From Shillito, J., and Matson, D. D.: Pediatrics, *41*:829–853, 1968. Reprinted with permission.)

Bilateral Lambdoid Synostosis

Bilateral lambdoid synostosis presents a flat, shallow occipital area. X-ray changes will establish the diagnosis. Particularly in Towne's view, the lambdoid sutures will be seen clearly in cases of positional molding or occipital flattening due to a family trait. In bilateral lambdoid synostosis these sutures will not be visible over their entire length and will be replaced by denser bone at least over part of the suture's normal position.

Multiple Suture Closures

Multiple suture closures may produce a striking appearance as shown in the child in Figure 25–12. This 1-week-old had only the squamosal and metopic sutures and the remnant of an anterior fontanelle patent. X-rays suggested that brain growth had been directed toward the anterior and posterior fontanelles and both squamosal regions (Fig. 25–13). Following staged and repeated operations, this child has developed normally, and her postoperative appearance is shown in Figure 25–18.

Total Synostosis

In theory, total synostosis should present as a small but normally shaped head, for if any suture remains patent, or has even a portion of its length patent, the brain will grow in that direction with resultant asymmetry. Total synostosis has not been seen in infancy at the Children's Hospital Medical Center in Boston. Several older children have come to attention, because of either papilledema, mental retardation, concomitant deformities of the face, or head trauma that necessitated skull x-rays, whose skulls were approximately normal in shape, who showed no evidence of cranial sutures by x-ray, but who had varying degrees of Lukenschädel (window skull) and the "beaten silver" appearance associated with chronic increased intracranial pressure, either current or previous.[14] The head size may be within normal limits. Mental function can in some cases be normal or nearly so. By what mechanism these skulls have grown is not clear.

TREATMENT

Goal

The goal of therapy is to provide between the involved bones an artificial separation that will function as would a normal suture during the period of brain growth and disappear thereafter. Placement of the artificial suture should duplicate normal suture location to permit anatomical restoration of normal contour; morcellation procedures without regard to suture pattern are unnecessary and less desirable; greater rapidity of spread and more prolonged function probably occurs at a single craniectomy site than would be possible at multiple narrower skull defects. Furthermore, the application of polyethylene film, or other suitable material, is easier if duplication of the normal suture is achieved surgically.[9]

Ideally operation should be done immediately upon diagnosis. It should be done as soon after birth as one considers the operation tolerable with negligible risk. Early operation is desirable in order to remove the constriction as soon as possible and gain maximal benefit from the corrective influence of the growing brain. By a few weeks of age the child's total blood volume has increased significantly, reducing the consequences of blood loss that invariably accompanies the operation. In cases involving one or two sutures, operation has been advised at 4 to 6 weeks of age. When many sutures are involved and pressure is also a problem, operation as early as 1 week of age has been successful (see Fig. 25–12).

General Principles

Scissors or saw cuts of the cranium heal promptly. Wider craniectomies are sealed very soon by new bone regenerating from the dura.[10] Chemical cauterization of the dura might jeopardize the underlying brain if the dura should leak and might excessively delay ultimate bone regeneration with its necessary protection.[2] Wrapping the craniectomy edges with an inert film has retarded sealing of the surgical defect adequately to achieve or approximate the ideal without preventing ultimate complete healing, which is desirable. Even with the method of using the inert film on the edge of the craniectomy, one sagittal synostosis patient required cranioplasty in the first decade of life because his schoolmates found they could percuss his motor cortex through an unhealed parasagittal craniectomy and temporarily paralyze his contralateral leg![16]

A craniectomy about 1 cm in width provides adequate room to manipulate the polyethylene film and to control small areas of dural bleeding without difficulty. Such bony cuts should extend across adjacent normal sutures. Both the outer and inner leaves of film are 1 cm wide. It is prepared by wrapping the unsterile film about the edges of a malleable abdominal retractor, tying it in position, and boiling the assembly for 20 minutes. This procedure will mold the film by heat in a folded position for ease in application, and also provides adequate sterilization. As a further precaution, the film on its retractor can be packaged in transparent sleeves for gas sterilization, after which the film is kept on the shelf for several weeks before use. If a shallow groove is cut into the abdominal retractor 1 cm from its edges, removal of the film is facilitated; the scrub nurse can easily pass a knife blade along the four grooves and remove two folded strips of film (Fig. 25–14). Commercially available strips of

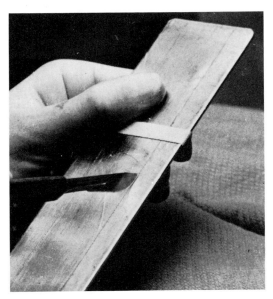

FIGURE 25–14 Cutting polyethylene film for use on craniectomy margins. Note groove in retractor.

Silastic material now on the market are thicker and under infants' scalps, therefore, a bit less desirable, although they should be equally effective.

The film is held to the bone by specially made tantalum clips or, if these are unavailable, by punching holes in the bone edges and passing 0000 silk sutures around the film and through the holes.[8] When the craniectomy lies in front of the hair line, it is desirable to use sutures to avoid the small lump produced by a tantalum clip, noticeable beneath the infant's thin scalp.

Scalp closure is with 0000 silk sutures, interrupted and inverted in the galeal area, and interrupted in the scalp. The use of a small tape dressing allows one to be more immediately aware of any subgaleal accumulation of blood postoperatively than if a full head dressing is applied.

Operation may be undertaken with acceptable risk if strict attention is paid to several important principles of surgery in the newborn.[17] Positioning to prevent pressure marks, maintenance of body temperature, and prompt and adequate replacement by intravenous catheter of blood loss during and after the operation are most important. Since a foreign body is left in the skull, meticulous attention to aseptic operative technique is necessary. Postoperative accumulation of blood in the subgaleal space is best handled by careful aspiration using a styleted needle, rather than by open drainage, to minimize the possibility of contamination. Such blood losses must be anticipated and replaced promptly. Determination of hematocrit is advisable in the recovery room and at six-hour intervals for the next 18 hours; then twice daily until accumulation has stopped and the hematocrit is stable.

Operative Technique

Metopic Craniectomy

The child should be positioned face up. The entire scalp is clipped and the anterior half shaved after induction of anesthesia. Incision is coronal, ear to ear, to just above the zygoma on each side, thus avoiding risk to the facial nerve, and just behind the hair line. It is wise to mark the hair line before shaving an infant's head, for determining the position of the hair line is somewhat difficult after shaving. Intradermal lidocaine (Xylocaine) 0.5 per cent with epinephrine 1:200,000 greatly facilitates hemostasis in the scalp. Small hemostats and spring skin clips are used, the latter on the anterior skin edge to prevent heavy hemostats from resting on the child's face.

The scalp is reflected over the face, down to each orbital rim and to the nasion. Pericranium is stripped from the ridged area and from the supraorbital area for a distance adequate to avoid the estimated final position of the polyethylene film.

Starting at the anterior fontanelle, if present, or at a small midline burr hole made just anterior to the coronal suture, the midline ridge is removed with various rongeurs down to the nasion. Just above the nasion there are invariably several small dural veins that connect the sagittal sinus to the bone, and these can cause embarrassing or even dangerous bleeding. They must be anticipated, and thorough hemostasis of both bony and dural bleeders must be maintained every centimeter of the way down to this region to prevent excessive blood loss during this short period of the operation.

Any residual thickening of the edges of this 1 cm craniectomy can be removed with a surgical air drill by using a cylindrical bit and simply shaving the outer table of the bone off until the bone edge appears to be of normal thickness. The bone is very vascular and should be waxed after every few strokes of the drill.

Next, a linear cut a few millimeters wide is made from both coronal sutures to the midline directly above the orbit using small rongeurs, a DeVilbiss rongeur or, in older children, a Gigli saw. It is not difficult inadvertently to tear the dura during this maneuver and the use of progressively smaller rongeurs, with the dura under direct vision and retracted slightly, is recommended. Any dural rents must be sutured to prevent persistent leak or pseudomeningocele formation. Waxing these bone edges can be facilitated by either depressing or slightly elevating the now rather mobile frontal bones.

Polyethylene film is placed over both edges of each flap of bone and secured with 0000 silk placed through small holes punched with a Cone punch.

Coronal Craniectomy

Position, preparation, and incision are identical to those of metopic craniectomy. In unilateral closure, the incision can be stopped above the uninvolved lateral canthus. After stripping pericranium from the intended site, the craniectomy is started by using the fontanelle, if present. The soft tissue attachment to the bone is incised after depressing the fontanelle and cutting carefully into and just under the bone edge with a No. 15 blade. The dura can then be elevated from the bone and the separation extended sharply an adequate distance both before and behind the coronal suture site to permit later application of polyethylene film.

In infants, rongeurs are easily used to create the craniectomy, which follows the line of the skin incision to the temporal region. Here it is essential to find the squamosal suture, which may be quite low. The squamosal suture can be identified by its adherence to the pericranium and to the dura, and after rongeuring across it, one can easily demonstrate motion of the bones around it. If the coronal craniectomy is directed too far anteriorly, the squamosal suture may not be encountered at all.

Next, the sphenoid wing or "keel" is identified on the inner table of the frontal bone. It has been our custom to remove the "keel" after careful retraction of surrounding dura and to wax its stump carefully. It is felt that this may allow forward migration of the temporal lobe and further improvement in the appearance of the forehead.

If the infant has shown marked depressions of the frontal areas supraorbitally, cuts are made just above the orbits as in metopic synostosis.

Sagittal Craniectomy

Here, two approaches are available, each utilizing a midline scalp incision. For over 30 years, the Children's Hospital Medical Center in Boston has made use of bilateral parasagittal craniectomies; others advocate a single midline craniectomy.[7] Both give good results. Parasagittal craniectomies make unnecessary the stripping of dura from bone directly over the sagittal sinus, with the attendant risk of tearing it. Although it is true that in the absence of the sagittal suture there will be no adherence to the bone, most infants, nonetheless, have some residual patent portions of this suture, and in this area the risk of sinus bleeding is real. Parasagittal craniectomies also leave bony protection over the sagittal sinus, which becomes more important if the operation should be done about the time a child becomes ambulatory, for then he is much more likely to strike this area forcibly than is an infant. Parasagittal craniectomies have given good results, and possibly the presence of four bone edges improves the chance of keeping the surgical defects open for an adequate period. Inexplicably, there will sometimes develop a prominence of the anterior end of the midline strip of bone just behind the coronal suture. This is undesirable, although it usually disappears gradually with age. This is not seen when a midline craniectomy is used.

Parasagittal Craniectomy

For this operation, it is best to put the child in the prone position in a horseshoe headrest. The majority of the patients have maximum involvement posteriorly where access is severely limited by a supine position. Without meticulous attention to details during positioning and preparing, and without frequent repositioning of the head during the operation, pressure necrosis of the forehead scalp will almost certainly occur. The headrest should be properly angled along its long axis to put equal pressure on the two frontal bosses and the two malar eminences, thus distributing the pressure as widely as possible. No lumps in the padding of the headrest can be tolerated. No fluid of any kind should wet the headrest; it must be covered with a towel during the skin preparation, and this towel removed and replaced with a dry one before final draping. A plastic adherent drape applied to the dried skin will protect the face and headrest during the operation. On cue from the anesthetist, as he watches to be sure the endotracheal tube is not dislodged, the infant's head is lifted by the operator just enough to clear the headrest for a few seconds every 15 minutes from the time the baby is first positioned until the operation is over. Because of the risk of placing the

eyes on the headrest during these maneuvers, it is wise to tape them shut before placing the child prone.

After making the skin incision and applying self-retaining retractors, it is best to work alternately on the left and right sides of the midline, covering the opposite side with moist gauze in the interim. This minimizes the exposed area and reduces the rate of blood loss with each step, since better control of a limited area can be achieved.

The site of each craniectomy is planned by estimating the width of the polyethylene film and plotting its medial edge 1 cm from the midline. The pericranium must be incised far enough laterally to avoid the lateral film strip; usually 5 cm from the midline is necessary.

The pericranium is stripped one side at a time, from above downward, to facilitate waxing of the bone. Electrocautery is often necessary on the infant's skull, either alone or to facilitate by its heating effect the retention of bone wax.

It may be possible, especially in small infants, to enter the epidural space beside the fontanelle with a No. 15 blade, elevate the dura, and rongeur out the craniectomy. If not, three burr holes will facilitate the use of a Gigli saw. One each is placed in the parietal bone adjacent to the coronal and lambdoid sutures, and the third halfway between these two. Rongeurs are used to extend the craniectomy across each adjacent suture. The dura must be separated from these sutures far enough medially and laterally to accept the film strip. The film is easily stapled or sewed to the bone in three places, securing it to the parietal bones but allowing it to project into the occipital and frontal extensions of the craniectomies.

Midline Sagittal Craniectomy

In midline craniectomies, the lateral position can be used for the child, since a less wide exposure is necessary. This avoids pressure necrosis, the pitfall of the prone position. A further factor in favor of the midline operation is its relative brevity and its smaller blood loss, both intraoperatively and postoperatively. The pericranial stripping is less wide, 2 cm from the midline on each side. The outer layer of the fontanelle should also be removed to prevent fusion anteriorly. A midline strip of bone is then removed after entering the epidural space either with a knife or through a burr hole. Note again adherence of the dura only to any existing normal portions of the suture.

Ordinarily a full-length craniectomy is done, removing these apparently normal segments of suture. However, in one or two infants with synostosis involving only a few centimeters of suture, a limited craniectomy, leaving normal suture behind, has corrected the deformity completely (Fig. 25–15).

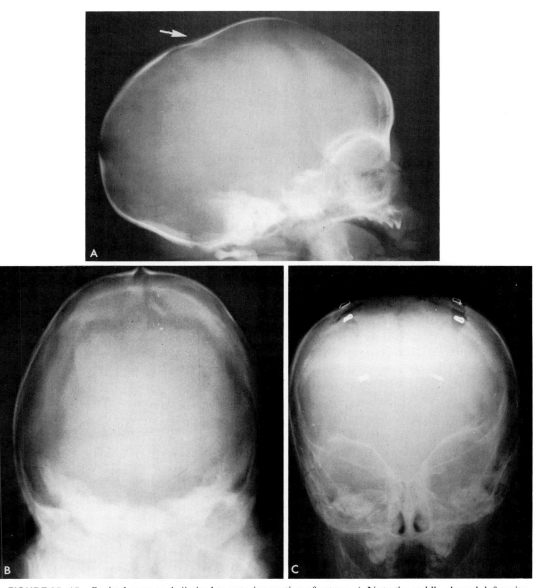

FIGURE 25–15 Sagittal synostosis limited to anterior portion of suture. *A*. Note the saddle-shaped deformity. *B*. Properly angled anteroposterior view showed this to be a synostosed area of the sagittal suture. *C*. Midline craniectomy of this portion resulted in a very satisfactory spread as shown by x-ray and disappearance of deformity clinically.

Lambdoid Craniectomy

The child should be in the prone position and all precautions necessary in the face-down position should be observed. Incision is planned from the posterior end of the sagittal suture to the posterior end of the squamosal suture. This is determined by x-ray or palpation over the involved side, or sides. After stripping 4 cm of pericranium, a burr hole is placed parasagittally to avoid entering the sinus. Rongeurs usually provide the most expeditious means of making the craniectomy. The sagittal suture must be crossed, and the squamosal suture must be identified and crossed. This demands adequate exposure laterally and prompt control of the nearby mastoid emissary vein, which is usually entered.

Multiple Sutures

Craniectomy techniques are as already detailed when multiple closures are treated. The planning of incisions and the staging of procedures can be summarized as follows:

Metopic and coronal synostosis — coronal incision, one stage

Coronal and sagittal — coronal and sagittal incisions, two stages

Sagittal and lambdoid — posterior parietal ear to ear and sagittal incisions, two stages

All sutures — coronal and posterior parietal ear to ear incisions, two stages

In this last situation, anterior halves of sagittal (or bilateral parasagittal) and squamosal craniectomies can be done using the coronal incision, and the posterior halves completed in the second stage, using the posterior incision. The operations are separated by at least one week.

Other combinations can be dealt with by utilizing these incisions as necessary.

If metopic and bilateral coronal synostosis coexist, the frontal bones can actually be removed, their edges lined with film, and the bones then sutured lightly back in place with 0000 silk.[13]

Mortality and Morbidity Rates

In a series of 519 surgically treated patients at the Children's Hospital Medical

TABLE 25-1. MORBIDITY (519 PATIENTS, 689 OPERATIONS)*

Number	Complication	Rate (Per Cent)
PERMANENT COMPLICATIONS		0.58
3	Scars, forehead, from pressure of head rest	
SERIOUS CORRECTABLE COMPLICATIONS		7.5
2	Major anesthetic	
7	Wound sepsis requiring reoperation	
4	Hematomas requiring reoperation	
2	Necrosis, isolated sagittal bone strip	
5	Dural tear, CSF accumulation requiring reoperation	
6	Tantalum clip eroding through scalp	
2	Cranioplasty necessary, persistent defect	
2	Cardiac problems	
1	Wound dehiscence	
1	Septicemia	
1	Seizure	
6	Multiple complications	
MINOR COMPLICATIONS		5.6
8	Minor anesthetic	
2	Wound sepsis, no reoperation	
8	Temporary pressure marks	
1	Late sepsis, no reoperation	
4	Late hematoma, due to trauma	
1	Minor irritation around clip	
4	Dural tear, CSF accumulation, no reoperation	
1	Edema, scalp and face, marked	
71	Total complications	14

*Morbidity rates are based upon the risk per patient, not the risk per operation. Although the overall complication rate is 14 per cent, note that only 0.58 per cent—three patients—had any permanent undesirable complications. (From Shillito, J., and Matson, D. D.: Pediatrics, 41:829–853, 1968. Reprinted with permission.)

Center in Boston, over a 36-year period, there were two deaths, with a risk of 0.39 per cent.[17] One infant died because of an unsuspected bleeding tendency; a second died of cardiac arrest probably related to inadequate rate of blood replacement. Complications that produced lasting sequelae numbered only three, at a rate of 0.58 per cent. All were significant areas of pressure necrosis of the scalp of the forehead resulting from the face-down position during parasagittal craniectomy. Total morbidity rate was 14 per cent, in about half of which cases complications could be considered serious. Except for the facial pressure scars, however, all complications were correctable (Table 25–1).

RESULTS OF OPERATION

The cosmetic improvement can be qualitated, but is not easily quantitated. The ef-

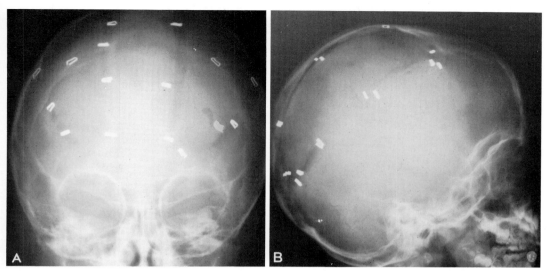

FIGURE 25–16 Sagittal synostosis. Postoperative x-rays on patient in Figures 25–3 and 25–4. Films were taken three years and nine months after operation. Note that the 1 cm wide craniectomies have spread markedly, *A*, and head is now quite round, *B*. (From Shillito, J., and Matson, D. D.: Pediatrics, *41*:829–853, 1968. Reprinted with permission.)

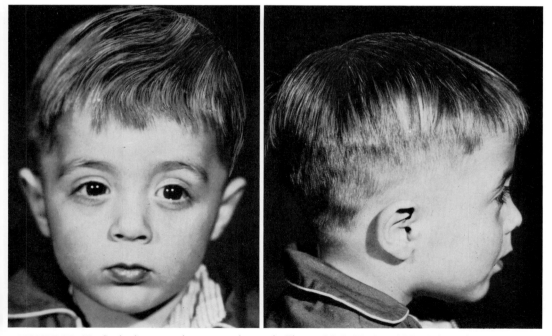

FIGURE 25–17 Sagittal synostosis, same patient as in Figures 25–3, 25–4, and 25–16, here shown at 2 years and 3 months of age. Operation was performed at 6 weeks of age. Now over 12 years old, this boy is considered completely normal. (From Shillito, J., and Matson, D. D.: Pediatrics, *41*:829–853, 1968. Reprinted with permission.)

TABLE 25–2. NECESSITY FOR REOPERATION*

SUTURE INVOLVEMENT	NUMBER OF PATIENTS OPERATED UPON	NUMBER OF PATIENTS REOPERATED UPON	PER CENT REQUIRING REOPERATION
Metopic	18	0	0
Lambdoid, one or both	12	0	0
Sagittal	287	18	6.3
Coronal, one	66	4	6.0
Coronal, both	59	18	30.5
Multiple	77	29	38.0
Overall	519	69	13.3

*Criteria have included: evidence of fusion of craniectomies in a child with multiple synostosis, evidence of return of increased intracranial pressure in a child with multiple synostosis, and evidence of fusion of craniectomies for any suture closure when subsequent brain growth could produce significant further cosmetic improvement. Reoperation for sagittal synostosis was frequently done before polyethylene film was used; more recently it has usually been unnecessary. Note the high incidence of reoperation in bilateral coronal and multiple synostosis. (From Shillito, J., and Matson, D. D.: Pediatrics, *41*:829–853, 1968. Reprinted with permission.)

Better cosmetic results follow early operation, ideally that performed within the first few weeks after birth. Satisfaction varies with the suture involved. The sagittal case operated upon early usually develops a normally shaped head, and reoperation for fusion is rarely done (Figs. 25–15, 25–16, and 25–17). Craniectomies for coronal synostosis do not spread as markedly as those for sagittal, perhaps because of a tethering effect of the nearby base of the skull. Reoperation is more frequent in this group (Table 25–2). Usually reoperation is necessary when many sutures are involved. When re-fusion occurs in multiple sutures, the problem is not only cosmetic, but involves increasing intracranial pressure. Follow-up at six-month intervals by clinical examination and by x-ray, after new bone has formed, is frequent enough to detect re-fusion. The infant shown in Figure 25–12 underwent a two-stage operation at 1 and 3 weeks of age, and re-fusion dictated reoperation at 18 months of age, when the two stages were repeated. The ultimate outcome has been most gratifying (Fig. 25–18).

fect on brain function, however, cannot even be estimated, since by operation on any given child, the control study for that child is lost.

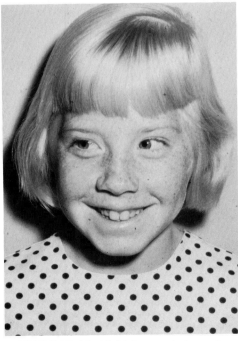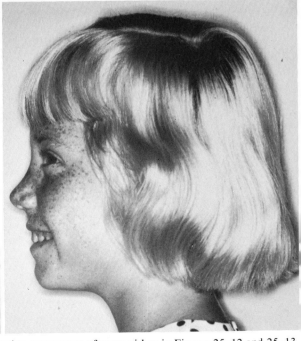

FIGURE 25–18 Multiple synostosis, postoperative appearance of same girl as in Figures 25–12 and 25–13. She is here 10 years old, has been getting excellent grades in school, and is considered normal. (*Left,* from Matson, D. D.: Neurosurgery of Infancy and Childhood. 2nd Ed. Springfield, Ill., Charles C Thomas, 1969. *Right,* from Shillito, J., and Matson, D. D.: Pediatrics, *41*:829–853, 1968. Reprinted with permission.)

***TABLE** 25-3. COSMETIC RESULT**

| SUTURE CATEGORY | WORSE | NO CHANGE (PER CENT) | IMPROVED | | | INADEQUATE FOLLOW-UP (PER CENT) |
			Slight (Per Cent)	*Suboptimal* (Per Cent)	*Optimal* (Per Cent)	
Metopic	0	5	0	14	33	48
Sagittal	0	2	1	21	52	23
One or both coronals	0	1	0	18	62	19
One or both lambdoids	0	0	0	8	53	39
Multiple	0	5	1	26	40	28
Overall	0	2	1	21	52	24
Total improved (Per cent)				74		

*No patients have been made worse since the adoption of current operative techniques. Those showing no improvement are children operated upon later in life; slight improvement is that detectable by x-ray examination but not apparent clinically. Suboptimal improvement indicates children operated upon later than desired. Optimal improvement indicates a result that produces an essentially normal contour of the skull. Facial appearance in Crouzon's syndrome and orbital involvement in coronal synostosis are expected. Inadequate cosmetic follow-up includes any child not followed for more than six weeks, or any child in whose hospital record either no adequate statement is made or no photograph is available. Note that 74 per cent were considered to have been improved even though only 36 per cent of the children were operated upon during the first six weeks of life (see Fig. 25-2). (From Shillito, J., and Matson, D. D.: Pediatrics, *41*:829–853. Reprinted with permission.)

Cosmetic result, even when only 36 per cent of the children in one series underwent surgery within the desired six weeks of birth, is shown in Table 25-3.[17]

INDICATIONS FOR REOPERATION

If one is certain that the craniectomy is sealed and the child still has considerable brain growth to anticipate, cosmetic improvement will continue if the craniectomy is reopened (Fig. 25-2). In multiple synostosis, if signs of increased intracranial pressure appear, reoperation is indicated, even when further cosmetic change can be only slight. Thus, a child only 18 months old with a re-fused coronal craniectomy will probably benefit from reoperation. A patient with re-fused coronal, sagittal, and

FIGURE 25-19 Typical growth curve of the head of a child with sagittal synostosis. In several cases in which accurate records have been kept by the pediatrician, growth rate of the head has been found to exceed normal preoperatively, as the head elongates. After bilateral parasagittal craniectomies the head begins to assume a more spherical contour and its growth rate as determined by its circumference becomes less than normal. Theoretically, recurrence of the excessive growth rate should indicate fusion of the surgical defects. This has not yet occurred in our experience. (From Shillito, J., and Matson, D. D.: Pediatrics, *41*:829–843, 1968. Reprinted with permission.)

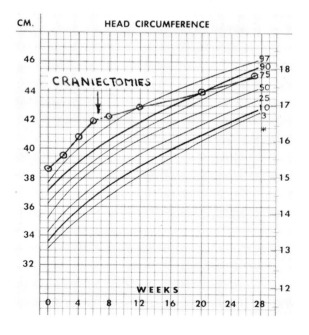

lambdoid sutures at 4 years of age, with any signs of increased intracranial pressure, would deserve consideration of further surgery.

In closure of a single or a limited number of sutures, when intracranial pressure remains normal, there is difficulty in determining when bony bridging has occurred. The head circumference curve in sagittal synostosis is interesting and should be a reliable indicator if re-fusion has occurred, although return of the abnormally rapid rate of increase in head circumference has yet to be documented since this phenomenon was noted (Fig. 25–19).[17] Progressive widening of a craniectomy is reassuring evidence that it is still patent. Tantalum clips help in this situation by serving as bench marks; skull projections must be identical to insure valid comparison. The radiological appearance of the junction between new and old bone is important, but may be misleading and suggest fusion, which subsequent widening belies. The presence of new bone does not in itself indicate fusion. A line resembling a normal suture will, rarely, appear in the new bone of a craniectomy and persist. In each patient, gains yet to be realized and improvement already achieved must be weighed carefully in making any decision regarding reoperation.

FACTS AND FALLACIES

Primary craniosynostosis is by definition a congenital defect involving the membranous bones of the skull appearing in utero, where it has been documented radiographically. There is no evidence that abnormality of the underlying brain causes primary synostosis. It can be diagnosed at birth by clinical and radiographic criteria. The synostotic suture may be abnormal over only a *part* of its length. This phenomenon may be one of the factors that delay diagnosis, since the roentgenographic appearance of the portion of this suture visualized by conventional projections may be falsely reassuring. Since the adjacent membranous bones are effectively tethered when only a small portion of the suture is absent, the remaining normal portions of the sutures will be obliterated progressively and prematurely, as they would in an adult when brain growth ceases. This phenomenon accounts for the fallacy that primary synostosis develops after birth; it will, rather, *progress* after birth.

The anterior fontanelle in one series was patent in about half the cases with synostosis of any or a combination of the four adjacent sutures.[17] Therefore, the presence of the anterior fontanelle does not rule out primary craniosynostosis, and conversely, early disappearance of the fontanelle does not in itself indicate craniosynostosis. Nevertheless, radiological investigation may be indicated when a physician feels that the fontanelle has closed too soon; this is the only reliable way to rule out craniosynostosis. Rarely, an anterior fontanelle bone will further confuse the diagnosis until x-rays are made.

The phenomenon of total synostosis is even less well understood. True microcephaly resulting from primary total craniosynostosis with mental retardation caused by constriction of an otherwise normal brain, has not been seen in this center. Several children with premature absence of all cranial sutures have had heads normal in circumference and not much deformed in shape, and skulls indicating previous increased intracranial pressure. This group deserves further study.

It has been repeatedly shown that early and proper surgical intervention will remove or significantly lessen cranial deformities due to primary craniosynostosis.[1, 17–19] The operative risk is justified by the cosmetic results alone and can be acceptably small if certain principles are respected.

REFERENCES

1. Anderson, F. M., and Geiger, L.: Craniosynostosis: A survey of 204 cases. J. Neurosurg., 22:229–240, 1965.
2. Anderson, F. M., and Johnson, F. L.: Craniosynostosis. A modification in surgical therapy. Surgery, 40:961–970, 1956.
3. Anderson, H., and Gomes, S. P.: Clinocephaly. Acta Paediat. Scand., 57:294–296, 1968.
4. Apert, E.: De l'acrocéphalosyndactylie. Bull. Soc. Méd. Paris, 23:1310–1331, 1906.
5. Coppoletta, J. M., and Wolbach, S. B.: Body length and organ weights. Amer. J. Path., 9:55–70, 1933.
6. Crouzon, Q.: Dysostose cranio-faciale héréditaire. Bull. Soc. Méd. Hôp. Paris, 33:545–555, 1912.

7. Davis, C. H., Jr., Alexander, E., Jr., and Kelly, D. L., Jr.: Treatment of craniosynostosis. J. Neurosurg., *30*:630–636, 1969.

8. Fowler, F. D., and Matson, D. D.: A new method for applying polyethylene film to the skull in the treatment of craniosynostosis. J. Neurosurg., *14*:584–586, 1957.

9. Ingraham, F. D., Alexander, E., Jr., and Matson, D. D.: Polyethylene, a new synthetic plastic for use in surgery. J.A.M.A., *135*:82–87, 1947.

10. Ingraham, F. D., Matson, D. D., and Alexander, E., Jr.: Experimental observations in the treatment of craniosynostosis. Surgery, *23*:252–268, 1948.

11. Kloss, J. L.: Craniosynostosis secondary to ventriculoatrial shunt. Amer. J. Dis. Child., *116*:315–317, 1968.

12. Laitinen, L.: Craniosynostosis, premature fusion of the cranial sutures. Ann. Paediat. Fenn., suppl. 6, Vol. 2, 1956.

13. Matson, D. D.: Surgical treatment of congenital anomalies of the coronal and metopic sutures. J. Neurosurg., *17*:413–417, 1960.

14. Matson, D. D.: Neurosurgery of Infancy and Childhood. 2nd Ed. Springfield, Ill., Charles C Thomas, 1969.

15. Shillito, J., Jr.: New suture in a site of craniectomy for synostosis. In progress.

16. Shillito, J., Jr., and Matson, D. D.: Sagittal synostosis: Indications for operation. J. Pediat., *59*:789–790, 1961.

17. Shillito, J., Jr., and Matson, D. D.: Craniosynostosis: A review of 519 surgical patients. Pediatrics, *41*:829–853, 1968.

18. Till, K.: Craniosynostosis. Develop. Med. Child Neurol., *8*:212–213, 1966.

19. Youmans, J. R.: Neurosurgically correctible congenital anomalies. J. Mississippi Med. Ass., *5*:77–83, 1964.

26

ANOMALIES OF THE CRANIOVERTEBRAL JUNCTION

The bony malformations at the cranio-vertebral junction consist of basilar impression, platybasia, distortion of the foramen magnum, and fusion (assimilation) of the first cervical vertebra with the foramen magnum, the latter sometimes resulting in anterior dislocation of C1 and C2. In addition, there may be fusion between other cervical vertebrae to constitute the Klippel-Feil or short-neck syndrome. In the English language, early articles on the subject appeared in 1931, in 1934, and in 1939, and a comprehensive review of the foreign literature by List was published in 1941.[5, 7, 11, 21] These malformations may be associated with dilatation of the spinal canal, with occult spina bifida, and occasionally with anterior spina bifida (hemivertebra). The external contours that may indicate the presence of these bony anomalies are a short neck, limited mobility of the cervical spine, a low posterior hair line, head tilt, Sprengel's deformity, scoliosis, webbing of the upper trapezia, a large head, and occasionally prognathism. Neurological symptoms develop in later life and are caused, not solely by the bony malformation, but by its long-continued effect on the associated hindbrain malformation. This is further demonstrated by the fact that similar symptoms and hindbrain malformations occur in patients with no structural changes in the bones.

The most common malformation of nervous tissue at the craniovertebral junc-tion is a congenital hindbrain hernia varying in degree from the typical Arnold-Chiari malformation to a mild herniation of the cerebellar tonsils. These herniations frequently are associated with an imperforate rhombic roof and with syringomyelia and syringobulbia.[13] Other anomalies are the Dandy-Walker malformation and the so-called arachnoid cysts at the foramina of Magendie and Luschka.[15] When these malformations of nervous tissue occur in the absence of changes in the bony configuration, the symptoms frequently are attributed to multiple sclerosis.

BONY MALFORMATIONS

Basilar Impression

As the name implies, in basilar impression the normally convex base of the skull about the foramen magnum is pushed inward, carrying with it the dens and the first cervical vertebra. Although the cause in most instances is present at birth, the deformity, per se, develops after birth. It results from the upright posture, which causes the relatively heavy head to settle downward on the cervical spine as does a pumpkin softening on a fence post. Fusion of cervical vertebrae to each other or to the occiput, when present, is an identifying mark of congenital basilar impression. However, this skull deformity is never present in the newborn and, therefore, is not truly congenital. It is known that bone-softening disorders such as Paget's disease, osteogenesis imperfecta, osteo-

W. J. GARDNER

malacia, hyperparathyroidism, and rickets may result in acquired basilar impression, the shape of which does not differ from that in the congenital form, except that it never is accompanied by bony fusion.[14] Radiological evidence has shown that basilar impression is progressive in Paget's disease and in osteogenesis imperfecta, but progression has not been demonstrated in the congenital form because the bone has acquired adult hardness before the diagnosis is suspected.[27]

The Mechanism

As the subhuman mammal gradually assumed the upright posture, his spine, which was designed by nature as a flexible horizontal beam, was converted to a vertical column with the head perched on top. Along with the assumption of this phylogenetically abnormal posture, the brain progressively increased in weight, while the relative thickness of the skull diminished. Fond mothers encourage their infants to assume the upright posture at a time when the head is still disproportionately large and the skull thin and malleable (Fig. 26–1). Calculation shows that a sphere (and consequently a head) 12 cm in diameter weighs 73 per cent more than one of 10 cm. A corresponding enlargement of the head in the newborn may result from compensated hydrocephalus and be readily overlooked.

In contrast, the infant with uncompensated hydrocephalus, hindbrain hernia, and myelocele seldom assumes the upright posture in early infancy, so that his heavy head is not exposed to these stresses until later. Like the adult with congenital basilar impression, the infant with myelocele may have hydromyelia and fused vertebrae, and always a dilated spinal canal with spina bifida. In this infant the foramen magnum is dilated, whereas in basilar impression it becomes narrowed as the base of the skull is pushed inward. The mechanics of narrowing of the foramen magnum is illustrated in the accompanying illustration (Fig. 26–2).

Platybasia

The interior of the human skull is roughly spherical, except that anterior to the foramen magnum there is a deep crosswise indentation formed in the coronal plane by the petrous pyramids and in the sagittal plane by the angle between the clivus and the base of the anterior fossa. The terms basilar impression and platybasia are frequently used interchangeably, although as

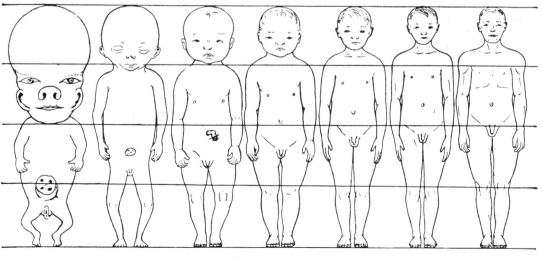

2mo. fetal   **4**mo. fetal   Newborn   2 yr.   6 yr.   12 yr.   25 yr.

FIGURE 26–1 Prenatal and postnatal stages illustrating the relatively large size of the head in infancy and childhood. (Redrawn from Scammon. In Patten, B. M.: Human Embryology. 2nd Ed. New York, McGraw-Hill Book Co., Reprinted with permission of the author and publisher.)

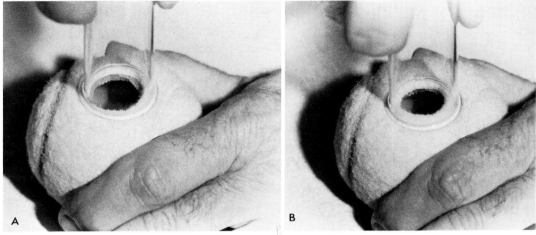

FIGURE 26-2 The mechanics of narrowing of the foramen magnum. Note how the hole in the tennis ball narrows as it is pushed inward by the pressure of the test tube. *A.* Before. *B.* After.

defined by Schüller, the latter is determined solely by the width of this angle.[29] The term platybasia (flat base), therefore, should be restricted to a widening of the basal angle, the top normal being 143 degrees.[31] It represents a pushing inward of the anterior rim of the foramen magnum with the sellar region acting as a hinge. It is merely one feature of basilar impression that need not be considered separately. Unfortunately, the clivus may be difficult to demonstrate roentgenographically because of superimposition of the petrous bones. Lateral tomograms yield better definition of these planes, as well as of the dens and the posterior and the anterior rims of the foramen magnum (lower end of the clivus). In basilar impression, and especially when there is widening of the basal angle, the body of C1 is higher than its lamina. The abnormal tilting of C1 (Bull's angle) may result in compensatory cervical lordosis to give the same outward appearance as a short cervical spine.[6] Widening of the basal angle also may result from increased intracranial pressure in utero caused by closure of cranial sutures. The mechanism in this case is similar to the elimination of a dent in a ping-pong ball when its contents is expanded by heating.

Assimilation of C1

The term is used to indicate fusion of the first cervical vertebra to the foramen magnum.[5] Assimilation is encountered only in the congenital form of basilar impression and, if incomplete, may be demonstrable only by tomography. This fusion results in fixation of the occipitoatlantoid joint. As a result, this joint can no longer contribute to the nodding movement of the head, in which case the atlantoaxial (C1–C2) joint, designed primarily for rotation, may take on some function of flexion. This abnormal movement, beginning early in life, causes the dens to tilt away from the body of C1 because of yielding of the immature transverse ligament, which normally restrains it. With exaggerated flexion, whether voluntary, accidental, or produced passively under anesthesia, this posterior tilting of the dens may cause serious compression of the medulla. This is more likely to occur if the foramen magnum is small, as in basilar impression. Since flexion is essential in positioning the patient, a lateral film should be made before operating.

The fusion of C1 to the foramen magnum, as well as the fusion of vertebrae at a lower level, has been attributed to faulty metameric segmentation (Fig. 26–3).[22] This term implies that the primitive bony segments, the sclerotomes, have failed to separate from one another. Inasmuch as they always originate as separate and distinct cell clusters during the somite stage, there cannot be a "failure of separation." When fusion is present, it has therefore occurred after the sclerotomes developed, but before

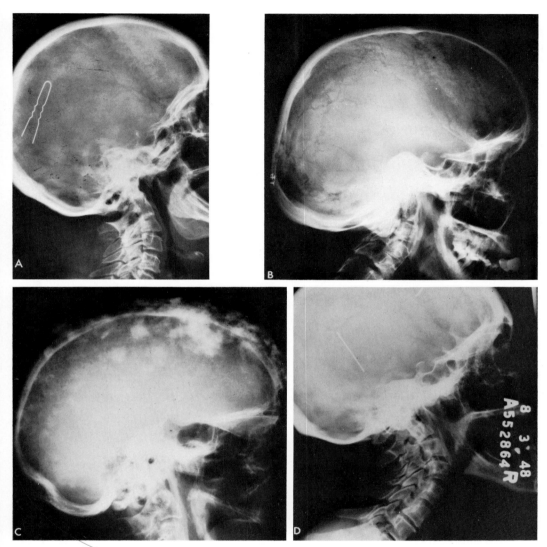

FIGURE 26–3 *A.* Basilar impression with occult spina bifida of C1, which is fused to the foramen magnum. There also is fusion between the bodies of C2 and C3. *B.* Severe congenital basilar impression. The entire body of C2 is above a line drawn between the posterior end of the hard palate and the lowest portion of the occipital bone. *C.* Acquired basilar impression due to Paget's disease. Note how the shape resembles that in congenital basilar impression. *D.* Basilar impression wih platybasia associated with a wide cervical canal and exaggerated lordosis.

they laid down cartilage. In the Klippel-Feil syndrome, the short canal usually is dilated and bifid, indicating that the bony fusion is the result of coalescence of adjoining sclerotomes because of overdistention; the transverse stretching causes a simultaneous shortening of the neural tube. This mechanism is beautifully illustrated in the roentgenograms in Feller and Sternberg's article on the Klippel-Feil syndrome.[12] They show that hemivertebrae may accompany this syndrome to constitute anterior as well as posterior spina bifida, anomalies that also are present in myelocele and in syringomyelia.

Roentgenographic Technique

Ideally, every lateral film of the skull should include the cervical spine. When

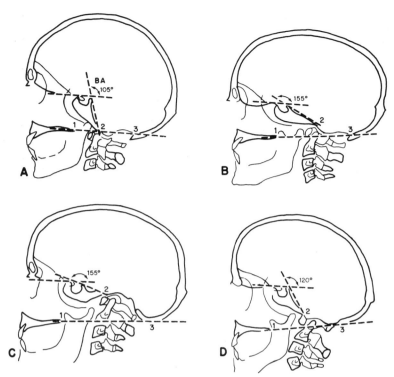

FIGURE 26–4 (1) The posterior end of the hard palate. (2) End of clivus—anterior rim of foramen magnum. (3) Posterior rim of foramen magnum. In *A* and *B* the horizontal line represents Chamberlain's line. In *C* and *D* it represents McGregor's line. *A*. Normal skull. Basal angle is normal (105 degrees). Chamberlain's line connecting 1 and 3 passes through 2. The tip of the odontoid process is below the line. *B*. Platybasia—basal angle is increased (155 degrees). Point 2 and tip of odontoid process are situated above Chamberlain's line. In this case the basilar impression has tilted the clivus and affected only the anterior rim of the foramen magnum. *C*. Basilar impression—basal angle is enlarged (155 degrees). Marked invagination of basiocciput with point 2 and tip of odontoid process well above McGregor's line. Note the upward tilting of C1 (Bull's angle). The occipital bone curves upward to the posterior rim of the foramen magnum. *D*. Assimilation of C1 to the foramen magnum. Basal angle may be normal (120 degrees). Point 2 and tip of odontoid process are situated above McGregor's line. Tilting of C2 widens the space between the laminae of C1 and C2, with posterior tilting of the odontoid and increased cervical lordosis. (Redrawn from Kahn, E., et al.: Correlative Neurosurgery. 2nd Ed. Springfield, Ill., Charles C Thomas, 1969.)

basilar impression is suspected, the central ray is directed through the foramen magnum, employing a long focal distance. The patient is erect and facing forward with the casette resting on his shoulder. It is impossible to obtain a satisfactory lateral film of the craniovertebral junction with the patient horizontal and the head turned to the side. It is just as illogical to make the exposure in this fashion as it would be to make a diagnostic x-ray of any other joint in a twisted position. If a satisfactory upright Bucky grid is not available, the lateral film of the skull may be made with the patient supine and a stationary grid in contact with the head and neck. Without exception, this lateral film should include the upper cervi-

cal spine because this relationship is so important in neurological diagnosis. If the sagittal diameter of the spinal canal below the level of C2 exceeds 17 mm, syringomyelia should be considered.[32]

The degree of basilar impression may be measured on the lateral film of the skull by one of two methods. With Chamberlain's method, a line is drawn from the posterior end of the hard palate to the posterior rim of the foramen magnum.[7] In the normal skull, this line usually will pass through the anterior rim of the foramen magnum constituted by the lower end of the clivus with the tip of the odontoid process below it. Since the anterior and posterior borders of the foramen magnum are difficult to demonstrate without tomography, McGregor's line is preferred to Chamberlain's.[24] This line is drawn from the posterior end of the hard palate to the lowest portion of the occipital bone (Fig. 26–4). The posterior rim of the foramen magnum, utilized in Chamberlain's method, is not a good reference point because it also is carried upward in basilar impression. This makes McGregor's line more informative, the upper limit of normal for the tip of the dens being 5 mm above the line. In severe basilar impression, the dens is obscured by the petrous bones, but its position is indicated by the body of C1, which is more readily seen. In this connection, it should be recalled that the upper portion of the dens develops embryologically from the body of C1. If assimilation is

suspected, tomography will help to identify it, and flexion and extension films will determine whether there is abnormal mobility of the dens.

On anteroposterior roentgenograms the degree of basilar impression is determined by drawing a line from one digastric groove to the other (interdigastric line of Fischgold [Fig. 26–5]). In the normal skull, this line crosses well above the level of the dens and of the occipitoatlantoid joints. In basilar impression, the tip of the dens and the occipital condyles approach this line or extend above it. Associated fusion of the occipitoatlantoid joints may be demonstrated in this view as well as an upward slanting of the petrous ridges as they proceed medially.

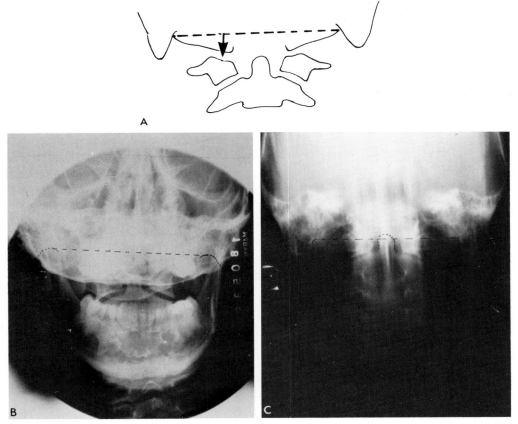

FIGURE 26–5 *A*. Interdigastric line of Fischgold is drawn between digastric grooves, which lie just medial to the bases of the mastoid processes. The distance from this line to the middle of the atlanto-occipital joint (*arrow*) is normally about 10 mm and decreases with basilar impression. *B*. Fischgold's line in the normal skull. *C*. A tomogram of a patient with basilar impression. The interdigastric line passes through the tip of the odontoid and the partly fused occipitoatlantoid joints. Note the upward tilt of the petrous bones.

MALFORMATIONS OF NERVOUS TISSUE

Congenital Hindbrain Hernia

The most common malformation of nervous tissue associated with the bony malformations just described is the congenital hindbrain hernia, generally referred to as the Arnold-Chiari malformation. This malformation was reported in detail by Chiari in 1891, when he described three degrees of herniation of the hindbrain "caused by hydrocephalus of the cerebrum."[8] Chiari's Type I deformity, now sometimes referred to as a pressure cone or occasionally as cerebellar ectopia, consists essentially of a herniation of the cerebellar tonsils through the foramen magnum. This Chiari found in an adult with hydrocephalus and hydromyelia. He described the more severe Type II in the case of an infant with hydrocephalus, myelocele, and hydromyelia. It consisted of a herniation of the inferior vermis, pons, medulla, and compressed fourth ventricle through the foramen magnum. There was a "steplike formation" (telescoping) of the elongated medulla opposite the lower end of the herniated cerebellum and a shortening of the cervical cord to compensate for the elongated brain stem. Three years later, Arnold gave an incidental and incomplete description of Chiari's Type II, and on this basis two of his students subsequently referred to it as the Arnold-Chiari malformation.[1, 30] In his third type, Chiari found the entire cerebellum herniated into a high cervical meningocele. This appears to have been a stillborn fetus, probably with severe Klippel-Feil syndrome, similar to those described by Feller and Sternberg.[12] This condition has acquired the name iniencephaly, and it likewise is accompanied by hydromyelia.[18] In Chiari's more frequently quoted second paper, he reported 14 cases of Type I, all in adults or adolescents, only one of whom had myelocele, and 7 cases of Type II, all in infants with myelocele.[9] Once more he stressed that both types were caused by hydrocephalus of the cerebrum and that Type II was merely a severe form of Type I. It is unfortunate that the term Arnold-Chiari malformation has become firmly established, since this term confuses the issue by referring only to Chiari's Type II and thus sets it apart from his Type I.

It is now known that in both adult and infantile forms of congenital hindbrain hernia, varying degrees of severity exist so that the shape of Type I gradually merges into that of Type II and vice versa. As was first described by Chiari, both types usually are associated with hydromyelia. In Type I, although the entire cerebellum is located lower than normal, only its tonsillar portion protrudes through the foramen magnum, and hydrocephalus, when present, is compensated. Associated with this tonsillar herniation in the adult, there frequently is a downward displacement of the brain stem, a telescoping of the cervicomedullary junction, upwardly slanting cervical nerve roots, and the obex of the fourth ventricle may extend into the cervical canal, just as in the infantile type.[15] In this case, the medulla is impacted in the foramen magnum along with the cerebellar tonsils. In both adult and infantile types, the foramina of the fourth ventricle are frequently bridged by a membrane representing an unperforated rhombic roof. Therefore, the only distinction between the congenital hindbrain hernia of the adult and that of the infant with myelocele is one of degree, although in the latter the cerebellar portion usually consists of vermis rather than tonsils (Fig. 26-6). The hindbrain herniation that results from posterior fossa tumor does not include the brain stem. In this case, the attachments of the mature dentate ligaments will prevent any tendency toward downward dislocation of the cervicomedullary junction.

Syringobulbia

Syringobulbia is a clinical, seldom an anatomical, diagnosis. With this clinical picture, the brain stem exposed at surgery does not appear cystic, although a deep median raphe, which is frequently disclosed on the floor of the fourth ventricle, presumably could connect with a collapsed syrinx. Such a deep raphe may involve the median longitudinal fasciculus. The symptoms of syringobulbia, including the paresis of the lower cranial nerves, usually are caused by the impaction of the hindbrain

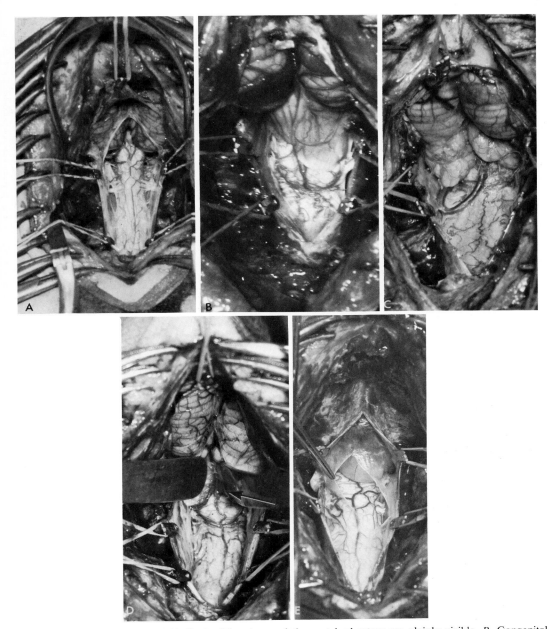

FIGURE 26–6 *A.* A normal hindbrain. The obex and the vertebral artery are plainly visible. *B.* Congenital hindbrain hernia in an adult. The right cerebellar tonsil is herniated farther than the left. Below its pale lower border a posterior bulging of the cervicomedullary junction may be seen. The upward slant of the second cervical nerve root is seen on the right side while the third pursues a normal downward course. *C.* The hindbrain hernia in syringomyelia is frequently accompanied by an elongated loop of the posterior-inferior cerebellar artery. *D.* An unperforated rhombic roof (*arrow*) bridges the foramen of Magendie. *E.* An unperforated rhombic roof may bulge to constitute the Dandy-Walker malformation, or as in this case, its two layers may separate to form an enclosed cyst separate from the arachnoid. This patient had syringomyelia.

hernia, rather than by cavitation of the brain stem as the name implies. However, one instance of true syringobulbia has been shown at operation to be a cephalad extension of a syringomyelic cavity associated with a Dandy-Walker malformation.[25]

Dandy-Walker Malformation

Contrary to common belief, the Dandy-Walker malformation is found not only in the hydrocephalic infant, but in some instances may be present in the adult with basilar impression and syringomyelia.[15] In the infant with Dandy-Walker malformation, the transverse sinus with the attached tentorium is too high; in the infant with Arnold-Chiari malformation it is too low.[19, 23] It remains to be shown that in the adult forms of these malformations, the transverse sinus is displaced in similar fashion. In the author's experience, such displacement has been investigated by angiography in only one instance of basilar impression. In this case, the position and course of the transverse sinus was characteristic of the Dandy-Walker malformation. In this malformation the posterior fossa is larger than normal and the bulging unperforated rhombic roof characteristically displaces the cerebellum in a cephalad direction. Since the foramina of Magendie and Luschka develop from a yielding of the rhombic roof, they really represent a single aperture, but normally they become separated from each other by the encroachment of the growing cerebellum. In cases in which the rhombic roof fails to perforate, it may be so freely permeable that the hydrocephalus of fetal life is completely compensated before delivery or shortly thereafter.

Arachnoid Cysts

Other anomalies of the hindbrain associated either with or without the bony anomalies already described are "arachnoid" cysts at the foramina of Magendie and Luschka.[16] These so-called cysts may be simple diverticula communicating with the fourth ventricle, and their attachments indicate that they represent an abortive form of the Dandy-Walker malformation. This is substantiated by the fact that, especially when found in children or adolescents, these membranes have an inner lining of ependyma and an outer layer of pia. They are not attached to the arachnoid, localizing signs are absent, and the protein content of the contained fluid shows it to be ventricular fluid. They may be encountered at the foramina of Luschka associated with a hindbrain hernia that squeezes shut the foramen of Magendie. Dorothy Russell described this combination in her case 19.[28] In some instances, the two layers of these membranes separate to form an enclosed cyst; in which case, the loculated fluid, though clear and colorless, may have a protein content considerably higher than that of the ventricle.[16] Choroid plexus may be attached to the medial surface of that portion of the cyst wall adjacent to the ventricle, but ependyma is usually lost as these encysted lesions age and enlarge progressively. When located at a foramen of Luschka, the enclosed cyst may produce the symptoms of an angle tumor. They are the most benign surgical lesions that occur in this area.

Syringomyelia

Associated with the congenital malformations of the hindbrain there usually is a cystic dilatation of the cervical cord that may be asymptomatic or may cause symptoms of syringomyelia. The syrinx is a dilatation or diverticulum of the central canal and is distended with ventricular fluid because it has maintained its connection with a partially obstructed fourth ventricle.[13] Beneath the obex, the upper end of the central canal is always patent and funnel-shaped. Such patency has not been demonstrated at operation except in association with a developmental anomaly of the hindbrain.

Symptomatology

The symptoms of these congenital malformations of the hindbrain are many and varied. They may implicate the cranial nerves, the cerebellum, the brain stem, or the spinal cord. Their late onset and disseminated character may lead to the diagnosis of multiple sclerosis. Long-standing elongation and compression of the appropriate cranial nerve may result in oculomotor palsies: trigeminal neuralgia, hemifacial spasm, impairment of hearing and taste, hoarseness, difficulty with deglutition, and spinal accessory or hypoglossal paresis.[14] There may be a cerebellar type of nystagmus and ataxia. Involvement of the brain stem may express itself in a horizontal, rotary or diagonal nystagmus, in a vertical down-beating nystagmus, in dissociated eye movements, and in oscillopsia in which the patient is conscious of the coarse nystagmoid movements.[10] There may be interruption of function of the medial longitudinal fasciculus, resulting in coarse horizontal nystagmus limited to the eye on the side toward which the gaze is directed. This sign is particularly likely to lead to the diagnosis of multiple sclerosis. Occipital headache is an expression of the impaction of hindbrain structures in the foramen magnum. It is a danger signal that may occur only with coughing or straining.

In many cases with hindbrain hernia, the symptoms are limited to the upper spinal cord and are characteristic of syringomyelia. They consist of dissociated sensory loss, particularly in the "shawl distribution" (i.e., scalp, neck, shoulders, arms, and upper thorax), but may also involve the face, torso, and lower extremities. Characteristically, there is atrophy of the small muscles of the hands, with weakness and loss of tendon reflexes in the arms. Scars resulting from burns are commonly seen and Charcot changes may develop in the shoulder joints.

Unilateral astereognosis is common in syringomyelia and indicates involvement of the cuneate nucleus. Contrary to popular belief, pain, particularly in the upper extremities, also is a frequent symptom. It is not dermatomal in distribution and may constitute the initial and only symptom of the syrinx. Sympathetic paralysis from involvement of a lateral column may be indicated by a unilateral loss of sweating. As the syrinx enlarges, long-tract signs develop in the lower extremities. Mirror movements in the upper extremities are occasionally seen and represent cross talk in the pyramidal decussation resulting from

its compression by the dens. The movements may not be typically "mirror." For instance, in one patient, flexion of the index finger caused simultaneous coarse fasciculations in the opposite triceps. Lesser degrees of bilateral synkinesis can be disclosed only by bilateral simultaneous electromyography.[2] Affecting the lower extremities, these associated muscular contractions usually escape detection, but were observed by List in his case 7.[21]

The symptoms of syringomyelia usually develop late and progress slowly, but in young adults the progression is more rapid. The symptoms may reach a plateau, but they never recede spontaneously. Since they may be simulated by an intramedullary tumor, the fallacy has developed that syringomyelia occasionally responds to radiation therapy. Because of the impaction of the hindbrain hernia, mild trauma may result in exacerbation of symptoms, transient quadriplegia, or sudden death.

Pneumoencephalography

In the absence of basilar impression, the diagnosis of these hindbrain anomalies may by confirmed by air study. With proper technique, the pneumoencephalogram characteristically will disclose a filling defect in the cisterna magna and, frequently, a failure of air to enter the ventricles.[20] Below the filling defect caused by the hindbrain hernia, the lateral film may show a collapse of the cystic cord (Fig. 26–7). This collapse occurs because withdrawal of the supporting fluid from the subarachnoid space permits the fluid within the syrinx to gravitate downward and to filter through its attenuated walls so that the upper portion is empty. This collapse can take place only in the anteroposterior direction because the distended cord is anchored laterally by the dentate ligaments. Pneumoencephalography will disclose no air in the ventricles in about 50 per cent of cases. If some air enters the lateral ventricles, they will appear to be dilated.[13]

Every air study in which a surgical lesion is anticipated should be performed in surgery by the neurosurgeon familiar with the case. The technique of pneumoencephalography is important. The injection of air

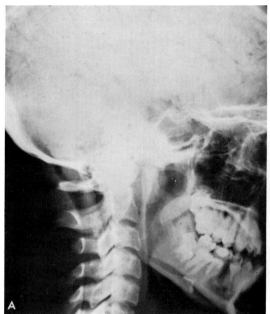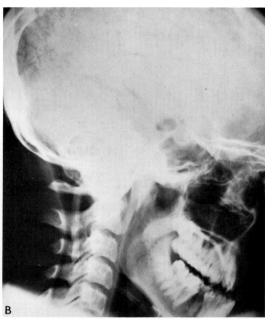

FIGURE 26-7 Pneumoencephalogram in syringomyelia. *A.* This early film shows no air in the ventricles. A hindbrain hernia is outlined in the cisterna magna, and below that the spinal cord is distended. *B.* A later film shows collapse of the distended cord with disappearance of the cerebellar hernia. The negative pressure in the syrinx transmitted to the ventricles caused the hernia to be withdrawn into the skull.

before removing fluid may reduce a congenital cerebellar hernia to the extent that it cannot be demonstrated on the film. Since the intracranial pressure is normal in syringomyelia despite the hernia, the exchange of fluid with air may be started without a preliminary air injection. The patient should be sitting with the head in acute flexion and fixed to the Bucky grid, so that a lateral film centering on the cisterna magna may be made *immediately* after the exchange of 20 ml. After this, the exchange may be continued at the operator's discretion. Acute flexion is necessary to render the cisterna magna more clearly visible by increasing the space between the lamina of C1 and the foramen magnum. This posture should be used with caution, however, if there is assimilation. The preliminary exchange must be carried out rapidly so as not to allow time for all of the injected air to enter the skull. For this reason general anesthesia, preferably thiopental (Pentothal), is employed.

Air is preferred to iophendylate (Pantopaque) because the latter will not differentiate a syrinx from an intramedullary tumor unless an effort is made to demonstrate a foraminal hernia. As the tonsils lie dorsal to the cervical cord, it may be necessary to remove the needle in order to place the patient in a supine position. Although seldom indicated, a small quantity of Pantopaque introduced into the lateral ventricle may be maneuvered into the fourth ventricle to demonstrate obstruction of the outlets and passage of the medium into the syrinx via the central canal. Arteriography may demonstrate an elongated loop of the posterior inferior cerebellar artery herniated through the foramen magnum, and the late venous phase may demonstrate an abnormal position of the transverse sinus.

Hydrodynamic Mechanism

The normal brain, being enclosed in a nonexpansible container, is a nonpulsating organ. Each cerebral pulse systole, therefore, is accompanied by a spurt of blood into the emerging veins, and by an accompanying spurt of ventricular fluid into the distensible spinal dural sac. Bering's studies have shown that within the ventricle the fluid pulse wave is a sharp spike that is reduced on reaching the cisterna magna and still further blunted at the lumbar level.[3, 4] This means that the distensibility of the spinal dural sac exerts a damping effect on the ventricular fluid pulse wave as it spurts from the fourth ventricle through the foramen magnum to pass down the spinal canal. This pulse wave, acting on the outer surface of the spinal cord, tends to close off its central canal. Conversely, if, as in fetal life, the ventricular fluid pulse wave does not escape freely, its water hammer effect is augmented and it will continue to be funneled into the central canal, causing it to gradually dilate. When, in addition, the foramen magnum is partly blocked by a cone-shaped hindbrain hernia, the intracranial subarachnoid pulse wave is superimposed on the intraventricular. The importance of the free escape of the fluid pulse wave from the rigid-walled intracranial cavity is suggested by the fact that the ventricles do not dilate in pseudotumor cerebri despite the increased intracranial pressure.[33]

When the hindbrain and upper spinal cord are exposed by a craniovertebral decompression in a subject in whom the fluid passageways are free, there is little or no visible pulsation of the nervous structures. However, if the ready escape of the intracranial fluid pulse wave is obstructed by a congenital hindbrain hernia, the impacted structures pulsate freely, moving caudally with each pulse systole and cephalad with its diastole. Because of this movement, the obstruction at the foramen magnum is more complete during systole, with resulting accentuation of the pulse wave in the intracranial fluid. The retraction of the hernia during diastole will permit fluid from the spinal canal to enter the cerebral subarachnoid spaces, as is also true of air injected during encephalography. To cause this intermittent blockage, the hindbrain hernia need not project below the foramen magnum to any significant degree, in which case the hernia may be overlooked after the dura is opened. Herniation should be suspected if at operation the vertebral arteries are obscured by overlying tonsils. Over the years, the to and fro movement of the impacted hernia results in damage to the involved structures, while the imprisoned ventricular fluid pulse wave may injure structures above the block by creating false diverticuli to constitute true syringobulbia.

Congenital hindbrain hernia develops during fetal life because the growing cerebellum expands in a posterior fossa too small to accommodate it. At this stage, the immature dentate ligaments are not able to prevent the medulla and upper cervical cord from taking part in this caudal dislocation. If severe, the hernia will cause a telescoping of the cervicomedullary junction sufficient to obstruct the central canal. This obstruction, although occurring in fetal life, requires time to develop so that the central canal below is dilated and usually remains so after its communication with the fourth ventricle is interrupted (noncommunicating hydromyelia). Because it develops during the stage of rapid cellular reproduction, this infantile hydromyelia is lined by ependyma and therefore is readily identified as a dilated central canal. If the hernia is less severe, the telescoping will be milder or nonexistent, so that the central canal remains a true diverticulum communicating with the fourth ventricle. Throughout life, it thus receives the impact of the augmented ventricular fluid pulse wave. The expansible spinal dural sac allows the central canal to expand and contract slightly with each pulse beat. Neurons, compared with neuroglia, are less able to resist this gentle long-continued water hammer effect, and eventually they succumb. Ependyma constitutes the first line of defense and is the first structure to disappear as the mature central canal continues to gradually dilate.

The upper part of the central canal, surrounded by impacted structures, cannot dilate significantly. However, below the impaction it dilates in response to the undamped ventricular fluid pulse wave. The posterior commissure yields first, while the anterior commissure remains intact and usually retains some of its ependymal covering. This indicates that the anatomical interruption of pain and temperature fibers occurs first in the gray matter lateral to the central canal rather than in the anterior commissure. Only thus can one explain the *unilateral* onset of dissociated sensory loss.

Where ependyma is lost, a diverticulum of the dilated central canal may develop and dissect longitudinally following the course of the long tracts. The communication between this diverticulum and the central canal may be small so that at most levels a cross-section will show a "true syrinx" paralleling the central canal with no apparent connection between them. The fluid in the syrinx is colorless; its protein content indicates its ventricular origin, and indigo carmine will enter it from the ventricle.

Our understanding of congenital hindbrain hernia and its resulting syringomyelia has been seriously delayed because the time-honored autopsy practice of removing the brain in one piece destroys the relationship between the area of pathological change and the surrounding bone and severs the communication between the fourth ventricle and the syrinx. In cases of suspected hindbrain hernia, the brain removal should be done, or at least supervised, by the clinician who is familiar with the case and therefore better able to anticipate the changes that must be investigated. It is essential that the cerebral hemispheres be removed first so as to expose the tentorium with the hindbrain in situ. Following this, a cervical laminectomy will permit removal of the hindbrain and cervical cord in one piece. Fixation of the structures by prior embalming is of great advantage.

It is now recognized that in the infant with congenital hindbrain hernia and myelocele, the transverse sinus with the attached tentorium is located much lower and closer to the foramen magnum than in the normal infant. Since the size of the

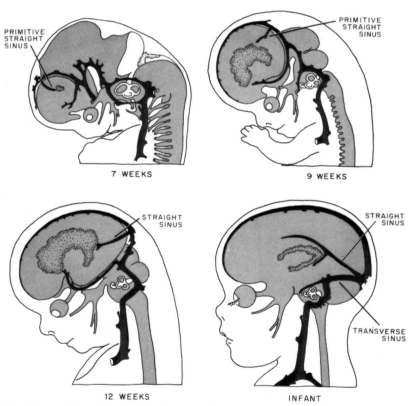

FIGURE 26–8 The straight and transverse sinuses with the attached tentorium originate far forward and are pushed posteriorly by the expanding forebrain. If they are pushed too far, the developing posterior fossa will be too small, as in the Arnold-Chiari malformation. If they are not pushed far enough, the fossa will be too large, as in the Dandy-Walker malformation. The relatively large size of the choroid plexus indicates its functional significance in this migration. (Redrawn from Padget, D., 1957; reproduced from J. Neurol. Neurosurg. Psychiat., *28*:247, 1965.)

posterior fossa is determined by the distance between the tentorium and the basilar process of the occipital bone, it may be encroached upon from above by a low tentorium or from below by basilar impression, or by a combination of both. Basilar impression, as has been shown, is always acquired postnatally, whereas an abnormally low position of the transverse sinus must of necessity have developed in intrauterine life. If the posterior fossa is much too small, the cerebellar portion of the hernia will consist of the earlier developing vermis, if less small, of the later developing tonsils. Although it remains to be demonstrated, a low attachment of the tentorium is the logical explanation of the congenital hindbrain hernia of adulthood, particularly when unaccompanied by basilar impression.

Padget's illustrations show that the anlage of the transverse sinus (and tentorium) arises far anteriorly and migrates posteriorly as the forebrain expands at the expense of the primitive hindbrain.[26] This excursion is almost complete by the twelfth week, at which time the forebrain still resembles a bag of water that contains a relatively enormous choroid plexus (Fig. 26–8). Although a choroid plexus appears first in the primitive fourth ventricle, it is quickly surpassed in size by that in the lateral ventricles. In view of this fact, it follows that excursion of the primitive transverse sinus is caused by fluid expansion of the forebrain resulting from the fluid pulse wave imparted by the rapidly enlarging anterior choroid plexus (Bering effect). In other words, the migration of the primitive transverse sinus is the result of hydrodynamic stresses, in which expansion of the forebrain competes with that of the hindbrain and the ultimate position of the sinus depends upon which wins.

Operative Technique

In basilar impression, the pushing inward of the foramen magnum handicaps the surgeon and necessitates adequate flexion of the head on the cervical spine. Therefore, before proceeding there must be assurance that the patient is breathing spontaneously. After positioning, a preoperative film of the craniocervical junction may be indicated to exclude posterior tilting of the dens. Before removal from the chair, a postoperative film may disclose air in lateral ventricles not previously delineated.

Since the cause of syringomyelia is not in the spinal cord but in the hindbrain, its treatment requires a midline exposure of the hindbrain. Incision of the syrinx treats the result, but does not correct the cause, nor does it relieve the impaction of the hindbrain hernia. Except in the case of a loculated cyst in the cerebellopontine angle, the surgical treatment of these malformations of the hindbrain is the same, whether or not they are associated with bony malformation. With the patient in the sitting position, through a midline incision, the laminae of the upper two cervical vertebrae are removed and the foramen magnum is enlarged posteriorly. It is neither necessary nor advisable to tap the lateral ventricle. If the exposure is performed with the patient prone, and particularly if preceded by a ventricular tap, a cerebellar hernia may be reduced and thus be overlooked. As the dura is opened in a linear fashion, the cerebellar tonsils will be found elongated and herniated into the foramen magnum so that the passageway between them and the medulla is squeezed shut by the impaction. This impaction is accentuated momentarily by the downward excursion of the tonsils occurring with each pulse systole. Occasionally it is necessary to remove additional laminae to decompress the tips of the herniated tonsils. The cerebellar hernia will be seen to interfere with the escape of the ventricular fluid pulse wave and to create a partial subarachnoid block at the foramen magnum, particularly during the pulse systole. The subarachnoid block is relieved by enlarging the foramen magnum, and the ventricular block by dissecting open the passageway between the cerebellar tonsils and the medulla. If the arachnoid is not adherent to the hernia, it will bulge after the dura is opened and create the false impression of a cisterna magna of normal size.

Because the neurological surgeon seldom has occasion to expose these structures when they are normal, the following observations are recommended to better define the pathological process. As soon as the posterior rim of the foramen magnum is removed, a suture or other suitable marker is placed on the outer layer of the dura to indicate its previous position. This reference point will enable the surgeon subsequently to measure the degree of downward displacement of the cerebellar tonsils and of the obex. After opening the dura, the presence or absence of posterior buckling of the cervicomedullary junction should be noted. The tonsils then may be separated gently to see whether the foramen of Magendie is bridged by a membrane, representing a failure of perforation of the rhombic roof. Exploration with a nerve hook beneath the obex will demonstrate patency of the upper end of the cervical canal. The depth of the median raphe should be noted and also the course of the upper cervical nerve roots as they proceed to their foramina of exit. Herniated tonsils, if not adherent, will drift apart after the dura is opened, with spontaneous release of the obstruction of the foramen. Therefore, if the foramen of Magendie appears patent, the edges of the dural incision should be reapproximated to determine whether this will squeeze it shut. The exposed portion of the cervical cord should be inspected for distention, fluctuation, or evidence of collapse, but the bony opening should not be extended downward for the sole purpose of demonstrating the suspected syrinx.

If the foramen of Magendie is bridged by a membrane, it must of course be excised. If the patient is young, this membrane may still have remnants of ependyma lining its ventricular surface. Separation of the cerebellar tonsils will reveal a funnel-shaped upper end of the central canal beneath the obex, frequently with a deep median raphe leading into it. This funnel-shaped entrance should be plugged with a bit of muscle in order to close off the central canal from the fourth ventricle. This should be done regardless of whether the symptoms suggest syringomyelia. Because the slippery muscle plug may be dislodged during postoperative straining or vomiting, a knot of silk suture material of adequate size may be used in its place. A syrinx opening onto the floor of the fourth ventricle, or a cystic brain stem has not been identified at operation in any of the author's cases. However, the sitting position of the patient will collapse a bulbar syrinx, which then could readily be overlooked, particularly if originating in a deep median raphe.

In concluding the operation, it is essential that the incised dura be left open, for if it is closed, the foramen of Magendie once more will be squeezed shut by the reimpaction of the hindbrain hernia. The edges of the dural incision, therefore, are sutured back to the spinal muscles at the foramen magnum, and a diamond-shaped patch of dural substitute is sewn in place in order to enlarge the diameter of the dural sac at this critical level. This important step also improves convalescence by preventing free access to the subarachnoid space of protein laden interstitial fluid, which otherwise is continually washed from the raw surface of the nuchal muscles by the fluid pulsations. Such access is indicated by spinal fluid protein levels up to 600 mg per 100 ml, persisting in some cases for weeks after operation. The presence of such excessive amounts of protein has been shown to impair cerebrospinal fluid absorption, which may reactivate a compensated hydrocephalus and necessitate a shunting procedure.[17] For the same reason, frequent spinal punctures are advisable to remove bloody spinal fluid during the early postoperative period. The subarachnoid injection of 40 to 80 mg of methylprednisolone (Depo-Medrol) will help prevent arachnoiditis from this source.

Precautions

It is neither necessary nor advisable to carry the laminectomy low enough to expose the syrinx. Extensive laminectomy sometimes has been followed by a severe flexion deformity of the cervical spine, presumably because of faulty innervation of the nuchal muscles. Amputation of the herniated tonsils is risky and leads to adhesions that may defeat the purpose of the operation. If the herniated tonsils are densely adherent, an attempt to separate them may damage the blood supply of the medulla. In this case, an incision should be made through the lower portion of the vermis in order to open the fourth ventricle and allow the escape of the imprisoned ventricular fluid pulse wave. A large muscle plug may then be placed in the pocket formed by the closed caudal end of the fourth ventricle. Extreme gentleness, meticulous hemostasis, and a small but adequate bony opening are essential. In rare instances, a delayed subarachnoid or intramedullary hemorrhage has occurred and has been attributed to the decompression of congenitally inadequate vessel walls. The presence of a dense band of adhesions binding the cerebellar tonsils to the brain stem offers a poorer prognosis. Attempts to remove them will usually result in interruption of blood vessels that nourish the medulla. Application of a G-suit eliminates the risk of postural hypotension and air embolism in the sitting position.

Case Selection and Prognosis

Surgery is advised only in patients whose symptoms are progressing, in whom occipital headaches are severe, or in whom quadriplegia has followed trauma. Longstanding neurological deficits, with the exception of ataxia, are seldom benefited. With the present operative technique, it is appropriate to tell a patient that there probably will be no progression of his symptoms after operation and probably there will be improvement of those symptoms that have developed most recently.

In a series of 74 patients operated upon for syringomyelia, there was prompt improvement in some of the symptoms in 52, no change in 11, worsening in 6, and 5 did not survive the operation.[13] Of the preoperative symptoms, subjective numbness, dissociated sensory loss and pain were most likely to be improved, although motor power, astereognosis, ataxia, and bulbar palsies were benefited in some.

REFERENCES

1. Arnold, J.: Myelocyste, Transposition von Gewebskeimen und Sympodie. Beitr. Path. Anat., 16:1–28, 1894.
2. Baird, P. A., Robinson, G. C., and Buckler, W. S.: Klippel-Feil syndrome. A study of mirror movement detected by electromyography. Amer. J. Dis. Child., 113:546–551, 1967.
3. Bering, E. A., Jr.: Choroid plexus and arterial pulsation of cerebrospinal fluid; demonstration of choroid plexuses as cerebrospinal fluid pump. A.M.A. Arch. Neurol. Psychiat., 73:165–172, 1955.
4. Bering, E. A., Jr.: Circulation of the cerebrospinal fluid. Demonstration of the choroid plexuses as the generator of the force for flow of fluid and ventricular enlargement. J. Neurosurg., 19:405–413, 1962.
5. Bezi, I.: Assimilation of atlas and compression of medulla: clinical significance and pathology of torticollis and localized chronic arthritis deformans of spine: Report of case. Arch. Path., 12:333–357, 1931.
6. Bull, J. W. D., Nixon, W. L. B., Pratt, R. T. C., and Robinson, P. K.: Paget's disease of the skull and secondary basilar impression. Brain, 82:10–22, 1959.
7. Chamberlain, W. E.: Basilar impression (platybasia): A bizarre developmental anomaly of the occipital bone and upper cervical spine with striking and misleading neurologic manifestations. Yale J. Biol. Med., 11:487–496, 1939.
8. Chiari, H.: Über Veränderungen des Kleinhirns infolge von Hydrocephalie des Grosshirns. Deutsche. Med. Wschr., 17:1172–1175, 1891.
9. Chiari, H.: Über die Veränderungen des Kleinhirns, der Pons und der Medulla oblongata infolge von congenitaler Hydrocephalie des Grosshirns. Denkschr. Akad. Wissensch. Wien, 63:71–116, 1895.
10. Cogan, D. G.: Down-beat nystagmus. Arch. Ophth., 80:757–786, 1968.
11. Ebenius, B.: The roentgen appearance in four cases of basilar impression. Acta Radiol., 15:652–656, 1934.
12. Feller, A., and Sternberg, H.: Zur Kenntnis der Fehlbildungen der Wirbelsaule; die anatomischen Grundlagen des Kurzhalses (Klippel-Feilschen Syndroms). Virchow Arch. Path. Anat., 285:112–139, 1932.
13. Gardner, W. J.: Hydrodynamic mechanism of syringomyelia: Its relationship to myelocele. J. Neurol. Neurosurg. Psychiat., 28:247–259, 1965.
14. Gardner, W. J., and Dohn, D. F.: Trigeminal neuralgia—hemifacial spasm—Paget's disease; significance of this association. Brain, 89:555–562, 1966.
15. Gardner, W. J., Abdullah, A. F., and McCormack, L. J.: The varying expressions of embryonal atresia of the fourth ventricle in adults: Arnold-Chiari malformation, Dandy-Walker syndrome, arachnoid cyst of the cerebellum, and syringomyelia. J. Neurosurg., 14:591–605, 1957.
16. Gardner, W. J., McCormack, L. J., and Dohn, D. F.: Embryonal atresia of the fourth ventricle: the cause of "arachnoid cyst" of the cerebellopontine angle. J. Neurosurg., 17:226–237, 1960.
17. Gardner, W. J., Spitler, D. K., and Whitten, C.: Increased intracranial pressure caused by increased protein content in the cerebrospinal fluid; an explanation of papilledema in certain cases of small intracranial and intraspinal tumors, and in the Guillain-Barré syndrome. New Eng. J. Med., 250:932–936, 1954.
18. Gilmour, J. R.: Essential identity of Klippel-Feil syndrome and iniencephaly. J. Path. Bact., 53:117–131, 1941.
19. Greenfield, J. G.: *In* Blackwood, W., Mc-

Menemey, W. H., Meyer, A., Norman, R. M., and Russell, D. S.: Neuropathology. 2nd Ed. London, Arnold, 1963.

20. Greenwald, E. M., Eugenio, M., Hughes, C. R., and Gardner, W. J.: The importance of the air shadow of the cisterna magna in encephalographic diagnosis. Radiology, *71*:695–701, 1958.

21. List, C. F.: Neurologic syndromes accompanying developmental anomalies of occipital bone, atlas and axis. Arch. Neurol. Psychiat., *45*: 577–616, 1941.

22. List, C. F.: Developmental anomalies of the craniovertebral border. Chapter 20, *In* Kahn, E., Crosby, E., and Schneider, T., eds.: Correlative Neurosurgery. 2nd Ed. Springfield, Ill., Charles C Thomas, 1969.

23. Matson, D. D.: Prenatal obstruction of the fourth ventricle. Amer. J. Roentgen., *76*:499–506, 1956.

24. McGregor, M.: Significance of certain measurements of skull in diagnosis of basilar impression. Brit. J. Radiol., *21*:171–181, 1948.

25. Newton, E. J.: Syringomyelia as a manifestation of defective fourth ventricular drainage. Ann. Roy. Coll. Surg. Eng., *44*:199–213, 1967.

26. Padget, D. H.: Development of cranial venous system in man from viewpoint of comparative anatomy. Carnegie Inst. Publication 611, Washington, 1957, pp. 79–140.

27. Ray, B. S.: Platybasia with involvement of central nervous system. Ann. Surg., *116*:231–250, 1942.

28. Russell, D. S.: Observations on the pathology of hydrocephalus. Med. Res. Counc. Spec. Rep. Ser., No. 265, 1949.

29. Schüller, A.: Zur Roentgen-Diagnose der basalen Impression des Schadels. Wien. med. Wchnschr., *61*:2593–2599, 1911.

30. Schwalbe, E., and Gredig, M.: Über Entwicklungsstörungen der Kleinhirns, Hirnstamms und Halsmarks bei Spina bifida. Beitr. Path. Anat., *40*:133–194, 1907.

31. Taveras, J. M., and Wood, E. H.: Diagnostic Neuroradiology. Baltimore, Williams & Wilkins Co., 1964.

32. Wells, C. E., Spillane, J. D., and Bligh, A. S.: The cervical spinal canal in syringomyelia. Brain, *82*:23–40, 1959.

33. Wilson, D. H., and Gardner, W. J.: Benign intracranial hypertension with particular reference to its occurrence in fat young women. Canad. Med. A. J., *95*:102–105, 1966.

27

LEPTOMENINGEAL CYSTS

Leptomeningeal or arachnoid cysts are benign thin-walled cysts lying in relation to or enclosed by the subarachnoid space, filled with clear fluid, located in general near primary fissures and spinal fluid cisterns of the cerebral cortex and cerebellum, and associated with varying degrees of cerebral tissue loss by compression. They are benign lesions — recognition and treatment are followed by good results.

Cystic lesions of the surface of the brain have been known and described sporadically in the literature for nearly 150 years. However, the etiology and pathogenesis have been obscure in most cases, and their classification therefore unsatisfactory. Four major types may be recognized: developmental anomalies of the meninges, meningeal cysts secondary to inflammation, post-traumatic leptomeningeal cysts, and ependymal cysts of the brain.

DEVELOPMENTAL ANOMALIES OF THE MENINGES

Starkman studied three cases of noninfectious cysts of the leptomeninges and, on the basis of sections taken at the junction of the cyst and normal arachnoid, proposed that the cysts result from a maldevelopment of the perimedullary mesh, with the sequestration of an enclosed chamber within the arachnoid membrane.[5] The developing fluid-filled subarachnoid space would be between it and the cortex, and a true intra-arachnoid cyst would be formed. It was further conjectured that these cysts may communicate with the subarachnoid space

and be expanded by a pumping action of the spinal fluid. Robinson, on the other hand, believed that the cysts are secondary to agenesis of the brain.[4] Whatever the etiology, the cysts characteristically lie beneath the arachnoid. The most common location is in the sylvian fissure, where there is compression of the underlying frontal and temporal opercula, with the island of Reil being brought into view. Other common locations are: the interhemispheral fissure, the cerebral convexity, the base of the brain, and over the midline of the cerebellum in the posterior fossa (Fig. 27–1). The transparent cyst walls do not show evidence of inflammation or hemorrhage. The cysts are usually filled with clear spinal fluid, although occasionally xanthochromic fluid of high protein content may be found. The underlying brain

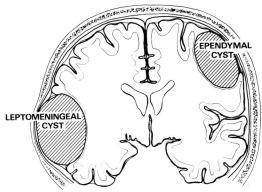

FIGURE 27–1 Leptomeningeal and ependymal cysts: The leptomeningeal cyst arises outside the pia, between the layers of the leptomeninges. It displaces dura and bone outward and pia and brain inward. The ependymal cyst lies beneath the pia and does not displace surface vessels, leptomeninges, dura, or bone. For characteristic locations and other features see text.

F. P. GOLDSTEIN
C. E. BRACKETT

may be perfectly normal, it may be compressed, or it may be atrophic and gliotic.

The signs and symptoms depend upon the location of the cyst. In early life the presentation may be that of a generalized enlargement of the head with symptoms and signs of increased intracranial pressure.[1] Those in the sylvian fissure give rise to headache, seizures, and occasionally focal neurological signs. Headache is more common when the leptomeningeal cyst is associated with the presence of hydrocephalus. Posterior fossa cysts are apt to produce nystagmus, unsteadiness of gait, and increased intracranial pressure. The clinical course is prolonged unless bleeding into the cyst follows trauma, in which case a previously asymptomatic cyst may rapidly become symptomatic.

Since the cysts are of long standing and may enlarge slowly, a significant proportion of them may be asymptomatic. The cysts located in the sylvian fissure cause thinning of the temporal bone and enlargement of the temporal fossa, forward protrusion of the greater wing and elevation of the lesser wing of the sphenoid bone, depression of the middle fossa, and erosion of the sella turcica. The electroencephalogram may show decreased activity over the area of the cyst. The diagnosis is established by carotid angiography, which shows the typical findings of an avascular sylvian mass. Cysts in other locations are less apt to cause focal bony changes. Those lying in the interhemispheric fissure may produce focal avascular deformities on the arteriogram. Those in the posterior fossa frequently produce aqueductal obstruction or displacement, depending upon their location. Differential diagnosis includes chronic subdural hematoma or hygroma, which may be separated by their different appearance on the arteriogram; cystic tumors of the brain, which are separated by the distinctive long-standing bony changes; and other types of leptomeningeal cysts, the differential diagnosis of which may be difficult.

Although these cysts can be drained by intermittent puncture, the treatment of choice is appropriate craniotomy, exposure and biopsy of the cyst, and resection of the outer cyst wall. Stripping of the cyst wall is usually not indicated. Recurrence may require a shunting procedure. These are benign lesions, and the prognosis with surgical treatment is excellent.

POSTINFECTIOUS LEPTOMENINGEAL CYSTS

These cysts follow meningitis in which circumscribed areas of the meninges are walled off by adhesions and a cyst is formed. This type would, on many occasions, be difficult to differentiate from those just described. Both developmental and postinfectious cysts may be multiple, are common in early life, and may cause generalized enlargement of the head. Adhesions may wall off any of the spinal fluid cisterns: e.g., chiasmal, basal, ambient, or medullary. The cysts lie in the subarachnoid space as space-occupying lesions.

Treatment of postinfectious cysts is similar to those of developmental cysts. The eradication of multiple cysts may be difficult.

POST-TRAUMATIC LEPTOMENINGEAL CYSTS

Post-traumatic leptomeningeal cysts are discussed separately in Chapter 52 in the section on Trauma.

EPENDYMAL CYSTS OF THE BRAIN

Ependymal cysts characteristically lie within the substance of the brain, usually the cerebral cortex, and are commonly located near the midline in the parasagittal position. The cysts are large and smooth-walled with a thin membrane, through which can be seen the clear contents of the cyst. Normal arteries and veins may traverse the cyst wall, which appears entirely similar to that of the previously described leptomeningeal cyst (Fig. 27–1). At craniotomy, however, careful biopsy of the cyst wall may reveal typical ependymal cells with all their histological characteristics. These ependymal cysts are presumed to arise from displaced remnants of ependyma. They are not connected with the ventricular system. Jakubiak et al., in reporting their experience with four cases, reviewed the hypotheses regarding the formation of these interesting lesions.[3] From the clinical point of view they present as benign intracerebral space-occupying lesions frequently associated wih seizures, hemiparesis, and signs and symptoms of increased intracranial pressure. They are commonly not associated with erosion of the overlying bone, and the picture in the pneumoencephalogram or arteriogram is that of a cystic intracerebral lesion. Therapy consists of exposure by appropriate craniotomy and excision of the cyst wall. Results following the operation are good.

REFERENCES

1. Anderson, F. M., and Landing, B. H.: Cerebral arachnoid cysts in infants. J. Pediat., *69*:88–96, 1966.
2. Gruszkiewicz, J., and Peyser, E.: Supratentorial arachnoidal cyst associated with hydrocephalus. J. Neurol. Neurosurg. Psychiat., *28*:438–441, 1965.
3. Jakubiak, P., Dunsmore, R. H., and Beckett, R. S.: Supratentorial brain cysts. J. Neurosurg., *28*: 129–136, 1968.
4. Robinson, R. G.: Local bulging of the skull and external hydrocephalus due to cerebral agenesis. Brit. J. Radiol., *31*:691–700, 1958.
5. Starkman, S. P., Brown, T. C., and Linell, E. A.: Cerebral arachnoid cysts. J. Neuropath. Exp. Neurol., *17*:484–500, 1958.

INDEX

In this index page numbers set in *italics* indicate illustrations or, when followed by *(t)*, tables. Drugs are indexed under their generic names when dosage or action or special use is given. The abbreviation vs. is used to indicate differential diagnosis.

Bacitracin *(Continued)*
  intrathecal, via lumbar puncture, *310(t)*
  wound irrigation with, in craniotomy, 540
  in spinal operations, 548
Bacteria, in infection in multiple injury, 872
  culture of, 903
  in septic shock, 884
Bacterial endocarditis, aneurysm from, in
  subarachnoid hemorrhage, 712
Bacterial meningitis, 1550. See also *Meningitis.*
  cerebrospinal fluid in, 309, *319(t)*
  coma from, 52
  postoperative, 2002
Bailey-Cushing classification of gliomas, 1298–
  1300, *1299, 1303(t),* 1341
Balance, in flocculonodular syndrome, 22
  in Schiebe's deafness, 417
  otological testing of, 410
  ventrolateral thalamotomy and, in Parkinson's
  disease, 1854
Ballismus. See *Hemiballism.*
Barbiturates, cerebral blood flow and, 669
  cerebral metabolism and, 524
  electroencephalographic activation by, 336
  in angiography, 90
  in general anesthesia, 514
  in post-traumatic epilepsy, 1038
  in psychogenic pain, 1641
  overdose of, electroencephalogram in, 344, *345*
  pain perception tests with, 1625
Barrier phenomena, in tumor chemotherapy, 1491
Basal approach, craniotomy, 543
Basal ganglia, 8
  calcification in, in skull films, *81*
Basilar artery, aneurysms of, 787–806
  angiography in, 159, *159*
  intracranial repair of, *791, 792, 792*
    bifurcation of, 793, *793(t), 793–797*
    trunk of, 798, *798(t), 798–800*
    ligation in, 790
  as collateral channel, 660
  normal radiological anatomy of, 122, *123, 125,*
    129, *130*
  occlusion of, signs and symptoms of, 699
  thrombosis of, angiography in, 152, *154*
Basilar fractures, of skull, 1013–1022, *1014, 1015,*
  1017–1019
    mechanism of, 971
    post-traumatic pain in, 1652
Basilar impression, 628, *629, 630*
  operative technique in, 641
  radiology in, 631, *632*
Basilar invagination, spinal roentgenograms in,
  235, *239*
Basilar vein, normal radiological anatomy of, 138
Battle's sign, in basilar skull fractures, 1013, 1016
BCNU, in tumor chemotherapy, 1499
  vincristine and, independent toxicity of, 1496
"Bedside manner," in psychogenic pain, 1639
Beevor's sign, in thoracic disc protrusion, 1188
  in thoracolumbar spinal cord lesions, 1086
Behavior, brain injury and, 1040, 1047
  care-soliciting, in psychogenic pain, 1642
  clinical diagnosis and, in child, 40–41
    in frontal lobe syndrome, *13,* 14
  disorders of, vs. cerebral hemisphere tumor, 1364

Behavior *(Continued)*
  limbic system in, 1887
    lateral circuit of, 1893, *1894*
  model in, 423
  psychological evaluation of, 424–428
    tests for, 428–432, *429,* 1040
Békésy audiometry, 415
  in acoustic neuroma, 1437, *1438*
  in eighth nerve deafness, 419, *420*
  in inner ear deafness, 417, *418*
Bell's palsy, clinical diagnosis of, 21
Benadryl. See *Diphenhydramine.*
Benedikt's syndrome, 21
Benign paroxysmal positional vertigo, 1033
Benzalkonium chloride, preoperative skin
  preparation with, 530
Benzedrine. See *Amphetamine.*
Benzhexol, in Parkinson's disease, 1841
Benztropine, in Parkinson's disease, 1841
Bergstrand classification of gliomas, 1341
Berry aneurysm, 709, *711(t),* 712–714, *712, 713(t)*
Beta rhythm, electroencephalographic, 342, *343,*
  345
Bethanechol, in postoperative urinary retention,
  1997
  in sensory and motor paralytic bladder, 1942
  supersensitivity test with, 1936
Bicarbonate, acid-base regulation and, 895
  normal levels of, 891
Biceps brachii muscle, in brachial plexus
  injury, 1116
Bielschowsky head tilt test, 386
Bimedial lobotomy, 1886
Biopsy, brain, complications of, 1972
  in cerebral hemisphere tumors, 1373
  in cryohypophysectomy, 1912
  in orbital tumors, 1287
Bipedicle flaps, scalp, *916,* 921
Biperiden, in Parkinson's disease, 1841
Bipolar cautery, in intracranial aneurysm repair,
  740, 759
  in microneurosurgical procedures, 555
  spinal cord tumor removal, 1527
Birth defects, 588–607. See also names of specific
  conditions.
Birth injury, cervical nerve root, 1060
Bladder, autonomous neurogenic, 27, 1938, *1938,*
  1943
  drainage of, types of, 1939
  innervation of, 1931
  motor paralytic, 1936, *1937,* 1942
  neurogenic dysfunction of, clinical diagnosis of, 27
    disc prolapse and, 1944
    in myelomeningocele, 598
    management of, 1938–1943, *1942*
    neurolytic nerve block and, 1732
    postoperative, 1997
    types of, 1936–1938, *1936–1938*
  pain in, 1698, 1700
  radiology of, 1933, *1934*
  reflex neurogenic, 1937–1938, *1937,* 1943
  sensory paralytic, 1936, *1936,* 1942
  uninhibited neurogenic, 27, 1937, *1937,* 1942
Blastomycosis, of spine, 1582
Bleeding. See *Hemorrhage* and *Subarachnoid
  hemorrhage.*

Brain stem (*Continued*)
  in trigeminal neuralgia, 1663
  lesions of, clinical diagnosis of, 47, 49
    optokinetic nystagmus in, 394
  tumors of, in children, 1481, 1486
    operative removal of, 1478
    symptoms of, 1467
  uncal herniation and, 951
  viral encephalitis of, 1557
Breast, carcinoma of, hormone dependency of, 1901
    hypophysectomy in, 1902–1904
      surgical, 1915, *1915(t)*
      results of, 1923
  metastatic to spine, radiology of, 255
  pain in, 1698
Breathing. See *Respiration*.
Bretylium, in hypothermia, 1458
Brissaud's syndrome, 21
Bromouridine, in tumor chemotherapy, 1500
Bronchopneumonia, postoperative, 1989
Bronchospasm, postoperative, 1988
Brown-Séquard syndrome, 30
Brucellosis, anterior cervical approach in, 1219
Bruising. See *Contusion*.
Bruit, in arteriovenous malformations of spinal
    cord, 854
  in carotid-cavernous fistula, 813
Bubble manometer, in intracranial pressure
    measurement, 446
Buckling, arterial, angiography in, 145–146, *145*
BUdR. See *Bromouridine*.
Buffer base, acid-base regulation and, 895
Bulbar nerve palsy, clinical diagnosis of, 22
Burns, electrical, peripheral nerve injury in, 1094
  intraoperative, 1960
  scalp, 912, *914, 915*
Bursitis, vs. cervical disc rupture, 1204
Bursting fracture, cervical, 1054, *1054*

Caffeine, cerebral blood flow and, *674(t)*
Caffey's disease, skull in, 1262
Calcification, skull films showing, extracalvarial, 57
    59
  in sellar tumors, 1421
  in thoracic disc protrusion, 1188
  pathological, 78, *79(t), 80, 81*
  physiological, 65, *68*
    displaced, 74, *75*
  vascular, in extracranial arterial occlusion, 702
  tumor, in meningioma, 1401, *1401*
Calcium, in multiple injury, 898
  in neurogenic bladder dysfunction, 1939
  in renal failure, 890
  normal levels of, 891
  urinary, hypophysectomy and, 1903
Calcium chloride, in cardiac arrest, 876, 1968
Callosomarginal artery, tumor displacement of, 164,
    165
Caloric test(s), in acoustic neuroma, 1436
  in coma, 49
  in post-traumatic dizziness, 1033
Calvarium, stereotaxic landmarks from, 1795, *1794–
    1797*
Campotomy, in Parkinson's disease, 1847

Cancer. See also *Carcinoma*.
  posterior rhizotomy in, 1742
  surgical hypophysectomy in, 1915, *1915(t)*
    results of, 1923
  thalamotomy in, 1785
  visceral pain in, 1697–1699
Capillaries, in arteriovenous malformations, of brain,
    827
  of spinal cord, 852
  in increased intracranial pressure, 453
Capping, of end-bulb neuroma, 1704, *1704(t)*, 1737
Carbamazepine, in trigeminal neuralgia, 1666, 1675
Carbohydrate metabolism, of cerebral hemisphere
    tumors, 1353
Carbon dioxide. See also *Carbon dioxide tension*.
  cerebral blood flow and, 664–667, *665, 666(t)*
    autoregulation of, 658, 669
    in increased intracranial pressure, 453
  monitoring of, air embolism and, 1965
    in anesthesia, 522
    in extracranial arterial occlusion, 706
  pneumoencephalography with, 216
  therapy with, in postoperative hiccough, 1998
    to increase cerebral blood flow, 686
Carbon dioxide tension, in anesthesia, cerebral
    blood flow and, 669
    passive hyperventilation and, 516
  controlled ventilation and, in respiratory arrest,
    871
  in acid-base regulation, 895
  in intracerebral steal phenomenon, 680
  intracranial pressure and, 448
    in pressure waves, 460
  respiration and, in coma, 46
    in increased intracranial pressure, 474
Carbonic acid, measurement of, 895
Carbonic anhydrase inhibitor, cerebral blood flow
    and, *673(t)*
Carcinoma. See also *Cancer*.
  breast, hypophysectomy and, 1901–1904, 1915,
    1915(t), 1923
  cephalic pain in, 1649
  cerebral edema and increased intracranial pres-
    sure in, 463
  cerebral hemisphere, 1352
  cytogenetic studies of, 1306
  in skull film, *75, 85*
  lung, apical, vs. cervical disc rupture, 1204
  meningeal, 1397, 1470
    cerebrospinal fluid in, *318(t)*, 1471
  nasopharyngeal and paranasal sinus, *75*, 1249–
    1253, *1250, 1251*
  nerve block in, 1649, 1728, 1729
  orbital, *1280(t), 1288(t), 1293*
  peripheral nerve, 1542
  prostate, hypophysectomy and, 1901, 1904
  radiotherapy in, 1507, 1536
  skull, *1244, 1245, 1245*
  spinal cord, 1516, 1536
  visceral pain in, 1697–1699
Cardiac arrest, in multiple injury, 875–877
  intraoperative, 1967
  postoperative, 1990
Cardiac massage, 875, 1967
Cardiac output, in induced hypothermia, 520
Cardiac pacing, in induced hypotension, 519

Celiac plexus block, diagnostic, 1725
  neurolytic, 1725, 1735
Cell(s), growth cycle of, in tumor chemotherapy,
  1492, *1492–1494*
  in cerebrospinal fluid, *315(t)*, 316, *318–319(t)*
Central cord syndrome, in cervical spine injury,
  1059
  in tentorial herniation, 951
Central beam aligned stereotaxic instruments,
  1812
Central pain, thalamotomy in, 1784
Cephalhematoma, 1253, *1254*
  skull film in, 77, 78, *79*
Cephalic pain, 1646–1661. Se also *Pain.*
Cerebellar ataxia, clinical diagnosis of, 9
  in meningioma, 1400
  in posterior fossa tumors, 1467
  rehabilitation in, 2016
Cerebellar ectopia, 634.
Cerebellar frame, for spinal operation, 545
Cerebellar hemisphere syndrome, clinical diagnosis
  of, 22
Cerebellopontine angle, anatomy of, 1440
  mass lesions of, vs. acoustic neuroma, *1452–
    1455*, *1453–1455*
  meningioma of, *1389(t)*, 1407
    pathology of, 1469
  Pantopaque examination of, 226, *227*
  tumors of, clinical diagnosis of, 21
    headache in, 1467, 1659
    in glossopharyngeal neuralgia, 1683
    postoperative problems in, 1479
    vs. trigeminal neuralgia, 1665
Cerebellum, agenesis of, 604
  astrocytoma of, in children, 1483–1485
    radiotherapy of, 1506
  edema of, postoperative, 1479
  function of, clinical examination of, 5, 22
    in infancy and childhood, 42
    in acoustic neuroma, 1437
    in posterior fossa lesions, 22, 1467
  hemorrhage into, 844–851, *844(t), 845*
  lesions of, equilibrium in, 410
  medulloblastoma of, in children, 1481
  sarcoma of, in children, 1483
  spinal cord tumors and, 1515
  tuberculoma of, 1570
  tumors of, operative removal of, 1477
    pathology of, 1468
    vs. cerebral hemisphere tumor, 1363
    vs. trigeminal neuralgia, 1665
Cerebral abscess. See Also *Abscess.*
  angiography in, 179, 1553, *1554*
  vs. cerebral hemisphere tumor, 1363
Cerebral angiography, 88–204. See also *Angiography.*
Cerebral arteries. See *Anterior cerebral artery* and
  Middle cerebral artery and *Posterior cerebral
  artery.*
Cerebral atrophy, cranioplasty in, 995, *996*
Cerebral blood flow, 651–697. See also *Blood flow,
  cerebral.*
Cerebral cicatrix, in epilepsy, 1869
Cerebral contusion, 956–959, *956, 957*
  angiography in, 196
Cerebral edema. See *Edema, cerebral.*

Cerebral embolism. See also *Air embolism.*
  in extracranial arterial occlusion, 700, 707
  reactive depression and psychogenic pain after,
    1633, 1634
Cerebral hemisphere(s), astrocytoma of, *1343,
  1344(t)*, 1345, *1345, 1347, 1355(t)*
  bilateral depression of, reflex eye movements in,
    49
  dermoid and epidermoid cysts of, 1350
  diseases of, optokinetic nystagmus in, 394
  dominance of, rehabilitation and, 2017
    tumor symptoms and, *1355(t), 1356(t)*, 1358
  ependymoma of, *1343, 1344(t), 1345*, 1347,
    1355(t), 1380
  glioblastoma of, *1343, 1344(t)*, 1345, *1345, 1347,
    1355(t)*
    psychological tests in, 433–435, *435*
  gliomas of, mixed, *1344(t)*, 1347, *1355(t), 1356(t)*
    secondary, 1353
  in physiology and pathology of consciousness, 45
  lipoma of, 79, *1351*, 1352
  medulloblastoma of, *1343, 1344(t), 1345*, 1347,
    1355(t), 1380
  metastatic carcinoma of, 1352
  metastatic malignant melanoma of, 1352
  microgliomatosis of, *1344(t)*, 1347, *1355(t)*
  oligodendroglioma of, *1343, 1344(t), 1345*, 1346,
    1355(t)
  teratoma of, 1351
  tuberculoma of, 1570, *1569–1574*
  tumors of, 1340–1387. See also names of specific
    tumors.
    biochemistry of, 1353
    chemotherapy in, 1381
    classification of, 1340
    diagnosis of, 1362
    immunotherapy in, 1381
    intraventricular, 1348
    pathology of, 1342
    postoperative care in, 1382, *1382*
    prognosis in, 1383
    psychological tests in, 433–437, *435, 436*
    radiotherapy in, 1379
    recurrence in, 1381
    symptoms and signs of, 1354, *1355(t), 1356(t)*
    treatment of, 1373
Cerebral palsy, ventrolateral thalamotomy in, 1860
Cerebral sclerosis, diffuse, clinical diagnosis of, 37
  multiple. See *Multiple sclerosis.*
  tuberous, genetic factors in, 1304
Cerebrospinal fluid, 308–324
  absorption of, test for, 581
  cells in, *315(t)*, 316, *318–319(t)*
  circulation of, hindbrain anomalies and, 638–641,
    640
    hydrocephalus and, 559, *560*, 581, *582, 583*
  collection of, 314
    prior to pneumoencephalography, 208
  drainage of, in excision of arteriovenous malfor-
    mation of brain, 834
    in surgical hypophysectomy, 1920
  drug administration into, in tumor chemotherapy,
    1497
  glucose in, *315(t)*, 317, *318–319(t)*
  in abscess, cranial, 1548, 1549
    spinal cord, 1575, 1577

Muscle(s) *(Continued)*
  smooth, sympathectomy and, 1766
  spasm of. See *Muscle spasm.*
Muscle relaxants, in lumbar disc disease, 1173
  in nitrous oxide anesthesia, 513
  in post-traumatic headache, 1034
Muscle spasm, in cervical disc rupture, 1198
  in lumbar disc disease, 1176
  in lumbar spinal cord injury, 1087
  in paraplegia, spinal pain in, 1692
  in temporomandibular joint pain, 1651
    neurolytic nerve block in, 1735
    post-traumatic headache and, 1026
Mutism, vs. aphasia, 13
Myasthenia gravis, ocular motility in, 391
Mycosis. See *Fungus.*
Mydriasis, pupillary, traumatic, 382
Myelin sheath, in entrapment syndromes, 1142
Myelitis, transverse, clinical diagnosis of, 29
  viral, 1557
Myelography, 257–283
  air, 265
  anesthesia for, 515
  appearance of specific lesions in, 265, *265–282*
  cisternal, 264, *264.* See also *Cisternography.*
  contrast agents for, 257
    nerve root damage from, 1689
  in achondroplasia, 1181
  in arteriovenous malformations, of spinal cord,
    854
  in cauda equina compression, 1182
  in cervical disc rupture, 1201–1203, *1201–1203*
    anterior operative approach and, 1226
  in cervical injury, 1052
  in diastematomyelia, 601
  in hyperextension-hyperflexion injury, 1080
  in lumbar disc disease, 1171
  in spina bifida occulta, 590
  in spinal cord abscess, extradural, 1575, *1575*
    intramedullary, 1577, *1578*
  in spinal cord tumors, 1520, *1521–1524*
    in children, 1533
  in spondylolysis, 1180
  in thoracic disc protrusion, 1188
  in tuberculosis of spine, 1581
  in viral encephalitis, 1560
  radionuclide tracers in, 301
  reaction to, postoperative, 2004
  technique of, 258, *259–263*
Myeloma, multiple, in skull film, *85*
  metastatic, of skull, 1248, *1248*
Myelomeningocele, 592–599, *592–596, 598*
  autonomous neurogenic bladder in, 598, 1943
  operative repair of, 597
    intubation in, 544
    posterior approach in, 545
  roentgenograms of spine in, 237, *243*
Myelopathy, clinical manifestations of, *35(t)*
  in radiotherapy of spinal cord, 1536
Myelotomy, Bishoff's, in painful paraplegia, 1692
Myerson's reflex, in Parkinson's disease, 1838
Myocardial infarction, postoperative, 1991
Myoclonus, 1862
  oculopalatopharyngeal, 395
Myofascial pain, nerve block in, diagnostic, 1725
  therapeutic, 1728

Myoglobinuria, in crush injury, 887
Myoneural junction, ocular motility and, 391–393,
  392
Myopathy. See *Muscle(s), disease of.*

Naffziger jugular compression test, in hyper-
    extension-hyperflexion injury, 1079
  in lumbar disc disease, 1170
Nalline. See *n-Allylnormorphine.*
Narcoanalysis, in psychogenic pain, 1640
Narcotics, contraindicated, in hyperextension-
    hyperflexion injury, 1081
  in post-traumatic headache, 1034
  in neuroleptanalgesia, 513
  in pain, 1688
    after neurolytic nerve block, 1733
    after spinal operations, 548
  intoxication with, pupils in, 48
Narrow spinal canal, congenital, 1180–1182
Nasal bones, fractures of, 928–930, *929, 930*
    frontal orbital lacrimal ethmoid and, 931–933,
    932–934
Nasociliary nerve, orbital anatomy of, 1278
Nasogastric tube feeding, diet for, 502
  in multiple injury, 899–901
  postoperative pneumonia and, 1989
Nasopharynx, carcinoma of, pain in, 1649
    skull and, 1249–1253, *1250, 1251*
  tumors of, in glossopharyngeal neuralgia, 1683
    vs. trigeminal neuralgia, 1665
Nausea, in cerebral hemisphere tumor, 1354
  in increased intracranial pressure, 468
Neck, clinical examination of, 5
Neck, malignant disease of, thalamotomy in, 1785
  pain in, in failed disc syndrome, 1690
  trauma to, angiography in, 179
Neck compression test, in hyperextension-
    hyperflexion injury, 1079
Necrosis, aseptic, bone, intraoperative, 1970
  liver, postoperative, 2000
  radiation, of skull, 1256
  spinal cord, in thoracic disc protrusion, 1191
  tissue, postoperative, 1982
Necrotizing encephalitis, 1556, 1560
Needle aspiration, in brain abscess, 1553
  in cardiac tamponade, 874
Needle biopsy, in cerebral hemisphere tumors, 1373
Needle electrode examination, electromyographic,
  359–361, *359*
Needles, for lumbar puncture, 311
  for myelography, 258
  for pneumoencephalography, 207
  for ventriculography, 231
  for vertebral angiography, 110, 112
Negative stress, in cerebral trauma and
  impairment of consciousness, 942
Negro, arterial anomalies in, carotid and
    vertebral, 148
  normal variation in, carotid, 113
Nembutal. See *Pentobarbital sodium.*
Neomycin-polymyxin B sulfate irrigant, in
  neurogenic bladder dysfunction, 1939
Neoplasms. See *Tumors.*

Petroclinoid ligament, in skull films, 66, *68*
Petrosal sinuses, normal radiological anatomy of, 135
Petrosal vein, in acoustic neuroma, *1447, 1448,*
 1449
pH. See *Acid-base balance.*
Phakomatoses, genetic factors in, 1304
Phantom limb pain, body image and, 1618
 in paraplegia, 1691
 operative treatment of, *1706(t),* 1710
 rehabilitation and, 1136
 thalamotomy in, 1784
Phantom target stereotaxic instrument, 1811, *1812*
Pharynx, anterior cervical approach and, 1218
 complications of, 1215, 1222
Phenobarbital, dosage in renal failure, 891
 in angiography, 90
 in epilepsy, postoperative, 1877
  post-traumatic, 1038
 in nonoperative aneurysm management, 729
Phenol, in neurolytic nerve block, 1729
 in neurogenic bladder dysfunction, 1941
 in pelvic cancer, 1699
 in peripheral neuralgia, 1708
 in spasticity, 2014
 injection technique for, 1732, *1733*
 results of, *1734(t)*
Phenolsulfonphthalein excretion test, 1933
Phenoperidine, in neuroleptanalgesia, 513
Phenothiazines, electroencephalographic activation
  by, 336
 in etiology of Parkinson's disease, 1839
 in psychogenic pain, 1641
Phenoxybenzamine, cerebral blood flow and, *673(t)*
 in hypovolemic shock, 883
Phenylephrine, cerebral blood flow and, *672(t)*
 in extracranial arterial occlusion, 706
 in neurogenic shock, 884
Pheochromocytoma, 1541
Phlebitis, intravenous therapy and, 2001
Phlebotomy, in fluid volume excess, 893
Phoria, latent ocular deviation, 384
Phosphorus-32, in brain scanning, in cerebral
  hemisphere tumors, 1368
"Photic driving," electroencephalographic, 335, *337,*
 338
Photography, operating microscope and, 553
Photophobia, 373, *373(t)*
Phrenic nerve, facial nerve anastomosis with, 1480
Physical examination. See *Examination.*
Physical therapy, in peripheral nerve injury, 1132
 in psychogenic pain, 1641
 rehabilitation and, 2013. See also *Rehabilitation.*
  center for, 2019
 spinal cord tumors and, 1533
Physiogenic pain, 1615, *1616(t)*
 amobarbital pain test and, 1625
 in psychogenic magnification, 1636
 thiopental pain test and, 1627
Pia, in trauma and state of consciousness, 937, 940
Picrotoxin, cerebral blood flow and, 671, *674(t)*
Picture Arrangement test, Wechsler, 428
Picture Completion test, Wechsler, 428
"Pie in the sky" visual field defect, 14
Pigmentation, meningeal, tumors and, 1396
Pilonidal sinus, vs. congenital dermal sinus, 603
Pineal body, in skull films, 66, 69, 74, *75*

Pineal body *(Continued)*
 tumors of, angiography in, 176
  pathology of, 1348
  posterior extension of, 1331, *1362*
  radiotherapy in, 1511
Pitressin. See *Vasopressin.*
Pituitary adenoma, 1412
 angiography in, 1423
 brain scan in, *291(t),* 294, *295*
 indications for operation in, 1425
 pathology of, 1415
 postoperative intracranial pressure waves in, 459,
  461
 radiotherapy in, 1430, 1508, *1509, 1510*
 sella in, in skull films, 70, *70, 74*
 symptoms of, 1413
Pituitary apoplexy, 1413
Pituitary extract, posterior cerebral blood flow and,
 674(t)
Pituitary gland, ablation of, 1901–1927. See also
  Hypophysectomy.
 cyst of, vs. empty sella syndrome, 1421
 function of, clinical evaluation of, 18
  preoperative evaluation of, 1951
   for stereotaxic hypophysectomy, 1912
 premedication for operation on, 527
 tumors of, 1412. See also *Pituitary adenoma.*
Planum spenoidale, in skull films, meningioma of,
 71, *73*
 normal variations of, 61, *62, 63*
Platybasia, 629, *632*
Pleural shunt, in cerebral hemisphere tumors, 1376
 in infantile hydrocephalus, 576
Plexus, brachial. See *Brachial plexus.*
 choroid. See *Choroid plexus.*
Plexus, pelvic, injuries of, 1124
Pneumoencephalography, 205–223
 anesthesia for, 207, 515, 638
  nitrous oxide in, 513
 aqueduct in, 211
 arteriovenous malformations of brain and, 830
 cisterns in, *206, 207, 209,* 211, 216
 complications in, 216, 1372, 1468
 equipment for, 207
 fractional, in brain stem tumors in children, 1486
  in stereotaxic landmark demonstration, 1794–
   1796, *1794–1796*
 in acoustic neuroma, 1449–1453, *1449–1453*
 in cerebral hemisphere tumors, 1370
 in epilepsy, 1872, *1873*
 in hydrocephalus, from posterior fossa tumor,
  1468
  infantile, 572
  normal-pressure, 580, *580*
 in hypertensive brain hemorrhage, 847
 in malformations of craniovertebral junction, 637,
  638
 in meningioma, 1402
 in orbital tumors, 1284, *1285*
 in sellar and parasellar tumors, 1423, *1423, 1424*
 in subarachnoid hemorrhage, 720
 positioning for, 208
 posterior fossa in, 213
 preparation of patient in, 205, *208(t)*
 technique in, 207, *209–213, 215, 217–222*
 ventricles in, 209, *209–213, 215, 217*